The Philadelphia Guide
Inpatient Pediatrics

Brief Table of Contents

The Philadelphia Guide

Inpatient Pediatrics

EDITORS

Gary Frank, MD, MS
Attending Physician, Divisions of
  General Pediatrics and Clinical
  Informatics
Al duPont Hospital for Children
Nemours Children's Clinic
Wilmington, DE

Marina Catallozzi, MD
Medical Director, Adolescent AIDS
  Program
The Children's Hospital at Montefiore
Assistant Professor, Section of
  Adolescent Medicine, Department
  of Pediatrics
The Albert Einstein College of Medicine
Bronx, NY

Samir S. Shah, MD
Attending Physician, Divisions of General
  Pediatrics and Infectious Diseases
The Children's Hospital of Philadelphia
Assistant Professor, Department of
  Pediatrics
University of Pennsylvania
School of Medicine
Philadelphia, PA

Lisa B. Zaoutis, MD
Director, Inpatient Pediatric Services
Division of General Pediatrics
The Children's Hospital of Philadelphia
Philadelphia, PA

LIPPINCOTT WILLIAMS & WILKINS
A **Wolters Kluwer** Company
Philadelphia • Baltimore • New York • London
Buenos Aires • Hong Kong • Sydney • Tokyo

351 West Camden Street
Baltimore, Maryland 21201-2436 USA

530 Walnut Street
Philadelphia, Pennsylvania 19106-3621 USA

The publisher is not responsible (as a matter of product liability, negligence, or otherwise) for any injury resulting from any material contained herein. This publication contains information relating to general principles of medical care which should not be construed as specific instructions for individual patients. Manufacturers' product information and package inserts should be reviewed for current information, including contraindications, dosages, and precautions.

Printed in China

Library of Congress Cataloging-in-Publication Data

The Philadelphia guide : inpatient pediatrics / editors, Gary Frank . . . [et al.].
   p. ; cm.
  Includes bibliographical references and index.
  ISBN-13: 978-1-4051-0428-9 (pbk. : alk. paper)
  ISBN-10: 1-4051-0428-7 (pbk. : alk. paper)   1. Pediatrics—Handbooks, manuals, etc.
  [DNLM: 1. Pediatrics—Handbooks. WS 39 P544 2005] I. Title: Inpatient pediatrics. II. Frank, Gary, 1971-
III. Children's Hospital of Philadelphia.

  RJ48.P485 2005
  618.92—dc22   2004029352

A catalogue record for this title is available from the British Library

Editor: Donna Balado
Managing Editor: Kathleen Scogna
Marketing Manager: Emilie Linkins

The publishers have made every effort to trace the copyright holders for borrowed material. If they have inadvertently overlooked any, they will be pleased to make the necessary arrangements at the first opportunity.

To purchase additional copies of this book call our customer service department at (800) 638-3030 or fax orders to (301) 824-7390. International customers should call (301) 714-2324.

Visiti *Lippincott Williams & Wilkins on the Internet: http://www.lww.com.* Lippincott Williams & Wilkins customer service representatives are available from 8:30 am to 6:00 pm, EST, Monday through Friday, for telephone access.

10 11 12 13 14 15

RRS1205

*To our mentors for sharing their
wisdom and knowledge*

*To our families for providing love and support
for all of our endeavors*

*To our patients for teaching us
and to their families for trusting us*

Acknowledgments

This work would not have been possible without the support of many individuals. First and foremost, we thank Dr. Stephen Ludwig for his wisdom, guidance, and encouragement. His dedication to medical education continues to inspire us. We appreciate the efforts of our Department Chair, Dr. Alan Cohen, and our Division Chiefs, Drs. Louis Bell, Paul Offit, and Don Schwarz, to create a stimulating learning environment. We thank our many colleagues who contributed their expertise in writing chapters for this book. Beverly Copland and Kate Heinle, our editors at Blackwell Publishing, demonstrated remarkable enthusiasm as this book developed. They have our sincere appreciation. We would also like to express our gratitude to the residents and fellows at The Children's Hospital of Philadelphia whose eagerness to learn makes teaching so rewarding.

TABLE OF CONTENTS

24. OTOLARYNGOLOGY
      Marc Eisen, MD, PhD,
      Steven D. Handler, MD, MBE

25. PROCEDURES
      Nicholas Tsarouhas, MD (with contribu-
      tions from Linda L. Brown, MD, Lauren
      Daly, MD, Reza Daugherty, MD, Marla J.
      Friedman, DO, Karen J. O'Connell, MD,
      Vivian Hwang, MD)

26. PSYCHIATRY
      Amy Kim, MD, Anthony L. Rostain, MD,
      MA

27. PULMONOLOGY
      David Hehir, MD, Michael F.
      Maraventano, MD, Suzanne Dawid, MD,
      PhD, Howard B. Panitch, MD

28. RHEUMATOLOGY
      Pamela G. Fitch, MD, Elise R. DeVore,
      MD, Jeffrey C. Klick, MD, Jon M.
      Burnham, MD

29. SURGERY
      Amy L. Winkelstein, MD, Mercedes
      Blackstone, MD, Suzanne Dawid, MD,
      PhD, Michael Nance, MD (with contribu-
      tions from James P. Franciosi, MD, MS,
      Leonard J. Levine, MD, Gary Frank,
      MD, MS)

ABOUT THE EDITORS

Gary Frank, MD, MS, FAAP, is a pediatrician at Alfred I duPont Hospital for Children, where he works primarily as an inpatient attending on a resident-based team. His non-clinical work is in the area of medical informatics, where he focuses on computerized provider order entry. He completed his residency at Children's Hospital of Philadelphia and attended medical school at the University of Pennsylvania School of Medicine. He has a Master of Science in Engineering Management from Stanford University and graduated from Dartmouth College with a Bachelor's degree in engineering.

Samir S. Shah, MD, completed a combined fellowship in Pediatric Infectious Diseases and Academic General Pediatrics at The Children's Hospital of Philadelphia. He is also pursuing a Master of Science degree in Clinical Epidemiology at the University of Pennsylvania School of Medicine. He graduated from Yale University School of Medicine and completed his pediatric residency training at The Children's Hospital of Philadelphia. He has received several teaching awards including Fellow Teacher of the Year and Faculty Teaching Honor Roll. His research interests include deriving clinical prediction rules to identify febrile children at high risk of invasive bacterial infection. He is editor or co-editor of several books, including *Blueprints Pediatric Infectious Diseases, Blueprints Infectious Diseases,* and *Pediatric Complaints and Diagnostic Dilemmas: A Case-Based Approach.* He also served as an associate editor for *Blueprints Pediatrics* (3rd edition).

Marina Catallozzi, MD, is an Assistant Professor in the Section of Adolescent Medicine at The Children's Hospital at Montefiore and the Albert Einstein College of Medicine. She is Medical Director of the Adolescent AIDS Program at Montefiore Hospital in the Bronx, New York, and a faculty member of the New York/New Jersey AIDS Education and Training Center. She is the co-Principal Investigator of the Adolescent AIDS Program's Adolescent Trials Network site. Dr. Catallozzi received her undergraduate and medical degrees from Brown University in Providence, Rhode Island. She completed her Pediatrics Residency, Chief Residency, and Adolescent Medicine Fellowship at The Children's Hospital of Philadelphia. Her research focuses on the relationship choices of adolescent women. She is also pursuing a Master of Science degree in Clinical Epidemiology at the University of Pennsylvania School of Medicine.

Lisa B. Zaoutis, MD, is currently Director of Inpatient Services for the Division of General Pediatrics at The Children's Hospital of Philadelphia. Her areas of particular interest include resident and nursing education and advancing General Pediatric Hospital Medicine as a recognized area of expertise in medical and nursing disciplines. She has received numerous teaching awards including Faculty Teacher of the Year from the residency programs at The Children's Hospital of Philadelphia and the Alfred I DuPont Hospital for Children and the Penn Pearls Teaching Award from the University of Pennsylvania School of Medicine.

CONTRIBUTORS

Asim Aminsharif Ahmed, MD
Clinical Fellow, Division of Pediatric
Infectious Diseases
Children's Hospital Boston
Harvard Medical School
Boston, MA

Kristin Andolaro, RD, LDN
Clinical Dietitian
Division of Pediatric Nephrology
The Children's Hospital of Philadelphia
Philadelphia, PA

Sarah C. Armstrong, MD
General Pediatrician
Jai Medical Center Clinical Staff
Department of Pediatrics
Johns Hopkins Hospital
Baltimore, MD

Jessica Arvay-Nezu, RD, CSP, LDN
Staff Pediatric Dietitian
The Children's Hospital of Philadelphia
Philadelphia, PA

Denise M. Bell, MD
Clinical Instructor, Department of Pediatrics
University of Pennsylvania School of Medicine
Philadelphia, PA

Louis M. Bell, MD
Professor of Pediatrics
University of Pennsylvania School of Medicine
Chief, Division of General Pediatrics
Attending Physician, Infectious Diseases
The Children's Hospital of Philadelphia
Philadelphia, PA

Suzanne Beno, MD, FRCPC
Division of Emergency Medicine
Department of Pediatrics
The Children's Hospital of Philadelphia
Philadelphia, PA

Peter H. Berman, MD
Professor, Neurology and Pediatrics
University of Pennsylvania School of Medicine
Senior Neurologist
The Children's Hospital of Philadelphia
Philadelphia, PA

Andrea A. Berry, MD
Instructor, Department of Pediatrics
University of Pennsylvania School of Medicine
Resident, Department of Pediatrics
The Children's Hospital of Philadelphia
Philadelphia, PA

Mercedes Blackstone, MD
Pediatrics Resident
The Children's Hospital of Philadelphia
Philadelphia, PA

Susan Boyden, MS, RD, LDN
Clinical Dietitian
The Children's Hospital of Philadelphia
Philadelphia, PA

Darla J. Bradshaw, RD, CNSD, LDN
Nutrition Support Dietitian
Pediatric Intensive Care Unit
The Children's Hospital of Philadelphia
Philadelphia, PA

Linda L. Brown, MD
Assistant Professor of Pediatrics
Yale University School of Medicine
Division of Pediatric Emergency Medicine
Yale-New Haven Children's Hospital
New Haven, CT

Cagla Bulgun, RD, LDN
Formula Room Manager, Neonatal Dietitian
The Children's Hospital of Philadelphia
Philadelphia, PA

Jon M. Burnham, MD
Assistant Professor
Department of Pediatrics
University of Pennsylvania School of Medicine
Attending Physician
Divisions of Rheumatology and General Pediatrics
The Children's Hospital of Philadelphia
Philadelphia, PA

Manish J. Butte, MD, PhD
Clinical Fellow, Division of Immunology
Children's Hospital Boston
Harvard Medical School
Boston, MA

Diane P. Calello, MD
Instructor of Pediatrics
University of Pennsylvania School of Medicine
Fellow, Pediatric Emergency Medicine and
Toxicology
The Children's Hospital of Philadelphia
Philadelphia, PA

John Casey, MD, CM
Assistant Professor of Pediatrics
Division of Neonatology
University of Connecticut Health Center
Farmington, CT

Nicole Celona-Jacobs, MS, RD, CDE
Program Coordinator of "Treatment Options
for Type 2 Diabetes in Adolescents and
Youth" Study
TODAY Study at The Children's Hospital
of Denver
Denver, CO

Rebecca Collier, MD
Hospitalist, Division of General Pediatrics
and Neonatology
The Children's Hospital of Philadelphia
Philadelphia, PA

Andrea Dahlman, MD
Instructor in Pediatrics
University of Pennsylvania School of Medicine
Pediatric Resident
The Children's Hospital of Philadelphia
Philadelphia, PA

Lauren Daly, MD
Attending Physician, Division of Emergency
Medicine
Alfred I. duPont Hospital for Children
Nemours Children's Clinic
Wilmington, DE

Reza Daugherty, MD
Instructor in Pediatrics
University of Pennsylvania School of Medicine
Fellow, Pediatric Emergency Medicine
The Children's Hospital of Philadelphia
Philadelphia, PA

Stefanie L. Davidson, MD
Assistant Clinical Professor
University of Pennsylvania School of Medicine
Instructor, Ophthalmology
The Children's Hospital of Philadelphia
Philadelphia, PA

Suzanne Dawid, MD, PhD
Fellow, Division of Infectious Diseases
The Children's Hospital of Philadelphia
Philadelphia, PA

Matthew Deardorff, MD, PhD
Pediatrics Resident
The Children's Hospital of Philadelphia
Philadelphia, PA

Ralph J. DeBerardinis, MD, PhD
Fellow, Medical Genetics
The Children's Hospital of Philadelphia
Philadelphia, PA

Elise R. DeVore, MD
Fellow in Adolescent Medicine
Children's Hospital Boston
Boston, MA

Dennis J. Dlugos, MD
Assistant Professor of Neurology
and Pediatrics
University of Pennsylvania School of Medicine
Attending Neurologist
The Children's Hospital of Philadelphia
Philadelphia, PA

Marc Eisen, MD, PhD
Assistant Instructor, Department
of Otorhinolaryngology
University of Pennsylvania School of Medicine
Resident in Otorhinolaryngology
University of Pennsylvania Medical Center
Philadelphia, PA

Lori Enriquez, RD, CSP, CNSP, LDN
Clinical Dietitian
The Children's Hospital of Philadelphia
Philadelphia, PA

Kristen A. Feemster, MD, MPH
Pediatric Resident Physician
The Children's Hospital of Philadelphia
Philadelphia, PA

Can Ficicioglu, MD, PhD
Assistant Professor of Pediatrics
University of Pennsylvania School of Medicine
Attending Physician in Metabolism
The Children's Hospital of Philadelphia
Philadelphia, PA

Pamela G. Fitch, MD
Pediatrics Resident
The Children's Hospital of Philadelphia
Philadelphia, PA

John M. Flynn, MD
Associate Professor of Orthopaedic Surgery
University of Pennsylvania School of Medicine
Orthopaedic Surgeon
The Children's Hospital of Philadelphia
Philadelphia, PA

James P. Franciosi, MD, MS
Pediatrics Resident
The Children's Hospital of Philadelphia
Philadelphia, PA

Christy L. Frantz, RD, LDN
Ketogenic Dietitian, Department of Neurology
The Children's Hospital of Philadelphia
Philadelphia, PA

Heather Morein French, MD
Pediatric Resident
The Children's Hospital of Philadelphia
Philadelphia, PA

Marla J. Friedman, DO
Attending Physician, Pediatric
Emergency Medicine
Miami Children's Hospital
Miami, FL

Rose C. Graham-Maar, MD
Clinical Instructor, Department of Pediatrics
University of Pennsylvania School of Medicine
Fellow, Division of Gastroenterology
and Nutrition
The Children's Hospital of Philadelphia
Philadelphia, PA

Rhonda M. Graves, MD
Clinical Instructor, Pediatrics
University of Pennsylvania School of Medicine
Chief Resident, Pediatrics
The Children's Hospital of Philadelphia
Philadelphia, PA

Adda Grimberg, MD, FAAP
Assistant Professor, Pediatrics
University of Pennsylvania School of Medicine
Attending Physician, Division of Pediatric
Endocrinology
The Children's Hospital of Philadelphia
Philadelphia, PA

Steven D. Handler, MD, MBE
Professor, Otorhinolaryngology: Head
and Neck Surgery
University of Pennsylvania School of Medicine
Associate Director, Pediatric
Otorhinolaryngology
The Children's Hospital of Philadelphia
Philadelphia, PA

Maria D. Hanna, MS, RD, LDN
Clinical Nutritionist
Department of Clinical Nutrition
The Children's Hospital of Philadelphia
Philadelphia, PA

Mary Catherine Harris, MD
Associate Professor of Pediatrics
University of Pennsylvania School of Medicine
Attending Neonatologist
The Children's Hospital of Philadelphia
Philadelphia, PA

David Hehir, MD
Fellow, Pediatric Cardiology and Critical
Care Medicine
University of Pennsylvania School of Medicine
The Children's Hospital of Philadelphia
Philadelphia, PA

Fred M. Henretig, MD
Professor of Pediatrics and Emergency
Medicine
University of Pennsylvania School of Medicine
Director, Section of Clinical Toxicology
The Children's Hospital of Philadelphia
Philadelphia, PA

Francis M. Hoe, MD
Fellow, Pediatric Endocrinology
Division of Endocrinology
The Children's Hospital of Philadelphia
Philadelphia, PA

Trevor L. Hoffman, MD, PhD
Fellow, Genetics
University of Pennsylvania School of Medicine
The Children's Hospital of Philadelphia
Philadelphia, PA

Jimmy W. Huh, MD
Assistant Professor of Anesthesia
and Pediatrics
University of Pennsylvania School of Medicine
Attending Physician, Division of Critical Care
The Children's Hospital of Philadelphia
Philadelphia, PA

Jennifer Minarcik Hwang, MD, MHS
Chief Resident, Pediatric Residency Program
The Children's Hospital of Philadelphia
Philadelphia, PA

Vivian Hwang, MD
Attending Physician, Department
of Emergency Medicine
INOVA Fairfax Hospital
Falls Church, VA

Malaka B. Jackson, MD
Fellow, Division of Endocrinology
The Children's Hospital of Philadelphia
Philadelphia, PA

Mark D. Joffe, MD
Associate Professor of Pediatrics
Director, Community Pediatric Medicine
The Children's Hospital of Philadelphia
University of Pennsylvania School of Medicine
Philadelphia, PA

Megan Johnston-Mullen, MS, RD, LDN
Clinical Nutritionist
Division of Gastroenterology and Nutrition
The Children's Hospital of Philadelphia
Philadelphia, PA

Paige Kaplan, MBBCh
Professor of Pediatrics
University of Pennsylvania School of Medicine
Section Chief, Metabolic Diseases
The Children's Hospital of Philadelphia
Philadelphia, PA

Melanie Katrinak, RD, LDN
Clinical Dietitian, Clinical Nutrition
The Children's Hospital of Philadelphia
Philadelphia, PA

Sarah D. Kelly, MS, RD, LDN
Endocrine Dietitian, Diabetes Center
for Children
The Children's Hospital of Philadelphia
Philadelphia, PA

Leslie S. Kersun, MD
Instructor, Division of Oncology
Department of Pediatrics
The Children's Hospital of Philadelphia
Philadelphia, PA

Amy Kim, MD
Fellow, Child and Adolescent Psychiatry
The Children's Hospital of Philadelphia
Philadelphia, PA

Samantha Zucker Kim, RD, CNSD, CDE, LDN
Clinical Dietitian
The Children's Hospital of Philadelphia
Philadelphia, PA

Jeffrey C. Klick, MD
Resident Physician, General Pediatrics
The Children's Hospital of Philadelphia
Philadelphia, PA

Ian Krantz, MD
Assistant Professor of Pediatrics
Division of Human Genetics
The Children's Hospital of Philadelphia
University of Pennsylvania School of Medicine
Philadelphia, PA

Christine T. Lauren, MD
Chief Resident
Pediatric Residency Program
The Children's Hospital of Philadelphia
Philadelphia, PA

Laura Lawler, MD
Pediatric Hospitalist Physician
Christiana Care Health Services
Newark, DE

Rachelle Lessen, MS, RD, IBCLC, LDN
Clinical Nutritionist/Lactation Consultant
The Children's Hospital of Philadelphia
Philadelphia, PA

Leonard J. Levine, MD
Instructor, Pediatrics
University of Pennsylvania School of Medicine
Fellow, Adolescent Medicine
The Children's Hospital of Philadelphia
Philadelphia, PA

Stephen Ludwig, MD
Professor of Pediatrics and Emergency
Medicine
University of Pennsylvania School of Medicine
Associate Chair for Medical Education
The Children's Hospital of Philadelphia
Philadelphia, PA

Michael F. Maraventano, MD
Pediatrics Resident
The Children's Hospital of Philadelphia
Philadelphia, PA

Maria R. Mascarenhas, MBBS
Associate Professor of Pediatrics
University of Pennsylvania School of Medicine
Chief, Nutrition Section
Division of Gastroenterology and Nutrition
The Children's Hospital of Philadelphia
Philadelphia, PA

Erin E. McGintee, MD
Fellow, Allergy and Immunology
The Children's Hospital of Philadelphia
Philadelphia, PA

Charles P. McKay, MD
Assistant Professor of Pediatrics
Thomas Jefferson University
Philadelphia, PA
Director, Bone and Mineral Program
Alfred I. duPont Hospital for Children
Wilmington, DE

Nancy Moore, RD, LDN
Clinical Dietitian
Clinical Nutrition
The Children's Hospital of Philadelphia
Philadelphia, PA

Sogol Mostoufi-Moab, MD
Pediatrics Endocrinology Fellow
The Children's Hospital of Philadelphia
Philadelphia, PA

Monica Nagle, RD, CNSD, LDN
Clinical Dietitian, Department of Clinical
Nutrition
The Children's Hospital of Philadelphia
Philadelphia, PA

Michael L. Nance, MD
Associate Professor of Surgery
University of Pennsylvania
Templeton Endowed Chair in Pediatric Trauma
The Children's Hospital of Philadelphia
Philadelphia, PA

Jason G. Newland, MD
Fellow, Infectious Diseases
The Children's Hospital of Philadelphia
Philadelphia, PA
Research Fellow, Pediatric Infectious Disease
Society
St. Jude's Children's Research Hospital
Memphis, TN

Karen J. O'Connell, MD
Instructor of Pediatrics
University of Pennsylvania School of Medicine
Fellow, Pediatric Emergency Medicine
The Children's Hospital of Philadelphia
Philadelphia, PA

Deborah Palmer, MD
Resident, Department of Pediatrics
University of Pennsylvania School of Medicine
The Children's Hospital of Philadelphia
Philadelphia, PA

Howard B. Panitch, MD
Associate Professor of Pediatrics
University of Pennsylvania School of Medicine
Attending Physician, Division of Pulmonary
Medicine
The Children's Hospital of Philadelphia
Philadelphia, PA

Sara K. Pasquali, MD
Resident in Pediatrics
The Children's Hospital of Philadelphia
Philadelphia, PA

Nicholas A. Pawlowski, MD
Associate Professor of Pediatrics
University of Pennsylvania School of Medicine
Allergy Chief
The Children's Hospital of Philadelphia
Philadelphia, PA

Irma Payan, RN, CRNP
Pediatric Nurse Practitioner
The Children's Hospital of Philadelphia
Division of Child Development, Rehabilitation,
and Metabolic Disease
Department of Pediatrics
Philadelphia, PA

David A. Piccoli, MD
Nutrition Biesecker Professor of Pediatrics
University of Pennsylvania School of Medicine
Chief, Division of Gastroenterology
and Nutrition
The Children's Hospital of Philadelphia
Philadelphia, PA

Annapurna Poduri, MD
Fellow in Epilepsy and Clinical
Neurophysiology
Children's Hospital Boston
Boston, MA

Leslie Raffini, MD
Assistant Professor of Pediatrics
University of Pennsylvania School of Medicine
Attending Hematologist
The Children's Hospital of Philadelphia
Philadelphia, PA

Jennifer Ranalli, RD, CNSD, LDN
Oncology Dietitian, Clinical Nutrition
The Children's Hospital of Philadelphia
Philadelphia, PA

Larry A. Rhodes, MD
Associate Professor of Pediatrics
University of Pennsylvania School of Medicine
Director of Electrophysiology
The Children's Hospital of Philadelphia
Philadelphia, PA

Megan Robinson, MS, RD, CDE, LDN
Clinical Dietitian
The Children's Hospital of Philadelphia
Philadelphia, PA

Anthony L. Rostain, MD, MA
Associate Professor of Psychiatry
and Pediatrics
University of Pennsylvania School of Medicine
Attending Physician
The Children's Hospital of Philadelphia
Philadelphia, PA

Richard M. Rutstein, MD
Associate Professor of Pediatrics
University of Pennsylvania School of Medicine
Medical Director, Special Immunology Service
The Children's Hospital of Philadelphia
Philadelphia, PA

Judit Saenz-Badillos, MD
Pediatrics Resident
The Children's Hospital of Philadelphia
Philadelphia, PA

Ann E. Salerno, MD
Fellow, Division of Nephrology
University of Pennsylvania School of Medicine
The Children's Hospital of Philadelphia
Philadelphia, PA

Donald F. Schwarz, MD, MPH
Vice Chairman, Department of Pediatrics
University of Pennsylvania School of Medicine
Chief, Craig-Dalsimer Division of Adolescent
Medicine
The Children's Hospital of Philadelphia
Philadelphia, PA

Alix Seif, MD, MPH
Pediatrics Resident
The Children's Hospital of Philadelphia
Philadelphia, PA

Sarbattama Sen, MD
Pediatrics Resident, General Pediatrics
The Children's Hospital of Philadelphia
Philadelphia, PA

Snehal N. Shah, MD
Epidemic Intelligence Service Officer
Division of Parasitic Diseases
National Center for Infectious Diseases
Centers for Disease Control and Prevention
Atlanta, GA

Renée A. Shellhaas, MD
Fellow, Division of Neurology
The Children's Hospital of Philadelphia
Philadelphia, PA

Nicholas B. Slamon, MD
Fellow, Critical Care Medicine
Alfred I. duPont Hospital for Children
Wilmington, DE

Neal Sondheimer, MD, PhD
Instructor of Pediatrics
University of Pennsylvania School of Medicine
Fellow, Metabolism and Genetics
The Children's Hospital of Philadelphia
Philadelphia, PA

Vijay Srinivasan, MD
Fellow, Health Services
Center for Outcomes Research
University of Pennsylvania School of Medicine
Fellow, Critical Care Medicine
The Children's Hospital of Philadelphia
Philadelphia, PA

Kathleen E. Sullivan, MD, PhD
Associate Professor of Pediatrics
University of Pennsylvania School of Medicine
Associate Physician
The Children's Hospital of Philadelphia
Philadelphia, PA

Gihan I. Tennekoon, MD
Professor of Neurology
University of Pennsylvania School of Medicine
Attending Physician
The Children's Hospital of Philadelphia
Philadelphia, PA

Rebecca Thomas, RD, LDN
Clinical Dietitian, Department
of Clinical Nutrition
The Children's Hospital of Philadelphia
Philadelphia, PA

Nicholas Tsarouhas, MD
Associate Professor of Clinical Pediatrics
University of Pennsylvania School of Medicine
Attending Physician, Emergency Medicine
Medical Director, Section of Transport
Medicine
The Children's Hospital of Philadelphia
Philadelphia, PA

Brenda Waber, RD, CSP, CNSD, LDN
Neonatal Dietitian, Department of Clinical
Nutrition
The Children's Hospital of Philadelphia
Philadelphia, PA

Michelle Verona Williams, MS, RD, CNSD
Dietitian, Department of Biochemical Genetics
The Children's Hospital of Philadelphia
Philadelphia, PA

Amy L. Winkelstein, MD
Instructor of Pediatrics
University of Pennsylvania School of Medicine
Chief Resident, Department of Pediatrics
The Children's Hospital of Philadelphia
Philadelphia, PA

Char Witmer, MD
Fellow, Hematology and Oncology
The Children's Hospital of Philadelphia
Philadelphia, PA

Joanne N. Wood, MD
Pediatric Resident
The Children's Hospital of Philadelphia
Philadelphia, PA

Krishna Wood, MD
Instructor
University of Pennsylvania School of Medicine
Pediatric Resident
The Children's Hospital of Philadelphia
Philadelphia, PA

Albert C. Yan, MD
Assistant Professor of Pediatrics and
Dermatology
University of Pennsylvania School of Medicine
Section Chief, Pediatric Dermatology
The Children's Hospital of Philadelphia
Philadelphia, PA

Colleen Yanni, MS, RD, LDN
Clinical Dietitian, Department of Clinical
Nutrition
The Children's Hospital of Philadelphia
Philadelphia, PA

Theoklis E. Zaoutis, MD
Assistant Professor, Department of Pediatrics
University of Pennsylvania School of Medicine
Director, Antimicrobial Stewardship Program
Division of Infectious Diseases
The Children's Hospital of Philadelphia
Philadelphia, PA

REVIEWERS

Emery H. Chang, MD
Resident, Department of Internal Medicine and Pediatrics
Tulane University
New Orleans, LA

Jennifer K. Clark, MD
Resident, Medicine/Pediatrics
Medical University of South Carolina
Charleston, SC

David Gloss, MD, MPH&TM
Class of 2004
Tulane University
New Orleans, LA

Richard H. Ko, MD, MHS
Resident, Pediatrics
University of California, San Francisco
San Francisco, CA

Peter J. Mc Guire, MS, MD
House Officer
Department of Pediatrics/Human Genetics
Mt. Sinai Medical Center
New York, NY

Tara Miller, MD
Resident, Pediatrics
Texas Children's Hospital
Ben Taub General Hospital
Houston, TX

Breck Nichols, MD, MPH
PGY-4 Resident, Medicine-Pediatrics
Los Angeles County—USC Medical Center
Los Angeles, CA

Joseph Scafidi, DO
Resident, Department of Pediatrics
The University Children's Hospital
University of Medicine and Dentistry, New Jersey
Newark, NJ

PREFACE

The Philadelphia Guide: Inpatient Pediatrics concisely yet comprehensively covers over 350 of the most commonly encountered pediatric medical conditions. The four editors, along with over one hundred fellows, attendings, residents, and pediatric specialists, have collaborated to provide a fresh new approach to inpatient pediatric care, guided by the combined expertise of skilled clinicians and teachers.

Caring for children in the inpatient setting is a challenging task in the constantly evolving field of pediatrics. The breadth of medical knowledge required to care for these increasingly complex patients is growing rapidly. Therefore, there is a great need for a clinically focused, easy-to-use manual to guide practitioners in making complicated diagnostic and therapeutic decisions.

Designed to be an invaluable resource on the wards *The Philadelphia Guide: Inpatient Pediatrics* features:
• 30 chapters addressing all of the major pediatric specialties
• Practical diagnostic strategies
• Extensive differential diagnosis suggestions
• Up-to-date, accurate treatment and management guidelines
• Alphabetical organization within chapters for rapid access
• Structured format with consistent headings throughout
• Classic and current evidence-based resources
• Convenient size to fit in white coat pockets

Three helpful appendices cover normal vital signs, neonatal codes, and PALS algorithms, and convenient tables on the inside covers allow for rapid access to pediatric dosages for emergency, airway, and rapid sequence intubation medications, as well as defibrillation and cardioversion.

A formulary was omitted (with the understanding that most institutions provide pediatric dosing guidelines) to allow for highly detailed coverage of treatment and management options, while still maintaining a manageable pocket size.

To ensure that this book met the needs of residents and housestaff in pediatrics, it was extensively reviewed prior to publication, and guided by the reviewers detailed feedback. They felt, as we hope you will, that *The Philadelphia Guide: Inpatient Pediatrics* provides them with the vital information necessary to make management decisions in the care of children.

As many clinicians are involved in the care of children, this book is ideal for practitioners of all levels, from students to attendings, physician assistants, nurse practitioners, pediatric nurses, and health practitioners from all disciplines involved in the care of children in the inpatient setting.

The goal of this book is to provide a single reference with sufficient detail to guide diagnostic and therapeutic decisions for a wide range of conditions. We believe that the consistent format, detailed focus on diagnosis and management, and comprehensive coverage of topics have accomplished that goal, enabling you to give the best care possible to your patients. We hope you think so, too.

Gary Frank, MD, MS
Samir S. Shah, MD
Lisa B. Zaoutis, MD
Marina Catallozzi, MD
Philadelphia, PA
June 2005

FOREWORD

Having practiced pediatric medicine over the last 35 years, I have witnessed remarkable changes and innovations. There have been incredible medical advances in equipment, medications, surgical procedures, non-medication therapies and most importantly in the elucidation and understanding of human disease. At the start of my career there were no desk top or handheld computers in regular use, nor were there any Computed Tomography (CT) scans or Magnetic Resonance Imaging (MRI) devices. We had only rudimentary knowledge of the human genome. There were only a small number of medications that we still use today. For example, major psychotropic medications were just beginning to be developed and used, and there were no second or third generation cephalosporins nor were there any inhaled agents such as albuterol. There were no laws protecting children from abuse. Indeed, the many changes that have occurred over the last three or four decades have been extraordinary and the rate of change in the future portends to be even more rapid.

Amidst all the innovations noted above, one area in which there has been relatively little change has been in the way the practice of medicine has been transmitted from one generation to the next. Medical education is still based on an apprenticeship model, much as it has been for centuries. In teaching both the art and science of medicine, we have relied on the method of a more experienced physician taking a novice by the hand and passing on the necessary knowledge, skills and professional attitudes. "See one—do one—teach one" has been the prevalent methodology since the times of Hippocrates of Cos (469–370 BC). Hippocrates is often recognized as the father of modern western medicine for two reasons. First of all, he believed in and demonstrated the scientific basis of illness and healing. Prior to his era the existing belief was that illness was inflicted from the gods and a matter of random circumstance. Hippocrates invoked scientific explanations and treatments. Secondly, and perhaps more importantly, Hippocrates was known for his writing and teaching medicine to his young followers. Even to this day, on the Isle of Cos, one can visit the Site of the Plane Tree of Hippocrates. This is the place where Hippocrates, the great teacher, sat in the shade of a large tree and instructed his eager and devoted students. The oath still taken by most graduating medical students stresses the duty and devotion to passing on the knowledge and skill set to others.

The Philadelphia Guide: Inpatient Pediatrics has very much followed in the ancient, but still relevant, traditions of our profession. It has been written by a talented group of young pediatricians who have recently completed their training at The Children's Hospital of Philadelphia and the Alfred I. DuPont Hospital for Children. The editors determined a need for a book that would help them and those they instruct to make day to day decisions about pediatric care on the in-patient units of their hospitals. In writing this guide, they have attempted to fill that educational need. In preparing the text, they sought counsel and guidance from those from whom they had learned their craft. The reader will note that each chapter has been prepared by young physicians who were guided and supervised by a faculty mentor. The result is a volume that is both practical and fresh in its approach yet sage in experience. The classic method of apprenticeship still lives not only in our everyday teaching methods but in the construction of this manual. In due time the young writers and editors whose names fill the pages that follow will help others and thus the perpetuation of our profession. So it was and so it will be. Having worked closely with each of the book's editors and with almost every chapter author, I am optimistic about the future of pediatrics. The contributors are all outstanding people and skilled pediatricians. Now they are teachers who are contributing to the medical education of others. With most facets of medicine being ever changing I rejoice in those things that will never change.

Stephen Ludwig, MD
Philadelphia, PA
February 2005

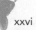

Krishna Wood, MD, Leonard J. Levine, MD, Marina Catallozzi, MD, Donald F. Schwarz, MD, MPH

ANOREXIA NERVOSA

DSM-IV criteria for anorexia nervosa are summarized below:
- Body weight less than 85% ideal body weight (IBW)
- Intense fear of gaining weight
- Disturbance in the way in which one's body weight or shape is experienced
- Amenorrhea or the absence of at least three consecutive menstrual cycles
- *Restricting type*: during the episode of anorexia nervosa, the person has not regularly engaged in binge-eating or purging behavior (self-induced vomiting, use of laxatives/diuretics/enemas)
- *Binge eating/Purging type*: during the episode of anorexia nervosa, the person has regularly engaged in binge eating or purging behavior

Epidemiology
- 1% of adolescent females; female:male = 20:1
- Age at presentation ranges from 10 to 25 years
- Increasing incidence in adolescent males, nonwhite populations, and lower socioeconomic groups; more common among individuals involved in sports or activities where size and body shape impact their success
- Bimodal age of onset at 14 and 18 years corresponding with life transitions (i.e., puberty, moving from high school to college or work)
- Mortality rates range from 0% to 20% (usually because of cardiac complications)

Etiology
- *Genetic*: increased risk in first-degree relatives with an eating disorder
- *Neurotransmitters*: serotonin and its relationship to hunger and satiety
- *Psychologic*: theories range from perfectionism, identity conflicts, history of abuse, negative comments from others about weight or appearance, enmeshed families, and sociocultural influences

Clinical Manifestations
- Menstrual disorders are the most common presentation.
- Frequently, patients do not have complaints, but family members are concerned about significant weight loss, secondary amenorrhea, dizziness, lack of energy, gastrointestinal complaints (constipation), and/or pale skin.
- Depending on amount of weight loss, clinical findings can range from normal to findings of orthostasis, bradycardia, hypothermia, hypotension, dry skin, lanugo hair, thinning hair, brittle nails, peripheral edema, acrocyanosis, and findings suggestive of purging such as eroded tooth enamel, scars on knuckles, or parotid enlargement.
- External evidence of self-harm, such as scars from cutting on the extremities

Diagnostics
- Must consider the differential diagnosis for weight loss and exclude malabsorption and catabolic states
- Clinical information is vital. Questions should focus on disordered thinking and behavior. Screening questions (such as the SCOFF, Martin et al., 1999) can be helpful:
  - Do you make yourself *sick* because you feel uncomfortably full?
  - Do you worry you have lost *control* over how much you eat?

Table 1.1: Laboratory Studies in Anorexia Nervosa

Study	Rationale/Interpretation
Serum chemistries	Hyponatremia—water loading or inappropriate regulation of ADH Hypophosphatemia—severe malnutrition Hypokalemic, hypochloremic metabolic alkalosis—vomiting Acidosis—laxative abuse Hypoglycemia High blood urea nitrogen and creatinine—dehydration +/− purging
Complete blood cell count	High hemoglobin—dehydration Anemia—chronic disease and/or iron deficiency Leukopenia and thrombocytopenia
Liver function tests (including prealbumin)	Prealbumin and albumin—evaluate nutritional status Abnormal liver enzymes—fatty liver infiltration
Cholesterol, triglycerides	Elevated due to abnormal lipoprotein metabolism
ESR	Normal to low in anorexia
Urinalysis	Low specific gravity—water loading
Morning cortisol level	Rule out adrenal insufficiency
Thyroid function tests	Euthyroid sick sinus syndrome—normal or low thyroid-stimulating hormone and normal thyroxine Rule out hyper- or hypothyroidism
β-HCG	Rule out pregnancy
Prolactin	Rule out prolactinoma
LH and FSH	Rule out ovarian failure

ADH, antidiuretic hormone; ESR, erythrocyte sedimentation rate; FSH, follicle-stimulating hormone; HCG, human chorionic gonadotropin; LH, luteinizing hormone.

- Have you recently lost more than *one* stone (6.3 kg [14 lb]) in a 3-month period?
- Do you believe yourself to be *fat* when others say you are too thin?
- Would you say that *food* dominates your life?

Give one point for every yes; scores of 2 or more indicate anorexia nervosa or bulimia

- Laboratory studies are not diagnostic of anorexia nervosa. Table 1.1 suggests tests to obtain in the initial assessment of a patient suspected of having anorexia nervosa. Further tests should be ordered based on clinical suspicion for other diseases.
- *ECG*: indicated for bradycardia less than 50 bpm to rule out prolonged QTc or dysrhythmias. Low voltage, ST segment depression, conduction abnormalities, etc., may be seen.
- *DEXA*: evaluate bone density in patients who are amenorrheic greater than 6 months.
- *Imaging*: chest x-ray, brain magnetic resonance imaging, barium enema, upper gastrointestinal series with small bowel follow-through, etc., should be considered based on clinical situation.

Management
- *Indications for inpatient treatment:*
- Weight less than 75% IBW, persistent weight loss, or acute food refusal

- Significant vital sign abnormalities (bradycardia with heart rate less than 40 bpm, hypotension, symptomatic orthostasis, or hypothermia)
- Acute medical disorders secondary to malnutrition (dehydration, electrolyte abnormalities, seizures, cardiac dysrhythmias) or acute psychiatric emergencies (suicidal ideation, psychosis)
- Consistent inability to promote health maintenance (uncontrollable binging and purging, failure of outpatient treatment)

- *Interdisciplinary team*: consisting of a physician, dietician or nutritionist, and mental health professional that generates a coordinated consistent plan of care and is available for team meetings with patient and family
- *Fluids/Electrolytes/Nutrition*:
  - Correction of dehydration
  - Blind weights with the patient wearing only a gown at same time and on the same scale each day are best. Expected rate of weight gain is 0.9 to 1.4 kg (2 to 3 lb) per week.
- *Refeeding syndrome*: constellation of cardiac, neurologic, and hematologic complications as phosphate shifts from extracellular to intracellular compartments in patients with total body phosphate depletion secondary to malnutrition
  - Pathophysiology: catabolic→anabolic state→energy used as adenosine triphosphate (ATP)→ phosphorus→erythrocyte 2,3 diphosphoglycerate (2,3 DPG)→tissue hypoxia
  - Risk factors: moderate to severe anorexia (less than 10% below IBW)
  - Prevention: slow refeeding with or without phosphorous supplementation (in patients with normal renal function)
  - Monitoring: telemetry, frequent vital signs, and electrolytes especially phosphorus, potassium, and magnesium
  - Clinical manifestations: cardiac arrest, delirium, congestive heart failure
- *Cardiovascular*: telemetry for patients with significant bradycardia, dysrhythmias, and electrolyte abnormalities until resolution of conditions
- *Gastrointestinal*: control of constipation with stool softeners (avoid laxatives). Metoclopramide may be helpful with bloating and constipation secondary to delayed gastric emptying.
- *Endocrinology*:
  - Osteopenia: weight gain is best therapy; a multivitamin with 400 IU of vitamin D and 1200-1500 mg/day of elemental calcium is recommended. Estrogen or estrogen/progestin replacement therapy should be considered.
  - Amenorrhea: menses will resume with adequate weight gain and improved nutritional status; no hormonal therapy required
- *Psychiatry*:
  - Safety and compliance: 1:1 observation by qualified staff with experience with eating disorders is required, especially in the beginning of treatment.
  - Mental status abnormalities improve with correction of malnourished state. Most interventions should begin after patient is medically stable.
  - Psychotherapy: cognitive behavioral therapy is the most effective form of therapy.
  - Pharmacotherapy: indicated only for treatment of comorbid disorders (i.e., depression, obsessive compulsive disorder)

DYSFUNCTIONAL UTERINE BLEEDING

Bleeding from the uterine endometrium unrelated to an anatomic lesion. Abnormal bleeding can be identified as menstrual cycles that occur less than 21 or more than 45 days apart, bleeding lasting more than 8 days, or blood loss greater than 80 mL.

Etiology
- Anovulatory cycles (over 75% of cases)
- Immature hypothalamic-pituitary-ovarian axis→no luteinizing hormone (LH) surge→failure to ovulate each month
- Can occur first few years after menarche

- No ovulation→estrogen unopposed because no corpus luteum or progesterone secretion→ continuously stimulated endometrium without stromal support→lining outgrows blood supply→ endometrium breaks down with variable shedding, necrosis, and irregular bleeding

Differential Diagnosis
- Anovulatory cycles: immaturity of hypothalamic-pituitary-ovarian axis
- Pregnancy: ectopic, threatened or incomplete abortion, placenta previa, hydatidiform mole
- Infection: vaginitis (e.g., *Trichomonas*), cervicitis (e.g., gonorrhea, *Chlamydia*), endometritis, salpingitis, pelvic inflammatory disease
- Endocrinopathy causing anovulation: thyroid disease (hypothyroidism, hyperthyroidism), hyperprolactinemia (e.g., prolactinoma, pituitary tumors), adrenal disorders (e.g., Addison disease, Cushing disease), polycystic ovarian syndrome
- Systemic disease causing anovulation: chronic renal failure, systemic lupus erythematosus
- Bleeding disorder: thrombocytopenia (e.g., idiopathic thrombocytopenic purpura), defects in platelet function, coagulation disorder (e.g., von Willebrand disease)
- Medications: direct effect on hemostasis (e.g., warfarin, chemotherapeutic agents), indirect effect by altering hormone levels (e.g., breakthrough bleeding with hormonal contraception)
- Trauma: laceration to vaginal mucosa or cervix
- Foreign body: retained tampon or condom
- Endometriosis: chronic pelvic pain, severe dysmenorrhea, dyspareunia
- Structural abnormalities (rare): uterine polyps, myoma, cervical hemangioma, arteriovenous malformation, neoplasm

Clinical Manifestations
- Physical exam may be unremarkable, especially if due to anovulatory cycles
- May have evidence of anemia (e.g., pallor, lethargy) or hypovolemia
- Headaches, visual changes, nipple discharge (suggestive of prolactinoma)
- Symptoms associated with thyroid disease (diarrhea or constipation, palpitations, skin changes, heat or cold intolerance) or other chronic diseases

Diagnostics
Clinical Assessment
- Menstrual history: age of menarche, interval between menses, duration of flow, frequency of tampon/pad changes, with or without cramping (cramping often is a marker for ovulatory cycles due to progesterone secretion), last menstrual period
- Other important history: abdominal pain, trauma, sexual activity, medications used, easy bleeding or bruising
- Family history: menstrual irregularities, bleeding disorders, or polycystic ovarian syndrome
- Symptoms of anemia (e.g., dizziness or lightheadedness)
- Assess hemodynamic stability
- Special attention to: nutritional status, visual fields (i.e., pituitary lesions), thyroid size, breast exam (for galactorrhea), evidence of androgen excess (hirsutism, acne), ecchymoses or petechiae, Sexual Maturity Rating
- Pelvic exam if ever been sexually active (including bimanual exam)

Studies
- Pregnancy test: on every adolescent female presenting with vaginal bleeding
- Complete blood count with differential
- Sexually transmitted disease (STD) testing: wet prep for *Trichomonas*, gonococcus, *Chlamydia* cultures, or nuclear DNA testing (urine or cervical swabs)
- PT/PTT
- Depending on history, may also consider thyroid-stimulating hormone, prolactin level, LH, follicle-stimulating hormone, serum androgens (e.g., free testosterone, dehydroepiandrosterone-S, androstenedione)
- Pelvic ultrasound (if mass palpated on bimanual exam or if concerned for structural abnormalities)

Management
- Depends on severity of bleeding and degree of anemia
- Hormonal therapy is the mainstay of treatment: usually oral contraceptive pill (OCP) used to provide hemostasis (estrogen) and to stabilize the endometrium (progesterone)
  - Address underlying pathology (e.g., infection, endocrinopathy)
- Adjunct management: menstrual diaries, iron supplementation, NSAIDs
- Mild dysfunctional uterine bleeding (DUB) (hemoglobin greater than 12, no active bleeding)
  - Prolonged menses or shortened cycles
  - Reassurance and observation
- Moderate DUB (hemoglobin 10 to 12 WITHOUT active bleeding): combined OCP with 30–35 µg ethinyl estradiol (EE) plus progestin
  - One pill daily for 6 months, then re-evaluate
  - If estrogen contraindicated, use oral progesterone only: medroxyprogesterone acetate 10 mg orally for 10 days, repeat monthly
- Moderate DUB (hemoglobin 10 to 12 WITH active bleeding)
  - Combined OCP
  - One pill four times daily for 4 days, then three times daily for 3 days, then twice daily for 2 days, then once daily
- Severe DUB (hemoglobin less than 10 WITH active bleeding)
  - Combined OCP with higher dose of estrogen (50 µg EE)
  - If not tolerating oral medications or if hemodynamically unstable, can use high-dose conjugated estrogen (Premarin) given intravenously every 4 hours up to 24 hours to control bleeding, then add oral progesterone or switch to OCP as soon as possible to avoid heavy estrogen withdrawal bleed.
  - Give antiemetics when estrogen given in multiple doses per day. Table 1.2 lists antiemetics.
  - Blood transfusions are rarely necessary in the management of DUB.

EMERGENCY CONTRACEPTION

Indications
- Contraceptive failure (i.e., broken condom, greater than two missed oral contraceptive pills); unprotected intercourse; sexual assault; 72 hours or less since aforementioned event

Contraindications
- Pregnancy; hypersensitivity to components; undiagnosed genital bleeding; migraine with focal neurologic deficit; thromboembolic disease (combined emergency contraception [EC])

Table 1.2: Anti-Emetic Medications

Medication	Dosage
Over The Counter	
Dimenhydrinate (*Dramamine*)	50 mg: 1–2 tabs 30–60 min before first EC dose; repeat q 4–6 hr prn (no more than 8 tabs in 24 hr)
Diphenhydramine (*Benadryl*)	25 mg: 1–2 tabs 1 hr before first EC dose; repeat q 4–6 hr prn
Meclizine (*Antivert*)	25 mg: 1–2 tabs 1 hr before first EC dose; repeat once in 24 hr prn
Prescription Only	
Promethazine (*Phenergan*)	25 mg: 1 tab or suppository 30–60 min before first EC dose; repeat q 4–6 hr prn

EC, emergency contraception; prn, as needed.

Table 1.3: Emergency Contraception Regimens*

Regimen Name	Pills per Dose/Color (Repeat once in 12 hrs)	Advantages of Regimen†	Disadvantages of Regimen
Yuzpe Regimen (Combined Estrogen/Progestin)			
Preven *Ovral, Ogestrel* *Alesse, Levlite* *Aviane* *Nordette, Levlen* *Levora, Lo/Ovral* *Low-Ogestrel* *Triphasil, Tri-Levlen, Trivora*	2 blue 2 white 5 pink 5 orange 4 light-orange 4 white 4 yellow 4 pink	• 75% efficacy • *Preven* comes with patient info book and urine pregnancy test • Patient may already have OCPs • Established safety/efficacy • Can continue as contraception	• 72-hr window • Side effects including nausea/vomiting common
Progestin Only			
Plan B *Ovrette*	1 white 20 yellow	• 89% efficacy • *Plan B* comes with patient info kit • More effective than combined • Less side effects	• 72-hr window
IUD	NA	• 99% efficacy • Can be inserted up to 5 days after unprotected sex • Can continue as contraception	• Contraindicated for those with or at risk of STDs, other pelvic infections, anatomic anomalies, and in immuno-compromised patients • Not highly recommended in teens

*Most effective when given in first 12 hours of unprotected sex.
†Applies to medications with a particular regimen unless specifically noted.
IUD, intrauterine device; NA, not applicable; OCPs, oral contraceptive pills; STDs, sexually transmitted diseases.

Mechanism of Action
- Prevention or delay of ovulation
- Impairment of corpus luteum
- Creation of unfavorable environment for implantation in endometrium

Adverse Effects
- Occur mostly with combined EC: nausea/vomiting; dizziness; fatigue; breast tenderness

Safety
- Short course of therapy leads to few complications
- May be prescribed without an office visit, and pharmacists in some states may provide without doctor's prescription

Anticipatory Guidance
- Table 1.3 lists EC regimens
- *Nausea/vomiting*: common in combined regimen; prescribe anti-emetic; refer to Table 1.2.
- *Effect on menstrual cycle*: next menses may be early or late but should come within 21 days
- *Effect on pregnancy*: hormonal EC does not affect established pregnancy or lead to birth anomalies
- *Follow-up*: not required but recommended for contraceptive counseling and/or pregnancy testing if no menses in 21 days

PELVIC INFLAMMATORY DISEASE

Clinical condition referring to the infection and inflammation of some or all of the upper genital tract including endometritis, salpingitis, tubo-ovarian abscess, and pelvic peritonitis. Pelvic inflammatory disease (PID) is a common and morbid complication of some sexually transmitted infections (STIs), in particular *Chlamydia trachomatis* (most commonly) and *Neisseria gonorrhoeae*.

Epidemiology
- Affects 8% of US women during reproductive years with more than 1 million US women having an episode of PID per year
- Major cause of ectopic pregnancies and chronic pelvic pain

Etiology
- Micro-organisms spread from the lower (cervix) to the upper (uterus, fallopian tubes, etc.) genital tract
- Thought to be a polymicrobial infection most commonly caused by STIs (*C. trachomatis* and *N. gonorrhoeae*), but can include the vaginal flora (anaerobes, *Gardnerella vaginalis*, *Haemophilus influenzae*, *Streptococcus agalactiae*, enteric gram-negative organisms), genital mycoplasmas, *Mycoplasma tuberculosis*, cytomegalovirus, and *Ureaplasma urealyticum*
- Previous episode of PID predisposes to another episode because of prior injury
- Pathogenesis is a complicated and poorly understood process involving interactions between genetics, immunology, and bacterial virulence factors
- Sexually active women younger than 25 years old are most at risk because the immature cervix is more likely to be infected with an STI.
- Higher risk of developing PID if higher number of sex partners

Clinical Manifestations
- Symptoms can range from none to severe.
- Lower abdominal pain is the most common presentation.
- Can also see fever, abnormal vaginal discharge, dyspareunia, dysuria, dysfunctional uterine bleeding, right upper quadrant pain (consistent with perihepatitis or Fitz-Hugh-Curtis syndrome secondary to capsular inflammation)

Diagnostics

- In 2002, the Centers for Disease Control (CDC) changed the diagnostic criteria for PID to improve the sensitivity and specificity of the diagnosis, lower the threshold for treatment, and decrease the sequelae.
- *Minimum criteria*: uterine or adnexal tenderness, cervical motion tenderness
- *Additional criteria to increase specificity*: WBCs on vaginal wet preparation, abnormal cervical or vaginal mucopurulent discharge, temperature (oral) greater than 38.3°C, elevated erythrocyte sedimentation rate or C-reactive protein, laboratory documentation of cervical infection with *C. trachomatis* or *N. gonorrhoeae*.
- PID is unlikely if the cervical discharge appears normal or no WBCs are found on the wet preparation of the vaginal secretions.
- More specific criteria for the diagnosis of PID include endometrial biopsy with evidence of endometritis, transvaginal ultrasound, or MRI demonstrating thickened tubes with or without free pelvic fluid or tubo-ovarian complex or abscess.
- Laparoscopy is the gold standard, but is not frequently warranted.

Management

- Regardless of laboratory results, treatment for PID must include coverage of *C. trachomatis*, *N. gonorrhoeae*, anaerobes, gram-negative organisms, and streptococci.
- Treatment should begin as soon as the diagnosis is made and should take into consideration availability, cost, and patient acceptance.
- Criteria for hospitalization: pregnancy; failure to improve with oral therapy; failure to follow or tolerate outpatient oral therapy; severe illness evidenced by nausea, vomiting, or high fever; tubo-ovarian abscess (TOA); inability to rule out a surgical abdomen
- *Parenteral regimens (adapted from the CDC 2002 STD treatment guidelines)*:
  - *Regimen A*: cefotetan 2 g IV every 12 hours OR cefoxitin 2 g IV every 6 hours PLUS doxycycline 100 mg orally (preferable because of pain with infusion and same bioavailability) or IV every 12 hours; discontinue IV therapy 24 hours after clinical improvement and complete 14 days of doxycycline; for TOA, can add clindamycin or metronidazole for increased anaerobic coverage
  - *Regimen B*: clindamycin 900 mg IV every 8 hours PLUS gentamicin loading dose IV or IM (2 mg/kg of body weight) followed by a maintenance dose (1.5 mg/kg) every 8 hours; can use single daily dose of gentamicin; discontinue IV therapy 24 hours after clinical improvement and complete 14 days of doxycycline 100 mg orally twice a day or clindamycin 450 mg orally four times a day (clindamycin has better anaerobic coverage for a TOA)
  - Alternative parenteral regimens exist but have not been as well studied.
- *Oral regimens (adapted from the CDC 2002 STD treatment guidelines)*:
  - *Regimen A*: ofloxacin 400 mg orally twice a day for 14 days OR levofloxacin 500 mg orally once daily for 14 days WITH OR WITHOUT metronidazole 500 mg orally twice a day for 14 days
  - *Regimen B*: ceftriaxone 250 mg IM in a single dose OR cefoxitin 2 g IM in a single dose and probenecid 1 g orally administered concurrently in a single dose or other parenteral third-generation cephalosporin (ceftizoxime or cefotaxime) PLUS doxycycline 100 mg orally twice a day for 14 days WITH OR WITHOUT metronidazole 500 mg orally twice a day for 14 days
  - Alternative oral regimens exist but have not been as well studied
- Expect clinical improvement within 3 days of initiating treatment; if no improvement, patient may require hospitalization, additional testing, or surgical intervention
- Partners who have had sexual contact with the patient during the 60 days before symptoms occurred should be treated empirically for *C. trachomatis* and *N. gonorrhoeae*.
- Prevent PID by screening high-risk women, treating any suspected PID, avoiding douching, treating bacterial vaginosis (because of the association with PID), and promoting condom use.

Resources

Bravender T, Emans SJ. Menstrual disorders: dysfunctional uterine bleeding. Pediatr Clin North Am 1999;46:545–553.

Burstein GR, Workowski KA. Sexually transmitted diseases treatment guidelines. Curr Opin Pediatr 2003;15:391–397.

Catallozzi M, et al. Sexually transmitted diseases. In: Schwartz MW, ed. Clinical Handbook of Pediatrics, 3rd ed. Philadelphia: WB Saunders, 2003.

Centers for Disease Control and Prevention. Sexually transmitted diseases treatment guidelines 2002. MMWR 2002;51(RR-6):48–52.

Centers for Disease Control and Prevention. STD prevention: pelvic inflammatory disease. Available at: http://www.cdc.gov/std/PID/STDFact-PID.htm. Accessed Nov. 16, 2004.

Clark LR, et al. Care of the adolescent patient with anorexia nervosa. JCOM 2000;7:65–70.

Committee on Adolescence. Identifying and treating eating disorders. Pediatrics 2003;111:204–211.

Diagnostic and Statistical Manual of Mental Disorders, 4th ed. Washington DC: American Psychiatric Association, 2000.

Emans SJ. Delayed puberty and menstrual irregularities. In: Emans SJ, Laufer MR, Goldstein DP, eds. Pediatric and Adolescent Gynecology, 4th ed. Philadelphia: Lippincott-Raven, 1998:163–262.

Forman SF. Eating disorders: Epidemiology, pathogenesis, and clinical features. Available at: www.uptodate.com; 2002:1–13. Accessed November 16, 2004.

Forman SF. Treatment of anorexia nervosa and bulimia nervosa. Available at: www.uptodate.com; 2002:1–7. Accessed November 16, 2004.

Hillman JK. "Just dieting" or an eating disorder? A practical guide for the clinician. Adolesc Health Update 2001;13:1–8.

Levine LJ, Catallozzi M, Schwarz DF. An adolescent with vaginal bleeding. Pediatric Case Rev 2003;3:83–90.

Mehler PS. Diagnosis and care of patients with anorexia nervosa in primary care settings. Ann Intern Med 2001;134:1048–1059.

Mitan LAP, Slap GB. Dysfunctional uterine bleeding. In: Neinstein S, ed. Adolescent Health Care: A Practical Guide, 4th ed. Philadelphia: Lippincott, Williams & Wilkins, 2002:966–972.

Morgan JF, Lacey JH. The SCOFF questionnaire: a new screening tool for anorexia nervosa. West J Med 2000;172:164–165.

Murphy B, Manning Y. An introduction to anorexia nervosa and bulimia nervosa. Nurs Standard 2003;18:45–52, 54–55.

Neinstein LS, ed. Adolescent Health Care, A Practical Guide, 4th ed. Philadelphia: Lippincott, Williams & Wilkins, 2002.

Peipert JF. Genital chlamydial infections. N Engl J Med 2003;349:2424–2430.

Polaneczky M. Oral contraceptives: Part I. Adolesc Health Update 2002;14:1–8.

Polaneczky M. Oral contraceptives: Part II. Adolesc Health Update 2002;15:1–7.

Simms I, Stephenson JM. Pelvic inflammatory disease epidemiology: what do we know and what do we need to know? Sex Transm Infect 2000;76:80–87.

Rimsza ME. Dysfunctional uterine bleeding. Pediatr Rev 2002;23:227–232.

Rosenblum J, Forman S. Evidence-based treatment of eating disorders. Curr Opin Pediatr 2002;14:379–383.

Wellbery C. Emergency contraception. Arch Fam Med 2000;9:642–646.

ANAPHYLAXIS

Anaphylaxis is an acute, potentially life-threatening systemic allergic reaction due to release of vasoactive substances from mast cells and basophils after an interaction of an allergen with cell-bound IgE.

Epidemiology
• Prevalence in United States: ~1% to 15%

Etiology
• Major causes: *foods* (seafood, nuts, legumes, eggs, milk, grains, mold-containing foods); *drugs* (antibiotics, chemotherapy, muscle relaxants, blood products, contrast dyes); *latex; insect stings* (especially hymenoptera)
• Occasionally exercise-induced or idiopathic

Differential Diagnosis
• Arrhythmia, myocardial infarction, aspiration, poisoning, pulmonary embolism, pneumothorax, status asthmaticus, seizure, stroke, head trauma, vasovagal reaction, hypoglycemia, hereditary angioedema, serum sickness, carcinoid syndrome, pheochromocytoma

Pathophysiology
• Initial exposure to antigen induces IgE-mediated sensitivity. Subsequent exposure to antigen results in antigen-antibody reaction with massive release of mediators including histamine, arachidonic acid derivatives, kinins, and platelet-activating factor from basophils and mast cells.
• Symptoms result from the action of mediators on tissue receptors throughout the body.
• Mast cells can also be activated by complement proteins C3a, C4a, and C5a, which are by-products of the complement cascade, termed anaphylatoxins.
• *Anaphylactoid* reactions refer to non–IgE-mediated mast cell degranulation.

Clinical Manifestations
• Symptoms usually begin within 30 minutes of exposure, and usually resolve within hours (in surviving patients).
• Occasionally biphasic or protracted
• Symptoms include feeling of doom; tingling of mouth or face; malaise, weakness, dizziness; chest tightness, dyspnea; anxiety, apprehension, mental status changes; sweating; pruritus, flushing; palpitations; headache; dysphagia; nasal congestion, sneezing, rhinorrhea; abdominal cramping, diarrhea, vomiting
• On exam: diaphoresis; flushing, urticaria, angioedema; oropharyngeal and laryngeal edema; stridor, wheezing, retractions; pulsus paradoxus; seizures, loss of consciousness
• May rapidly progress to hypotension, tachycardia, arrhythmias, cardiac arrest, and death

Diagnostics
• Usually a clinical diagnosis; increased plasma tryptase concentration useful if obtained within 4 hours of event

Management
• Remember ABCs, including supplemental oxygen
• Epinephrine 1:1000, 0.01 mL/kg (maximum 0.5 mL) IM; may repeat every 15 minutes
• Nebulized albuterol 0.01–0.05 mL/kg of 0.5% solution every 15 minutes as needed

- Nebulized racemic epinephrine 0.25–0.5 mL of 2.25% solution
- Diphenhydramine 1 mg/kg IM or IV every 6 hours (maximum 300 mg/day)
- Ranitidine 1 mg/kg IM or IV (max 50 mg) every 6 hours
- Solumedrol 2 mg/kg IV initially, then 1 mg/kg IV every 6 hours
- Trendelenburg position
- Rapid IV normal saline for hypotension unimproved with epinephrine
- Severe cases require endotracheal intubation and pressor support (for example, dopamine, norepinephrine, or phenylephrine for continued hypotension)

ASTHMA

Asthma is a diffuse, obstructive, chronic inflammatory disease of large and small airways punctuated by acute exacerbations. This section addresses acute asthma exacerbation.

Epidemiology
- Affects approximately 7% of children younger than 17 years of age
- Eighty percent to 90% present by 4 to 5 years of age
- Prevalence higher in African Americans and Hispanics, inner-city youth

Differential Diagnosis of Recurrent Wheezing
- *Anatomic:* extrinsic (e.g., vascular ring, lymphadenopathy, tumor) or intrinsic (e.g., foreign body, tracheomalacia, bronchial adenoma, congestive heart failure, pulmonary sequestration) to airway
- *Inflammatory/infectious:* poorly controlled asthma, bronchial papilloma, atypical pneumonia, hypersensitivity pneumonitis, pulmonary hemosiderosis, alpha 1-antitrypsin, gastroesophageal reflux
- *Genetic/metabolic:* cystic fibrosis, primary immune deficiency, alpha 1-antitrypsin deficiency, sarcoidosis, hypocalcemia
- *Mimics of wheezing:* vocal cord dysfunction, laryngomalacia

Pathophysiology
- Allergic and non-specific stimuli may trigger exacerbation (examples of triggers include upper airway infections; smoke; inhaled allergens such as pet dander, dust mites, or pollen; chemical sprays; exercise; aspirin)
- Mast cells in airway mucosa release mediators (histamine, leukotrienes, platelet-activating factor) that cause bronchoconstriction, hypersecretion of mucus, airway edema, epithelial desquamation, and infiltration of inflammatory cells
- Early immune response: bronchoconstriction
- Late-phase reaction (6 to 8 hours later): continued airway hyperresponsiveness with inflammatory cell infiltration
- Airway obstruction with nonuniform ventilation and atelectasis leads to ventilation/perfusion (V/Q) mismatch. Hyperinflation leads to decreased compliance and increased work of breathing. Increased intrathoracic pressure impairs venous return and reduces cardiac output.

Clinical Manifestations
- Onset may be acute or gradual, depending on trigger.
- Tight, nonproductive cough that is often worse at night
- Wheeze, shortness of breath
- May have abdominal pain and/or vomiting
- On exam: wheezing; decreased breath sounds; prolonged expiratory phase; accessory muscle use; cyanosis; tachypnea; tachycardia; increase in anterior-posterior diameter of chest wall; pulsus paradoxus; nasal flaring; palpable liver and spleen secondary to hyperinflation; increased nasal secretions, mucosal swelling, sinusitis, or nasal polyps; atopic dermatitis

Diagnostics
Clinical
- History of recurrent coughing and/or wheezing, or history of atopy in patient or family members supports the diagnosis
- Diagnosis is supported by response to bronchodilators

Spirometry
- Establish airflow obstruction: forced expiratory volume in 1 second (FEV_1) less than 80% predicted, FEV_1/forced vital capacity (FVC) less than 65% lower limit of normal
- Establish reversibility with inhaled bronchodilator: FEV_1 should increase greater than 12% (not possible in children younger than 5 years of age)

Laboratory
- Blood or sputum eosinophilia is suggestive, but not diagnostic.
- Elevated serum IgE with asthma symptoms supports diagnosis.
- ABG should be obtained in severe exacerbations: initial findings include low pO_2 and low pCO_2. Later findings of high pCO_2 and low pH are ominous signs of respiratory failure.

Radiographic
- Chest x-ray: findings may include hyperinflation, peribronchial thickening, atelectasis, and pneumothorax.

Other Studies
- Skin testing or RAST testing to identify potential triggers
- Methacholine challenge: response to bronchodilator after inhalation of methacholine suggests asthma
- Exercise testing: running while breathing cold, dry air results in bronchoconstriction in virtually all asthmatics

Management (Acute Exacerbation)
- Short-acting inhaled beta-2 agonists (e.g., albuterol MDI or nebulized)
- Inhaled anticholinergics: ipratropium bromide (0.25–0.5 mg nebulized, every 20 to 30 minutes mixed with initial albuterol treatments, then every 2 to 6 hours) has additive effect with beta-agonists. In emergency department (ED), ipratropium reduces likelihood of admission; once hospitalized, no reduction in length of hospital stay.
- Systemic corticosteroids for moderate to severe exacerbations: prednisone (2–4 mg/kg/day divided twice daily for 5 days, maximum 80 mg/day) or dexamethasone orally or IV (0.6 mg/kg initially and repeated 12 to 18 hours later, maximum 16 mg/dose)
- Frequent reassessment of respiratory status
- *Consider admission:* persistent respiratory distress; SaO_2 less than 91%; peak flow rate less than 50% of predicted levels; underlying high-risk factors (e.g., congenital heart disease, neuromuscular disease, cystic fibrosis), ED visit in previous 24 hours.
- Additional interventions in cases of *status asthmaticus:*
  - Pulse oximetry monitoring, supplemental oxygen
  - Consider CBC, serum electrolytes, and blood gas
  - Continuous nebulized albuterol (10–20 mg/hr)
- If severely ill, consider:
  - Epinephrine SC (0.01 mL/kg of 1:1000 solution, maximum 0.5 mL)
  - Magnesium sulfate (25 mg/kg, max 2 g) IV
  - Terbutaline SC (0.01 mg/kg, max 0.4 mg) or IV (2–10 μg/kg bolus, then 0.08–0.4 μg/kg/min and titrate up to max of 6 μg/kg/min)
- See Table 2.1 for asthma classification and discharge management. For additional information on the diagnosis and long-term management of asthma in children, please refer to guidelines such as the National Asthma Education and Prevention Program (NAEPP) Expert Panel Report Guidelines (http://www.nhlbi.nih.gov/guidelines/asthma/asthgdln.pdf)

Table 2.1: Potential Long-Term Strategies for Management of Asthma

Severity	Symptoms/PEF*	Medications
Mild Intermittent	≤ 2 d/wk or ≤ 2 nights/mo or PEF ≥ 80%	None daily
Mild Persistent	≥ 2 d/wk but < 1/d or > 2 nights/mo or PEF ≥ 80%	Inhaled steroid (low dose); +/– leukotriene receptor antagonist or cromolyn
Moderate Persistent	Daily or > 1 night/wk or PEF 60%–80%	Inhaled steroid (low dose) + long-acting inhaled beta agonist OR Inhaled steroid (medium dose); +/– leukotriene receptor antagonist
Severe Persistent	Continual and frequent nighttime or PEF ≤ 60%	Inhaled steroid (high dose) + long-acting inhaled beta 2 agonist

PEF, peak expiratory flow rate.
(Adapted from NAEPP Expert Panel Report: Guidelines for the Diagnosis and Management of Asthma—Update on Selected Topics 2002. NIH publication no. 02-5075; originally printed June, 2002.)

SERUM SICKNESS

Serum sickness is a vasculitis secondary to a type III hypersensitivity reaction in response to a foreign antigen. The term "serum sickness" is often applied to hypersensitivity reactions involving multiple mechanisms.

Differential Diagnosis
• Urticaria/angioedema, mononucleosis, viral infections, group A streptococcal infection, juvenile rheumatoid arthritis, systemic lupus erythematosus, acute rheumatic fever, erythema multiforme, Henoch-Schönlein purpura

Etiology
• Most commonly seen with drug hypersensitivities

Pathophysiology
• Type III hypersensitivity or immune-complex disease
• Antibodies form 1 to 3 weeks after exposure to antigen. Antigen-antibody complexes form and deposit in small blood vessels throughout the body.
• Immune complexes activate complement, causing neutrophil aggregation. Aggregated neutrophils release toxic granules, leading to tissue damage.

Clinical Manifestations
• Onset usually 1 to 3 weeks after antigen exposure
• Signs and symptoms: fever; rash (urticaria, erythema of palms and soles is serpiginous, may be purpuric); edema and flushing of face and neck; myalgias, arthralgias, polyarticular arthritis; severe pruritus; abdominal cramping and diarrhea
• Rare complications: carditis, glomerulonephritis, Guillain-Barré syndrome, peripheral neuritis

Diagnostics
• Thrombocytopenia, leukocytosis, or leukopenia
• May see mild proteinuria, hemoglobinuria, hematuria

- Plasma cells on peripheral smear
- Elevated ESR, sheep cell agglutinin titer, C3a anaphylatoxin
- C3, C4 levels depressed
- May find specific serum antibodies directed at offending antigen
- Immunofluorescence studies of skin lesions may reveal immune complex deposits

Management
- Aspirin, NSAIDs, and antihistamines; hospitalization only in severe cases
- Corticosteroids for severe disease (1–2 mg/kg/day divided three times daily, for 7 to 10 days then tapered over 3 to 4 weeks)
- Plasmapheresis indicated for refractory cases

URTICARIA/ANGIOEDEMA

Urticaria **is an allergic symptom complex consisting of erythematous, blanching, raised pruritic skin lesions, often with central pallor.** *Angioedema,* **a more severe form of urticaria, involves submucosal and subcutaneous tissues, as well as other organ systems, especially respiratory and gastrointestinal.**

Epidemiology
- Occurs in up to 20% of the population

Etiology
- Ingestions (food, drugs); inhalations (pollens, pet dander); injections (drugs, insect stings, blood transfusions)
- Infections: certain viruses, bacteria, parasites
- Skin contact: plant or animal substances, topical drugs
- Physical exposures: cold, sun, exercise, dermatographism
- Other diseases: vasculitides, serum-sickness, malignancy
- Other etiologies: hereditary angioedema, episodic angioedema with eosinophilia, cholinergic urticaria, chronic urticaria, psychogenic urticaria

Pathophysiology
- IgE-mediated: antigen binds to mast cell or basophil-bound IgE antibody, resulting in release of inflammatory mediators.
- Non–IgE-mediated: C3a, C5a, some drugs (e.g., codeine, ciprofloxacin), and physical factors (cold, heat, pressure, sunlight) activate mast cells
- Autoimmune urticaria: IgG autoantibodies directed at IgE bound to mast cells
- Mast cell activation releases histamine, which increases vasodilation, vascular permeability, and neurologic reflexes (leads to characteristic "wheal and flare")

Clinical Manifestations
- Individual wheals appear in one area for 20 minutes to 3 hours, disappear and then reappear in another area.
- Episodes typically last 24 to 48 hours, rarely up to 6 weeks.

Diagnostics
- Largely a clinical diagnosis. Skin testing is only helpful when specific food or drug allergies are identified.
- Skin biopsy is recommended when individual urticarial lesions last longer than 24 hours to exclude urticarial vasculitis.

Management
- Antihistamines for 48 to 72 hours (e.g., loratidine cetirizine, hydroxyzine, diphenhydramine) for primary management
- Subcutaneous epinephrine 1:1000, 0.01 mL/kg (maximum 0.3 mL) may be used in severe cases for acute relief.

- Combining both an H1 (hydroxyzine) and H2 (ranitidine) antihistamine may be of use in cases of chronic urticaria.
- Cyproheptadine: prophylaxis for cold-induced urticaria
- Chronic urticaria has been treated with both corticosteroids and low-dose cyclosporine with limited success.
- Autoimmune chronic urticaria is treated with intravenous immune globulin and/or plasmapheresis.

Resources

Atkinson TP, Kaliner MA. Anaphylaxis. Med Clin North Am 1992;76:841–855.

Behrman R, et al., eds. Nelson Textbook of Pediatrics. 16th ed. Philadelphia: WB Saunders, 2000.

Craven D, Kercsmar CM, Myers TR, et al. Ipratropium bromide plus nebulized albuterol for the treatment of hospitalized children with acute asthma. J Pediatr 2001;138:51–58.

Fleishr GR, Ludwig S. Textbook of Pediatric Emergency Medicine. 4th ed. Philadelphia: Lippincott, Williams and Wilkins, 2000.

Freeman T. Anaphylaxis: diagnosis and treatment. Primary Care Clin Office Pract 1998;25:809–817.

Huston DP, Bressler RB. Urticaria and angioedema. Med Clin North Am 1992;76:805–840.

Neugut AI, Ghatak AT, Miller RL. Anaphylaxis in the United States: an investigation into its epidemiology. Arch Intern Med 2001;161:15–21.

Platt R, Dreis MW, Kennedy DL, Kuritsky JN. Serum sickness-like reactions to amoxicillin, cefaclor, cephalex-in, and trimethoprim-sulfamethoxazole. J Infect Dis 1988;158:474–477.

Analgesia and Sedation   3

Suzanne Beno, MD, FRCPC, Jimmy W. Huh, MD

Analgesia

Analgesia is the diminution or elimination of pain in the conscious patient.

- Even neonates demonstrate behavioral and hormonal changes in response to painful procedures.
- Children do not have to understand the meaning of pain to experience pain.
- Preemptive analgesia may decrease post-injury opioid requirements.

ASSESSMENT OF PAIN

- *Infants* have physiologic and behavioral responses to pain:
  - Increased blood pressure, respiratory rate, heart rate
  - Crying, diaphoresis, flushing
  - Facial expressions, body movements
- *Preschoolers*:
  - OUCHER scale combines numeric and faces scales, making it appropriate for young children; available at www.oucher.org.
  - FACES scale: The child is asked to point to the face that best describes his/her own pain (Figure 3.1).
- *School age or adolescent*:
  - Self-report: verbal numeric pain rating scale. Pain is rated from 1 to 10.

LOCAL ANESTHESIA

Eutectic Mixture of Local Anesthetics (EMLA)
- 2.5% Lidocaine/2.5% Prilocaine
- Apply to intact skin; complete anesthesia in 60 to 90 minutes
- Use for blood drawing, bone marrow, lumbar puncture in non-emergent settings
- May use ELA-max for faster onset: topical lidocaine only; anesthesia in 30 minutes
- Contraindications: methemoglobinemia, age less than 1 month

Lidocaine, Epinephrine, Tetracaine (LET)
- Used for dermal lacerations; apply to open wound
- Contraindications: areas supplied by end-arteries (digits, pinna, nose, penis)

Tetracaine, Adrenaline, Cocaine (TAC)
- Contraindications: areas supplied by end-arteries, mucous membranes, or adjacent areas, patients taking MAO inhibitors

Viscous Lidocaine
- For children who can expectorate
- Combine with diphenhydramine and Maalox in equal parts (1:1:1) to create magic mouthwash (can also exclude lidocaine if mouth sores create a concern for systemic absorption)
- Usual dose: 15 mL of undiluted mixture; maximum dose is 4.5 mg/kg or 300 mg of lidocaine component (up to every 3 hours). Smaller amounts work well.

Lidocaine Jelly
- Used for nasogastric tube placement and urethral catheterizations

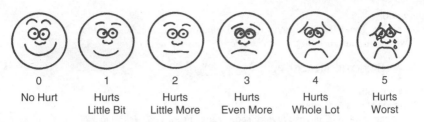

0	1	2	3	4	5
No Hurt	Hurts Little Bit	Hurts Little More	Hurts Even More	Hurts Whole Lot	Hurts Worst

Figure 3.1 Wong-Baker FACES Scale for Pain Assessment. (Reprinted with permission from Wong DL, Hockenberry-Eaton M, Wilson D, et al. Wong's Essentials of Pediatric Nursing. 6th ed. St. Louis: Mosby, 2001:1301.)

Injectable Local Anesthetic
- Buffer with 1 mL (1 meq/mL) $NaHCO_3$ per 9 mL lidocaine or 1 mL $NaHCO_3$ per 20 mL bupivacaine to reduce pain associated with injection.
- Enhance efficacy and duration by using in combination with epinephrine.
- Contraindicated in areas supplied by end arteries

NARCOTIC ANALGESICS

- Doses are listed as equianalgesic doses
- All narcotics can be reversed with naloxone hydrochloride (Narcan) 0.01 mg/kg IV/IM/SC/ETT; naloxone can be repeated every 2 minutes as needed to maximum of 10 mg

Codeine
- 0.5–1.0 mg/kg/dose orally (PO) with onset in 30 to 60 minutes; duration: 3 to 4 hours
- Synergistic with acetaminophen
- Side effects: nausea, emesis, constipation

Fentanyl
- 0.001 mg/kg/dose IV with onset in 1 to 2 minutes; duration: 0.5 to 1 hour
- 0.001 mg/kg/dose transdermal with onset in 12 minutes; duration: 2 to 3 hours
- 0.01 mg/kg/dose transmucosal with onset in 15 minutes
- Watch for chest wall rigidity with high doses and rapid push, which can be reversed with naloxone or neuromuscular paralysis/endotracheal intubation.

Hydromorphone
- 0.015 mg/kg/dose IV/SC with onset in 5 to 10 minutes; duration: 3 to 4 hours
- 0.02–0.08 mg/kg/dose PO with onset in 30 to 60 minutes (usual adult dose 2 mg); duration: 3 to 4 hours
- May cause nausea and pruritus (less than morphine)

Meperidine
- 1.0 mg/kg/dose IV with onset in 5 to 10 minutes; duration: 3 to 4 hours
- 1.5–2.0 mg/kg/dose PO with onset in 30 to 60 minutes; duration: 2 to 4 hours
- Side effects: tachycardia, seizures, worsens bronchospasm

Methadone
- 0.1 mg/kg/dose IV with onset in 5 to 10 minutes; duration: 4 to 24 hours
- 0.1 mg/kg/dose PO with onset in 30 to 60 minutes; duration: 4 to 24 hours
- Commonly used as an opioid taper

Morphine
- 0.1 mg/kg/dose IV with onset in 5 to 10 minutes; duration: 3 to 4 hours
- 0.1–0.2 mg/kg/dose IM/SC with onset in 10 to 30 minutes; duration: 4 to 5 hours
- 0.2–0.5 mg/kg/dose PO with onset in 30 to 60 minutes; duration 4 to 5 hours
- Side effects: nausea, sedation, pruritus, constipation, seizures (neonates)

Oxycodone
- 0.1 mg/kg/dose PO with onset in 30 to 60 minutes; duration: 3 to 6 hours
- Fewer gastrointestinal effects than codeine

NON-NARCOTIC ANALGESICS

Acetaminophen
- Antipyretic; weak analgesic
- Side effects: hepatic necrosis (overdosage), renal insufficiency (chronic use)
- Usual dose: 10–15 mg/kg PO or rectally every 4 to 6 hours; adult dose: 325 mg–1 g/dose
- Maximum dose: 4 g/day (adult); 5 doses (2.6 g)/day (peds)

Nonsteroidal Anti-inflammatory Drugs
- Useful for inflammatory pain
- Side effects: platelet inhibition, gastrointestinal irritation, nephrotoxicity
- Ibuprofen: 5–10 mg/kg PO every 6 to 8 hours with maximum 40 mg/kg/day
- Ketorolac: 0.5 mg/kg/dose IV/IM every 6 hours with maximum 30 mg every 6 hours
- Naproxen: 5–10 mg/kg/dose PO every 8 to 12 hours with maximum 1000 mg/day

Aspirin
- Used for specific indications only in children (e.g., Kawasaki disease)
- 10–15 mg/kg/dose PO with max of 4 g/day (adult) or 60–80 mg/kg/day
- Side effects: Reye's syndrome, avoid in children with varicella or influenza

NON-PHARMACOLOGIC METHODS OF ANALGESIA

- Distraction, music, play

PATIENT CONTROLLED ANALGESIA (PCA)

- Indicated for acute/chronic pain of known etiology as well as preemptive pain management.
- Route: IV, SC, or epidural/spinal
- Dosing for PCA:
  - *Morphine:* basal 10–20 µg/kg/hr; bolus 10–20 µg/kg; lockout 8 to 10 minutes, four to six boluses per hour; maximum dose per hour: 100–150 µg/kg
  - *Hydromorphone:* basal 3–4 µg/kg/hr; bolus 3–4 µg/kg/hr; lockout 8 to 10 minutes, four to six boluses per hour; maximum dose per hour 15–20 µg/kg
  - *Fentanyl:* basal 0.25–1 µg/kg/hr; bolus 0.25–1 µg/kg; lockout 8 to 10 minutes, 2 to 3 boluses per hour; maximum dose per hour 2 µg/kg

Sedation

Sedation is a continuum:
- *Conscious Sedation:* a medically controlled state of depressed consciousness; patient retains ability to maintain a patent airway; patient has purposeful responses to physical stimulation or verbal command; patient maintains protective airway reflexes.
- *Deep Sedation:* a medically controlled state of depressed consciousness or unconsciousness; patient has partial or complete loss of protective airway reflexes; patient has purposeful responses to physical stimulation or verbal command.
- *General Anesthesia:* medically controlled state of unconsciousness with loss of protective reflexes, inability to maintain patent airway and loss of purposeful response.

PREPARATION FOR SEDATION

- NPO Guidelines (American Society of Anesthesiology [ASA]):
  - No oral liquids for 2 hours before if younger than 2 years old or 4 hours if older than 3 years old
  - Avoidance of milk/solids 8 hours before procedure
  - Emergency: delay if possible or use lightest possible level of sedation

- Necessary History: medical history; last solid and liquid oral intake; recent illness; medication or drug use; pertinent family history; allergies and adverse reactions
- ASA Classification: I: Normal; II: Mild systemic disease; III: Severe systemic disease; IV: Severe systemic disease that is a constant threat to life; V: Moribund, operative intervention critical to survival
- Physical exam: age, weight, vital signs, oxygen saturation, absence of head injury, cardiovascular exam, lung exam, neurologic exam, mental status
- Equipment: appropriately sized positive pressure oxygen delivery system; suction apparatus including catheters (Tonsil, Yankauer); age-appropriate blood pressure cuff and oxygen saturation monitor; crash cart with age-appropriate drugs and equipment
- Monitoring:
  - Continuous pulse oximetry and heart rate monitoring
  - Vital signs with blood pressure every 15 minutes for conscious sedation and every 5 minutes for deep sedation

PRE-PROCEDURE SEDATION SUGGESTIONS

Radiology (CT and MRI) in Patient 6 Weeks to 3 Years Old
- 6 weeks to 3 years old is most likely age requiring sedation.
- Need for relative immobility but not analgesia
- Chloral hydrate PO: 60–75 mg/kg/dose (1/2 dose for neonates) 30 to 60 minutes before procedure; repeat 1/2 dose 30 minutes after initial. Maximum 2 g.
- Pentobarbital 2–6 mg/kg slow IV push with titration to response:
  - Give in increments of 1–2 mg/kg IV.
  - Time to sedation is 2 to 5 minutes and time to recovery is 1 hour.
- Midazolam is unreliable in producing sedation with immobility.
- Young infants often can be swaddled and may not require sedation.

Lumbar Puncture
- Infants younger than 2 months not routinely sedated for this procedure.
- Midazolam 0.2 mg/kg IV given 3 to 5 minutes before lumbar puncture significantly decreases anxiety in older children.

Fracture Reduction/Joint Relocation/Incision and Drainage/Burn Debridement/Central Venous Line/Chest Tubes
- Option 1: Midazolam IV (0.05–0.1 mg/kg with maximum dose of 2 mg) plus Fentanyl (1–2 μg/kg)
- Option 2: Ketamine (0.5–2 mg/kg) slow IV push. Use atropine with ketamine to decrease secretions.
- When using combination of sedative/analgesic, start with lowest dose possible.

Post Procedure
- *Discharge criteria:* vital signs within 15% of admission readings; ambulatory for age without assistance; tolerates oral challenge

Resources

Burg J. Pediatrics/sedation. Available at www.emedicine.com, 2002; vol 3, no. 1.

Fleisher G, Ludwig S, ed. Textbook of Pediatric Emergency Medicine. 4th ed. Philadelphia: Lippincott, Williams & Wilkins; 2000.

Jew R. Pharmacy Handbook and Formulary, 2003–2004. Hudson, Ohio: Lexi-Comp; 2003.

Kennedy RM, Luhmann JD. The "ouchless emergency department" getting closer: advances in decreasing distress during painful procedures in the emergency department. Pediatr Clin North Am 1999;46:1215–1241.

Sagarin MJ, et al. Rapid sequence intubation for pediatric emergency airway management. Pediatr Emerg Care 2002;18:417–423.

Wong DL, Hockenberry-Eaton M, Wilson D, et al. Wong's Essentials of Pediatric Nursing. 6th ed. St. Louis: Mosby, 2001:1301.

Yaster M, et al. Pediatric Pain Management and Sedation Handbook. St. Louis: Mosby, 1997.

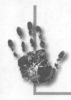

CALCULATIONS   4

Gary Frank, MD, MS

ALVEOLAR–ARTERIAL OXYGEN GRADIENT (A-a GRADIENT)

$$\text{A-a gradient} = PAO_2 - PaO_2$$
$$PAO_2 = FiO_2\,(P_{atm} - P_{H20}) - (PaCo_2/R)$$

PAO_2 = Partial pressure of alveolar oxygen in mm Hg
PaO_2 = Partial pressure of arterial oxygen in mm Hg
FiO_2 = Fraction of oxygen in inspired air (0.21 in room air)
P_{atm} = Partial pressure of the atmosphere (~760 mm Hg at sea level)
P_{H20} = Partial pressure of water vapor (~47 mm Hg at 37°C)
$PaCO_2$ = Partial pressure of carbon dioxide
R = Respiratory quotient (~0.8)
- To calculate A-a gradient, obtain ABG, preferably with patient on room air or 100% FiO_2 to obtain measured values (PaO_2 and $PaCO_2$)
- Normal gradient: 20 to 65 mm Hg on 100% O_2; 5 to 20 mm Hg on room air
- Hypoxia due to hypoventilation alone has a normal A-a gradient.
- If A-a gradient is increased, check if supplemental O_2 corrects PaO_2:
  - PaO_2 corrects: asthma or other conditions associated with ventilation-perfusion mismatch
  - PaO_2 does not correct: shunt

ABSOLUTE NEUTROPHIL COUNT

$$ANC = WBC \times (Polys/100 + Bands/100)$$

WBC = White blood cell count in cells/mm^3
Polys = Percentage of polymorphonuclear neutrophils
Bands = Percentage of band forms
- Neutropenia generally defined as absolute neutrophil count (ANC) less than 1500 cells/mm^3
- Severe neutropenia (ANC < 500 cells/mm^3) associated with high risk of infection

ANION GAP (SERUM)

$$\text{Serum Anion Gap} = [Na^+] - ([Cl^-] + [HCO_3^-])$$

$[Na^+]$ = Serum concentration of sodium in mEq/L
$[Cl^-]$ = Serum concentration of chloride in mEq/L
$[HCO_3^-]$ = Serum concentration of bicarbonate in mEq/L
- Normal anion gap is 8 to 12 mEq/L
- Acidosis with elevated anion gap may be due to MUD PILES: Methanol, Uremia, Diabetic ketoacidosis, Paraldehyde or Phenformin, Iron tablets or Infection or INH, Lactic acidosis, Ethanol or Ethylene glycol, Salicylates

BIOSTATISTICS

	Disease Present	Disease Absent
Test Positive	A	B
Test Negative	C	D

$Sensitivity = A/(A + C)$
$Specificity = D/(B + D)$
$Positive\ Predictive\ Value = A/(A + B)$
$Negative\ Predictive\ Value = D/(C + D)$

BODY MASS INDEX

$$Body\ Mass\ Index = weight/height^2$$

Weight in kilograms
Height in meters
• Adult values: normal is 18 to 25; overweight is 25 to 30; obese is greater than 30
• Pediatric norms vary by age

BODY SURFACE AREA (MOSTELLER METHOD)

$$Body\ Surface\ Area = \sqrt{weight \times height/3600}$$

Body Surface Area in meters^2
Weight in kilograms
Height in centimeters
• Used to calculate dosages for certain medications
• Other formulas have been derived by DuBois and others

CONVERSIONS

Degrees Fahrenheit = 1.8 × degrees Celsius + 32   1 atmosphere = 760 mm Hg
1 inch = 2.54 centimeters   1 teaspoon = 5 milliliters
1 tablespoon = 15 milliliters   1 kilogram = 2.2 pounds
1 fluid ounce = 30 milliliters   1 dry ounce = 30 grams

CORRECTED QT INTERVAL

$$Corrected\ QT\ Interval = \frac{QT}{\sqrt{RR\ preceding}}$$

QT = Measured QT interval in seconds
RR = Preceding RR interval in seconds
• Corrected QT interval (QTc) greater than 0.44 seconds is concerning for long QT syndrome
• Certain electrolyte abnormalities and medications may increase the QTc

CORRECTED SERUM CALCIUM (FOR LOW ALBUMIN)

$$Corrected\ Serum\ Calcium = (ALB_n - ALB_p) \times 0.8 + Ca_p$$

ALB_n = Normal plasma albumin concentration = 4.0 g/dL
ALB_p = Measured plasma albumin concentration in g/dL
Ca_p = Measured plasma calcium concentration in mg/dL
• Corrects the measured plasma calcium concentration for hypoalbuminemia
• Measuring an ionized calcium level may be more accurate

CORRECTED SERUM SODIUM (FOR HYPERGLYCEMIA)

$$Corrected\ Serum\ Sodium = Na_p + (GL_p - 100) \times 1.6/100$$

Na_p = Measured plasma sodium concentration in mmol/L
GL_p = Measured plasma glucose concentration in mg/dL

- Hyperglycemia causes a "pseudohyponatremia" due to the shift of water from the intracellular space to the extracellular space.

CREATININE CLEARANCE (FROM TIMED URINE COLLECTION)

$$CrCl = (U_{Cr} \times U_{Vol})/(P_{Cr} \times T_{min})$$
$$Corrected\ CrCl = CrCl \times 1.73/BSA$$

CrCl = Creatinine clearance in mL/min
Corrected CrCl = Corrected to a body surface area of 1.73 m^2 in mL/min/1.73 m^2
U_{Cr} = Urine creatinine in mg/dL
U_{Vol} = Urine volume in mL
P_{Cr} = Plasma creatinine concentration in mg/dL
T_{min} = Time of urine collection in minutes
- Represents volume of plasma cleared of creatinine per unit time
- Creatinine is freely filtered, not reabsorbed, and minimally secreted by the kidneys. Thus, creatinine clearance is an estimate of glomerular filtration.

CREATININE CLEARANCE (SCHWARTZ METHOD)

$$CrCl = K \times Height/P_{Cr}$$

CrCl = Creatinine clearance in mL/min
K = 0.33 for low birth weight infants; 0.45 for term infants; 0.55 for children; 0.55 for adolescent girls; 0.7 for adolescent boys
Height in centimeters
P_{Cr} = Plasma creatinine concentration in mg/dL

FRACTIONAL EXCRETION OF SODIUM

$$Fractional\ Excretion\ of\ Sodium = 100 \times (U_{Na} \times P_{Cr})/(U_{Cr} \times P_{Na})$$

U_{Na} = Urine sodium concentration in meq/L
P_{Cr} = Plasma creatinine concentration in mg/dL
U_{Cr} = Urine creatinine concentration in mg/dL
P_{Na} = Plasma sodium concentration in meq/L
- Fractional excretion of sodium less than 1.0% concerning for prerenal state (and other etiologies)
- Fractional excretion of sodium greater than 2.0% concerning for acute tubular necrosis (and other etiologies)

FREE WATER DEFICIT

$$FWD = 0.6 \times weight \times (Na_p/140 - 1)$$

FWD in liters
Weight in kilograms
Na_p = Measured plasma sodium concentration in meq/L
- Used to determine the amount of free water needed to treat hypernatremia

GLOMERULAR FILTRATION RATE (SCHWARTZ FORMULA)

$$GFR = K \times Height/P_{Cr}$$

Glomerular filtration rate (GFR) in mL/min/1.73 m^2
K = 0.35 (preterm infant), 0.45 (term infant), 0.55 (girls and prepubertal boys), 0.70 (postpubertal boys)

Height in cm
P_{Cr} = Plasma creatinine concentration in mg/dL
- One of a number of methods for estimating and/or measuring GFR
- GFR can be used to screen for kidney disease, follow disease progression, confirm need for definitive treatment (e.g., dialysis, transplantation), and help determine appropriate medication doses for patients with kidney disease.

GLUCOSE INFUSION RATE

$$GIR = \%glucose \times Rate_{daily}/144 = (\%glucose \times Rate_{hourly})/(6 \times Weight)$$

Glucose infusion rate (GIR) in mg/kg/min
%glucose = Percent glucose in intravenous fluid (e.g., D10W contains 10% glucose)
$Rate_{daily}$ = Fluid administration rate in mL/kg/day
$Rate_{hourly}$ = Fluid administration rate in mL/hour
Weight in kg
- Used in the management of hypoglycemia, especially in neonates
- Glucose utilization of healthy neonates is approximately 5–8 mg/kg/min.

MEAN ARTERIAL PRESSURE

$$\text{Mean Arterial Pressure} = (\text{Systolic Pressure} + 2 \times \text{Diastolic Pressure})/3$$

- Based on assumption that diastole lasts approximately twice as long as systole

OSMOLALITY (SERUM)

$$\text{Calculated Serum Osmolality} = (2 \times Na) + (GLC/18) + (BUN/2.8)$$

Na = Serum sodium concentration in mEq/L
GLC = Serum glucose concentration in mg/dL
BUN = Serum urea nitrogen concentration in mg/dl
- Normal serum osmolality is approximately 285 to 295 mOsm/L.
- If the measured serum osmolality is more than 10 mOsm/L above the calculated serum osmolality, consider causes for an osmolal gap such as mannitol, ethanol, methanol, and ethylene glycol.

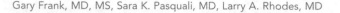

Gary Frank, MD, MS, Sara K. Pasquali, MD, Larry A. Rhodes, MD

Congenital Heart Disease

AORTIC STENOSIS

A form of acyanotic congenital heart disease in which obstruction of the left ventricular outflow tract leads to a systolic pressure gradient between the left ventricle (LV) and the aorta.

- *Aortic Valve Stenosis:* most common form of aortic stenosis; frequently due to bicuspid aortic valve; identified in up to 2% of adults
- *Subvalvular Stenosis:* due to fibromuscular ring or shelf below the aortic valve; may be associated with malalignment ventricular septal defect (VSD) or aortic coarctation
- *Supravalvular Stenosis:* least common form of aortic stenosis; may be localized or diffuse; may be associated with Williams syndrome

Epidemiology
- 3% to 6% of congenital heart defects; male:female = 4:1

Pathophysiology
- *Critical aortic stenosis:* high pressure gradients across the aortic valve may result in left ventricular (LV) failure, low cardiac output, and pulmonary edema.
- As cardiac output increases with growth during childhood, the pressure gradient may increase.
- Abnormal diastolic filling is due to LV hypertrophy.

Clinical Manifestations
- Often asymptomatic in infancy
- Symptoms depend on severity and location of obstruction; May present with irritability, paleness, tachycardia, tachypnea, retractions, rales
- Congestive heart failure (CHF) is most common in neonates with critical disease or in adults with untreated disease.
- Valve calcifications may lead to worsening disease in adults.
- Occasional ventricular arrhythmias and sudden death may occur.
- On exam: early systolic ejection click at the apex; harsh systolic murmur at the base radiates to the neck; palpable left ventricular lift; precordial systolic thrill at base

Diagnostics
- *Chest x-ray:* may show evidence of LV hypertrophy
- *ECG:* may show evidence of LV hypertrophy or LV strain in severe disease
- *Echocardiography:* defines anatomy and hemodynamic severity of the lesion
- *Cardiac catheterization:* occasionally used to establish severity and measure pressure gradient across aortic valve

Management
Medical
- Prostaglandin E_1 (PGE_1) dilates the ductus arteriosus to augment systemic circulation in severely ill neonates.
- Digoxin: consider for patients with poor cardiac output or LV hypertrophy.
- Antibiotic prophylaxis against bacterial endocarditis is necessary during invasive procedures.
- Exercise avoidance is mandatory in severe disease.

Surgical
- *Aortic Valve Stenosis:* percutaneous balloon aortic valvuloplasty; surgical valvotomy; aortic valve replacement with prosthetic valve, aortic homograft, or pulmonary autograft (Ross procedure)
- *Subaortic Stenosis:* surgical removal of fibromuscular shelf or ring
- *Supravalvular Stenosis:* prosthesis to widen or repair stenotic segment

ATRIAL SEPTAL DEFECT

A form of acyanotic congenital heart disease characterized by openings in the atrial septum at one of the following four locations:

- Ostium secundum: located at site of foramen ovale; 50% to 70% of all atrial septal defects (ASDs)
- Ostium primum: located low in the septum; atrioventricular (AV) valve often involved
- Sinus venosus: located high in the septum near the superior vena cava; associated with anomalous pulmonary venous return
- ASD of the inferior vena cava: least common

Epidemiology
- 5% to 10% of congenital heart disease; female:male = 2:1; 1 in 1500 live births

Pathophysiology
- Small defects may close spontaneously.
- Magnitude of left-to-right shunt depends on size of the defect and pulmonary and systemic vascular resistance.
- May lead to right atrial and right ventricular volume overload; rarely, pulmonary vascular disease develops.

Clinical Manifestations
- Often asymptomatic; may not present until adulthood
- May present as heart murmur in 3- to 5-year-old patients
- Occasionally presents in childhood with fatigue, dyspnea, respiratory infections, and CHF
- CHF is more common if the ASD is associated with another defect.
- Atrial dysrhythmias including fibrillation and supraventricular tachycardia are more common in adults.
- Pulmonary hypertension is more common in adults.
- Paradoxical emboli may occur.
- On exam: S_1 is loud or normal; S_2 is widely split and fixed; prominent right ventricular cardiac impulse; midsystolic pulmonary ejection murmur; diastolic murmur at left lower sternal border may represent flow across the tricuspid valve if pulmonary:systemic flow ratio (Qp:Qs) is greater than 2:1

Diagnostics
- *Chest x-ray:* right atrial enlargement, right ventricular hypertrophy (RVH), dilated pulmonary artery, increased pulmonary vasculature
- *ECG:* right axis deviation and RVH
- *Echocardiography:* reveals location, size, and associated anomalies
- *Cardiac catheterization:* may be used to confirm presence of the defect and determine pulmonary:systemic flow ratio (Qp:Qs)

Management
Medical
- Prophylactic antibiotics are recommended before oropharyngeal surgical procedures.
- CHF is managed with digoxin and diuretics.
- Occasional arrhythmias may require medical management.
- Secundum ASDs close spontaneously in ~40% of patients.

Surgical
- Usually recommended if pulmonary:systemic flow ratio (Qp:Qs) is greater than 2:1, patient is symptomatic, or ASD is moderate or large in size.
- Uncomplicated ASDs are often closed between 2 and 4 years of age.
- Traditionally, the defect is sutured or a patch is applied, often under cardiopulmonary bypass. Recently, a variety of closure devices that are deployed by transvenous catheterization have gained popularity.

COARCTATION OF THE AORTA

A form of acyanotic congenital heart disease in which there is narrowing of the aorta, most commonly just beyond the origin of the left subclavian artery.

- May occur in isolation or in association with other cardiac defects and/or non-cardiac birth defects.

Epidemiology
- 5% to 8% of congenital heart defects; male:female = 2:1
- Often associated with Turner syndrome

Pathophysiology
- Degree of symptoms depends on severity of coarctation.
- LV outflow tract obstruction leads to LV hypertrophy and increased systolic pressures.
- Decreased blood flow to lower extremities may occur, especially after closure of the ductus arteriosus.
- In severe disease, LV dysfunction may lead to pulmonary edema and low output cardiac failure.
- An extensive collateral circulation may develop.

Clinical Manifestations
- Neonates: may present in the first 3 weeks of life, especially after closure of the ductus arteriosus, with tachypnea, poor feeding, diaphoresis, congestive heart failure, cardiogenic shock, and/or decreased femoral pulses.
- Older children: upper extremity hypertension and claudication.
- On exam: decreased or absent femoral pulses; systolic murmur at left sternal border between third and fourth intercostal space radiating to left infrascapular area; ejection click if bicuspid aortic valve is present

Diagnostics
- Four-extremity blood pressures (BPs): differential in BP (>10 mm Hg) between right upper extremity and lower extremities
- *Chest x-ray:* rib notching noted in children over 6 years of age
- *ECG:* LV hypertrophy and possible left atrial enlargement in older children; right ventricular hypertrophy in neonates.
- *Echocardiography:* reveals segment of coarctation and associated anomalies
- *Cardiac catheterization:* may be performed to delineate affected segment and identify collateral circulation
- *MRI:* may help define lesion and identify collateral vessels; used for serial follow-up

Management
Medical
- In severely affected neonates, PGE_1 (0.03–0.1 µg/kg/min) maintains patency of ductus to help provide distal perfusion.
- Digoxin and diuretics as necessary to manage heart failure
- Rebound hypertension is common in the immediate postoperative period and may require antihypertensive medication.

Surgical
- Timing depends on age of diagnosis, severity of disease, and related defects.
- Multiple approaches include percutaneous balloon angioplasty, end-to-end anastomosis, subclavian flap repair, prosthetic patch, bypass graft, endovascular stent

ENDOCARDIAL CUSHION DEFECT

A form of acyanotic congenital heart disease in which there is malformation of the endocardial cushion resulting in defects in the interatrial and/or interventricular septum. Defects may be partial (e.g., ostium primum atrial septal defect, common atrium, posterior ventricular septal defect, cleft mitral valve) or complete (e.g., complete atrioventricular canal).

- *Complete atrioventricular canal:* one large atrioventricular valve, which usually has five leaflets.

Epidemiology
- 4% to 5% of congenital heart disease; 0.19 in 1000 live births
- 30% of children with complete endocardial cushion defects have Down syndrome; 20% to 25% of children with Down syndrome have endocardial cushion defects.

Pathophysiology
- Varying degrees of left-to-right shunt result in congestive heart failure and recurrent pneumonias. The hemodynamics depend on the specific location of the defect, the degree of shunting, and valvular incompetence.

Clinical Manifestations
- May present with failure to thrive, tachypnea, tachycardia, respiratory infections, and/or congestive heart failure
- Untreated defects may lead to Eisenmenger syndrome (irreversible pulmonary arterial hypertension resulting from long-standing excessive pulmonary blood flow).
- Physical exam findings depend on the extent of the lesion and may include: hyperdynamic precordium with palpable thrill at left lower sternal border; accentuated pulmonic component of S_2; variable systolic murmur may be inaudible or grade 3–4/6 and holosystolic; signs of CHF

Diagnostics
Findings depend on the extent of the lesion and may include:
- *Chest x-ray:* cardiomegaly, pulmonary vascular congestion, prominent main pulmonary artery
- *ECG:* left or superior deviation of QRS axis (–40 to –150 degrees), ventricular hypertrophy (right and/or left), prolonged PR interval
- *Echocardiography:* helps define size of the defects, size of the ventricles, and anatomy of the valve
- *Cardiac catheterization:* usually reserved for patients with complete atrioventricular canal; may be used to evaluate pulmonary hypertension and to look for additional ventricular septal defects (VSDs)

Management
Medical
- Endocarditis prophylaxis
- Anticongestive medications: digoxin, diuretics, ACE inhibitors

Surgical
- Definitive surgical treatment may be necessary before one year of age to prevent irreversible pulmonary hypertension.
- Palliative pulmonary artery banding is usually reserved for cases in which more definitive surgical options are contraindicated.

HYPOPLASTIC LEFT HEART SYNDROME

A form of cyanotic congenital heart disease characterized by underdevelopment of the left ventricle and ascending aorta. The mitral and aortic valves are atretic or critically stenosed. Systemic circulation is dependent on a patent ductus arteriosus (PDA).

Epidemiology

- 1% of congenital heart disease
- Most common cause of cardiac death in the first month of life
- Chromosomal abnormalities in up to 25% of patients

Pathophysiology

- Blood returning from the lungs passes through a patent foramen ovale or an atrial septal defect into the right atrium and right ventricle. If a VSD is present and the aortic valve is not completely stenotic, a small amount of blood may enter the aorta directly. Otherwise, there is complete mixing of systemic and pulmonary blood, which enters the pulmonary artery and passes through a PDA into the systemic circulation. As pulmonary vascular resistance decreases and the PDA closes, systemic output decreases and a metabolic acidosis ensues. Alternatively, if pulmonary vascular resistance remains high and the PDA is open, poor pulmonary blood flow may lead to severe hypoxemia.

Clinical Manifestations

- While the majority of patients present shortly after birth, some present after 48 hours of life as the ductus arteriosus closes.
- Cyanosis, dyspnea, poor feeding, CHF, hepatomegaly, poor perfusion, decreased peripheral pulses, shock
- On exam: right parasternal lift; single, loud S_2; soft, nonspecific systolic ejection murmur

Diagnostics

- *Prenatal ultrasound:* allows for antenatal diagnosis, counseling, and time to consider treatment options
- *Chest x-ray:* cardiomegaly, pulmonary venous congestion, pulmonary edema
- *ECG:* right ventricular hypertrophy
- *Echocardiography:* defines anatomy
- *Cardiac catheterization:* unnecessary if echocardiogram is diagnostic

Management

Medical

- Without intervention, hypoplastic left heart syndrome (HLHS) is fatal within the first month of life.
- PGE_1 maintains ductal patency and systemic perfusion (initial dose: 0.05–0.1 µg/kg/min).
- Metabolic acidosis may be treated with sodium bicarbonate.
- Ratio of pulmonary vascular resistance (PVR) to systemic vascular resistance (SVR) is actively managed to assure adequate oxygenation and systemic output. Generally, SaO_2 greater than 70% is adequate and SaO_2 greater than 90% is undesirable because it indicates pulmonary overcirculation. *Supplemental oxygen is usually NOT required.*
- Increased PaO_2 and decreased $PaCO_2$ both lead to decreased PVR. Thus, mechanical ventilation, sedation, and nitrogen can all be used to control the PVR:SVR ratio.

Surgical

- *Norwood Procedure:* a three-staged surgical repair of HLHS. Survival after all three stages is approximately 50%.
- *Orthotopic Heart Transplantation:* still preferred at some centers; requires lifelong immunomodulatory therapy; shortage of available donors

TETRALOGY OF FALLOT

A form of cyanotic congenital heart disease resulting from a malaligned infundibular septum and characterized by 1) overriding aorta; 2) right ventricular outflow tract obstruction (RVOTO); 3) malalignment VSD; 4) right ventricular hypertrophy

- *Paroxysmal Hypercyanotic Attacks ("TET spells")* are
  - Characterized by the sudden onset of increased cyanosis, dyspnea, and change in mental status (often with irritability)

- Due to sudden increased ratio of pulmonary to systemic vascular resistance resulting in increased shunting and reduction in pulmonary blood flow
- May lead to severe hypoxemia, metabolic acidosis, and death
- Onset generally between 2 and 9 months of age

Epidemiology
- 5% to 7% of congenital heart disease; incidence: 1 in 2700
- 15% of patients with TOF have DiGeorge syndrome; 50% of patients with DiGeorge syndrome have TOF

Pathophysiology
- Pulmonary valve annulus has variable size and helps determine degree of RVOTO.
- Severity of symptoms determined by degree of RVOTO (related to subvalvular pulmonary stenosis) and right-to-left shunt; degree of shunt depends on pulmonary vascular resistance, systemic vascular resistance, and presence of a patent ductus arteriosus.
- VSD is usually large and unrestrictive.
- Mild cases may have imperceptible cyanosis ("pink tet").

Clinical Manifestations
- Cyanosis in most patients by 1 year of age; dyspnea with exertion; clubbing
- Tendency to assume a "knee-to-chest" or squatting position
- Paroxysmal hypercyanotic attacks ("tet" spells)
- On exam: right ventricular impulse and systolic thrill palpable along left sternal border; harsh systolic ejection murmur at left sternal border; single second heart sound

Diagnostics
- *Chest x-ray:* "boot-shaped" heart, clear lung fields, possible right aortic arch
- *ECG:* right axis deviation, right ventricular hypertrophy, dominant R wave or RSR' pattern in precordial leads
- *Echocardiography:* overriding and enlarged aorta, aortic-septal discontinuity, narrowed right ventricular outflow tract, hypoplastic pulmonary arteries, VSD
- *Cardiac catheterization:* often necessary to assess magnitude of right-to-left shunt and to define the anatomy and associated anomalies

Management
"TET" Spells
- Remove restrictive clothing, calm patient, and place in knee-chest position.
- Oxygen
- Morphine
- Phenylephrine or IV beta-blocker rarely required

Medical
- In neonates, avoid stressors such as cold, and monitor blood glucose levels.
- If RVOTO is severe, infants may be dependent on a patent ductus arteriosus; consider PGE$_1$ (initial dose: 0.1 µg/kg/min).
- Oral propranolol may decrease frequency and severity of "tet" spells.

Surgical
- *Palliative Surgery*: systemic-to-pulmonary artery shunt (e.g., modified Blalock-Taussig shunt) can augment pulmonary blood flow in severely affected infants.
- *Total Surgical Correction*: often done during infancy.

TOTAL ANOMALOUS PULMONARY VENOUS RETURN

A form of cyanotic congenital heart disease in which the pulmonary veins drain anomalously into systemic veins. There are four types of total anomalous pulmonary venous return (TAPVR):

1. *Supracardiac:* pulmonary veins course superiorly to a "vertical vein," which drains into the innominate vein. Blood then flows to the superior vena cava and the right atrium.

2. *Cardiac:* pulmonary veins insert directly into the coronary sinus and right atrium.

3. *Infracardiac:* pulmonary veins course inferiorly through a descending vein, which drains into the portal system. Blood then flows to the hepatic veins, inferior vena cava, and right atrium. Pulmonary venous obstruction may occur at the diaphragm.

4. *Mixed:* combination of other types.

Epidemiology
• 1% to 2% of congenital heart defects; male > female

Pathophysiology
• Because pulmonary venous return enters systemic venous circulation, mixing through an atrial septal defect or a patent foramen ovale must occur for survival.
• Right atrial, ventricular and pulmonary artery dilation are common due to volume overload.
• If pulmonary venous obstruction exists (common with infracardiac TAPVR), pulmonary congestion and hypertension develop. In this case, neonates will be cyanotic and show early signs of respiratory distress.
• If there is no pulmonary venous obstruction and the atrial septal defect is not restrictive, then oxygen saturations above 90% are common. These patients are still at risk for right heart failure.

Clinical Manifestations
• If pulmonary venous obstruction exists, patients present at 24 to 48 hours of life with cyanosis, tachypnea, and tachycardia.
• If pulmonary venous obstruction does not exist, patients present with mild cyanosis, failure to thrive, dyspnea, and/or congestive heart failure.
• *With pulmonary venous obstruction:* single, loud S_2; gallop; faint or no murmur
• *Without pulmonary venous obstruction:* increased right ventricular impulse; S_2 widely split and fixed; characteristic quadruple or quintuple rhythm; 2/6 to 3/6 systolic ejection murmur at left upper sternal border; mid-diastolic rumble at left lower sternal border

Diagnostics
• *Chest x-ray:* if pulmonary venous obstruction exists, pulmonary edema is seen. If pulmonary venous obstruction does not exist, cardiomegaly is seen.
• *ECG:* right ventricular hypertrophy
• *Echocardiography:* large right ventricle, compressed left ventricle, atrial septal defect, or patent foramen ovale
• *MRI:* may be used to confirm diagnosis and help define anatomy
• *Cardiac catheterization and angiography:* helps define anatomy, ratio of pulmonary to systemic flow, and degree of pulmonary hypertension

Management
• Supplemental oxygen
• Treat congestive heart failure with digoxin and diuretics
• Correction of metabolic acidosis
• PGE_1 may improve mixing by maintaining patency of the ductus arteriosus. PGE_1 may also decrease venous obstruction in infracardiac TAPVR by maintaining patency of the ductus venosus. However, PGE_1 carries a risk of worsening pulmonary congestion by increasing left to right shunt through a patent ductus arteriosus.
• Goal of surgery is to redirect pulmonary venous return to the left atrium.

TRANSPOSITION OF THE GREAT ARTERIES

A form of cyanotic congenital heart disease whereby the aorta arises from the morphological right ventricle and the pulmonary artery arises from the morphological left ventricle.

• The most common form is dextra-transposition of the great arteries (d-TGA) in which the aorta is anterior and to the right of the pulmonary artery.

- In type 1 TGA, the ventricular septum is intact.
- In type 2 TGA, a ventricular septal defect exists. Varying degrees of pulmonary stenosis and pulmonary vascular obstruction may also exist.

Epidemiology
- 5% of congenital heart disease; male:female = 3:1
- More common in infants of diabetic mothers

Pathophysiology
- TGA results in two parallel circuits such that deoxygenated blood is carried by the aorta to the body, while oxygenated blood is carried by the pulmonary artery to the lungs.
- To sustain life, mixing must occur through an associated patent ductus arteriosus, ventricular septal defect, or atrial septal defect.
- Balanced bidirectional shunting must occur or one of the parallel circuits would become depleted.
- If untreated, TGA is usually fatal in the neonatal period.

Clinical Manifestations
- Dyspnea and cyanosis from birth, progressive respiratory distress, feeding intolerance, congestive heart failure
- On exam: often, no murmur is appreciated; murmur of ventricular septal defect may be noted; single, loud S_2

Diagnostics
- *Hyperoxia Test:* 100% oxygen is administered via oxyhood for 10 minutes. If PaO_2 increases above 100 mm Hg, parenchymal lung disease is suspected, whereas a PaO_2 less than 50 indicates cyanotic heart disease. Alternatively, an increase in PaO_2 of less than 10 to 30 mm Hg indicates congenital heart disease.
- *Chest x-ray:* mild cardiomegaly, "egg-on-a-string" appearance of cardiac silhouette, pulmonary vascular congestion
- *ECG:* right axis deviation, right ventricular hypertrophy, right atrial enlargement
- *Echocardiography:* confirms anatomy and associated defects; helps estimate degree of mixing
- *Cardiac catheterization:* confirms anatomic defect; angiogram may be used to define coronary anatomy; may be accompanied by balloon atrial septostomy as initial palliative procedure

Management
Medical
- PGE_1: dilates the ductus arteriosus in order to augment mixing (initial dose: 0.05 μg/kg/min)
- Sodium bicarbonate: for severe metabolic acidosis
- Oxygen
- Digoxin
- Diuretics
- Iron (if anemic)

Surgical
- *Balloon Atrial Septostomy (Rashkind Procedure):* increases interatrial mixing; may stabilize the ill neonate before definitive treatment
- *Arterial Switch Operation (ASO):* restores left ventricle as the systemic pump
- *Atrial Switch Operation (Mustard or Senning technique):* risk of late right ventricular failure

TRICUSPID ATRESIA

A form of cyanotic congenital heart disease in which there is no outlet from the right atrium to the right ventricle. The entire systemic blood flow enters the left atrium via a patent foramen ovale or an atrial septal defect.

Epidemiology
- 1% of congenital heart defects

Pathophysiology

- In the absence of a VSD, there is a small or absent right ventricle (i.e., hypoplastic right heart syndrome, pulmonary atresia with intact ventricular septum).
- In the presence of a VSD, right ventricular function depends on the size of the VSD and the degree of pulmonary stenosis.
- If there is transposition of the great arteries, left ventricular blood enters the pulmonary artery and causes pulmonary edema.
- Pulmonary blood flow may be dependent on a patent ductus arteriosus.

Clinical Manifestations

- Most patients present by 2 months of age with cyanosis and tachypnea.
- Occasionally, patients with transposition of the great arteries develop pulmonary overcirculation and present with congestive heart failure.
- Rarely, older patients present with cyanosis, dyspnea on exertion, polycythemia, and easy fatigability.
- On exam: may have holosystolic murmur at left sternal border; single S_2; increased left ventricular impulse

Diagnostics

- *Chest x-ray:* may see pulmonary undercirculation or overcirculation
- *ECG:* left axis deviation, right atrial enlargement, left ventricular hypertrophy
- *Echocardiography:* absent tricuspid valve, small or absent right ventricle, large left ventricle
- *Cardiac catheterization:* helps define anatomy, size of ventricular septal defect, and pulmonary:systemic flow ratio

Management

Medical
- PGE_1 in severely cyanotic infants (e.g., no VSD) maintains patency of ductus arteriosus and promotes pulmonary blood flow.
- Treatment of congestive heart failure may be necessary in patients with high pulmonary flow

Surgical
- If pulmonary blood flow is diminished, initial palliative procedures may include balloon atrial septostomy, Blalock-Taussig shunt, or surgical septectomy.
- If pulmonary blood flow is increased, pulmonary arterial banding may be beneficial.
- Definitive surgical correction is beyond the scope of this chapter.

TRUNCUS ARTERIOSUS

A form of cyanotic congenital heart disease in which a single arterial trunk arising from the heart supplies the pulmonary, systemic, and coronary circulations:

- One semilunar valve with two to seven septal leaflets, which may be stenotic or regurgitant
- Large ventricular septal defect
- Four subtypes based on the origin of the pulmonary arteries:
  - Type 1: main pulmonary artery arises from the base of the trunk and then divides into right and left pulmonary arteries
  - Type 2: separate origins of the right and left pulmonary arteries from the posterior aspect of the trunk
  - Type 3: separate origins of the right and left pulmonary arteries from the lateral aspects of the trunk
  - Type 4: a form of pulmonary atresia in which pulmonary circulation is derived from multiple, small arteries arising from the descending aorta

Epidemiology

- 1% to 3% of congenital heart defects
- May be associated with DiGeorge syndrome

Pathophysiology
- Because blood leaves the heart through a single trunk, complete mixing occurs and cyanosis may be minimal.
- Degree of arterial oxygen saturation depends on the ratio of systemic to pulmonary vascular resistance.
- As pulmonary vascular resistance decreases postnatally, pulmonary blood flow increases and heart failure often develops.
- Associated anomalies may include truncal stenosis, truncal insufficiency, and interrupted aortic arch.

Clinical Manifestations
- May present with mild cyanosis, CHF, poor growth
- Features of DiGeorge syndrome
- On physical exam: bounding pulses; systolic ejection click; single S_2; harsh systolic murmur; diastolic decrescendo murmur if truncal insufficiency

Diagnostics
- *Chest x-ray:* cardiomegaly, boot-shaped heart, pulmonary congestion, possible right aortic arch
- *ECG:* left ventricular hypertrophy, right ventricular hypertrophy
- *Echocardiography:* VSD; single great artery; helps define origin of pulmonary arteries
- *Cardiac catheterization:* may provide additional information about pulmonary vasculature and other VSDs

Management
Medical
- Goal of medical management is to treat CHF.
- Diuretics, digoxin, and ACE inhibitors are mainstays of therapy.

Surgical
- Definitive management requires surgical intervention.
- A patch closure of the VSD is performed.
- A conduit from the right ventricle to the pulmonary arteries may incorporate a pulmonary valve homograft.
- In the past, surgical banding of pulmonary arteries was used in an attempt to limit pulmonary overcirculation

VENTRICULAR SEPTAL DEFECT

A form of acyanotic congenital heart disease characterized by an opening in the ventricular septum in one of four locations:

1. *Perimembranous:* defect involving the membranous septum beneath the aortic valve; 70% of VSDs
2. *Muscular (trabecular):* defect within the muscular septum between the left and right ventricles; often involves multiple, small defects which may be difficult to repair surgically; 5% to 20% of VSDs
3. *Outlet (supracristal, subpulmonary, conoseptal, subarterial):* defect beneath the pulmonic valve which communicates with the RV outflow tract; 5% to 7% of VSDs
4. *Inlet:* located posteriorly and inferiorly to perimembranous VSDs; 5% to 8% of VSDs; often associated with endocardial cushion defects
- VSDs are classified as tiny, small, moderate, large, or very large:
  - Small VSDs are less than 3 mm; large VSDs are about the same size as the aortic valve annulus (10 mm in a newborn)

Epidemiology
- Two to six per 1000 live births; 25% of congenital heart disease
- Most common form of congenital heart disease

Pathophysiology

- Small defects (restrictive) are not usually hemodynamically significant.
- Large defects (unrestrictive) allow significant left-to-right shunting, which may lead to pulmonary overcirculation, compromise of systemic cardiac output, and CHF.
- Large, unrepaired defects often lead to pulmonary vascular obstructive disease and Eisenmenger's syndrome.
- Complications include pulmonary vascular obstruction, RV outflow tract obstruction, aortic regurgitation, and endocarditis.

Clinical Manifestations

- May be asymptomatic
- Symptomatic VSDs often present at 4 to 6 weeks of age as pulmonary vascular resistance decreases and may present with dyspnea, poor growth, feeding difficulties, sweating, fatigue, CHF
- VSDs are often silent in the newborn period while pulmonary vascular resistance is similar to systemic vascular resistance.
- Physical exam findings vary depending on size and location of the VSD as well as the degree of pulmonary vascular resistance and may include: loud, harsh, blowing holosystolic murmur at left lower sternal border (LLSB); palpable thrill at LLSB with parasternal lift and apical thrust; S_3 may be present. Small defects may be associated with loud murmurs.

Diagnostics

- *Chest x-ray:* may be normal or may reveal cardiomegaly and increased pulmonary vasculature
- *ECG:* may be normal or may reveal evidence of left ventricular hypertrophy, left atrial hypertrophy, and biventricular hypertrophy
- *Echocardiography:* reveals the size and location of the VSD
- *Cardiac catheterization:* may be performed in complicated cases

Management

Medical

- Small VSDs are often well tolerated.
- Approximately 70% of VSDs close spontaneously. Small, muscular defects are most likely to close spontaneously.
- Antibiotic prophylaxis should be provided for dental visits, oral surgery, and instrumentation of the gastrointestinal and genitourinary tracts.
- If signs of CHF, consider diuretics, ACE inhibitors and digoxin

Surgical

- Indications for surgery include uncontrolled CHF, pulmonary hypertension, and significant left-to-right shunt (pulmonary:systemic flow ratio (Qp:Qs) > 2:1)
- Direct surgical repair under cardiopulmonary bypass may incorporate a Dacron patch.
- Pulmonary arterial palliative banding is usually reserved for complicated cases and premature infants.
- Surgical complications include cardiac dysrhythmias (especially right bundle branch block), residual shunt, myocardial dysfunction, respiratory complications, and central nervous system complications.

SURGERIES FOR CONGENITAL HEART DISEASE

Arterial Switch Operation (of Jatene)

- *Indication:* transposition of the great arteries
- *Definition:* the coronary arteries are reimplanted into the pulmonary artery (neoaorta). The pulmonary artery and aorta are transected, switched, and reanastamosed.

Balloon Valvuloplasty

- *Indication:* pulmonary valve stenosis, aortic valve stenosis
- *Definition:* a sausage-shaped balloon is placed through the affected valve and inflated to relieve obstruction at the valve.

Blalock-Taussig Shunt
- *Indication:* tetralogy of Fallot, tricuspid atresia, pulmonary atresia
- *Definition:* direct anastomosis of the subclavian artery to the ipsilateral pulmonary artery, thereby creating a systemic to pulmonary shunt

Blalock-Taussig Shunt, Modified
- *Indication:* tetralogy of Fallot, tricuspid atresia
- *Definition:* a Gortex graft connects the subclavian artery to the ipsilateral pulmonary artery, thereby creating a systemic to pulmonary shunt.

Fontan Procedure
- *Indication:* tricuspid atresia, transposition of the great arteries, single ventricle
- *Definition:* conduit from right atrium to pulmonary artery. Many versions exist including fenestrated Fontan, total cavo-pulmonary connection, and partial or Hemi Fontan.

Glenn Shunt, Classic
- *Indication:* augmentation of pulmonary blood flow
- *Definition:* anastomosis between the transected right pulmonary artery and the side of the superior vena cava, which is ligated distal to the anastomosis.

Glenn Shunt, Bidirectional
- *Indication:* augmentation of pulmonary blood flow
- *Definition:* direct end-to-side anastomosis of transected superior vena cava to undivided right pulmonary artery, allowing blood flow to both lungs.

Mustard Procedure
- *Indication:* transposition of the great arteries
- *Definition:* use of pericardial or prosthetic baffles to divert pulmonary venous blood to the right ventricle and systemic venous blood to the left ventricle.

Norwood Procedure
- *Indication:* hypoplastic left heart syndrome
- *Definition:* a three-staged repair:
  - Stage 1 (neonatal period): reconstruction of the hypoplastic aorta using the main pulmonary artery, placement of a Blalock-Taussig shunt (systemic to pulmonary artery shunt), and removal of the atrial septum
  - Stage 2 (6 months): connection of the superior vena cava to the right pulmonary artery (Hemi-Fontan)
  - Stage 3 (18 months): connection of the inferior vena cava to the right pulmonary artery (Fontan)

Park Atrial Septostomy
- *Indication:* transposition of the great arteries, tricuspid atresia, pulmonary atresia with intact ventricular septum
- *Definition:* creation of a defect in the interatrial septum with a blade-tipped catheter.

Pulmonary Artery Banding
- *Indication:* coarctation of the aorta with VSD, truncus arteriosus, tricuspid atresia, single ventricle, complicated ventricular septal defect
- *Definition:* constriction of the pulmonary artery to reduce pulmonary blood flow

Rashkind Balloon Atrial Septostomy
- *Indication:* transposition of the great arteries, tricuspid atresia, pulmonary atresia with intact ventricular septum
- *Definition:* a balloon catheter is placed through the foramen ovale or existing atrial septal defect into the left atrium. It is inflated and rapidly pulled back into the right atrium, thereby creating a large opening in the atrial septum to improve mixing.

Ross Procedure
- *Indication:* aortic stenosis
- *Definition:* replacement of diseased aortic valve with patient's own pulmonary valve. A homograft is placed into the position of the pulmonary valve, and the coronary arteries are reimplanted into the graft.

Senning Procedure
- *Indication:* transposition of the great arteries
- *Definition:* use of the atrial septal flap and right atrial free wall as baffles to divert pulmonary venous blood to the right ventricle and systemic venous blood to the left ventricle.

Acquired Heart Disease

CONGESTIVE HEART FAILURE

CHF occurs when oxygen delivery by the heart is insufficient to meet the metabolic and circulatory demands of the body.

Etiology
- *Congenital Cardiac Causes of CHF:* atrioventricular septal defect, coarctation of the aorta, critical aortic or pulmonary stenosis, patent ductus arteriosus, transposition of the great arteries, tricuspid atresia, hypoplastic left heart syndrome, truncus arteriosus, ventricular septal defect, total anomalous pulmonary venous return
- *Acquired Cardiac Causes of CHF:* arrhythmias, Kawasaki disease, viral myocarditis, rheumatic heart disease, metabolic disorder, muscular dystrophy, chemotherapy (e.g., doxorubicin), idiopathic dilated cardiomyopathy
- *Non-cardiac Causes of CHF:* acute hypertension, anemia, hyperthyroidism, obstructive sleep apnea

Clinical Manifestations
- *Infants:* failure to thrive, increased work of breathing, feeding difficulties, excessive perspiration
- *Children and adolescents:* shortness of breath, reduced exercise tolerance, peripheral edema, cough, orthopnea
- On exam: hepatomegaly, puffy eyelids, swollen feet, rales, tachypnea, tachycardia, gallop rhythm

Diagnostics
- *Chest x-ray:* helps assess degree of cardiomegaly and pulmonary edema
- *ECG:* may demonstrate cardiomegaly or rhythm disturbances
- *Echocardiography:* helps define congenital heart defects, ventricular size, ventricular function, and shortening fraction (normally 28% to 40%)

Management
- *General measures:* oxygen; salt restriction; treatment of precipitating factors such as fever, anemia, infection, hypertension, and arrhythmias
- *Diuretics:*
  - *Loop diuretics* (e.g., furosemide) are considered first-line therapy for CHF. Electrolyte abnormalities (e.g., hypokalemia, hypochloremia) are common.
  - *Thiazide diuretics* (e.g., chlorothiazide, hydrochlorothiazide) work at the distal tubule and are often used to complement loop diuretics.
  - *Spironolactone* is potassium sparing and is often used in combination with loop or thiazide diuretics.
- *Digoxin* increases cardiac contractility; toxicities include bradycardia, heart block, and ventricular arrhythmias.
- *Afterload Reducing Agents:*
  - Reduction in afterload results in increased stroke volume and improved cardiac output.
  - *ACE Inhibitors* (e.g., captopril, enalapril): reduce peripheral vascular resistance by blocking the conversion of angiotensin I to angiotensin II. ACE inhibitors are also thought to have a positive effect on myocardial remodeling.

- *Intravenous agents* such as milrinone, nitroprusside, and hydralazine are usually reserved for intensive care unit (ICU) patients.
- *Intravenous Inotropic Agents:* dopamine, dobutamine, isoproterenol, and milrinone are generally reserved for ICU patients.

ENDOCARDITIS

Infection/inflammation of the cardiac endothelium with an associated immune response.

Epidemiology
- Incidence is increasing due to IV drug use, survivors of cardiac surgery, patients taking immunosuppressants, and chronic IV catheters.
- More common with congenital heart disease associated with a steep pressure gradient: patent ductus arteriosus, restrictive ventricular septal defect, left-sided valvular disease, systemic-pulmonary communications

Etiology
- *Common organisms: Streptococcus viridans* (~50%); *Staphylococcus aureus* (~30%)
- *Other organisms:* e.g., fungal, HACEK group (*Haemophilus* spp, *Actinobacillus actinomycetemcomitans, Cardiobacterium hominis, Eikenella corrodens, Kingella* spp)
- *Common associations:* congenital heart disease: *S. aureus;* dental procedures: *S. viridans;* bowel/GU surgery: *group D Strep;* IV drug use: *Pseudomonas* spp., *Serratia* spp; cardiac surgery: *Candida* spp

Pathophysiology
- Turbulent blood flow damages the endothelium.
- Damaged site serves as nidus for adherence of bacteria.
- Platelets and fibrin form a vegetation that may embolize.
- Immune response produces systemic symptoms.

Clinical Manifestations
- Fevers, chills, night sweats, dyspnea, arthralgias, central nervous system manifestations, chest/abdominal pain
- On exam: tachycardia; new or changing murmur; splenomegaly; manifestations of heart failure; Roth spots (pale retinal lesions surrounded by hemorrhage); Janeway lesions (flat, painless, on palms and soles); Osler nodes (painful nodes on pads of fingers and toes)

Diagnostics
- Blood cultures drawn from two separate sites
- Elevated erythrocyte sedimentation rate and C-reactive protein
- Leukocytosis, anemia, hypogammaglobulinemia
- Echocardiography: can detect vegetations greater than 2–3 mm; may detect valvular dysfunction; transesophageal echocardiography is more sensitive.

Modified Duke Criteria
- *Major criteria:* positive blood culture (typical microorganism from two different blood cultures; enterococcus without primary focus; positive serology for Q fever) or echocardiographic evidence
- *Minor criteria:* predisposing condition, temperature greater than 38.0°C, vascular or immunologic phenomena on physical exam, laboratory studies suggestive of infection
- *Definite endocarditis:* pathologic diagnosis, 2 major, 1 major and 3 minor, or 5 minor
- *Possible endocarditis:* 1 major and 1 minor or 3 minor
- *Rejected:* alternate diagnosis accounts for symptoms, resolution of manifestations with ≤ 4 days of antibiotic therapy, or no pathologic evidence at surgery

Management
Empiric therapies based on American Heart Association guidelines (therapy may be tailored based on susceptibilities):
- *S. viridans:* penicillin G for 4 to 6 weeks
- *S. aureus:* nafcillin for 6 to 8 weeks

- HACEK group: third generation cephalosporin
- Culture negative: nafcillin and gentamicin
- Fungal: amphotericin B; surgery often indicated
- Indications for surgery: intracardiac abscess, severe valvular regurgitation, CHF, infected prosthetic material
- Outcome: most relapses occur in 1 to 8 weeks after therapy; mortality is 20% to 25% with antibiotics; serious morbidity (e.g., CHF, systemic, or pulmonary emboli) in 50% to 60% of patients

ENDOCARDITIS PROPHYLAXIS

According to the 1997 recommendations of the American Heart Association, cardiac conditions are categorized as high-risk, moderate-risk, and negligible-risk for bacterial endocarditis (Adapted from Dajani AS, et al. Prevention of Bacterial Endocarditis: Recommendations of the American Heart Association. JAMA 1997;277:1794–1801.):

- *High-Risk:* prosthetic cardiac valve (including bioprosthetic and homograft); previous bacterial endocarditis; complex cyanotic congenital heart disease; surgically constructed systemic pulmonary shunt or conduit
- *Moderate-Risk:* most other congenital cardiac malformations; acquired valvular dysfunction (e.g., rheumatic heart disease); hypertrophic cardiomyopathy; mitral valve prolapse with valvular regurgitation and/or thickened leaflets
- *Negligible-Risk (prophylaxis unnecessary):* isolated secundum ASD; surgical repair of ASD, VSD, or PDA (without residua beyond 6 months); previous coronary artery bypass graft surgery; mitral valve prolapse without regurgitation; physiological, functional, or innocent heart murmurs; previous Kawasaki disease without valvular dysfunction; previous rheumatic fever without valvular dysfunction; cardiac pacemakers and implanted defibrillators

Prophylaxis Recommendations
Dental and Oral Procedures
- Prophylaxis recommended for patients at high or moderate risk
- Antiseptic mouthrinse (e.g., chlorhexidine 15 mL just before procedure)
- Amoxicillin 1 hour before procedure (50 mg/kg, max = 2 g)
- Clindamycin is an acceptable alternative to amoxicillin

Genitourinary and Non-esophageal Gastrointestinal Procedures
- *High-Risk:* Ampicillin (50 mg/kg IM/IV, max = 2 g) and gentamicin (1.5 mg/kg, max = 120 mg) within 30 minutes of start of procedure; 6 hours later, give ampicillin (25 mg/kg IM/IV, max = 1 g) or amoxicillin (25 mg/kg PO, maximum = 1 g)
- *High-Risk, allergic to ampicillin/amoxicillin:* Vancomycin (20 mg/kg IV, max = 1.0 g) over 1 to 2 hours plus gentamicin (1.5 mg/kg IV/IM, max = 120 mg); complete within 30 minutes of start of procedure.
- *Moderate-Risk:* Amoxicillin (50 mg/kg PO, maximum = 2 g) 1 hour before procedure, or ampicillin (50 mg/kg IM/IV, maximum = 2.0 g) within 30 minutes of start of procedure.
- *Moderate-Risk, allergic to ampicillin/amoxicillin:* Vancomycin (20 mg/kg IV, maximum = 1.0 g) over 1 to 2 hours; complete within 30 minutes of start of procedure.

MYOCARDITIS

Myocarditis is inflammation of the myocardium with myocellular necrosis.

Epidemiology
- Typically sporadic, but occasionally epidemic
- Infants usually have more acute and fulminant course
- Has been implicated in sudden infant death syndrome

Etiology
- Viral is most common (e.g., coxsackievirus, adenovirus)
- Other infectious agents: bacterial, fungal, parasitic, *Borrelia burgdorferi*
- *Trypanosoma cruzi* (Chagas disease) and *Clostridium diphtheriae* are common outside the United States.
- Collagen vascular disease
- Immune mediated: Kawasaki disease, rheumatic fever
- Toxin induced (e.g., cocaine)
- Giant cell myocarditis: rare, but often severe and fatal

Pathophysiology
- Involves damage to the myocardium from the initial infection, as well as the subsequent immune response
- May result in dilated cardiomyopathy

Clinical Manifestations
- Often preceded by a flu-like illness
- May present with new onset congestive heart failure or arrhythmias
- Dyspnea, exercise intolerance, fevers
- May be acute and fulminant or chronic
- On exam: fever, tachycardia, tachypnea, gallop, signs of congestive heart failure, murmur of mitral insufficiency

Diagnostics
- *Chest x-ray:* cardiomegaly +/– pulmonary edema
- *ECG:* tachycardia, low QRS voltages, ST/T-wave changes, arrhythmias
- *Echocardiography:* enlarged chambers, impaired LV function, mitral regurgitation
- *Laboratory studies:* ESR, CRP, cardiac enzymes, serum viral titers, Lyme titers
- *Endomyocardial biopsy:* gold standard for diagnosis. Viral polymerase chain reaction (PCR) on biopsy sample is more sensitive than serum PCR.

Management
Medical
- *Congestive Heart Failure:* ACE inhibitors, digoxin, diuretics. Inotropic agents should be used with caution, because the damaged myocardium is more sensitive to arrhythmias.
- *Immunosuppression may be appropriate depending on etiology:* IVIG (2 g/kg over 24 hours), steroids, cyclosporin, others
- *Outcome:* approximately one third recover, one third have residual dysfunction, and one third develop chronic CHF requiring transplant; mortality up to 75% in neonates
Surgical
- Transplant is often necessary.
- LVAD (left ventricular assist device) and ECMO (extra-corporeal membrane oxygenation) may be used as a bridge to transplant.

PERICARDITIS

Pericarditis is defined as inflammation of the pericardium.

Epidemiology
- Infectious type is more common in younger children
- Incidence slightly higher in males

Etiology
- Viral: echovirus and coxsackie B most common
- Bacterial, including *Mycoplasma tuberculosis*
- Collagen vascular: rheumatoid arthritis, lupus
- Uremia
- Neoplastic or radiation induced

- Drug-induced (e.g., procainamide, hydralazine)
- *Post-pericardiotomy syndrome*: seen in ~10% of children 1 to 4 weeks after cardiac surgery

Pathophysiology
- Deposits of infectious material or an inflammatory infiltrate results in an immune response and leads to changes in pericardial membrane function.
- A pericardial effusion may result if altered hydrostatic and/or oncotic pressure leads to fluid accumulation.
- *Tamponade:* an increase in intrapericardial pressure results in restriction of ventricular filling and a decrease in cardiac output.
- *Constrictive pericarditis* is the late result of earlier pericarditis and is characterized by a thick, fibrotic, calcified pericardium.
- *Post-pericardiotomy syndrome:* a nonspecific hypersensitivity reaction after manipulation of the pericardial space

Clinical Manifestations
- Fever, dyspnea
- Chest pain often radiates to the back or left shoulder, is worse with lying down, and is alleviated by leaning forward.
- On exam: fever, tachypnea, tachycardia, friction rub, muffled heart sounds (if an effusion is present)
- With tamponade, may have signs of CHF, *pulsus paradoxus* (exaggerated decrease in systolic BP by greater than 10 mm Hg with inspiration), or *Kussmaul's sign* (paradoxical rise in jugular venous pressure during inspiration).

Diagnostics
- *Chest x-ray:* cardiomegaly with "water bottle" appearance if effusion present
- *ECG:* tachycardia, diffuse ST elevation, T-wave inversion; may see *electrical alternans* if effusion present (variation of QRS axis with each beat due to movement of the heart within the pericardial fluid)
- *Echocardiogram:* with effusion, will see fluid in the pericardial space. In tamponade: RV collapse in early diastole, atrial collapse in end-diastole and early systole

Management
- *Viral:* usually self-limited. Treatment includes rest, analgesia, anti-inflammatory medications.
- *Bacterial:* open drainage and aggressive antibiotic therapy
- *Collagen vascular:* steroids and salicylates often used
- *Post-pericardiotomy:* rest, aspirin
- *Constrictive pericarditis:* pericardial stripping
- *Pericardiocentesis:* indications include hemodynamic compromise, bacterial pericarditis, and as a diagnostic aid; send pericardial fluid for cell count, culture, and cytology; complications can include arrhythmias and hemopericardium.

Electrocardiography

PRECORDIAL LEAD PLACEMENT

V1: 4th ICS, RSB
V2: 4th ICS, LSB
V3: Equidistant between V2 and V4
V4: 5th ICS, left MCL
V5: Horizontal to V4, left AAL
V6: Horizontal to V4, left MAL
V3R, V4R, V5R, V6R: Mirror image to V3, V4, V5, and V6 on the right side of the chest.

Note: ICS = intercostal space, RSB = right sternal border, LSB = left sternal border, MCL = midclavicular line, AAL = anterior axillary line, MAL = midaxillary line, MCL = midclavicular line

RATE

- On a standard ECG, paper moves at 25 mm/sec.
- Each small square is 1 mm (0.04 sec) and each large square is 5 mm (0.2 sec) (Figure 5.1)
- Heart rate can be estimated by counting the number of large boxes between QRS intervals where 1 box = 300 bpm, 2 boxes = 150 bpm, 3 boxes = 100 bpm, 4 boxes = 75 bpm, 5 boxes = 60 bpm, and 6 boxes = 50 bpm.

RHYTHM

- The cardiac rhythm may be determined by examining the rhythm strip that appears at the bottom of a standard 12-lead ECG.

AXIS

- The QRS axis represents the net direction of electrical activity during ventricular systole (Figure 5.2 and Table 5.1)

P WAVE

- Represents sinus node depolarization (Figure 5.1)
- Best seen in leads II and V_1
- In children, P-wave is normally less than 2.5 mm tall and 0.10 seconds in duration
- Tall P-waves may represent right atrial enlargement whereas wide P-waves may represent left atrial enlargement

PR INTERVAL

- From beginning of P-wave to beginning of QRS complex
- Refer to Table 5.2 for PR Interval Norms

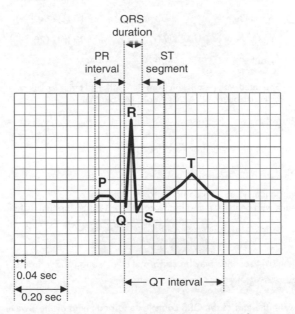

Figure 5.1   Segments and Intervals. (Modified with permission from Awtry EH, et al. Blueprints Cardiology. 2nd ed. Boston: Blackwell Publishing, 2006: Figure 3.2.)

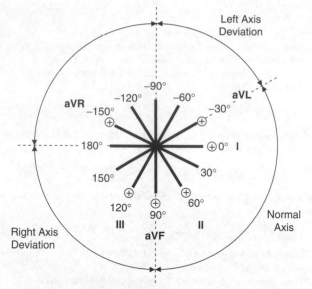

Figure 5.2   Axis.

Table 5.1: Normal QRS Axis by Age		
Age	Mean (Degrees)	Range (Degrees)
1 wk–1 mo	+110	+30 to +180
1–3 mo	+70	+10 to +125
3 mo–3 yr	+60	+10 to +110
> 3 yr	+60	+20 to +120
Adult	+50	−30 to +105

(Reprinted with permission from Park MK. Pediatric Cardiology
for Practitioners. 4th ed. St. Louis: Mosby, 2002.)

QRS COMPLEX

- Represents ventricular depolarization (see Table 5.2)

QT INTERVAL

- Measured from beginning of QRS complex to end of T-wave
- QT interval varies with heart rate and is corrected by Bazett's formula as follows:

$$QT_c = \frac{QT}{\sqrt{RR \text{ preceding}}}$$

- QTc greater than 0.44 seconds may be abnormal (see "Long QT Syndrome")

ST SEGMENT

- Segment between the end of the QRS complex and beginning of the T-wave
- Displacement by more than 1 to 2 mm from the isoelectric line may represent myocardial injury, pericarditis, or a repolarization abnormality

Table 5.2: QRS Duration Norms and PR Interval Norms in Seconds

Age	QRS Duration Norms Mean	QRS Duration Norms Upper Limit	PR Interval Norms Mean	PR Interval Norms Upper Limit
0–1 mo	0.05	0.065	0.09–0.10	0.11–0.12
1–6 mo	0.05	0.07	0.09–0.11	0.11–0.14
6 mo–1 yr	0.05	0.07	0.10–0.11	0.11–0.14
1–3 yr	0.06	0.07	0.10–0.12	0.12–0.15
3–8 yr	0.07	0.08	0.12–0.15	0.14–0.17
8–12 yr	0.07	0.09	0.14–0.16	0.15–0.18
12–16 yr	0.07	0.10	0.15–0.16	0.16–0.19
Adult	0.08	0.10	0.15–0.17	0.17–0.21

Reprinted with permission from Park M, Guntheroth WG. How to Read Pediatric ECGs. 3rd ed. St Louis: Mosby, 1992.

T WAVE

- Represents ventricular repolarization
- Normally upright in leads I and II and inverted in aVR
- Abnormalities may represent ischemia or electrolyte abnormalities

LEFT VENTRICULAR HYPERTROPHY, ECG SIGNS

- Left axis deviation (Table 5.3)
- R-wave in I, II, III, aVL, V5, or V6 greater than upper limit of normal
- S-wave in V1 or V2 greater than upper limit of normal
- Signs of volume overload: Q-wave in V5 and V6 5 mm or greater and tall, symmetric T-waves
- Signs of strain: inverted T-waves in leads I or aVF, V5-V6

Table 5.3: R and S Voltage Norms in V_1 and V_6: Mean (Upper Limit) in mm

Age	R in V_1	R in V_6	S in V_1	S in V_6
0–1 mo	15 (25)	6 (21)	10 (20)	4 (12)
1–6 mo	11 (20)	10 (20)	7 (18)	2 (7)
6 mo–1 yr	10 (20)	13 (20)	8 (16)	2 (6)
1–3 yr	9 (18)	12 (24)	13 (27)	2 (6)
3–8 yr	7 (18)	14 (24)	14 (30)	1 (5)
8–12 yr	6 (16)	14 (24)	16 (26)	1 (4)
12–16 yr	5 (16)	14 (22)	15 (24)	1 (5)
Young adult	3 (14)	10 (21)	10 (23)	1 (13)

Reprinted with permission from Park M, Guntheroth WG. How to Read Pediatric ECGs. 3rd ed. St Louis: Mosby, 1992.

RIGHT VENTRICULAR HYPERTROPHY, ECG SIGNS

- Right axis deviation
- R-wave in V1, V2, or aVR greater than upper limit of normal
- S-wave in I or V6 greater than upper limit of normal
- Q-wave in V1
- Signs of strain: T axis outside normal range (0 to –90 degrees), inverted in V1

Arrhythmias

ATRIAL FIBRILLATION

An ectopic atrial foci leads to an extremely fast atrial rate (350 to 600 bpm). The ventricular response is usually fast (greater than 100 bpm) and "irregularly irregular." The fast, disorganized ventricular response may lead to decreased cardiac output. Atrial fibrillation is much more common in adults than in children.

Etiology
- Structural heart disease, dilated atria, myocarditis, digitalis toxicity, cardiac surgery

Management
- For sustained atrial fibrillation (>48 hours), consider anticoagulation with warfarin or heparin and echocardiogram to look for thrombus.
- Digoxin with or without beta-blockers may control the ventricular rate.
- Termination of atrial fibrillation may be achieved through direct current cardioversion (especially in unstable patients) or with antiarrhythmic medications (e.g., amiodarone)

ATRIAL FLUTTER

An intra-atrial reentrant circuit leads to a rapid atrial rate around 300 bpm with a characteristic sawtooth pattern on ECG. Because the ventricles cannot respond at 300 bpm, there is often 2:1, 3:1, or 4:1 block.

Etiology
- Structural heart disease, myocarditis, digitalis toxicity, cardiac surgery, dilated atria with mitral insufficiency

Management
- To prevent thromboembolism, consider anticoagulation with warfarin or heparin before cardioversion.
- Vagal maneuvers or adenosine may produce a temporary slowing of the heart rate, but do not terminate the rhythm.
- Procainamide or amiodarone may terminate the rhythm.
- Digoxin slows the ventricular rate by increasing the AV block.
- Direct current cardioversion often restores normal sinus rhythm.

ATRIOVENTRICULAR BLOCK

AV block ("heart block") occurs when conduction through the atrioventricular node is impaired.

First-Degree AV Block
- *Definition:* PR interval above the upper limit of normal for age
- *Etiology:* rheumatic fever, cardiomyopathy, atrial septal defect, Ebstein's anomaly, infectious diseases, ischemic heart disease, hyperkalemia, digitalis toxicity, other medications
- *Management:* generally asymptomatic and does not require treatment.

Second-Degree AV Block, Mobitz Type I (Wenckebach)
- *Definition:* progressive lengthening of PR interval with eventual dropped beat
- *Etiology:* myocarditis, cardiomyopathy, myocardial infarction, congenital heart defect, cardiac surgery, digitalis toxicity, other medications
- *Management:* usually does not progress and does not require treatment

Second-Degree AV Block, Mobitz Type II
- *Definition:* normal PR intervals are followed by episodes of heart block (i.e., P-wave is not conducted to the ventricles)
- *Etiology:* myocarditis, cardiomyopathy, myocardial infarction, congenital heart defect, cardiac surgery, digitalis toxicity, other medications
- *Management:* may progress to complete heart block; may require pacemaker

Third-Degree AV Block
- *Definition:* complete dissociation of atrial and ventricular activity (i.e., no relationship between P-wave and QRS complex)
- *Etiology:* isolated anomaly, maternal SLE, Sjorgen syndrome, congenital heart defect, cardiac surgery, myocarditis, endocarditis, Lyme carditis, acute rheumatic fever, cardiomyopathy, myocardial infarction, certain drug overdoses
- *Management:* patients are often unstable and may require transcutaneous pacing, atropine, or isoproterenol. A transvenous or permanent pacemaker is often required.

LONG QT SYNDROME

A cardiac repolarization abnormality characterized by prolongation of the QT interval, which can result in torsades de pointes and sudden cardiac death.

- Corrected QT interval is calculated by Bazett's formula:

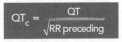

$$QT_c = \frac{QT}{\sqrt{RR \text{ preceding}}}$$

Etiology
Hereditary Causes of Long QT Syndrome
- *Jervell-Lange-Nielsen Syndrome:* autosomal recessive, congenital deafness
- *Romano-Ward Syndrome:* autosomal dominant transmission, normal hearing
- Sporadic mutations in potassium and sodium channels

Acquired Causes of a Prolonged QT Interval
- *Electrolyte Abnormalities:* hypokalemia, hypomagnesemia, hypocalcemia
- *Drugs:* antiarrhythmics, tricyclic antidepressants, erythromycin, antihistamines, phenothiazine, cocaine, organophosphates
- *Other:* stroke, subarachnoid hemorrhage, myocardial ischemia, liquid protein diets

Pathophysiology
- Lengthening of ventricular repolarization leads to R on T phenomena and precipitation of torsades de pointes.
- Congenital long QT syndrome is due to mutations in the transmembrane sodium or potassium ion channels responsible for cardiac repolarization.

Clinical Manifestations
- Often presents with unexplained syncope or sudden cardiac death brought on by exercise or fright
- May present with presyncope, seizures, dizziness, and palpitations

Diagnostics
- *Family History:* long QT syndrome or unexplained sudden cardiac death
- *ECG:* increased QTc, torsades de pointes, T-wave alternans, notched T-waves, low resting heart rate

- *Corrected QT interval:* QTc greater than 440 milliseconds is suspicious and QTc greater than 460 milliseconds is concerning
- *Exercise Stress Test:* prolongation of QTc seen with exercise
- *24 Holter Monitor:* may demonstrate arrhythmia

Management
Short Term
- Immediate cardioversion of torsades de pointes
- Magnesium bolus and infusion
- Maintain high normal level of potassium
- Temporary cardiac pacing
- Withdrawal of offending drugs
- Correction of electrolyte abnormalities
- Isoproterenol in cases of acquired long QT

Long Term
- Beta-blockers
- Left thoracic sympathectomy
- Permanent pacemaker and cardioverter-defibrillator
- May have to avoid sports and stressful activities

PREMATURE ATRIAL CONTRACTION

An atrial beat arising from an ectopic stimulus in the left or right atrium, which occurs before the next normal sinus beat is due.

- The P-wave has a different shape than the normal sinus P-wave.
- If the PAC is conducted, the QRS complex is generally the same as the QRS complex of preceding beats.
- Occasionally, the PAC is conducted aberrantly through the ventricles causing a wide QRS complex.
- If the PAC reaches the AV node while it is still refractory, the PAC may not be conducted to the ventricles.

Etiology
- PACs are very common in normal people and do not necessarily indicate the presence of disease.
- Other causes: emotional stress, hyperthyroidism, caffeine, structural heart disease, medications (epinephrine, theophylline)

Management
- Medical management generally not required if PACs are an isolated finding

PREMATURE VENTRICULAR CONTRACTION

A premature ventricular contraction (PVC) is a ventricular beat arising from an ectopic ventricular stimulus, which occurs before the next normal sinus beat is due.

- Wide QRS complex (greater than 0.08 seconds in infants, greater than 0.12 seconds in children)
- Two PVCs in a row are called a "couplet" or a "pair."
- Three PVCs in a row define ventricular tachycardia.
- PVCs may be uniform indicating they arise from a single focus.
- Multiform PVCs may arise from different foci or from the same focus and often signify underlying heart disease.
- *R on T Phenomenon*: when PVCs occur during the T-wave of the preceding beat, they may precipitate ventricular tachycardia or ventricular fibrillation.

Etiology
- PVCs often occur in normal hearts.
- Other causes: anxiety, caffeine, hypoxemia, sympathomimetics, myocardial infarction, electrolyte abnormalities, structural heart disease

Management

- PVCs are often benign and usually do not require treatment.
- Correction of underlying abnormalities (e.g., electrolyte abnormalities) may reduce the frequency of PVCs.
- Medications such as beta-blockers or anti-arrhythmics are occasionally considered.

SUPRAVENTRICULAR TACHYCARDIA

A reentrant supraventricular rhythm may occur when there are two conducting pathways, unidirectional block in one pathway, and slow conduction in the other pathway. Supraventricular tachycardia may also be due to an automatic atrial rhythm. The two most common forms of reentrant SVT are:

- Atrioventricular nodal reentry tachycardia (AVNRT): the AV node consists of a slow, posterior pathway and a fast, anterior pathway. Onset may be triggered by a premature atrial impulse, which reaches the AV node when the fast pathway is still refractory. The premature impulse conducts anterogradely through the slow pathway and then retrogradely through the fast pathway. AVNRT is more common in teens and young adults.
- Atrioventricular reentry tachycardia (AVRT): an accessory pathway exists outside of the AV node. Anterograde conduction typically occurs via the AV node and retrograde conduction via the accessory pathway (orthodromic). This results in a normal QRS complex. Anterograde conduction occasionally occurs via the accessory pathway and retrograde conduction via the AV node (antidromic). This results in a wide QRS complex, which may be difficult to differentiate from ventricular tachycardia. AVRT is common in Wolff-Parkinson-White (WPW) syndrome and is more common in infants and toddlers.

Clinical Manifestations

- Rapid, regular heart rate, usually 150 to 250 bpm
- Palpitations, syncope, near-syncope, lightheadedness, shortness of breath

Diagnostics

- *Laboratory studies:* consider electrolytes
- *Chest x-ray:* may show infection, cardiomyopathy, pulmonary edema
- *Echocardiogram:* if structural heart defect suspected
- *ECG during SVT:* heart rate 150 to 250 bpm, P-wave may be within or after QRS, typically narrow QRS, occasionally wide QRS.
- *ECG after termination of the SVT:* may show a delta wave (upsloping QRS complex) in WPW syndrome.
- *Adenosine:* may terminate the arrhythmia

Management

Short Term

- If unstable, direct current cardioversion: (0.5 J/kg increased in steps to 2 J/kg)
- Vagal maneuvers: ice to face, Valsalva, carotid sinus massage
- Adenosine by rapid IV push (initial dose 0.1 mg/kg [max 6 mg], increase by 0.05 mg/kg if unsuccessful to maximum of 0.35 mg/kg or 12 mg)
- Calcium channel blockers (avoid in infants less than 1 year old), class IC agents, digoxin (controversial), and amiodarone may also be effective.

Long Term

- Antiarrhythmic drug therapy: propranolol, verapamil, amiodarone, procainamide, quinidine, flecainide, digoxin
- Radiofrequency catheter ablation is often successful in ablating the accessory pathway
- No treatment is sometimes an acceptable alternative.
- Digoxin and calcium channel blockers are contraindicated in WPW syndrome.

SYNCOPE

Syncope is transient loss of consciousness and postural tone due to inadequate cerebral perfusion.

Epidemiology
- 15% of children and adolescents between ages 8 and 18 experience syncope.
- Unusual under age 6 except in the setting of seizure disorders, breath-holding, and cardiac abnormalities

Etiology
- *Neurocardiogenic syncope (vasodepressor, vasovagal):*
  - Most common type of syncope; may be provoked by increased vagal tone during micturition, defecation, cough, or hair brushing; may be provoked by peripheral vasodilation during "fight or flight" response, warm temperature, anxiety, or blood drawing.
  - Decreased cardiac filling leads to increased cardiac contractility and activation of stretch receptors. A reflex increase in vagal tone further compromises cardiac output, resulting in syncope.
- *Cardiac syncope:*
  - Dysrhythmias may include SVT, VT, heart block, WPW, long QT syndrome.
  - Outflow tract obstruction: hypertrophic obstructive cardiomyopathy, pulmonary hypertension
  - Inflow obstruction: restrictive cardiomyopathy, effusion
  - May be accompanied by brief seizure (*Stokes-Adams syndrome*)
- *Neuropsychiatric syncope:* seizures, migraines, hypoglycemia, "hysterical" syncope, hyperventilation (e.g., panic attack)

Clinical Manifestations
- Symptoms of "pre-syncope" may include diaphoresis, lightheadedness, palpitations, and tunnel vision.
- Cardiac symptoms may include palpitations, shortness of breath, chest pain, and color changes.
- Family history may be notable for sudden death, arrhythmias, congenital heart disease, seizures, metabolic disorders, and psychiatric history.
- Significant physical exam findings are uncommon in children.
- Vital signs may demonstrate orthostasis.
- Systolic ejection murmur that increases with Valsalva or standing is concerning for HOCM.
- Loud second heart sound may indicate pulmonary hypertension.

Diagnostics
- ECG recommended regardless of cardiac symptoms
- If concern for seizure activity or trauma: neurology referral, EEG, head CT
- If concern for cardiac disease: ECG, chest x-ray, echocardiogram, exercise stress test, Holter monitor
- Tilt table testing may help diagnose neurocardiogenic syncope.

Management
Acute Management
- Keep patient supine until fully recovered.
- For an arrhythmia, consider pharmacologic treatment, defibrillation, or cardioversion as per Pediatric Advanced Life Support protocols.

Cardiac Syncope
- Congenital heart disease present: treat underlying cause
- Arrhythmia present: may need internal defibrillator, medication, radiofrequency ablation in catheterization laboratory (e.g., WPW syndrome)
- Exercise stress test and electrophysiologic testing in catheterization laboratory may aid in diagnosis.

Neurocardiogenic Syncope
- Volume expansion: encourage fluid and salt intake
- Mineralocorticoids (e.g., Florinef) increase circulating volume and help maintain cerebral perfusion pressure. Efficacy is approximately 60% to 80%.
- Beta-blockers modify the abnormal feedback loop and prevent increased vagal output.

VENTRICULAR FIBRILLATION

An uncoordinated, chaotic ventricular rhythm with QRS complexes of varying size and shape. Ventricular fibrillation is a pulseless rhythm without effective cardiac output and is terminal unless an effective ventricular beat is restored.

Etiology
- Hyperkalemia, severe hypoxia, surgery, myocarditis, myocardial infarction
- Drugs and toxins: digitalis, quinidine, catecholamines, anesthetics

Management
- CPR, airway, oxygen, IV or IO access
- Defibrillate up to three times (2 J/kg, 4 J/kg, 4 J/kg) and then with 4 J/kg 30 to 60 seconds after each medication.
- Epinephrine (first dose: 0.1 mL/kg of 1:10,000 IV/IO or 0.1 mL/kg of 1:1000 via ETT; subsequent doses 0.1 mL/kg of 1:1000 IV/IO/ETT)
- Amiodarone (5 mg/kg IV/IO)
- Lidocaine (1 mg/kg IV/IO)

VENTRICULAR TACHYCARDIA

Ventricular tachycardia (VT) is defined as at least three premature ventricular beats in a row at a rate above 120 bpm (varies by age) characterized by wide QRS complexes.

- Sustained VT lasts longer than 30 seconds.

Etiology
- Cardiomyopathy, myocarditis, cardiac surgery, electrolyte abnormalities, drugs and toxins, long QT syndrome, anomalous left coronary artery

Management
Ventricular Tachycardia with Pulses
- Early cardiology consultation is recommended.
- The following medications may be considered: amiodarone (5 mg/kg IV over 20 to 60 minutes), procainamide (15 mg/kg over 30 to 60 minutes), or lidocaine (1 mg/kg over 2 to 4 minutes).
- If signs of shock are present, immediate synchronized cardioversion is indicated (0.5–1 J/kg initially, up to 2 J/kg).
- Magnesium (25 mg/kg over 10 to 20 minutes) is indicated if torsades de pointes is suspected.

Pulseless Ventricular Tachycardia
- CPR, airway, oxygen, IV or IO access
- Defibrillate up to three times (2 J/kg, 4 J/kg, 4 J/kg) and then with 4 J/kg 30 to 60 seconds after each medication.
- Epinephrine (first dose: 0.1 mL/kg of 1:10,000 IV/IO or 0.1 mL/kg of 1:1000 via ETT; subsequent doses 0.1 mL/kg of 1:1000 IV/IO/ETT)
- Amiodarone (5 mg/kg IV/IO)
- Lidocaine (1 mg/kg IV/IO)
- Magnesium (25 mg/kg over 10 to 20 minutes) is indicated if torsades de pointes is suspected.

WOLFF-PARKINSON-WHITE SYNDROME

A form of ventricular pre-excitation in which an accessory pathway bypasses the AV node leading to a variety of supraventricular tachyarrhythmias.

Epidemiology
- Affects 0.1% to 3% of general population
- Occasionally inherited in an autosomal dominant pattern
- May be associated with Ebstein anomaly or corrected transposition

Pathophysiology
- Atrial impulses bypass the AV node through the accessory pathway causing pre-excitation
- Paroxysmal supraventricular tachycardia (SVT) in WPW usually results from antegrade conduction through the AV node and retrograde conduction through the accessory pathway (orthodromic).
- Paroxysmal SVT may result from antegrade conduction through the accessory pathway and retrograde conduction through the AV node (antidromic). In this case, the QRS complex is wide and the rhythm may be difficult to distinguish from ventricular tachycardia.
- Patients are also at risk for atrial fibrillation, atrial flutter, and ventricular fibrillation (rare).

Clinical Manifestations
- Palpitations, dizziness, syncope, chest discomfort, shortness of breath

Diagnosis
- *Family History:* WPW, SVT, sudden cardiac death, unexplained early death (e.g., car accidents, drownings)
- *ECG:* shortening of the PR interval, widening of the QRS complex, slurred upstroke of the QRS complex (delta wave)

Management
- Vagal maneuvers such as ice to face, Valsalva, carotid sinus massage (hemodynamically stable patients)
- Adenosine: initial drug of choice (initial dose: 0.1 mg/kg IV; maximum 6 mg)
- Other potential agents: calcium channel antagonists, beta-blockers, digoxin, procainamide; however, caution should be used with digoxin and calcium channel blockers, which may increase the ventricular rate during atrial fibrillation and can lead to ventricular fibrillation.
- Radiofrequency catheter ablation is the treatment of choice in symptomatic and high-risk patients.

Resources

Congenital Heart Disease

Andrews R, Tulloh R, Sharland G, et al. Outcome of staged reconstructive surgery for hypoplastic left heart syndrome following antenatal diagnosis. Arch Dis Child 2001;85:474–477.

Behrman R, Kliegman R, Jenson H. Nelson Textbook of Pediatrics. 16th ed. Philadelphia: WB Saunders, 2000.

Blaustein AS, Ramanathan A. Tricuspid valve disease. Clinical evaluation, physiopathology, and management. Cardiol Clin 1998;16:551–572.

Braunwald E, ed. Heart Disease: A Textbook of Cardiovascular Medicine. 6th ed. Philadelphia: WB Saunders, 2001.

Driscoll DJ. Left-to-right shunt lesions. Pediatr Clin North Am 1999;46:355–368.

Fedderly RT. Left ventricular outflow obstruction. Pediatr Clin North Am 1999;46:369–384.

Fox RE, Crosson JE, Campbell AB. Radiological case of the month. Arch Pediatr Adolesc Med 2001;155:193–194.

Gatzoulis MA, Rigby ML, Shinebourne EA, Redington AN. Contemporary results of balloon valvuloplasty and surgical valvotomy for congenital aortic stenosis. Arch Dis Child 1995;73:66–69.

Grifka RG. Cyanotic congenital heart disease with increased pulmonary blood flow. Pediatr Clin North Am 1999;46:405–425.

Gutgesell HP, Barton DM, Elgin KM. Coarctation of the aorta in the neonate: associated conditions, management, and early outcome. Am J Cardiol 2001;88:457–459.

Haas G. Advances in pediatric cardiovascular surgery: anatomic reconstruction of the left ventricular outflow tract in transposition of the great arteries with pulmonic valve abnormalities. Curr Opin Pediatr 2000; 12:501–504.

Krovetz LJ. Spontaneous closure of ventricular septal defects. Am J Cardiol 1998;8:100–101.

Ledesma M, Alva C, Gomez FD, et al. Results of stenting for aortic coarctation. Am J Cardiol 2001;88:460–462.

McDaniel NL. Ventricular and atrial septal defects. Pediatr Rev 2001;22:265–270.

Momma K, Kondo C, Ando M, et al. Tetralogy of Fallot associated with chromosome 22q11 deletion. Am J Cardiol 1995;76:618–621.

Murphy JG, Gersh BJ, Mair DD, et al. Long-term outcome in patients undergoing surgical repair of tetralogy of Fallot. N Engl J Med 1993;329:593–599.

Nygren A, Sunnegardh J, Berggren H. Preoperative evaluation and surgery in isolated ventricular septal defects: a 21 year perspective. Heart 2000;83:198–204.

Park MK. Pediatric Cardiology for Practitioners. 4th ed. St. Louis: Mosby, 2002.

Rowland DG, Hammill WW, Allen HD, Gutgesell HP. Natural course of isolated pulmonary valve stenosis in infants and children utilizing Doppler echocardiography. Am J Cardiol 1997;79:344–349.

Salmon AP. Hypoplastic left heart syndrome—outcome and management. Arch Dis Child 2001;85:450–451.

Spitaels SE. Ebstein's anomaly of the tricuspid valve complexities and strategies. Cardiol Clin 2002;20:431.

Taeed R, Shim D, Kimball TR, et al. One-year follow-up of the amplatzer device to close atrial septal defects. Am J Cardiol 2001;87:116–118.

Turner SW, Hunter S, Wyllie JP. The natural history of ventricular septal defects. Arch Dis Child 1999;81:413–416.

Waldman JD, Wernly JA. Cyanotic congenital heart disease with decreased pulmonary blood flow in children. Pediatr Clin North Am 1999;46:385–404.

Acquired Heart Disease

Batra AS, Lewis AB. Acute myocarditis. Curr Opin Pediatr 2001;13:234–239.

Behrman R, Liegman H, Jenson H, ed. Nelson's Textbook of Pediatrics. 16th ed. Philadelphia: WB Saunders, 2000.

Brook MM. Pediatric bacterial endocarditis: treatment and prophylaxis. Pediatr Clin North Am 1999;46:275–286.

Dajani AS, Taubert KA, Wilson W, et al. Prevention of bacterial endocarditis: recommendations of the American Heart Association. JAMA 1997;277:1794–1801.

Kay JD, Colan SD, Graham TP Jr. Congestive heart failure in pediatric patients. Am Heart J 2001;142:923–928

Milazzo AS Jr, Li JS. Bacterial endocarditis in infants and children. Pediatr Infect Dis J 2001;20:799–801.

O'Laughlin MP. Congestive heart failure in children. Pediatr Clin North Am 1999;46:263–273.

Oakley CM. Myocarditis, pericarditis and other pericardial diseases. Heart 2000;84:449–454.

Park MK. Pediatric Cardiology for Practitioners. 4th ed. St. Louis: Mosby, 2002.

Shaddy RE. Optimizing treatment for chronic congestive heart failure in children. Crit Care Med 2001;9(suppl):s237–240.

Electrocardiography

Park M, Guntheroth WG. How to Read Pediatric ECGs. 3rd ed. St Louis: Mosby, 1992.

Park MK. Pediatric Cardiology for Practitioners. 4th ed. St Louis: Mosby, 2002.

Arrhythmias

Al-Khatib SM, Pritchett E. Clinical features of Wolff-Parkinson-White Syndrome. Am Heart J 1999;138:403–413.

Behrman R, Kliegman H, Jenson H, ed. Nelson's Textbook of Pediatrics. 16th ed. Philadelphia: WB Saunders, 2000.

Brady WJ Jr, Harrigan RA. Evaluation and management of bradyarrhythmias in the emergency department. Emerg Med Clin North Am 1998;16:361–388.

Braunwald E, ed. Heart Disease: a Textbook of Cardiovascular Medicine. 6th ed. Philadelphia: WB Saunders, 2001.

Goldberger AL. Clinical Electrocardiography: a Simplified Approach. 6th ed. St. Louis: Mosby, 1999.

Khan IA. Long QT syndrome: diagnosis and management. Am Heart J 2002;143:7–14.

Kugler JD, Danford DA. Management of infants, children, and adolescents with paroxysmal supraventricular tachycardia. J Pediatr 1996;120:324–338.

Lewis DA, Dhala A. Syncope in the pediatric patient. Pediatric Clin North Am 1999;46:205–219.

Park MK. Pediatric Cardiology for Practitioners. 4th ed. St. Louis: Mosby, 2002.

Rosner MH, Brady WJ Jr, Kefer MP, Martin ML. Electrocardiography in the patient with the Wolff-Parkinson-White syndrome: diagnostic and initial therapeutic issues. Am J Emerg Med 1999;17:705–714.

Tanel RE, Walsh EP. Syncope in the pediatric patient. Cardiol Clin 1997;15:277–294.

The American Heart Association in collaboration with the International Liaison Committee on Resuscitation. Guidelines 2000 for Cardiopulmonary Resuscitation and Emergency Cardiovascular Care. Part 10: pediatric advanced life support. Circulation 2000;102(suppl):I291–342.

Trohman RG. Supraventricular tachycardia: implications for the intensivist. Crit Care Med 2000;28(suppl):n129–135.

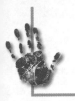

DERMATOLOGY 6

Sogol Mostoufi-Moab, MD, Albert C. Yan, MD

Blistering Disorders

NECROTIZING FASCIITIS

A rapidly progressive, acute, necrotizing life-threatening infection of the skin and sub-cutaneous tissue, usually associated with severe systemic toxicity.

- Can be rapidly fatal if not recognized and treated promptly

Epidemiology
- Risk factors: antecedent varicella infection; general debilitation following surgery or trauma

Etiology
- Common: ß-hemolytic group A *Streptococcus*
- Less common: *Staphylococcus aureus*, anaerobic streptococci, group B *Streptococcus*, *Proteus vulgaris*, and *Bacteroides fragilis*. In neutropenic patients, *Pseudomonas aeruginosa*. May be polymicrobial (especially with perineal involvement)

Differential Diagnosis
- Cellulitis, erysipelas, pyoderma, staphylococcal scalded skin syndrome, toxic shock syndrome, burns

Clinical Manifestations
- Cellulitis associated with fever, erythema, pain, and edema
- Rapid progression to central patches of bluish discoloration with or without blistering followed by ulceration, gangrene, and systemic toxicity that may include features of toxic shock syndrome

Diagnostics
- Clinical diagnosis requires high level of suspicion.
- Cultures of blood, skin, and deep tissue (biopsy)
- Skin biopsy reveals tissue necrosis.
- Leukocytosis, elevated CRP, ESR, and creatine kinase

Management
- Prompt surgical consultation and surgical debridement of necrotic tissue (delay results in higher mortality). Surgical re-exploration and repeat debridement 24 to 48 hours following initial debridement
- Broad spectrum antibiotics empirically (e.g., ampicillin-sulbactam, penicillin + clindamycin, ticarcillin-clavulanate, or imipenem). Adjust therapy based on culture results.
- Intravenous immunoglobulin may benefit patients with a toxic shock-like syndrome.
- Hyperbaric oxygen therapy may be helpful where available.
- Even in best circumstances, mortality can be as high as 20% to 30%.

STAPHYLOCOCCAL SCALDED SKIN SYNDROME

Staphylococcal scalded skin syndrome (SSSS) is a bacterial toxin–mediated exfoliative eruption characterized by areas of red skin and superficial desquamation, resembling skin that has been scalded.

Epidemiology

- Generally occurs in children who lack neutralizing antibodies to staphylococcal toxins, including children younger than 5 years of age, preterm infants, or older children and adults with renal impairment or immunosuppression.

Etiology

- Exfoliative toxins produced by staphylococci act as serine proteases and bind to a specific cell adhesion molecule (desmoglein-1) in the epidermis, causing superficial separation.

Differential Diagnosis

- Burns, toxic epidermal necrolysis, Kawasaki disease, toxic shock syndrome, toxin-mediated perineal erythema, erythema multiforme, Stevens-Johnson syndrome

Clinical Manifestations

- Fever (low-grade), malaise, irritability in a young child accompanied by a generalized erythematous, tender, scarlatiniform rash
- Erythema starts in intertriginous zones and perioral areas before generalizing.
- Mild to moderately tender skin
- Nikolsky sign: skin wrinkles and peels off with applied traction
- Areas of skin may denude revealing moist, red surfaces resembling burns.
- Involved areas eventually desquamate without scarring within 10 to 14 days.

Diagnostics

- Bacterial Gram stain and culture: identification of potential foci of infection is important. Most common areas include the nasopharynx, conjunctivae, blood; rarely, focal areas of impetigo or osteomyelitis may be associated. Toxin-induced blisters or areas of exfoliation, however, will generally be culture-negative.
- Skin biopsy: if necessary to differentiate from toxic epidermal necrolysis (TEN), skin biopsy for frozen section can be performed rapidly to differentiate superficial split within granular layer (SSSS) from deeper, full-thickness epidermal involvement (TEN).

Management

- Most patients have an excellent prognosis if identified and treated. Patients require supportive therapy and management of fluids and electrolytes.
- Parenteral antibiotics are recommended for extensive skin involvement or serious systemic disease. Use oxacillin, nafcillin, or cefazolin for empiric therapy. Clindamycin or cotrimoxazole may be necessary in areas with high prevalence of methicillin-resistant strains.
- Localized or limited involvement may respond to oral antibiotics: clindamycin, cotrimoxazole, dicloxacillin, cephalexin, amoxicillin-clavulanate
- Topical antibiotics and topical steroids are NOT indicated.
- Therapy should be continued for a minimum of 7 to 10 days.

STEVENS-JOHNSON SYNDROME AND TOXIC EPIDERMAL NECROLYSIS

Stevens-Johnson syndrome (SJS) and TEN occur together as part of a clinical spectrum. Although there are clinical similarities, erythema multiforme minor is a separate entity.

- SJS is an immunologically mediated mucocutaneous reaction involving typical targetoid lesions associated with erosive mucositis of two or more mucous membranes. Skin involvement is limited to 20% or less of body surface area (BSA).
- TEN: a life-threatening mucocutaneous reaction involving extensive (>20% BSA) skin sloughing often in association with mucous membrane erosions. This condition may evolve from pre-existing SJS.

Etiology

- Proposed mechanisms: circulating immune complexes and elaboration of circulating proapoptotic factors (Fas ligand)

- Most common drugs implicated: penicillin-related antibiotics, sulfonamides, and aromatic anticonvulsants (phenobarbital, phenytoin, carbamazepine)
- Occasionally occurs with *Mycoplasma pneumoniae* infection

Differential Diagnosis

- Exanthematous erythematous macules and papules: viral exanthems, urticaria, urticarial vasculitis, secondary syphilis
- Targetoid lesions: annular urticaria, figurate erythemas (e.g., erythema annulare centrifugum)
- Bullous lesions: bullous impetigo, linear IgA disease (chronic bullous dermatosis of childhood), childhood bullous pemphigoid, childhood pemphigus vulgaris
- Skin peeling and sloughing: SSSS, toxic shock syndrome, Kawasaki disease
- Mucositis: herpetic gingivostomatitis, aphthous stomatitis, pemphigus vulgaris

Clinical Manifestations

Stevens-Johnson Syndrome

- Primary lesions: atypical targetoid lesions (central area often violaceous or blistered, surrounded by a doughnut-shaped, elevated area of pallor and a peripheral rim of erythema); mucositis (oropharyngeal, conjunctivae, urethral, rectal; rarely, gastroesophageal and pulmonary epithelia may become involved) often results in pain, poor oral intake and dehydration.
- Severe involvement may result in cutaneous dyschromia and even scarring. Areas of mucous membrane involvement are at risk for scarring, adhesions, blindness, or strictures.
- Distribution: in contrast to classic acral distribution of erythema multiforme minor, lesions are more generalized and may concentrate more on the torso
- By definition, involves less than 20% of the BSA

Toxic Epidermal Necrolysis

- Primary lesions: tender, red areas of skin often on dependent areas (lower back, buttocks) but which may occur at any site; these red areas may blister or simply slough and typically show a positive Nikolsky sign.
- Mucositis in TEN may be as severe as in SJS with similar potential sequelae.
- Distribution: widespread, generalized process involving greater than 20% of the BSA
- Extensive full-thickness denudation of skin clinically resembles burned skin and predisposes patient to sepsis, fluid and electrolyte disturbances, and thermal instability.

Diagnostics

- Electrolyte disturbances (especially hyponatremia) occur as a result of dehydration and fluid losses.
- Usually a clinical diagnosis but skin biopsy can be helpful:
  - SJS: intense interface reaction along the dermal-epidermal junction with central necrosis or blister formation
  - TEN: can be performed as a frozen section and reveals full-thickness epidermal necrosis and a subepidermal split

Management

- Dermatologic consultation recommended
- Prompt discontinuation of etiologic drug (e.g., anticonvulsant) or treatment of etiologic underlying infection (e.g., *Mycoplasma*)
- Fluids, electrolytes, and nutritional issues are critical.
- Close surveillance for infection/sepsis
- For SJS, hospitalization recommended for fluid and electrolyte management
- For TEN, hospital admission to a burn center or intensive care setting experienced with management of TEN decreases morbidity and mortality.
- Skin: erosions require diligent wound care (saline or acetic acid soaks), topical antibiotics (bacitracin, silver sulfadiazine), systemic analgesia; if extensive as with TEN, care at a burn center is recommended.

- Appropriate consultation for mucous membrane involvement: eyes (ophthalmology); urethral (urology); gastroesophageal, intestinal, rectal (gastroenterology); pulmonary (pulmonology)
- Systemic steroids are of uncertain benefit. Short-term early use may moderate disease progression, but prolonged use is contraindicated.
- In case studies and series, intravenous immunoglobulin (IVIG) has been highly effective at arresting progression of the disease for both SJS and TEN. If vital organs (eye, gastrointestinal, respiratory) are at risk, use of IVIG 0.5 mg/kg/day for 4 days may be beneficial.

Exanthems

ACUTE URTICARIAL HYPERSENSITIVITY

An acute cutaneous reaction characterized by annular and polycyclic urticarial plaques (often called "urticarial multiforme").

Etiology
- Presumably occurs in response to medications (most commonly antibiotics) or as a post-viral phenomenon

Epidemiology
- Usually occurs in infants and younger children

Differential Diagnosis
- Serum sickness, erythema multiforme, viral exanthem (Tables 6.1, 6.2)

Clinical Manifestations
- Primary lesions: generalized annular and polycyclic urticarial lesions.
- Lesions may develop a purplish hue, but typically are evanescent, lasting less than 24 hours.
- Edema of hands, feet, and periocular areas common.
- Dermatographism: stroking of the skin results in urtication at the site
- Fever may be seen in association with underlying infection.

Diagnostics
- No specific diagnostic tests are indicated.

Management
- Discontinue potential causative medications.
- Antihistamines (e.g., diphenhydramine, hydroxyzine) should be administered at regularly scheduled intervals until patient responds to therapy.

Table 6.1: Comparison of Acute Urticarial Hypersensitivity and Erythema Multiforme Minor	
Acute Urticarial Hypersensitivity	**Erythema Multiforme Minor**
Annular, polycyclic urticarial lesions (centers are often white)	Targetoid lesions (centers are purple)
Lesions range from small to giant	Lesions are often small to medium-sized
Evanescent lesions (resolve within 24 hours)	Fixed lesions (lesions persist for up to 1 week)
Peripheral edema common	Peripheral edema not typically seen
Itching common	Itching uncommon
Responds to antihistamines and steroids	Possible response to steroids; no response to antihistamines

Table 6.2: Common Cutaneous Drug Reactions

Cutaneous Drug Reaction	Key Clinical Features	Commonly Associated Drugs	Treatment
Urticaria	Evanescent, itchy wheals lasting <24 hours; angioedema	Penicillin-based antibiotics; ACE inhibitors	Discontinue drug; start antihistamines
Morbilliform eruptions	Symmetrically distributed "measles-like" erythematous macules and papules; may be pruritic	Antibiotics such as penicillin and cotrimoxazole	Discontinuation of drug advised although in some patients, reaction may resolve if drug continued; antihistamines for pruritus
Erythema multiforme minor	Target lesions ("triple-color" phenomenon); mucositis (one mucous membrane)	Usually occurs with infections (e.g., herpes simplex) rather than drugs	Self-limited eruption; supportive care
Erythema multiforme major (Stevens-Johnson syndrome)	Atypical target lesions (may not have typical "triple-color" appearance); mucositis (2 or more mucous membranes) < 20% body surface area	Antibiotics (e.g., penicillins, sulfonamides); anticonvulsants (e.g., phenobarbital, phenytoin, carbamazepine)	Prompt discontinuation of drug. Early initiation of systemic steroids may be of benefit but use is controversial; severe cases may be successfully treated with IVIG; supportive care
Toxic epidermal necrolysis	Extensive areas of tender, red skin associated with skin sloughing and denudation; mucositis often present	Antibiotics such as penicillins and sulfonamides; anticonvulsants such as phenobarbital, phenytoin, carbamazepine, lamotrigine	Prompt discontinuation of drug. Early initiation of systemic steroids may be of benefit but use is controversial; severe cases may be successfully treated with IVIG; supportive care

(Continued)

Table 6.2: Common Cutaneous Drug Reactions (continued)

Cutaneous Drug Reaction	Key Clinical Features	Commonly Associated Drugs	Treatment
Fixed drug eruption	Solitary or limited eruption of well-defined red-brown tender lesions. Lesions often have a burning sensation and heal with dyschromia.	Oral contraceptives; NSAIDs; tetracyclines; anticonvulsants	Discontinuation of drug
Erythema nodosum	Tender erythematous nodules on lower extremities	Oral contraceptives	Discontinuation of drug; NSAIDs
DRESS (drug reaction with eosinophilia and systemic signs), includes anticonvulsant hypersensitivity syndrome	Exanthematous eruption associated with liver toxicity, eosinophilia, atypical lymphocytosis, late-onset thyroid dysfunction	Aromatic anticonvulsants (phenytoin, phenobarbital, carbamazepine); sulfonamide antibiotics; minocycline	Discontinuation of drug; systemic steroids; supportive care

- Consider adjunct H2-blockers: cimetidine, ranitidine
- Occasionally, systemic steroids can be helpful.
- The cutaneous urticarial reaction responds rapidly to antihistamines; the edema may respond more slowly.
- Self-limited

ERYTHEMA MULTIFORME (MINOR)

An immunologically mediated mucocutaneous eruption characterized by targetoid lesions with an acral predilection. The oral mucous membranes are commonly affected.

Epidemiology
- Affects older children and young adults most commonly

Etiology
- Erythema multiforme is a reactive phenomenon seen in response to a plethora of inciting agents including infectious agents, medications, inflammatory conditions, and environmental agents.
- Recurrent erythema multiforme minor is strongly associated with herpes simplex virus (HSV) infection and may occur a few days to a few weeks following HSV infection.

Differential Diagnosis
- Exanthematous erythematous macules and papules: viral exanthems, urticaria, urticarial vasculitis
- Targetoid lesions: annular urticaria, figurate erythemas (e.g., erythema annulare centrifugum)
- Mucositis: herpetic gingivostomatitis, aphthous stomatitis, pemphigus vulgaris

Clinical Manifestations
- Primary lesions: classic lesions are targetoid and show a "triple-color" phenomenon in which the central area is violaceous, the surrounding area is elevated with pallor, and the peripheral rim is erythematous.
- Mucositis: limited to one mucous membrane (usually the oral mucosa)
- Distribution: typically has an acral predilection symmetrically involving the arms and legs, palms and soles, with fewer lesions on the torso

Diagnostics
- Usually a clinical diagnosis though skin biopsy may help in atypical cases

Management
- Self-limited phenomenon, often requiring only supportive care
- Poor oral intake from mucositis may require intravenous rehydration or hyperalimentation.
- Antihistamines (diphenhydramine, hydroxyzine, cetirizine) may treat pruritus.
- Ophthalmologic consultation is recommended for ocular involvement.

Vascular Phenomena

COMPLICATED HEMANGIOMAS

Hemangiomas of infancy are common vascular tumors that undergo a stereotypical pattern of proliferation, stabilization (plateau), and gradual involution. Most hemangiomas require no therapy beyond active non-intervention and appropriate education regarding the natural history of these birthmarks. Complications may arise with certain hemangiomas occurring near vital structures, in certain anatomic locations, or in patients with multiple lesions (Table 6.3).

Epidemiology
- More common in female infants, preterm infants, multiple gestations, and in association with chorionic villus sampling and amniocentesis.
- Most complications with hemangiomas arise during the proliferative phase, during the first 6 to 9 months of life.

Table 6.3: Complications-Related to Hemangiomas

Predisposing Factor	Complication
Periocular location	Amblyopia
Nasal tip	Incomplete involution
Beard distribution	Airway involvement
Large facial, segmental pattern	PHACES syndrome
Midline prevertebral location	Spinal dysraphism
Perineal or perianal site	Ulceration
Multiple ≥ 6	Visceral hemangiomatosis
Large lesions	Mild thrombocytopenia NOT Kasabach-Merritt phenomenon

Etiology
- Most cases are sporadic without clear genetic predisposing factors.
- Hemangiomas of infancy share many similar cellular markers with placental tissue and may have a common precursor.

Differential Diagnosis
- Vascular malformations: venous malformations, arteriovenous malformations, lymphatic malformations
- Rapidly involuting congenital hemangioma: a congenital hemangioma that involutes rapidly (during the first year) and may result in cutaneous atrophy
- Non-involuting congenital hemangioma: a congenital hemangioma with overlying telangiectasia that does not involute
- Vascular-appearing tumors: lipoblastoma, fibrosarcoma or other soft-tissue sarcomas; these are often large, congenital lesions showing rapid growth, ulceration, and fixation to underlying tissue.

Clinical Manifestations
- Lesions are often not visible at birth and become manifest within the first 4 to 8 weeks after delivery. Lesions may begin as faint areas of macular erythema and then rapidly become elevated.
- Superficial lesions have a "strawberry" appearance. Deep lesions may appear soft and bluish without much superficial change. Mixed lesions may have features of both superficial and deep lesions.
- Lesions undergo proliferation and may grow rapidly during the first 6 to 9 months; they then plateau or stabilize until approximately 1 year of age. After 1 year of age, hemangiomas undergo slow, gradual involution with approximately 10% of lesions resolving each year.
- Most involute, but residua of telangiectasia or fibrofatty tissue may remain.
- Complications prompting admission may include rapidly growing periocular hemangiomas threatening vision that are unresponsive to systemic steroid therapy, symptomatic airway hemangiomas not responding to systemic steroid therapy, extensive ulcerated hemangiomas with secondary infection or sepsis, symptomatic visceral hemangiomatosis resulting in congestive heart failure, PHACES syndrome
- PHACES syndrome: large segmental facial hemangiomas in association with posterior fossa abnormalities, arterial anomalies, aortic coarctation, eye and midline sternal anomalies. Consider admission for symptomatic coarctation of the aorta, abnormal vasculature, or associated hydrocephalus or central nervous system malformations.

Diagnostics
- MRI may help delineate anatomic extent of orbital or airway hemangiomas, or help evaluate associated anomalies as in PHACES syndrome.
- Skin biopsy for atypical lesions may help rule out malignant tumors.

Management
- Periocular hemangiomas threatening vision:
  - Dermatology and ophthalmologic consultation
  - Consider systemic steroid therapy (2–3 mg/kg/day of prednisone or prednisolone) during the proliferative phase for those in danger of amblyopia. Monitor for steroid-related side effects.
  - Consider gastrointestinal prophylaxis with ranitidine or cimetidine
  - If steroids prove inadequate, consider surgical or more intensive pharmacologic intervention (interferon or vincristine)
- Symptomatic airway involvement:
  - Dermatology and ENT consultation
  - Consider systemic steroid therapy (2–3 mg/kg/day of prednisone or prednisolone) during proliferative phase if danger of airway occlusion
  - If steroids prove inadequate, consider surgical or more intensive pharmacologic intervention (interferon or vincristine)
- Ulcerated hemangiomas with superinfection:
  - Consider dermatology consultation
  - Soaks with tap water, saline, or acetic acid twice daily
  - Topical antibiotic therapy (topical mupirocin or topical metronidazole) and daily to twice-daily dressing changes with non-adherent dressings (Telfa or petrolatum gauze)
  - Systemic antibiotic therapy (antistaphylococcal)
  - Consider systemic steroids and pulsed dye laser therapy if recalcitrant
- Visceral hemangiomatosis:
  - Patients with 6 or more lesions may be at particular risk.
  - Hepatomegaly, splenomegaly, congestive heart failure may all indicate visceral hemangiomatosis. Hypothyroidism has occasionally been seen with liver hemangiomas.
  - Ultrasound or MRI may help delineate extent of involvement.
  - Systemic steroid therapy for symptomatic patients
  - Interventional radiologic embolization of selected lesions
- PHACES syndrome
  - Consultation: Dermatology, Cardiology, Ophthalmology, or Neurology
  - Imaging to delineate extent of systemic involvement
  - If anatomic extent involves periocular area (amblyopia risk) or the neck or lower face (airway risk), patients should be evaluated accordingly.

Resources

Blistering Disorders

American Academy of Pediatrics. Severe invasive group A streptococcal infections: a subject review. Pediatrics 1998;101:136–140.

Bachot N, Roujeau JC. Differential diagnosis of severe cutaneous drug eruptions. Am J Clin Dermatol 2003;4:561–572.

Clark P, Davidson D, Letts M, et al. Necrotizing fasciitis secondary to chickenpox infection in children. Can J Surg 2003;46:9–14.

Dahl PR, Perniciaro C, Holmkvist KA, et al. Fulminant group A streptococcal necrotizing fasciitis: clinical and pathologic findings in 7 patients. J Am Acad Dermatol 2002;47:489–492.

Ladhani S. Recent developments in staphylococcal scalded skin syndrome. Clin Microbiol Infect 2001;7:301–307.

Mascini EM, Janzse M, Schouls LM, et al. Penicillin and clindamycin differentially inhibit the production of pyrogenic exotoxins A and B by group A streptococci. Int J Antimicrob Agents 2001;18:395–398.

Metry DW, Jung P, Levy ML. Use of intravenous immunoglobulin in children with Stevens-Johnson syndrome and toxic epidermal necrolysis: seven cases and review of the literature. Pediatrics 2003;112:1430–1436.

Moss RL, Musemeche CA, Kosloske AM. Necrotizing fasciitis in children: prompt recognition and aggressive therapy improve survival. J Pediatr Surg 1996;31:1142–1146.

Exanthems

Forman R, Koren G, Shear NH. Erythema multiforme, Stevens-Johnson syndrome and toxic epidermal necrolysis in children: a review of 10 years' experience. Drug Safety 2002;25:965–972.

Leaute-Labreze C, Lamireau T, Chawki D, et al. Diagnosis, classification, and management of erythema multiforme and Stevens-Johnson syndrome. Arch Dis Child 2000;83:347–352.

Mortureux P, Leaute-Labreze C, Legrain-Lifermann V, et al. Acute urticaria in infancy and early childhood: a prospective study. Arch Dermatol 1998;134:319–323.

Tamayo-Sanchez L, Ruiz-Maldonado R, Laterza A. Acute annular urticaria in infants and children. Pediatr Dermatol 1997;14:231–234.

Vascular Phenomena

Garzon MC, Frieden IJ. Hemangiomas: when to worry. Pediatr Ann 2000;29:58–67.

Metry DW, Hebert AA. Benign cutaneous vascular tumors of infancy: when to worry, what to do. Arch Dermatol 2000;136:905–914.

Andrea Dahlman, MD, Mark D. Joffe, MD

Primary and Secondary Survey

This is a systematic approach to evaluating a critically ill child.

PRIMARY SURVEY (A-B-C-D-E)

A: Airway and Cervical Spine Stabilization
- Airway patency: assess for upper airway obstruction.
- Open airway with head-tilt/jaw-thrust maneuver (use jaw thrust for trauma).
- Use jaw-thrust maneuver if concern for neck injury.
- Clear debris: large bore (e.g., Yankauer) suction catheter
- C-spine immobilization (ensure proper collar size)
- Consider oral (length = distance from teeth to angle of jaw), nasopharyngeal (length = distance from angle of jaw to tip of nose), or laryngeal mask airway.
- Consider endotracheal intubation.

B: Breathing/Ventilation
- Assess breath sounds, chest rise, respiratory rate.
- Administer oxygen as needed.
- Consider bag-valve-mask ventilation.

C: Circulation
- Assess heart rate and rhythm, pulse, skin color, capillary refill.
- Establish IV access within 90 seconds or three attempts. Consider intraosseous access (if <8 years old) or central venous access.
- Consider 20 mL/kg of lactated Ringer's (LR) or normal saline (NS) over 5 to 15 minutes if signs of dehydration or shock.
- Consider chest compressions if cardiopulmonary arrest.

D: Disability (Rapid Neurologic Evaluation) and Dextrose
- Assess pupillary response.
- Assess mental status using the Glasgow Coma Scale (see Table 19.3) or AVPU system
- AVPU system: A: Alert; V: Responds to verbal stimuli; P: Responds to painful stimuli; U: Unresponsive
- Check bedside blood sugar.

E: Exposure/Decontamination
- Fully undress patient to evaluate for hidden injury.
- Environmental control
- Patient temperature: maintain normothermia to decrease metabolic needs

SECONDARY SURVEY

Physical Exam
- Complete physical exam from head to toe
- Remember the following important aspects:
  - Pupillary and funduscopic exam
  - Otoscopy to evaluate for hemotympanum

- Press on chest wall and pelvis to establish stability.
- Log roll the patient to assess for injuries to back. Evaluate the entire spine for step-offs or tenderness. Also, evaluate the axillae and perineum, and perform a rectal exam to evaluate tone and for blood.

AMPLE History
- A: Allergies; M: Medications; P: Past medical history; L: Last meal; E: Environments and events

Selected Topics in Emergency Medicine

BURNS

First-degree: redness and mild inflammatory response confined to epidermis; somewhat painful; heals in 3 to 5 days without scarring

Superficial second-degree: destruction of the epidermis and less than half of the dermis; blistering; pink-red color and moist appearance due to capillary network; edema due to increased capillary permeability

Deep second-degree: destruction of epidermis and greater than 50% of dermis; paler, drier appearance; speckled appearance due to thrombosed vessels; many weeks to heal and may need skin grafts

Third-degree or full-thickness: pale or charred color and leathery appearance; nontender due to destruction of cutaneous nerves; cannot re-epithelialize and only heals from periphery; most require skin grafting

Fourth-degree: full-thickness involving underlying fascia, muscle, or bone

Epidemiology
- Mechanism of injury tends to change with age:
  - *Infants:* bathing-related scalds, child abuse
  - *Toddlers:* hot liquid spills
  - *School-age:* playing with matches
  - *Adolescent:* volatile agents and high-voltage electric lines
- Six mechanisms of thermal injury: scalds, contact burns, fire, chemical, electrical, radiation

Pathophysiology
- Increased capillary permeability results in edema, third spacing, fluid loss, and hypovolemic shock.
- Inhalation injuries may result in airway damage, carbon monoxide poisoning, and diffuse lung injury.
- The inflammatory phase involves leukocyte infiltration, cytokine release, and complement activation. Epithelial cells undergo metaplasia to produce stratified squamous epithelial cells required for healing of skin. Neovascularization and fibroblast migration occur in 1 to 3 weeks.

Diagnostics
- ABG with co-oximetry: check for carbon monoxide poisoning (carboxyhemoglobin levels: toxic = 20% to 60%; lethal, > 60%)
- Follow serial electrolytes (rapid fluid shifts).
- Chest x-ray: may be normal initially, even with significant inhalation injury
- Determine percent body surface area (BSA) involved. In adolescents and adults, the "rule of 9s" can be used to estimate percent BSA (Table 7.1). In neonates and toddlers, the head comprises a larger percent BSA (Table 7.1).

Management
Initial Management
- Consider early intubation for those with airway injury, with smaller diameter ETT than usual for age.

Table 7.1: Percent Body Surface Area by Age

	Neonate	Toddler	Adolescent/Adult
Head	18%	15%	9%
One arm	8%	8%	9%
Front torso	20%	20%	18%
Back	20%	20%	18%
One leg	13%	15%	18%

- 100% oxygen, especially if carbon monoxide poisoning
- Vascular access: upper extremities in intact skin; no circumferential taping
- High ambient temperature to decrease heat loss
- Consider urinary catheter, nasogastric tube, tetanus toxoid

Fluid Therapy
- Initial bolus: 20 mL/kg of LR
- Crystalloid solutions (e.g., LR) are recommended during first 24 hours.
- Colloid solutions for volume expansion and preservation of serum oncotic pressure may be considered after 12 to 24 hours.
- Parkland fluid resuscitation formula:
  - 4 mL/kg/% body surface area with second- and third-degree burns
  - Give half in the first 8 hours and half in the next 16 hours
  - Underestimates evaporative loss and maintenance needs of young children
  - Add maintenance in children younger than 5 years old

Antibiotics
- Consider IV penicillin for first 3 to 5 days due to higher risk for streptococcal infections in children than adults

Burn Wound Care
- Premedicate with pain medication before wound care or dressing changes.
- Cover burns loosely with clean sheets until cardiorespiratory status is stabilized.
- If less than 2% BSA: topical petrolatum gauze
- If 2% or greater BSA: topical silver sulfadiazine cream (Silvadene) or bacitracin (especially to face). Mafenide acetate (Sulfamylon) is also effective but inhibits carbonic anhydrase, which may contribute to metabolic acidosis.
- Cleanse with large volumes of lukewarm sterile saline.
- Wipe away loose tissue with sterile gauze.
- Leave unruptured bullae intact unless in locations that are likely to rupture.
- Change dressings twice per day; leave face open.
- First degree: moisturize
- Partial-thickness: cleanse with mild soap and water, one-fourth strength povidone-iodine solution or saline alone.
- Escharotomy if absent flow or with extensive, full-thickness thoracic burns

Pain Control
- Cover burns with clean sheet to prevent exposure of sensory nerve receptors.
- After adequate circulation is established, consider narcotic analgesics (e.g., morphine 0.1–0.15 mg/kg).

Disposition
- Admit to hospital if: partial-thickness burns greater than 10% of BSA; full-thickness burns over 2% of BSA; location at high risk for disability (face, perineum, hands/feet, circumferential burn, overlying joints); concern that burns cannot be adequately cared for at home

CLOSED HEAD INJURY

Nonpenetrating Head Trauma

Pathophysiology

- *Epidural hematoma:* rapid accumulation of blood between dura and cranium; often due to laceration of middle meningeal artery secondary to skull fracture; may have initial loss of consciousness followed by lucid interval and then rapid deterioration.
- *Subdural hematoma:* due to tearing of an artery or bridging vein between dura and brain parenchyma
- *Shaken-baby syndrome:* acceleration-deceleration brain injury; may result in retinal hemorrhages, subdural hematomas, and subarachnoid blood; often there is no sign of external trauma, but can include an impact injury
- *Impact seizure:* occurs at time of minor head injury with quick return to baseline
- *Postconcussive blindness:* associated with injury to back of head; temporary loss of vision for minutes to hours and then normal vision returns

Clinical Manifestations

- Irritability, pallor, lethargy, emesis, headache, dizziness
- Examine head carefully for scalp hematoma or depressed skull fracture.
- Bruises around eyes (racoon's eyes), behind ear (battle sign), or hemotympanum may indicate basilar skull fracture.
- Pupillary exam to assess responsiveness and size, and exam of fundi to assess for papilledema or intraocular hemorrhage
- Signs of elevated intracranial pressure (ICP): irritability/headache, bulging fontanelle, bradycardia, hypertension, altered respiratory pattern, decreased level of consciousness, seizures

Diagnostics

- Try to determine the mechanism of injury and if there was loss of consciousness or seizure activity after the injury.
- *Skull films:* some role as a screening tool to determine need for head CT but negative skull films do not exclude intracranial injury; useful if skull fracture is suspected but no sign of intracranial injury (e.g., normal-appearing young infant with scalp contusion), if CT is unavailable, or if sedation is not indicated. Consider a skeletal survey if abuse is suspected.
- *CT scan of head:* recommended if change in mental status, focal neurologic abnormality, severe injury, concerning mechanism, or persistent symptoms such as vomiting, lethargy, or headache.

Management

- Goal is to prevent secondary injury and systemic insults, prevent increasing ICP, and detect lesions requiring surgery. Assume cervical spine injury and suspect other injuries until proven otherwise.
- *Mild head injury:* if thorough physical exam is unremarkable, patient may be discharged with instructions to watch for signs of increased ICP or hemorrhage (depression of mental status, progressive vomiting more than 4 hours post-trauma, visual disturbances, ataxia, seizures).
- *Moderate head injury:* requires prolonged observation in the emergency department or admission due to small chance of worsening cerebral edema and subsequent intracranial hemorrhage.
- *Severe head injury:*
  - Stabilize cervical spine
  - Administer supplemental oxygen
  - Insert two intravenous cannulas
  - Maintain intubated patients at a $PaCO_2$ of 35 to 40 mm Hg
  - Unless patient is hypovolemic, limit parenteral fluid to maximum of two thirds of daily maintenance rate.
  - Consider mannitol (0.5–1.0 g/kg of 20% solution) when acute herniation is suspected or proven; may also use 3% saline

- Consider seizure prophylaxis with diphenylhydantoin.
- Corticosteroids are generally not recommended.
- *Criteria for discharge from emergency department:* traumatic force not life-threatening; GCS 15; nonfocal neurologic exam; no significant symptoms; no history of prolonged loss of consciousness (or normal CT); no intracranial abnormalities on CT (if obtained); reliable caretakers who are able to return if necessary; no suspicion of abuse or neglect

CONCUSSION

Temporary and immediate post-traumatic impairment of neurologic function, which may be associated with confusion, loss of consciousness, and amnesia.

Pathophysiology
- Often from direct impact or rotational forces
- White matter fibers are sheared or stretched.
- Alteration of neurotransmitter levels, cerebral blood flow, and oxygen use
- *Second impact syndrome:* serious neurologic deterioration or death after second seemingly minor head impact (usually within days of initial injury). Impaired autoregulation of cerebral blood flow may be exacerbated by second impact, resulting in cerebral edema and a rapid increase in intracranial pressure.
- *Postconcussion syndrome:* symptoms of confusion, amnesia, headaches, or dizziness may persist for days or weeks.
- Subtle neuropsychiatric abnormalities persist longer than symptoms.

Diagnostics
- CT scan: usually normal; may find abnormalities in cerebrovascular autoregulation
- MRI: subtle evidence of brain contusion or diffuse axonal injury

Management
- No specific therapy required if normal mental status and physical exam
- Consider acetaminophen for headaches, but avoid narcotics, which may mask progression of symptoms.
- Review signs of progressing intracranial injury before discharge.

Guidelines for Returning to Competition Following Concussion
Grade 1 (mild)
- Definition: transient confusion; no loss of consciousness; mental status abnormalities for 15 minutes or less; no amnesia
- After first concussion: may return to play if asymptomatic for 15 minutes
- After second concussion: no sports activity until asymptomatic for 1 week

Grade 2 (moderate)
- Definition: transient confusion; mental status abnormalities for greater than 15 minutes; amnesia; no loss of consciousness
- After first concussion: no sports activity until asymptomatic for 1 week
- After second concussion: no sports activity until asymptomatic for 2 weeks

Grade 3 (severe)
- Definition: any loss of consciousness
- After first concussion: hospital evaluation; no sports activity until asymptomatic for 1 week if loss of consciousness was brief (seconds); no sports activity for 2 weeks if loss of consciousness was prolonged (minutes or longer).
- After second concussion, no sports activity until asymptomatic for 1 month.
- If any abnormality on CT or MRI: no sports activity for remainder of season and patient should be discouraged from any future return to contact sports.

DROWNING AND NEAR DROWNING

Drowning: death from asphyxia within 24 hours of submersion; may be immediate or after resuscitation

Near-drowning: survival of more than 24 hours

Epidemiology
• Fourth leading cause of death for children 19 years old and younger
• Residential swimming pool is most common site in industrialized countries

Pathophysiology
General
• Suffocation and asphyxia may occur with or without pulmonary aspiration after submersion in a liquid medium.
• During initial panic, laryngospasm is triggered by small amount of water entering the hypopharynx.
• Often, victim struggles violently and swallows copious water.
• Affected organs include the brain, lungs, heart, kidneys, hematologic and gastrointestinal systems. Patients are also at risk for bacteremia and sepsis due to breakdown of protective mucosal barriers.

Anoxic-Ischemic Injury
• Primary cause of mortality and morbidity is central nervous system (CNS) injury, with potential for irreversible injury after 3 to 5 minutes of hypoxemia.
• Loss of cerebral autoregulation and blood-brain barrier integrity leads to neuronal death, cytotoxic cerebral edema, and increased intracranial pressure. Hyperglycemia may exacerbate CNS injury.
• Myocardial hypoxemia at 3 to 4 minutes leads to circulatory failure.

Pulmonary Aspiration
• Even small volume may cause profound hypoxemia.
• Seawater is hypertonic and draws interstitial and intravascular fluid into alveoli, inactivates surfactant, increases alveolar surface tension, and causes atelectasis.
• Freshwater is hypotonic and washes out surfactant.
• Pulmonary vascular endothelium is damaged by hypoxia, ischemia, and aspiration resulting in increased vascular permeability, noncardiogenic pulmonary edema, and adult respiratory distress syndrome.

Fluid and Electrolyte Abnormalities
• Seawater drowning can cause intravascular volume depletion.
• Fresh water drowning may cause hyponatremia and hemolysis leading to hyperkalemia and hemoglobinuria.
• Diabetes insipidus may occur following CNS injury.
• Syndrome of inappropriate antidiuretic hormone secretion may occur due to pulmonary or CNS injury.

Diagnostics
• Chest x-ray: pulmonary edema with bilateral disseminated alveolar pattern or signs of aspiration; often normal initially
• ABG/oximtery: hypoxemia and metabolic acidosis
• CBC: concern for trauma/hemorrhage if significant anemia
• ECG: asystole, bradycardia, ventricular fibrillation, or ventricular tachycardia
• Consider bronchoscopy if foreign body is suspected.
• Consider neuroimaging if CNS injury is suspected.
• Hypoxic-ischemic injuries can lead to non-specific patterns of renal, hepatic, or pancreatic injury as well as disseminated intravascular coagulation.

Management

At the Scene

- Survey the scene
- Extrication and immediate CPR; follow ABCs
- Cervical spine precautions for child abuse, water sport accidents, unknown circumstances
- Consider endotracheal intubation and placement of nasogastric tube.

In the Hospital

- If patient arrives awake, alert, and fully responsive, observe for at least 8 to 12 hours before discharge.
- Consider continuous ECG monitoring, echocardiography, central venous pressure monitoring, and pulmonary artery catheter placement.
- Evaluate core temperature for evidence of hypothermia.
- Consider 0.5–1.0 mL/kg of 50% dextrose or 2–4 mL/kg of 10% dextrose if hypoglycemic.
- *Respiratory Management*:
  - Continuous positive airway pressure if alert and breathing spontaneously with mild-moderate hypoxemia
  - Consider supplemental oxygen, and either bag-mask ventilation or endotracheal intubation with goal $PaCO_2$ 35 to 40 mm Hg to avoid cerebral hypoperfusion.
  - Beta-2 agonist therapy if bronchospasm
  - Consider high-frequency ventilation and inhaled nitric oxide.
  - Controversial: surfactant therapy, partial liquid ventilation, extracorporeal life support, "defoaming" of pulmonary edema with butyl alcohol vapor
- *CNS Management:*
  - Mild head elevation if not hypotensive
  - Avoid hyper/hypoglycemia
  - Controversial: superoxide dismutase, lipid peroxidation inhibitors, calcium channel inhibitors, glutamate antagonists, barbiturates, and hypothermia
- Prophylactic antibiotics are not generally recommended. If there is evidence of systemic toxicity, hemodynamic instability, or signs/symptoms of pneumonia, consider empiric antibiotics (e.g., ticarcillin-clavulanate).
- Corticosteroids are not recommended.
- If gastrointestinal symptoms (bloody diarrhea), consider bowel rest, nasogastric suction, gastric pH control

HYPOTHERMIA

Body core temperature below 35°C

- *Frostnip:* firm, cold white area on the face, ears, or extremities; blistering and peeling over the next 24 to 72 hours; occasionally leaves mild hypersensitivity to cold for days or weeks
- *Immersion Foot (Trench Foot):* feet become cold, numb, pale, and edematous due to damp, poorly ventilated boots in cold weather; may develop tissue maceration and infection; prolonged autonomic disturbance causes increased sweating, pain, and hypersensitivity to temperature changes
- *Frostbite:* cold, hard, white anesthetic and numb areas; upon rewarming, area becomes blotchy, itchy, red, swollen, and painful; results range from normal to gangrene
- *Chilblain (Pernio):* erythematous, vesicular, ulcerative lesions due to vasoconstriction; often involves ears, tips of fingers and toes, and exposed parts of legs; may be itchy and painful with swelling and scabbing; may persist for 1 to 2 weeks or longer
- *Panniculitis (cold-induced fat necrosis):* red or purple-blue macular, papular, or nodular lesions; common; usually benign; may persist for 10 days to 3 weeks

Epidemiology

- Primary: accidental, homicidal, suicidal
- Secondary: complicates many systemic diseases

Pathophysiology
- Loss of body heat by conduction (e.g., wet clothing), convection (e.g., wind chill), radiation (e.g., exposure), or evaporation

Local Injury
- Ice crystals form between or within cells, interfering with the sodium pump and leading to rupture of cell membranes
- Clumping of red blood cells and platelets causes microembolism or thrombosis. Secondary neurovascular responses shunt blood away from affected areas leading to further damage.

Systemic Effects
- Due to fatigue and glycogen depletion, maximal heat production can only be sustained for a few hours. The basal metabolic rate increases two to five times, and oxygen consumption increases due to shivering thermogenesis.
- At 32°C to 37°C: vasoconstriction, shivering, nonshivering basal and endocrinologic thermogenesis
- At 24°C to 32°C: basal metabolic rate depressed without shivering
- Less than 24°C: mechanisms for heat conservation are inactive

Clinical Manifestations
- Fatigue, apathy, irritability, incoordination, clumsiness, dizziness, mental confusion
- *Core temperature afterdrop:* temperature declines after removal from cold due to equilibration across gradient and circulatory changes
- Cardiac: decreased mean arterial pressure and cardiac index; atrial and ventricular dysrhythmias; initial tachycardia then bradycardia due to decreased spontaneous depolarization of pacemaker cells
- Renal: diuresis
- Respiratory: decreased ciliary motility, noncardiogenic pulmonary edema
- Neurologic: cranial nerve signs may indicate central pontine myelinolysis
- Greater than 32°C: hyperactive reflexes, less than 32°C hypoactive reflexes, less than 26°C absent reflexes

Diagnostics
- Electrolytes: may reveal hyperkalemia, hypokalemia, elevated blood urea nitrogen and creatinine, hyperglycemia or hypoglycemia.
- ABG: higher oxygen and carbon dioxide levels and lower pH than actual values
- Hematocrit increases 2% for every 1°C decrease in temperature
- Amylase elevation
- ECG: upright ST segment in aVL, aVF, left precordial leads; prolongation of PR interval then QRS interval then QT interval as hypothermia worsens; at less than 32°C, J wave at junction of QRS complex

Management
Local Injury
- Avoid freeze and rethaw cycles because these can cause permanent tissue injury.
- Initially, warm the damaged area by rubbing against the unaffected hand, abdomen, or axilla.
- Consider rapid warming with water bath (temperature approximately 42°C to 45°C), warm/moist air or oxygen, heating pads, or thermal blankets.
- Provide anti-inflammatory and analgesic agents as needed.
- Keep area dry, open, and sterile.
- Consider excision or amputation only after prolonged observation with conservative therapy.

Systemic Symptoms
- Cardiac monitoring; intravenous and arterial catheters as needed
- Fluid resuscitation: heat fluids to 40°C to 42°C
- Consider endotracheal intubation. May need blind nasotracheal intubation if cold-induced trismus. Place nasogastric tube.

- Gastric or colonic irrigation with warm saline or peritoneal dialysis if severe hypothermia (effectiveness unknown)
- Control fluid, pH, blood pressure, oxygen
- Cardiopulmonary bypass when temperature less than 28°C
- Vasodilating agents: prazosin or phenoxybenzamine
- Anticoagulants: heparin, dextran (equivocal results)
- Oxygen helpful at high altitudes
- Indwelling bladder catheters to monitor urinary output and determine severity of vascular fluid shifts
- Consider low-dosage (2–5 ug/kg/min) dopamine infusions if hypotension does not respond to crystalloids and rewarming
- Consider adrenocortical insufficiency or steroid dependency if patient fails to rewarm.
- If less than 3 months of age, consider prophylactic antibiotics.

Resources

American Academy of Neurology. Practice parameter: the management of concussion in sports. Neurology 1997;48:581–585.

American Academy of Pediatrics. The management of minor closed head injury in children. Pediatrics1999;104:1407–1415.

American College of Surgeons. Advanced Trauma Life Support Program. Chicago: American College of Surgeons, 1997.

Behrman R, Kliegman R, Jenson H, eds. Nelson Textbook of Pediatrics. 17th ed. Philadelphia: Elsevier, 2004.

Ender PT, Dolan MJ. Pneumonia associated with near-drowning. Clin Infect Dis 1997;25:896–907.

Fleisher G, Ludwig S, eds. Textbook of Pediatric Emergency Medicine. 4th ed. Philadelphia: Lippincott, Williams & Wilkins, 2000.

Kelly JP, Rosenberg JH. The development of guidelines for the management of concussion in sports. J Head Trauma Rehabil 1998;13:53–65.

Marx JA, ed. Rosen's Emergency Medicine: Concepts and Clinical Practice. 5th ed. St. Louis: Mosby, 2002.

Monafo WW. Initial management of burns. N Engl J Med 1996;335:1581–1586.

Orlowski JP, Szpilman D. Drowning: rescue, resuscitation, and reanimation. Pediatr Clin North Am 2001;48:627–646.

Quayle KS, Jaffe DM, Kuppermann N, et al. Diagnostic testing for acute head injury in children: when are head computed tomography and skull radiographs indicated? Pediatrics 1997;99:1–8.

Schutzman SA, Barnes P, Duhaime AC, et al. Evaluation and management of children younger than two years old with apparently minor head trauma: proposed guidelines. Pediatrics 2001;107:983–993.

Wojtys EM, Hovda D, Landry G, et al. Concussion in sports. Am J Sports Med 1999;27:676–687.

Francis M. Hoe, MD, Malaka B. Jackson, MD,
Adda Grimberg, MD, FAAP

Diabetes Mellitus and Diabetic Ketoacidosis

DIABETES MELLITUS

Syndrome characterized by fasting and postprandial hyperglycemia. Diabetes mellitus encompasses a heterogeneous group of disorders including type 1 diabetes mellitus, type 2 diabetes mellitus, maturity onset diabetes of the young (MODY), and secondary diabetes mellitus.

Epidemiology
- *Type 1 diabetes mellitus:* onset predominantly in childhood, but may occur at any age; prevalence: 1.9 per 1000
- *Type 2 diabetes mellitus:* most prevalent among obese; in children, onset usually in mid-puberty; more frequent in African Americans, Hispanics, Pacific Islanders, Asians, and Pima Indians
- *MODY:* autosomal dominant inheritance; onset usually between 9 and 25 years of age

Etiology
- *Type 1:* autoimmune-mediated destruction of pancreatic islets in predisposed individuals (with certain HLAs) triggered by unknown agent
- *Type 2:* insulin resistance and relative insulin deficiency
- *MODY:* genetic defects in enzymes or nuclear transcription factors involved in the regulation of insulin secretion or pancreatic islet development
- *Other etiologies:* exocrine pancreatic diseases (cystic fibrosis, pancreatectomy, hemachromatosis); other endocrinopathies (acromegaly, Cushing disease, pheochromocytoma); drug or chemical induced (glucocorticoids, beta-blockers, phenytoin, asparaginase, cyclosporine, tacrolimus, vacor, pentamidine, diazoxide, nicotinic acid, thiazides); infections (cytomegalovirus, congenital rubella); genetic syndromes (Prader-Willi syndrome, Down syndrome, Turner syndrome, Klinefelter syndrome)

Pathophysiology
- Insulin deficiency and/or impaired insulin action results in the abnormal metabolism of carbohydrate, protein, and fat.
- *Type 1:* destruction of pancreatic β cells leads to insulin deficiency. Insulin deficiency results in excessive hepatic glucose production and impaired glucose utilization in muscle and fat leading to hyperglycemia, glucosuria and osmotic diuresis. Lipolysis and impaired lipid synthesis lead to elevated lipids, cholesterol, triglycerides, and free fatty acids, which are converted into ketones. Impaired utilization of glucose, excessive caloric losses in urine, increasing catabolism, and dehydration all lead to weight loss.
- *Type 2:* insulin resistance and inadequate insulin secretion result in relative insulin deficiency. Most patients have sufficient insulin to suppress lipolysis, ketogenesis, and metabolic acidosis.

Clinical Manifestations
- *Type 1:* polyuria; polydipsia; polyphagia; weight loss; secondary enuresis; weakness, lethargy; blurry vision; occasional pyogenic skin infections and in adolescent females, monilial vaginitis; frequently presents with ketosis, ketonuria, and DKA
- *Type 2:* overweight and obese; absent or mild polyuria and weight loss; acanthosis nigricans (velvety hyperpigmented patches in skin folds of neck, axilla, arms); glucosuria; usually no ketonuria; infrequently presents with DKA; may already have long-term complications at diagnosis

Diagnosis
- Criteria for diagnosis of diabetes mellitus: random plasma glucose greater than 200 mg/dL, OR fasting plasma glucose greater than 126 mg/dL, OR 2-hour plasma glucose during oral glucose tolerance test greater than 200 mg/dL. These abnormalities must be present on 2 different days OR in the presence of symptoms of diabetes (polyuria, polydipsia, weight loss).
- Urinalysis for glucose and ketones
- HgA1c: reflects average blood glucose concentration of preceding 2 to 3 months; index of long-term glycemic control. Target for diabetes control varies by age. HgA1c goal is 7.5% to 9% for children younger than 5 years of age and 6% to 7% for adolescents.
- *Type 1:* low fasting insulin and C-peptide levels; often positive β-cell autoantibodies
- *Type 2:* acanthosis nigricans; normal or elevated fasting insulin and C-peptide levels; no β-cell autoantibodies
- *MODY:* diabetes in at least three generations; autosomal dominant pattern of inheritance; diabetes before age 25 in at least one family member

Management
Seek consultation from a pediatric endocrinologist. The following recommendations are general guidelines used at the authors' institution (also see Diabetic Ketoacidosis section):

Long Term
- *Type 1:* daily requirement for exogenous insulin; monitor metabolic control; attention to dietary intake
- *Type 2:* weight management; increase daily physical activity and decrease sedentary activity; decrease caloric and fat intake; most require insulin or oral hypoglycemics (metformin, acarbose)
- Normalize blood glucose and HgA1c: self-monitoring of blood glucose; HbA_{1c} every 3 months
- Monitor for long-term complications:
  - Small vessels: retinopathy (regular ophthalmologic screening); nephropathy (regular screening for hypertension and microalbuminuria); neuropathy
  - Large vessels: atherosclerosis (regular screening for hyperlipidemia); ischemic heart disease; arterial obstruction with gangrene of extremities

Management of Ketosis (without Acidosis)
- If ill or hyperglycemic (>240 mg/dL), check for ketonuria
- Encourage oral hydration: 1 ounce/hr × "age"; if blood glucose level less than 180 mg/dL, drink carbohydrate containing fluids; if blood glucose 180 to 240 mg/dL, drink half carbohydrate containing and half sugar-free fluids; if blood glucose greater than 240 mg/dL, drink sugar-free fluids
- Provide extra short-acting insulin: 10% of total daily dose of insulin SC every 2 hours until ketosis resolves
- Monitor blood glucose and ketones in urine every 2 hours
- If signs and symptoms persist or worsen, suspect diabetic ketoacidosis (DKA)

Management during Infections
- Often require additional insulin (~110% to 120% total daily dose)
- If vomiting, omit short-acting insulin and reduce total daily dose of insulin by ~50%. If unable to tolerate fluids orally, admit for IV fluids with glucose (D10%/1/2 NS), insulin infusion (0.02–0.05 U/kg/hr), and monitoring of electrolytes and glucose.

Hypoglycemic Reactions
- Due to honeymoon phase, errors in insulin dose, reduction in oral intake, or increased physical activity
- Give simple carbohydrates (like juice, sugar-containing soda, cake icing, or glucose tablets); recheck blood glucose 20 minutes later, and repeat as necessary.
- If vomiting, combative, seizing, or losing consciousness, give glucagon 1 mg IM.

Insulin
- Subcutaneous injections: rotate sites to prevent fibrosis and lipodystrophic changes (Table 8.1).

Table 8.1: Insulin Pharmacodynamics

Type	Name	Onset (hr)	Peak (hr)	Effective duration (hr)	Maximal duration (hr)
Short-acting	Regular	0.5–1.0	2–3	3–6	4–6
	Lispro (Humalog)*	0.25–0.5	1–2	2–3	3–4
	Novolog†	<0.5	1	2–3	3–5
Intermediate-acting	NPH	2–4	4–10	10–16	14–18
	Lente	3–4	4–12	12–18	16–20
Long-acting	Ultralente	6–10		18–20	20–30
	Glargine (Lantus)‡		no peak	11 to > 24	
Premixed	Insulin 70/30 (70% NPH, 30% regular)	70% same as NPH above; 30% same as regular above			
	Insulin 75/25 (75% NPH, 25% Lispro)	75% same as NPH above; 25% same as Lispro above			

* Lispro: Usually given right before meal. Useful for infants and younger children where insulin dose determined by carbohydrates ingested and given after meal.
† Novolog: Similar to Lispro.
‡ Glargine: No peak, relatively constant concentration.

- Insulin pumps: short-acting insulin given as continuous subcutaneous infusion (basal) plus boluses with meals

DIABETIC KETOACIDOSIS

Hyperglycemia, ketonemia, and acidosis due to lack of insulin

Pathophysiology
- Hyperglycemia
- Ketoacidosis: ketones cause a metabolic acidosis with a compensatory respiratory alkalosis with rapid deep breathing (Kussmaul respirations). Acetoacetate is converted to acetone, giving the breath a fruity odor.
- Dehydration: glucosuria and ketonuria cause urinary water and electrolyte loss. Weight loss and dehydration ensue.
- Impaired consciousness: from dehydration, acidosis, hyperosmolality, and diminished cerebral oxygen utilization; may result in coma and death
- Acute stress of trauma or infection may worsen the metabolic derangements.

Diagnostics
- Hyperglycemia
- Metabolic acidosis (pH < 7.3 and HCO_3 < 15 mEq/L)
- Ketonemia and ketonuria
- Pseudohyponatremia:

$$\text{corrected } [Na^+] = \text{measured } [Na^+] + 1.6 \times [(\text{glucose} - 100)/100]$$

- Hyperkalemia: at risk for arrhythmias; consider ECG
- If sepsis is suspected, check blood and urine cultures.
- Leukocytosis and elevated serum amylase are common.

Management
- Consult endocrinology
- Recommend intensive care unit, especially if pH less than 7.0, age younger than 5 years, blood glucose greater than 1000 mg/dL, or altered mental status
- First, replete intravascular volume. Then, correct fluid deficit, electrolyte deficit, and acid-base status as below:

Fluid Management
- Replace fluid deficit: usually about 10% dehydrated
- Provide ongoing maintenance requirements
- Replace ongoing losses from osmotic diuresis
- Replacement schedule:
  - First hour: normal saline (0.9%) 10–20 cc/kg bolus; reassess cardiovascular status and repeat as necessary to prevent hypovolemic shock.
  - Initial 16 hours: half of fluid deficit + maintenance + ongoing losses (with normal saline); usually ~ twice maintenance rate + ongoing losses
  - Over next 32 hours: half of fluid deficit + maintenance + ongoing losses (with normal saline); usually ~1.5 × maintenance rate + ongoing losses
- Strict monitoring of input and output; bladder catheterization in obtunded and comatose patients

Electrolyte Management
- Glucose: monitor blood glucose every hour. Lower glucose by ~100 mg/dL/hr. When blood glucose less than 300 mg/dL, add glucose to fluids (dextrose 5%). Goal blood glucose is 100 to 180 mg/dL.
  - Two-bag system: one bag of fluids with no dextrose and another with 10% dextrose. By varying the rate of fluid from each, one can vary the dextrose infusion rate without changing electrolytes or total volume.
- Potassium: check serum potassium periodically. Patients are initially hyperkalemic due to acidosis; however, they are total body potassium depleted and become hypokalemic as acidosis improves and insulin and glucose are given.
  - If urinary output is adequate, add potassium to fluids: If potassium is normal, consider 40 mEq/L; may need as much as 60 to 80 mEq/L
  - Consider ECG: risk for life-threatening arrhythmia
- Phosphate depleted: substitute some chloride with phosphate in fluids

Insulin Therapy
- Insulin infusion: initially 0.1 U/kg/hr; as hyperglycemia and acidosis correct, consider decreasing infusion rate; continue infusion until pH and acidosis correct
- Check electrolytes and acid-base status every 2 to 4 hours.
- Switch to subcutaneous insulin regimen when DKA has resolved and patient is tolerating oral intake. See Table 8.1.

Metabolic Acidosis
- Corrects with insulin treatment
- Bicarbonate use is controversial.

Cerebral Edema
- Incidence (in DKA): ~1%; mortality rate: 40% to 90%
- Risk factors: younger than 5 years old, newly diagnosed diabetes, high serum glucose, severe acidosis, low pCO_2, true hyponatremia on presentation
- Management: reduce fluid rate; give mannitol 10–20 g/m^2 (1 g/kg) IV every 2 to 4 hours; hyperventilate

Hypothalamic-Pituitary-Adrenal Axis

ADRENAL INSUFFICIENCY

Deficient production of cortisol caused by lesions in the hypothalamus, or pituitary or adrenal gland

Etiology

- *Primary adrenal insufficiency* (Addison disease): autoimmune adrenalitis; autoimmune polyglandular syndromes; tuberculosis, HIV, fungal infections; Waterhouse-Friderichsen syndrome (adrenal hemorrhage associated with meningococcemia); adrenal thrombosis, infarction, or necrosis; congenital adrenal hyperplasia; adrenoleukodystrophy; primary xanthomatosis; hereditary unresponsiveness to adrenocorticotropic hormone (ACTH); metastatic carcinoma or lymphoma
- *Secondary adrenal insufficiency*: long-term glucocorticoid therapy; pituitary lesions; hypothalamic lesions; pituitary/hypothalamic surgery; head trauma; central nervous system (CNS) irradiation

Pathophysiology

- *Primary adrenal insufficiency*: lesion in the adrenal gland results in deficient cortisol production; low cortisol results in elevated ACTH and melanocyte stimulating hormone (MSH), resulting in hyperpigmentation; some diseases are also associated with varying degrees of mineralocorticoid and androgen deficiency or excess:
  - Mineralocorticoid (aldosterone) deficiency results in hyponatremia, hyperkalemia, acidosis, dehydration, and hypotension. Mineralocorticoid excess causes hypertension.
  - Androgen deficiency in females results in absence of secondary sexual characteristics: lack of pubic and axillary hair, acne, body odor. Androgen excess results in virilization, accelerated growth, increased muscle mass, acne, hirsutism, deep voice, and advanced bone age.
- *Secondary adrenal insufficiency*: lesion in the hypothalamus or pituitary results in insufficient ACTH to stimulate the adrenal gland to produce cortisol.

Clinical Manifestations

- *Signs and symptoms*: apathy, listlessness, fatigue, weakness; anorexia, weight loss; nausea/vomiting, diarrhea, abdominal pain; dizziness, orthostatic hypotension; salt craving; hyperpigmentation (in primary adrenal insufficiency); decreased axillary and pubic hair; hypovolemia; tachycardia
- *Acute adrenal insufficiency/crisis*: fever; confusion; hypotension; shock; death; precipitated by severe stress such as major illness, surgery, or trauma

Diagnostics

Suspect Adrenal Insufficiency

- Electrolyte abnormalities including hyponatremia, hypochloremia, hyperkalemia, acidosis, and hypoglycemia
- Random cortisol less than 18 µg/dL (common in normal individuals).

Diagnosis Confirmed by

- Elevated ACTH with low cortisol (primary adrenal insufficiency)
- *ACTH stimulation tests*: standard ACTH dose 250 µg IV (125 µg for infants). Measure cortisol at times 0, 30, and 60 minutes. Normally, ACTH stimulates adrenals to produce cortisol (>18 µg/dL). In primary adrenal insufficiency, there is minimal to no response. In secondary adrenal insufficiency, there may be some response. With adrenal understimulation and atrophy, cortisol may be deficient; consider low dose ACTH (1 µg) stimulation test.
- *Insulin-induced hypoglycemia*: hypoglycemia normally stimulates counter-regulatory hormones including ACTH and cortisol; risk of hypoglycemic seizures
- *Metyrapone test*: tests ability of pituitary gland to make ACTH and adrenal's ability to make steroid precursors in secondary adrenal insufficiency. Metyrapone inhibits 11-hydroxylase, an enzyme in the steroidogenesis pathway. Measure cortisol, ACTH, 11-deoxycortisol, and urinary 17-hydroxycorticosteroids
- *Corticotropin releasing hormone (CRH) testing*: give CRH 1 µg/kg IV and measure ACTH and cortisol response; tests ability of pituitary gland to make ACTH in secondary adrenal insufficiency

Other Studies

- Plasma renin activity: elevated in mineralocorticoid deficiency
- In primary adrenal insufficiency, consider abdominal ultrasound or CT to assess for adrenal hypertrophy or hemorrhage.
- In secondary adrenal insufficiency, consider MRI of the brain to assess for CNS lesions.

Management

- If adrenal insufficiency is suspected, consult endocrinology.
- In a stable patient with suspected adrenal insufficiency, send studies to confirm diagnosis before starting steroids. Steroid treatment will interfere with the interpretation of test results.
- Fluids: correct hypovolemia with normal saline intravenous fluid boluses.
- Glucocorticoids
  - *Replacement therapy*: hydrocortisone 10–15 mg/m^2/day orally (PO) divided three times daily
  - *Stress dosing*: for physiologic stress (febrile illnesses, vomiting, dental procedures, initial presentation) give hydrocortisone 45–60 mg/m^2/day PO every 8 hours (or IV every 4 hours). For severe stress (surgery, trauma, severe illness, or repeated emesis) give hydrocortisone 100 mg/m^2 IV/IM once followed by 100 mg/m^2/day IV.
  - *Glucocorticoid withdrawal*: if treated for less than 10 days, may discontinue therapy abruptly. If treated for greater than 2 weeks, the hypothalamic-pituitary-adrenal (HPA) axis may be suppressed and glucocorticoids should be tapered. Provide stress dose coverage until HPA axis recovers (up to 12 months).
- Mineralocorticoid replacement: for primary adrenal insufficiency with mineralocorticoid deficiency and salt-losing form of congenital adrenal hyperplasia (CAH), give 9α-fluorocortisol (Florinef) 0.05–0.2 mg PO daily. Some patients require salt replacement with sodium chloride.
- Medical alert identification bracelet

CONGENITAL ADRENAL HYPERPLASIA

Diseases due to defects in the steroidogenesis pathway in the adrenal gland

Etiology

- Autosomal recessive mutations of steroidogenesis pathway enzymes
- 21-hydroxylase deficiency; lipoid congenital adrenal hyperplasia; 3β-hydroxysteroid dehydrogenase deficiency; 17α–hydroxylase/17,20-lyase deficiency; 11β-hydroxylase deficiency

Epidemiology

- Incidence of 21-hydroxylase deficiency: 1:14,000 (causes 95% cases of CAH)

Pathophysiology

- Defective enzyme in steroidogenic pathway results in excess accumulation of precursors and deficiency of end products.
- Certain precursors and products have glucocorticoid (cortisol, corticosterone, aldosterone), mineralocorticoid (aldosterone, deoxycorticosterone, cortisol), and virilizing (dehydroepiandrosterone, androstenedione, testosterone, dihydrotestosterone) properties.

21-Hydroxylase Deficiency

- Cortisol deficiency: unable to convert 17-hydroxyprogesterone (17OHP) to 11-deoxycortisol; results in adrenal insufficiency
- Aldosterone deficiency: cannot convert progesterone to deoxycorticosterone; results in hyponatremia, hyperkalemia, acidosis, hypotension, shock, death
- Virilization: absence of cortisol feedback inhibition leads to increased ACTH, adrenal hyperplasia and increased steroidogenesis, accumulation of steroid precursors (especially 17OHP), increased testosterone, virilization in females, and accelerated skeletal maturation

Clinical Manifestations

- Clinical phenotype is dependent on specific genetic defect and pattern of excess and deficient steroids.
- 21-hydroxylase deficiency:
  - Salt-wasting CAH (with no 21-hydroxylase activity): ambiguous genitalia in newborn females; salt losing crisis within days or early weeks of life; lethargy; poor feeding; vomiting, diarrhea; dehydration; hyponatremia; hyperkalemia; acidosis; hypotension; shock; fatal if untreated

- Simple virilizing CAH (with mild defects in 21-hydroxylase): no salt-wasting; virilized females; clitoromegaly; fusion of labioscrotal folds; premature puberty in males; pubic, axillary, and facial hair; phallic growth with prepubertal testes; advanced bone age
- Nonclassical CAH: very mild form; mild to moderate hirsutism, virilization, menstrual irregularities; decreased fertility in adolescent and adult females

Diagnostics (21-Hydroxylase Deficiency)
- Diagnosis suggested by:
  - Abnormal newborn screen for 17OHP: >2000 ng/dL after 24 hours old; normally elevated in normal newborns less than 24 hours old; also elevated in premature and severely ill newborns; check 17OHP level with serum or plasma sample
  - Salt wasting episode
  - Ambiguous genitalia
  - Rapid growth and virilization of males
- Confirm diagnosis by ACTH stimulation:
  - ACTH 15 mcg/kg IV (max 0.25 mg)
  - Measure cortisol and 17OHP at 0, 30, and 60 minutes
  - Salt-losing and simple virilizing CAH: basal 17OHP greater than 2000 ng/dL; stimulated 17OHP greater than 5000 to 10,000 ng/dL; subnormal cortisol response
  - Nonclassical CAH: basal 17OHP normal to mildly elevated; stimulated 17OHP 1500 to greater than 10,000 ng/dL; normal cortisol response
- Other studies:
  - Electrolytes: hyponatremia, hyperkalemia in salt-losing CAH
  - Random cortisol if clinically ill
  - ACTH: elevated in severe forms of 21-hydroxylase deficiency and other forms of CAH with cortisol deficiency
  - Plasma renin activity: elevated due to mineralocorticoid deficiency
  - Random and ACTH stimulated levels of pregnenolone, progesterone, deoxycorticosterone, corticosterone, 18-hydroxycorticosterone, 17-hydroxypregnenolone, 11-deoxycortisol, DHEA, androstenedione, and testosterone; to distinguish from other forms of CAH and adrenal or testicular tumors
  - Consider genetic analysis for CYP21 (or 21-hydroxylase) mutation

Management
- Seek consultation from pediatric endocrinology
- Fluids: correct hypovolemia with normal saline intravenous fluid boluses. For salt-wasting CAH, give normal saline in IV fluids.
- Glucocorticoids: if stable, send studies to confirm diagnosis before starting steroids; physiologic replacement hydrocortisone 10–15 mg/m^2/day (PO divided three times daily/IV divided every 4 hours); initially require higher dose (stress dosing) to suppress HPA axis
- Stress dosing: for physiologic stress, including febrile illnesses and vomiting, give hydrocortisone 45–60 mg/m^2/day PO divided every 8 hours; for severe stress such as surgery, trauma, severe illness, or repeated emesis, give hydrocortisone 100 mg/m^2 IV/IM once followed by 100 mg/m^2/day divided every 4 hours; for non-classic CAH, treat only if symptomatic
- Mineralocorticoids (for salt-losing CAH): fludrocortisone (Florinef) 0.05–0.2 mg/day
- Salt (for salt-losing CAH): in newborns, NaCl 1–3 g (17–51 mEq) per day
- If ambiguous genitalia, seek consultation from psychology, pediatric surgery/urology, and genetics
- Medical alert identification

CUSHING SYNDROME

Syndrome resulting from chronic glucocorticoid excess

Etiology
- *Iatrogenic Cushing syndrome*: chronic exposure to supraphysiologic doses of ACTH or glucocorticoids

- *Cushing disease*: ACTH-secreting pituitary adenoma
- *Ectopic ACTH syndrome*: tumor (non-pituitary) that secretes ACTH; associated with neuroblastoma, pheochromocytoma, thymoma, bronchial and pancreatic carcinoma
- *Adrenal tumors*: adrenal adenoma and carcinoma; both secrete cortisol
- Multinodular adrenal hyperplasia: rare; secretes both cortisol and adrenal androgens

Epidemiology
- At younger than 7 years old, adrenal tumors most common
- At older than 7 years old, Cushing disease most common

Clinical Manifestations
- Weight gain, obesity (truncal), linear growth retardation, osteopenia
- Menstrual irregularities, hirsutism, hypertension, fatigue, precocious or delayed puberty, plethora, psychological disturbances, weakness, proximal muscle wasting, buffalo hump, headache
- Violaceous striae, easy bruising, ecchymoses, acne
- Hyperpigmentation (in ACTH-dependent Cushing syndrome)

Diagnosis
- Suspect if accelerated weight gain combined with stunted linear growth
- Diagnostic studies to determine if hypercortisolism is present:
  - *24-hour urinary free cortisol*: greater than 80 µg/m^2/day, greater than 40 µg/g of creatinine
  - *24-hour urinary 17-hydroxysteroid*: normal is 2–7 mg/g of creatinine
  - *Night-time salivary cortisol*: greater than 1 µg/dL at bedtime; greater than 0.27 µg/dL at midnight
  - *Overnight dexamethasone suppression test*: 15 µg/kg, max 1 mg; plasma cortisol greater than 5 µg/dL
- Additional studies
  - *Baseline cortisol*
  - *Baseline ACTH*: mild or equivocal elevation in Cushing disease; very high (100–1000 pg/mL) in ectopic ACTH syndrome; suppressed in adrenal tumors and multinodular adrenal hyperplasia
  - *Standard high-dose dexamethasone suppression test*: measure cortisol, ACTH, and 24-hour urinary excretion of 17 hydroxysteroid, 17 ketosteroids, free cortisol, and creatinine; obtain baseline for 2 days; then, give low-dose dexamethasone (20 µg/kg/d) for 2 days followed by high-dose dexamethasone (80 µg/kg/day) for 2 days. Normally, cortisol, ACTH, and urinary steroids are suppressed by low-dose dexamethasone. In Cushing disease, steroid levels are suppressed by high-dose dexamethasone (but not low dose). In ectopic ACTH syndrome and adrenal tumors, steroid levels are not suppressed by high-dose dexamethasone
  - *CRH stimulation test*: distinguishes between Cushing disease (ACTH and cortisol increase) and ectopic ACTH syndrome (ACTH and cortisol do not increase).
  - *Imaging*: head MRI (confirm pituitary adenoma in Cushing disease, poor sensitivity); adrenal CT or MRI (localization of adrenal tumors); chest and/or abdomen CT or MRI (for tumor in ectopic ACTH syndrome)
  - *Inferior petrosal sinus sampling (after CRH stimulation)*: compares ACTH levels from pituitary draining into the petrosal sinus vs. peripheral vein; distinguishes Cushing disease from ectopic ACTH syndrome

Management
- *Cushing disease*: transsphenoidal adenectomy
- *Ectopic ACTH syndrome*: surgical excision of tumor; if tumor not resectable, consider treatment with steroidogenesis inhibitors or bilateral adrenalectomy
- *Adrenal tumor*: unilateral adrenalectomy
- *Multinodular adrenal hyperplasia*: bilateral adrenalectomy

Thyroid Disease

CONGENITAL HYPERTHYROIDISM

Usually the result of maternal Graves disease (active or in remission), or maternal hypothyroidism.

Epidemiology
- Less than 2% of mothers with Graves disease give birth to an affected infant
- Female:male = 1:1

Pathophysiology
- Transplacental passage of thyrotropin receptor stimulating antibodies (TRSAb) (a maternally produced IgG₁) leads to excessive thyroid hormone production in the offspring.
- Concomitant transplacental passage of thyrotropin receptor blocking antibodies (TRBAb) and/or antithyroid medications can affect the onset, severity, and course.

Clinical Manifestations
- Prenatal: fetal tachycardia, goiter, intrauterine growth retardation
- Postnatal:
  - General appearance: irritable, hyperactive, anxious, flushed, diaphoretic, markedly decreased subcutaneous fat, voracious appetite
  - Vital signs: elevated temperature, blood pressure, heart rate, respiratory rate
  - Advanced bone age, craniosynostosis, frontal bossing, triangular facies, microcephaly, ventriculomegaly
- In severe cases: hepatosplenomegaly, jaundice, cardiac failure with severe hypertension, death
- Long-term morbidity can include: craniosynostosis, growth retardation, intellectual and developmental impairments, secondary central hypothyroidism

Diagnostics
- Elevated TRSAb, thyroxine (T4), and triiodothyronine (T3); low thyroid-stimulating hormone (TSH)

Management
- Methimazole or PTU (see Graves disease for dosing)
- One drop/day of saturated solution of potassium iodide (SSKI) at 48 mg iodide/drop can increase the rate of decrease in circulating thyroid hormone
- β-blockers if needed
- If decompensation, consider digoxin, IV fluids, corticosteroids
- Prognosis: remission is gradual, usually within 3 to 4 months of age

GRAVES DISEASE

An autoimmune disease that affects the thyroid, orbital tissue, and skin

Epidemiology
- Most common cause of hyperthyroidism in children
- Peak incidence in ages 10 to 15 years; female:male = 5:1
- Associated with other autoimmune disorders; most affected children have a positive family history for an autoimmune thyroid disease

Clinical Manifestations
- Endocrine: goiter of varying degrees, systemic symptoms of hyperthyroidism
- Ocular: exophthalmos, lid lag
- Cardiac: tachycardia, palpitations, cardiomegaly, systolic hypertension, elevated pulse pressure
- Respiratory: tachypnea

- Gastrointestinal: diarrhea, increased appetite without change in weight or with weight loss
- Musculoskeletal: linear growth acceleration, bone maturation
- Neurologic: tremors, proximal muscle weakness, tongue fasciculations
- Immunologic: lymphadenopathy, thymic enlargement, peripheral lymphocytosis, splenomegaly
- Psychiatric: emotional lability, hyperactivity
- *Thyroid Storm*: acute onset of hyperthermia and severe tachycardia that can progress rapidly to delirium, coma, and death

Pathophysiology
- TRSAb produced by plasma cells in the thyroid gland bind to TSH receptors, leading to excessive thyroid hormone release and follicular cell hyperplasia.
- Effects may be counterbalanced by the production of TRBAb.

Diagnostics
- Elevated T4, free T4, T3, free T3
- Low TSH, elevated thyroglobulin
- Positive thyroid peroxidase antibodies
- Positive TRSAb; disappearance predicts remission
- Reduced bone density, advanced bone age, craniosynostosis

Management
Medical Management
- Thionamide drugs (methimazole or propylthiouracil) block production of T3 and T4 (by inhibiting incorporation of inorganic iodide) and may suppress autoimmunity within the thyroid, thereby decreasing TRSAb levels. Methimazole (Tapazole) 0.25–1.0 mg/kg/day, once daily, or propylthiouracil (PTU) 5–10 mg/kg/day, divided three times daily
- Atenolol: for symptomatic relief of catecholamine-mediated symptoms

Radioiodine (I-131) thyroid ablation
- Alternative or adjuvant to medical or surgical therapy
- Complete effects may not be seen for 2 to 3 months, and subsequent hypothyroidism is common, necessitating lifelong T4 replacement.

Surgical Management
- Indicated if there is failure of medical therapy or concern for a coexisting carcinoma
- Subtotal thyroidectomy may be performed only after a euthyroid state has been achieved medically.

Other Selected Topics

CEREBRAL SALT WASTING

Renal sodium wasting associated with a CNS insult leading to hypovolemia and hyponatremia

Etiology
- Subarachnoid hemorrhage, neurosurgery, CNS tumor, meningitis, hydrocephalus, stroke, brain death

Pathophysiology
- Hypothesis: increased atrial or brain-derived natriuretic factor leads to renal sodium wasting, hypovolemia, and hyponatremia.

Clinical Manifestations
- Polyuria, hypovolemia, hypotension, nausea, vomiting, weakness, headache, lethargy, psychosis, coma, seizures
- Associated CNS insult

Diagnostics
- Diagnostic studies:
  - Hyponatremia with hypovolemia (if volume expanded, suspect syndrome of inappropriate antidiuretic hormone [SIADH])
  - Urine [Na] inappropriately elevated
- Other corroborative studies:
  - Plasma osmolality low with high urine osmolality
  - Atrial natriuretic peptide high
  - Plasma aldosterone and vasopressin decreased or normal
  - Creatinine clearance normal or decreased
  - Blood urea nitrogen (BUN) normal or increased
  - Renin normal or elevated
  - Body weight stable or decreased
  - Hypovolemia via central venous pressure monitoring or radioisotope dilution techniques

Management
- Treat underlying disorder
- Restore intravascular volume with NaCl and water: initially may need NaCl 150–450 mEq/L
- Acute hyponatremia or [Na] less than 120 mEq/L: rapid correction with 3% saline 6 cc/kg over 1 hour will increase [Na] by 5 mEq/L
- Chronic hyponatremia: correct [Na] by 0.5 mEq/L/hr or 12 mEq/L/day; with rapid correction, at risk for central pontine myelinolysis
- Monitor: vital signs, weight, intake and output, neurologic exam, serum and urine electrolytes
- Patients are at risk for developing other sodium disorders (diabetes insipidus [DI], [SIADH] secretion) and must be reevaluated with change in clinical status.

DIABETES INSIPIDUS

Excessive urinary loss of water caused by inability to produce or respond to vasopressin, also called antidiuretic hormone (ADH)

Etiology
Central DI
- CNS neoplasm; Sheehan syndrome (postpartum pituitary infarction resulting in hypopituitarism); congenital midline brain lesions; head trauma (basal skull fracture, fracture of sella turcica); neurosurgery in region of hypothalamus or pituitary; intraventricular hemorrhage; brain death
- Familial, autosomal dominant central diabetes insipidus
- Infiltrative diseases: Langerhans cell histiocytosis, lymphocytic hypophysitis, sarcoidosis
- Infectious diseases: viral encephalitis, bacterial meningitis (meningococcus, *Cryptococcus*, *Listeria*, toxoplasmosis), congenital cytomegalovirus, tuberculosis, histiocytosis, actinomycosis, Guillain-Barré syndrome
- Increased vasopressin metabolism by vasopressinase during pregnancy
- DIDMOAD (diabetes insipidus, diabetes mellitus, optic atrophy, deafness)
- Other: autoimmune diseases, drug-induced, idiopathic

Nephrogenic DI
- Most common is drug-induced: lithium, demeclocycline, foscarnet, clozapine, amphotericin, methicillin, rifampin
- Congenital, X-linked nephrogenic diabetes insipidus
- Congenital, autosomal recessive nephrogenic diabetes insipidus
- Hypercalcemia, hypokalemia
- Ureteral obstruction, chronic pyelonephritis, polycystic kidney disease, medullary cystic disease, renal dysplasia, chronic renal failure
- Sjögren syndrome, sarcoidosis, amyloidosis
- Sickle cell disease
- Primary polydipsia with mild nephrogenic DI

Pathophysiology
- *Central DI*: lesions in hypothalamus or pituitary result in lack of vasopressin synthesis and/or secretion. Without vasopressin, the renal collecting ducts are not stimulated to resorb water.
- *Nephrogenic DI*: due to abnormalities in the function and/or structure of the renal collecting ducts due to vasopressin receptor or aquaporin defects, injury to the epithelial cells of the collecting ducts, or diluted renal medullary interstitium from long-standing polydipsia or decreased sodium/protein intake.
- *Central and nephrogenic DI*: kidneys are not able to concentrate the urine leading to excessive urinary water loss, increased thirst, and polydipsia. If there is impaired thirst or no access to water, hypernatremia and a hyperosmolar state develop. If chronic, megabladder, hydroureter, and hydronephrosis may develop.

Clinical Manifestations
- Polyuria, nocturia, polydipsia (crave cold fluids, especially water)
- Hypernatremia and dehydration
- Coma and seizure (from severe hypernatremia)
- CNS neoplasm: symptoms of increased intracranial pressure (ICP)
- Hypothalamic tumors: growth failure, cachexia or obesity, fever, sleep disturbance, precocious puberty, emotional disorders
- Nephrogenic DI: chronic dehydration; infants exhibit irritability, poor feeding, water preference, vomiting, growth failure, intermittent high fevers; repeated episodes of dehydration result in brain damage, mental retardation, and abnormal behavior.

Diagnostics
Initial Studies
- Urine output high; urine osmolality low (50–300 mOsm/L)
- Serum osmolality high (see below); serum [Na] high
- Specific gravity low (1.001–1.010)

Diagnostic Studies
- Serum osmolality greater than 300 mOsm/L and urine osmolality less than 300 mOsm/L; unlikely DI if serum osmolality less than 270 mOsm/L or urine osmolality greater than 600 mOsm/L
- Water deprivation test if serum osmolality 270–300 mOsm/L:
  - Tests ability to concentrate urine by withholding fluid
  - Admit and consult endocrinology
  - Monitor serum and urine sodium and osmolality
  - Monitor frequent vital signs and weight for signs of dehydration.
  - In DI, serum osmolality greater than 300 mOsm and urine osmolality less than 600 mOsm
  - Also test response to vasopressin: central DI responds to vasopressin with decreased UOP and increased urine osmolality. Nephrogenic DI is resistant to vasopressin.

Other Studies
- Serum K^+, Ca^{2+}, glucose, and BUN
- Urine glucose and amino acids
- MRI of pituitary and hypothalamus
- Ultrasound to delineate urinary tract anatomy
- Test other anterior pituitary hormones: Langerhans cell histiocytosis associated with anterior pituitary deficits
- β-HCG for germinoma

Management
Initial Management
- Correct water deficit
  - If hypotensive, normal saline (NS) bolus
  - Water deficit = $0.6 \times$ weight $\times (1 - 140/[Na])$
  - Correct water deficit with D5 water

- Correct chronic hypernatremia slowly: lower plasma osmolality 1–2 mOsm/L/hr ([Na] by 0.5–1 mM/L/hr) over 48 hours to avoid cerebral edema
- Correct acute and symptomatic hypernatremia rapidly: if seizure, lower [Na] by 3–4 mM/L over 1 to 2 hours
- Treat ongoing urinary water losses
- Monitor intake and output
- Check frequent serum and urine electrolytes

Chronic Management
- Fluids alone:
  - When intact thirst mechanism and free access to fluids (especially in nephrogenic DI): patients should be PO ad lib
  - When thirst mechanism not intact and/or controlling volume of fluid intake (e.g., infants, postoperative patients): maintenance requirements = 1 L/m^2/day or 40 mL/m^2/hr (D5% 1/4 NS if IV); replace for urine output greater than 40 mL/m^2/hr with D5 water up to 2 L/m^2/day or 80 mL/m^2/hr
- Vasopressin and analogues for central DI:
  - Aqueous vasopressin IV (Pitressin): useful for acute DI, coma, surgery, or unable to use intranasal spray; requires frequent or continuous administration
  - Desmopressin (DDAVP): various routes (PO, intranasal aqueous solution, intranasal spray, parenteral)
- In nephrogenic DI
  - Fluids: 300–400 mL/kg/day
  - Salt restriction: Na less than 1 mM/day
  - Protein: 2 g/kg/day
  - Ensure adequate calories for growth
  - Thiazide diuretics: hydrochlorothiazide 2–4 mg/kg/day
  - Indomethacin: 2 mg/kg/day
  - Amiloride: 20 mg/1.73 m^2/day
  - High-dose desmopressin helpful for some

HYPOGLYCEMIA

Venous plasma glucose below 40 mg/dL or symptoms of hypoglycemia with plasma glucose below 60 mg/dL

Etiology
- Ketotic hypoglycemia: occurs after fasting 14 to 24 hours; presents at age 1 to 5 years, and usually resolves by age 10 years
- Neonates: transient hypoglycemia on first day of life, sepsis, polycythemia
- Drugs: alcohol intoxication, salicylate intoxication, beta-blocker
- Excess insulin: exogenous (diabetics, Munchausen by proxy syndrome); sulfonylurea ingestion; infant of a diabetic mother; perinatal stress–induced hyperinsulinism; congenital hyperinsulinism; Beckwith-Wiedemann syndrome; insulinoma
- Hormone deficiency: panhypopituitarism; growth hormone deficiency, ACTH or cortisol deficiency (see adrenal insufficiency)
- Inborn errors: glycogen storage diseases (GSD); fructose-1,6-diphosphatase deficiency; galactosemia; hereditary fructose intolerance; fatty acid oxidation and ketogenesis defect (medium-chain acyl-CoA dehydrogenase deficiency, HMG CoA synthase deficiency; HMG CoA lyase deficiency); disorders of amino acid metabolism (maple syrup urine disease, methylmalonic acidemia, tyrosinemia)
- Other: dumping syndrome, liver disease, Fanconi-Bickel syndrome, severe diarrhea, severe malnutrition, severe malaria, Jamaican vomiting sickness (from eating unripe ackee fruit of *Blighia spaida* tree), Reye syndrome

Pathophysiology

- Normally during fasting, insulin is suppressed and the counter-regulatory hormones (glucagon, cortisol, growth hormone, epinephrine) prevent hypoglycemia.
- Excess insulin or lack of counter-regulatory hormones results in hypoglycemia.
- Normal fasting adaptations involve hepatic glycogenolysis, hepatic gluconeogenesis, adipose tissue lipolysis, fatty acid oxidation and ketogenesis, and inhibition of glycogen synthesis. Defects in these metabolic pathways can result in hypoglycemia.
- Hyperinsulinism and defects in glycogenolysis result in hypoglycemia after a shorter fasting duration compared to defects in gluconeogenesis, hormone deficiencies, and fatty acid oxidation disorders.

Clinical Manifestations

- Symptoms due to activation of autonomic nervous system: diaphoresis, shakiness, tachycardia, anxiety, weakness, hunger, nausea, vomiting
- Symptoms due to neuroglycopenia: irritability, restlessness, headache, confusion, poor speech, poor concentration, altered level of consciousness, seizure, hypothermia, personality changes, bizarre behavior, sense of impending doom
- Additional symptoms in newborns: cyanotic episodes, apnea, respiratory distress, refusal to feed, brief myoclonic jerks

Diagnostics

- To determine etiology, obtain *critical laboratory tests* at time of hypoglycemia: plasma electrolytes (including bicarbonate), insulin, C-peptide, cortisol, growth hormone, ketones (beta-hydroxybutyrate and acetoacetate), free fatty acids, lactate, ammonia, total and free carnitine, acyl carnitine profile, IGFBP-1, urine ketones, and organic acids
- Laboratory results associated with specific etiologies:
  - Hyperinsulinism: inadequately suppressed insulin when hypoglycemic; low ketones, low free fatty acids when hypoglycemic; positive glycemic response to glucagon stimulation when hypoglycemic; elevated ammonia in glutamate dehydrogenase activation hyperinsulinism
  - Growth hormone deficiency: abnormal growth hormone provocative tests
  - ACTH/cortisol deficiency: see adrenal insufficiency
  - Glycogen storage diseases: lactic acidosis; abnormal fed glucagon stimulation test; hyperlipidemia, hyperuricemia, hypophosphatemia, anemia, microalbuminuria in GSD, type 1; neutropenia in GSD, type 1B
  - Fatty acid oxidation disorders: no serum or urine ketones, low serum carnitine

Management

- If awake and alert, give glucose orally
- If impaired consciousness, give D10 or D25 2–4 cc/kg IV
- Start continuous glucose (NG or IV)
- Consult endocrinologist and/or metabolism specialist
- Management of specific etiologies:
  - Hyperinsulinism: glucagon 1 mg IM/SQ/IV in emergency; diazoxide for perinatal stress induced hyperinsulinism and glutamate dehydrogenase hyperinsulinism; octreotide (high rate of tachyphylaxis); glucagon infusion (1 mg IV over 24 hours) as temporizing measure; pancreatectomy if persistent hypoglycemia
  - GSD, type 1: give pure glucose; avoid galactose and fructose (lactose and sucrose); frequent feeding and/or continuous nasogastric feeding; uncooked cornstarch may extend feeding interval; growth hormone replacement may also be necessary
  - ACTH/cortisol deficiency: hydrocortisone replacement (see Adrenal Insufficiency)
  - Dumping syndrome: acarbose; if acarbose fails, continuous feeding

RICKETS

Decreased or defective bone matrix mineralization secondary to decreased calcium and/or phosphorus availability for deposition of hydroxyapatite; usually involves the epiphysis and newly formed trabecular and cortical bone

Etiologies
- *Rickets of prematurity:* 30% of affected infants have birth weight <1000g
- *Vitamin D abnormalities:*
  - Nutritional deprivation: low dietary vitamin D intake with decreased sunlight exposure; malabsorption syndromes (celiac disease, biliary obstruction, gastric resection, cystic fibrosis with pancreatic insufficiency, and poor gastrointestinal absorption of fat-soluble vitamins); medications that interfere with vitamin D metabolism (cholestyramine, phenytoin, phenobarbital)
  - Metabolic errors: defects in hepatic vitamin D metabolism (rare); renal 25-OH-vitamin D3-1-hydroxylase deficiency (a.k.a., pseudovitamin D deficient rickets or vitamin D–dependent rickets type I); 1,25-dihydroxyvitamin D3–resistant rickets (a.k.a., vitamin D–dependent rickets type II; *VDR*)
- *Calcium deficiency:* nutritional deprivation, hypercalciuria
- *Phosphorus deficiency:*
  - Nutrition deprivation: low-birth-weight infants; use of aluminum-containing antacids
  - Familial hypophosphatemic rickets (FHR): most common form of rickets in North America; an X-linked dominant disorder; defect in renal tubular resorption of phosphorus
  - Renal tubular acidosis: primary, Fanconi syndrome, tyrosinemia type I
  - Oncogenic hypophosphatemic osteomalacia
  - Cadmium and lead excess
- *Bone mineralization inhibitors:* aluminum, bisphosphonates, fluoride
- *Hypophosphatasia:*
  - Decreased synthesis of bone, liver, and kidney alkaline phosphatase isoenzymes leads to an accumulation of mineralization inhibitors (e.g., pyrophosphate), preventing increase of phosphorus level necessary for hydroxyapatite formation
  - Avoid treatment with vitamin D due to increased potential for secondary hypercalcemia

Clinical Manifestations
- Presenting in first year of life: craniotabes, frontal bossing, cranial suture widening, flaring of wrists, rachitic rosary (beading or enlargement of the costochondral junctions), Harrison grooves
- Presenting after first year of life: genu varum (bow-leg deformity) in early childhood; genu valgum (knock-knee deformity) in late childhood; bone pain
- Other manifestations: increased sweating, dental abnormalities, muscle weakness, hypotonia, atelectasis, pneumonia, anemia

Diagnostics
- Alkaline phosphatase: mildly to markedly elevated
- Radiographic findings: osteopenia with pseudofracture lines; widening, flaring, cupping, or fraying of long bone metaphysis; rachitic rosary; flaring of the lower thoracic rib cage; in adolescence, rachitic changes of the iliac crest can be seen because it is the last to fuse.
- See Table 8.2

Management
Vitamin D Deficiency
- Vitamin D (ergocalciferol) 4000 IU PO daily for weeks to months or a single dose of 600,000 IU IM; decrease to 400 IU daily when healing rachitic lesions are seen on x-ray evaluation.
- 50 mg/kg/day of elemental calcium: prevents hypocalcemia secondary to bone matrix remineralization (i.e., "hungry bone" syndrome)

Renal 1-α-Hydroxylase Deficiency (Vitamin D–Dependent Rickets Type I)
- Calcitriol, 10–20 ng/kg/day

Hereditary 1,25-Vitamin D–Resistant Rickets (Vitamin D–Dependent Type II)
- High doses of calcitriol (6 µg/kg/day) and up to 3 g/day of elemental calcium should be tried in all affected patients: observe serial serum calcium, phosphate, alkaline phosphatase, creatinine,

| Table 8.2: Laboratory Findings in Major Causes of Rickets | | | | |
Finding	Calcium	Phosphorus	iPTH	Calcitriol
Anticonvulsant-induced	↓	↓	↑	NI, ↓
Calcium deficiency	↓↓	↓	↑	↑
FHR	NI	↓↓	NI	↓, NI
Phosphorus deficiency	NI, ↑	↓↓	↑	↓, NI
Renal 1-α hydroxylase deficiency	↓↓	↓↓	↑	↓↓↓
VDR gene defect	↓↓	↓↓	↑↑↑	↑↑↑
Vitamin D deficiency: Mild	NI, ↓	NI, ↓	NI	NI
Vitamin D deficiency: Severe	↓	↓	↑↑	↓

FHR, familial hypophosphatemic rickets; iPTH, intact PTH; calcitriol, 1,25-dihydroxyvitamin D3.
Adapted from Sperling M, ed. Pediatric Endocrinology. 2nd ed. Philadelphia: WB Saunders, 2002:647.

and parathyroid hormone; check urine calcium and creatinine excretion, skeletal films and renal ultrasound to evaluate for nephrocalcinosis.
- Refractory patients: continuous IV or intracaval administration of 0.4–1.4 g of elemental calcium/m²/day. After rickets have healed, maintain with 3.5–9 g of elemental calcium/m²/day.

Familial Hypophosphatemic Rickets
- Calcitriol, 20 ng/kg/d increased up to 60 ng/kg/day as needed
- Elemental phosphorus, 30–60 mg/kg/day divided four to six times/day
- If rickets recurs consider adding amiloride diuretic therapy to increase renal tubular calcium absorption

Chronic Renal Disease
- Decrease dietary phosphorus intake. Decrease dietary phosphorus absorption by giving calcium carbonate.
- Calcitriol as daily PO dose or as three-times weekly IV pulse
- Avoid aluminum-containing gels
- Occasionally requires parathyroidectomy

Calcium Deficiency
- Elemental calcium, 1000–1300 mg/day

Hypophosphatasia
- Currently no specific or effective therapy is available.
- Vitamin D administration should be avoided.
- Phosphate administration may heal rickets in mild cases.

SYNDROME OF INAPPROPRIATE ANTIDIURETIC HORMONE

Inappropriately elevated antidiuretic hormone (ADH; vasopressin) with low serum osmolality and expanded extracellular volume

Etiology
- CNS: meningitis, encephalitis, brain tumor, brain abscess, head trauma/surgery, CNS leukemia, subarachnoid hemorrhage, hydrocephalus, psychiatric disease, perinatal asphyxia, Guillain-Barré syndrome

- Infections: pneumonia, HIV/AIDS, tuberculosis, herpes zoster, respiratory syncytial virus, aspergillosis, infantile botulism
- Neoplasms: oat cell carcinoma; bronchial carcinoid; lymphoma; Ewing sarcoma; tumors of pancreas, duodenum, thymus, bladder, ureter
- Drugs: carbamazepine, lamotrigine, chlorpropamide, vinblastine, vincristine, tricyclic antidepressants
- Other: post-ictal period after generalized seizures, prolonged nausea, acute intermittent porphyria

Pathophysiology
- Inappropriate secretion of ADH by hypothalamus or ectopic secretion of ADH or ADH-like peptide
- ADH secretion is not inhibited by normal osmotic feedback mechanisms.
- ADH stimulates renal collecting ducts to resorb water leading to volume expansion, dilutional hyponatremia, and decreased serum osmolality.
- Hypo-osmolality may lead to swelling of cells and cerebral edema.

Clinical Manifestations
- Anorexia, nausea and vomiting, headache, weakness, irritability, personality changes, change in mental status, seizures

Diagnostics
- Low serum $[Na]^+$ and serum osmolality (<270 mOsm/L)
- High urine osmolality (>100 mOsm/L) and urine Na^+ (>20 mM/L), with hyperuricemia
- Other corroborative studies: low serum ADH level, serum K^+, Cl^-, and uric acid; plasma renin activity low; weight stable or increased; urine volume normal or decreased; blood volume normal or increased via central venous pressure or radioisotope dilution
- Rule out adrenal, thyroid, pituitary, and renal insufficiency
- Rule out diuretic use

Management
- Treat underlying disorder
- Frequent monitoring of vital signs, weight, intake and output, serum and urine electrolytes and osmolality
- Symptomatic hyponatremia (associated with seizures or coma):
  - Initially, increase [Na] by 10% (~10 mM) with 3% saline at 1–2 mL/kg/hr. If severe symptoms, increase rate to 4–6 mL/kg/hr.
  - Then, correct [Na] by 0.5 mM/L/hr or 12 mM/L/day
  - Lasix IV
  - Consider hemodialysis to remove excess water
  - Rapid correction (especially with chronic hyponatremia) has been associated with central pontine myelinolysis.
- Chronic management
  - Fluid restriction 1 L/m^2/day: obligatory renal solute load 500 mOsm/m^2/day excreted in 500 mL/m^2/day; insensible losses 500 mL/m^2/day
  - Demeclocycline: induces nephrogenic diabetes insipidus

TANNER STAGING

Used to define male and female pubertal development (Table 8.3).

Table 8.3: Tanner Staging

Males

	Testes	Penis
I	Prepubertal	Prepubertal
II	Testes enlarge, scrotum reddens and changes texture	Slight enlargement
III	Larger	Longer
IV	Scrotum darkens	Larger and wider with development of glans
V	Adult size	Adult size

Female breast development

I	Prepubertal
II	Breast and papilla elevated as small mound with palpable subareolar bud, areolar diameter increased
III	Enlargement and elevation of whole breast
IV	Areola and papilla form secondary areolar mound
V	Mature breast contour, nipple projects

Male and Female pubic hair development

I	None
II	Sparse, short, straight, at base of penis/at medial border of labia
III	Darker, longer, coarser, and curlier, sparsely over pubic bones
IV	Coarse, curly, resembles adult hair; but spares thighs
V	Adult distribution with inverse triangle pattern and spread to medial surface of thighs

Resources

Diabetes Mellitus and Diabetic Ketoacidosis

American Diabetes Association. Type 2 diabetes in children and adolescents. Diabetes Care 2000;23:381–389.

Glaser N, Barnett P, McCaslin I, et al. Risk factors for cerebral edema in children with diabetic ketoacidosis. N Engl J Med 2001;344:264–269.

Radovick S, ed. Pediatric Endocrinology: A Practical Clinical Guide. Totowa: Humana, 2003.

Sperling M, ed. Pediatric Endocrinology. 2nd ed. Philadelphia: WB Saunders, 2002.

The Diabetes Control and Complications Trial Research Group. The effect of intensive treatment of diabetes on the development and progression of long-term complications in insulin-dependent diabetes mellitus. N Engl J Med 1993;329:977–986.

Hypothalamic-Pituitary-Adrenal Axis

Arnaldi G, Angeli A, Atkinson AB, et al. Diagnosis and complications of Cushing's syndrome: a consensus statement. J Clin Endocrinol Metab 2003;88:5593–5602.

Behrman R, et al., eds. Nelson Textbook of Pediatrics. 16th ed. Philadelphia: WB Saunders, 2000.

Boscaro M, et al. Cushing's syndrome. Lancet 2001;357:783–791.

Magiakou M, Chrousos G. Cushing's syndrome in children and adolescents: current diagnostic and therapeutic strategies. J Endocrinol Invest 2002;25:181–194.

Oelkers W. Adrenal insufficiency. N Engl J Med 1996;335:1206–1212.

Speiser PW, White PC. Congenital adrenal hyperplasia. N Engl J Med 2003;349:776–788.

Joint LWPES/ESPE CAH Working Group. Consensus statement on 21-hydroxylase deficiency from the Lawson Wilkins Pediatric Endocrine Society and the European Society for Paediatric Endocrinology. J Clin Endocrinol Metab 2002;87:4048–4053.

Sperling M, ed. Pediatric Endocrinology. 2nd ed. Philadelphia: WB Saunders, 2002.

Thyroid Disease

Behrman R, et al., eds. Nelson Textbook of Pediatrics. 16th ed. Philadelphia: WB Saunders, 2000.

Lafranchi SH, Snyder DB, Sesser DE, et al. Follow-up of newborns with elevated screening T4 concentrations. J Pediatr 2003;143:296–301.

Palit TK, Miller CC III, Miltenburg DM. The efficacy of thyroidectomy for Graves' disease: a meta-analysis. J Surg Res 2000;90:161–165.

Radovick S, ed. Pediatric Endocrinology: A Practical Clinical Guide. Totowa: Humana, 2003.

Sperling M, ed. Pediatric Endocrinology. 2nd ed. Philadelphia: WB Saunders, 2002.

Other Selected Topics

Albanese A, Hindmarsh P, Stanhope R. Management of hyponatremia in patients with acute cerebral insults. Arch Dis Child 2001;85:246–251.

Baylis P, Cheetham T. Diabetes insipidus. Arch Dis Child 1998;79:84–89.

Behrman R, et al. eds. Nelson Textbook of Pediatrics. 16th ed. Philadelphia: WB Saunders, 2000.

de Lonlay-Debeney P, Poggi-Travert F, Fournet JC, et al. Clinical features of 52 neonates with hyperinsulism. N Engl J Med 1999;340:1169–1175.

Gartner LM, Greer FR. Prevention of rickets and vitamin D deficiency: new guidelines for vitamin D intake. Pediatrics 2003;111:908–910.

Kappy M, Ganong C. Cerebral salt wasting in children: the role of atrial natriuretic hormone. Adv Pediatr 1996;43:271–308.

Kumar S, Berl T. Sodium. Lancet. 1998;352:220–228.

Ng DD, Ferry RJ Jr, Kelly A, et al. Acarbose treatment of postprandial hypoglycemia in children after Nissen fundoplication. J Pediatr 2001;139:877–879.

Pogacar PR, Mahnke S, Rivkees SA. Management of central diabetes insipidus in infancy with low renal solute load formula and chlorothiazide. Curr Opin Pediatr 2000;12:405–411.

Rake JP, Visser G, Labrune P, et al. Glycogen storage disease type 1: diagnosis, management, clinical course and outcome. Eur J Pediatr 2002;161(suppl):s20–34.

Singer I, Oster JR, Fishman J. The management of diabetes insipidus in adults. Arch Intern Med 1997;157:1293–1301.

Sperling M, ed. Pediatric Endocrinology. 2nd ed. Philadelphia: WB Saunders, 2002.

Stanley CA. Hyperinsulinism in infants and children. Pediatr Clin of North Am 1997;44:363–374.

Stanley CA, Thornton PS, Ganguly A, et al. Preoperative evaluation of infants with focal or diffuse congenital hyperinsulinism by intravenous acute insulin response tests and selective pancreatic arterial calcium stimulation. J Clin Endocrinol Metab 2004;89:288–296.

Thacher TD, Fischer PR, Pettifor JM. The usefulness of clinical features to identify active rickets. Ann Trop Paediatr 2002;22:229–237.

Wharton B, Bishop N. Rickets. Lancet 2003;362:1389–1400.

FLUIDS AND ELECTROLYTES

Gary Frank, MD, MS, Vijay Srinivasan, MD, Lisa B. Zaoutis, MD

Fluid Therapy

MAINTENANCE FLUID THERAPY

Maintenance fluid requirements can be estimated by the Holliday-Segar method. Daily water requirements are calculated based on body weight and the assumption that each kilocalorie of energy metabolized results in the net consumption of 1 mL of water (Table 9.1). Water requirements form the basis for the estimated needs for sodium and potassium (Table 9.2). This method is not recommended for premature infants or term infants younger than 2 weeks of age.

- Dextrose-containing intravenous fluids are used to supply a portion of the caloric needs, to prevent hypoglycemia and starvation ketosis.
- Stock solutions containing 5% dextrose (D_5) are appropriate for most situations, but 10% dextrose (D_{10}) or higher is also available.
- Dextrose concentrations above 12.5% are usually reserved for central catheters, because the increased osmolality is irritating to peripheral veins.

Table 9.1: Estimate of Maintenance Fluid Requirements Based on Body Weight

Body Weight	Water Requirement	
	Daily	Hourly
1st 10 kg	100 mL/kg/day	4 mL/kg/ hr
2nd 10 kg	50 mL/kg/day	2 mL/kg/ hr
Weight above 20 kg	20 mL/kg/day	1 mL/kg/ hr

Sample Maintenance Fluid Calculation

Maintenance fluid, sodium, and potassium requirements for a 37-kg child:

Water Requirement:		
First 10 kg, give 100 mL/kg/day:	10 kg × 100 mL/kg/day = 1000 mL/day	
Second 10 kg, give 50 mL/kg/day:	10 kg × 50 mL/kg/day = 500 mL/day	
>20 kg give, 20 mL/kg/day:	17 kg × 20 mL/kg/day = 340 mL/day	
Total:	37 kg	1840 mL/day
OR		
First 10 kg, give 4 mL/kg/hr:	10 kg × 4 mL/kg/hr = 40 mL/hr	
Second 10 kg, give 2 mL/kg/hr:	10 kg × 2 mL/kg/hr = 20 mL/hr	
>20 kg give, 1 mL/kg/hr:	17 kg × 1 mL/kg/hr = 17 mL/hr	
Total:	37 kg	77 mL/hr

Sodium Requirement:

3 mEq/100 mL/day × 1840 mL/day = 55 mEq/day

$$\frac{55\ mEg/day}{1840\ mL/day} = \frac{Na^+}{1000\ mL}$$

$$Na^+ = 30\ mEq/L$$

- Note: normal saline solution (NSS) contains 0.9% NaCl or 154 mEq/L. In this case, a stock solution containing 0.22% NaCl (1/4 NSS) would provide 34 mEq NaCl/L.

Potassium Requirement:

2 mEq/100 mL/day × 1840 mL/day = 37 mEq/day

$$\frac{37\ mEg/day}{1840\ mL/day} = \frac{K^+}{1000\ mL}$$

$$K^+ = 20\ mEq/L$$

- The addition of 20 mEq/L of KCl would provide the approximate needs for potassium.

Therefore, an order for routine maintenance fluids for this child would be:

D_5/0.2% NaCl with 20 mEq KCl/L to run at 77 mL/hour.

- It can also be written as: D_5/1/4 NSS + 20 mEq KCl/L @ 77 mL/hour.

Standard (Stock) Solutions for Routine Maintenance Intravenous Fluids
D_5/0.2% NS with 20 mEq KCl/L is a good choice for maintenance fluid for most routine situations. Some other helpful guidelines:
- KCl is often added after the child's first void.
- D_{10} is often substituted for D_5 in premature infants and neonates due to their increased glucose requirements and diminished glycogen stores.
- Some clinicians routinely use D_5/0.45% NaCl for children that weigh more than 20 kg. The increased sodium concentration is not usually problematic, but exceeds the calculated daily sodium requirement using the Holliday-Segar method.
- KCl concentration in the IV solution is often reduced to 10 mEq/L to reduce irritation to the peripheral vein. This may be appropriate if additional (e.g., enteral) intake is occurring, or if it is anticipated that IV fluids alone will be used for only a limited time.
- Common stock intravenous fluids (IVFs) are listed in Table 9.3.

Table 9.2: Basic Electrolyte Requirements	
Electrolyte	Estimated Need (mEq/100 mL water)
Sodium	3
Potassium	2
Chloride	2

Table 9.3: Terminology and Conversions for Stock Intravenous Solutions

Stock Solution	Common Terminology	Dextrose Content (g/dL)	Sodium Chloride Content (mEq/L)
Dextose 5% in water	D_5W	5	0
Dextrose 10% in water	$D_{10}W$	10	0
Dextrose 5% in 0.9% NaCl	D_5/NSS	5	154
Dextrose 5% in 0.45% NaCl	D_5/½NSS	5	77
Dextrose 5% in 0.22% saline	D_5/¼NSS	5	34
Dextrose 5% in 0.22% NaCl with 20 mEq KCl/L	D_5/¼NSS + 20 mEq KCl/L	5	34
3% saline	"hypertonic" saline	0	513

NSS,1 Normal saline solution.

Exceptions to Standard Fluid Management
- Acute central nervous system (CNS) disorders (trauma, stroke, spinal cord lesions): consider limiting fluids to two thirds maintenance and watch for syndrome of inappropriate antidiuretic hormone (SIADH) secretion.
- Fever increases metabolic rate and therefore maintenance requirements go up (add ~10% for every °C increase > 38°C).
- Tachypnea: an additional 10% to 20% of maintenance is needed.
- Burns: increased needs based on percent body surface area involved.
- Anuria/oliguria: decrease to one third maintenance plus replace urine output.

Duration of Maintenance Fluid Therapy
- For durations > 2 to 3 days, consider enteral or parenteral nutrition.

REPLACEMENT FLUID THERAPY

Replacement therapy corrects pre-existing deficits (dehydration) and ongoing losses.

Dehydration
Consider both the extent of the dehydration and the overall balance of water and sodium that is created.
- If pre-illness weight is available, then calculate percent dehydration:

% dehydration = ((Pre-illness Weight − Current Weight)/Pre-illness Weight) × 100

- If pre-illness weight is not available, percent dehydration can be clinically assessed:
  - *Mild Dehydration (3% to 5%):* thirst, normal exam, reduced urine output
  - *Moderate Dehydration (6% to 10%):* tachycardia, dry mucosa, sunken eyes, delayed capillary refill, irritable, oliguria
  - *Severe Dehydration (11% to 15%):* thready pulses, low blood pressure, anuria, cold and mottled, lethargy
- In hyponatremic dehydration, the clinical findings are more pronounced, and therefore the degree of dehydration is less than the clinical picture suggests.

- In hypertonic dehydration, the clinical findings are less prominent and therefore the degree of dehydration is more severe than the clinical picture suggests. The skin is often described as "doughy."
- *Laboratory findings in dehydration:*
  - Elevation of serum creatinine and urea
  - Alteration of serum sodium, potassium, and bicarbonate
  - Increase in urine specific gravity (except with impaired renal concentration)
  - Elevation of blood cell counts (hemoconcentration)
- *Type of dehydration*
  - *Isonatremic* (serum Na^+ 130–150 mEq/L): loss of Na^+ and water in a balance that does not exceed the body's ability to maintain isonatremia
  - *Hyponatremic* (serum Na^+ < 130 mEq/L): retention or replacement of free water in the face of Na^+ salt and water losses.
  - *Hypernatremic* (serum Na^+ > 150 mEq/L): loss of free water in excess of Na^+- containing fluid

Ongoing Losses
- The gastrointestinal tract is a common source of ongoing losses from illness, or postoperative drainage. These ongoing losses are replaced with parenteral fluids, in volumes equivalent to the losses at a frequency that will avoid significant depletions (e.g., every 1 to 8 hours).
- The replacement fluid should contain electrolytes in concentrations that approximate the lost fluid. Some recommendations are listed in Table 9.4.

Oral Rehydration
- Consider oral rehydration if patient is hemodynamically stable and if there is no impairment of swallowing function
- Oral rehydration solutions (ORS) are best, with concentrations of electrolytes and carbohydrates that approximate the World Health Organization/UNICEF ORS product.
- Small volumes (e.g., 5 to 10 mL) frequently (e.g., every 5 to 10 minutes) are initiated, and increased slowly as tolerated.

Parenteral Rehydration
Phase I: Initial Stabilization
- Administer 20 mL / kg IVF bolus (NSS or lactated Ringer's) and repeat as needed. This will have three benefits:
  1. Temporarily restores intravascular volume and stabilizes hemodynamics
  2. Replaces pre-existing total body Na^+ and water deficits, which are present in isonatremic, hyponatremic, and hypernatremic dehydration
  3. Begins to normalize serum Na^+ levels in hyponatremic and hypernatremic dehydration

Phase II: After Initial Stabilization
This simplified approach is offered in situations of routine dehydration, with normal renal function, and evidence of clinical improvement.
- IVF typically used for maintenance (e.g., D_5/0.2% NS with 20 mEq KCl/L) can be started after completion of the initial stabilization.

Table 9.4: Replacement of Ongoing Fluid Losses	
Source	Replacement (1mL:1mL)
Gastric secretions	0.45% NSS + 10 mEq KCl/L
Diarrhea	0.2% NSS + 25 mEq KCl/L + 20 mEq $NaHCO_3$/L
Small intestine	0.45% NSS + 20 mEq KCl/L + 20 mEq $NaHCO_3$/L

- The rate of fluid administration during this phase is estimated at 1.25 to 1.5 times the calculated maintenance needs. This can be continued for the first 12 to 24 hours after completion of the initial stabilization.
- Increased maintenance requirements (e.g., fever) may warrant further increases in the IVF rate.
- Significant ongoing losses (e.g., continued vomiting and/or diarrhea) will require additional fluid replacement.
- Modifications to the rate and nature of the IVF should be guided by:
  - Urine output: goal = 1–2 mL/kg/hr
  - Urine specific gravity: goal = 1.005–1.015
  - Weight, vital signs, clinical appearance
  - Repeat serum electrolytes: if needed
  - Urine electrolytes: if abnormal renal function is suspected.

Phase III: Resolution
- Trials of oral/gastric feeds usually begin with clear liquids if vomiting is present.
- If vomiting is resolved, or not a factor, prompt advancement to regular diet is encouraged (including breast milk or infant formula).
- Avoid foods high in simple sugars (e.g., juices, sodas) that can worsen or prolong diarrheal symptoms.
- Wean IVF rate or hold IVF for short periods to encourage oral intake.

Electrolyte Abnormalities

HYPOCALCEMIA

Serum calcium concentration less than 8.0 mg/dL (<2.0 mmol/L), or serum ionized calcium level less than 1.13 mmol/L

Etiology
- Hypoparathyroidism: familial, DiGeorge syndrome, idiopathic, surgical
- Vitamin D deficiency: dietary deficiency, lack of sunlight, malabsorption
- Vitamin D resistance: familial hypophosphatemic rickets, Fanconi syndrome, renal tubular acidosis
- Other: renal insufficiency, diuretic abuse, hypoproteinemia, acute pancreatitis, magnesium deficiency.

Clinical Manifestations
- Vomiting, muscle weakness, irritability
- Severe: tetany, seizures, laryngospasm, prolonged QT interval
- Rickets: craniotabes, rachitic rosary, limb deformities (genu varum and valgum), thickened wrists and ankles

Management
- Management depends on underlying etiology. Initial diagnostics include:
  - Serum: electrolytes, calcium (total and ionized), BUN, creatinine, magnesium, phosphorus, protein, albumin, alkaline phosphatase, vitamin D levels, parathyroid hormone
  - Urine: calcium, phosphorus, pH, protein, glucose
  - Hand/wrist x-ray
  - Consider electrocardiogram
- If patient is hypoalbuminemic, correct total calcium (increase serum calcium by 0.8 mg/dL for each 1.0 g/dL that albumin is below normal) or measure ionized calcium level.
- For severe symptoms, consider intravenous calcium (e.g., calcium gluconate) replacement with cardiac monitoring.
- Once patient is stable, consider oral calcium replacement (e.g., calcium carbonate, calcium citrate).

- If patient is hypomagnesemic, replace magnesium (may be given IM).
- Depending on etiology, patient may need vitamin D replacement.

HYPERCALCEMIA

Serum calcium concentration greater than 11.0 mg/dL

Etiology
- Hyperparathyroidism, malignancy (bony metastases, ectopic parathyroid hormone production), immobilization, vitamin D intoxication, familial hypocalciuric hypercalcemia, hyperthyroidism, sarcoidosis, thiazide diuretics, milk-alkali syndrome

Clinical Manifestations
- Neurologic: headache, weakness, lethargy, change in mental status, coma, hyporeflexia, seizures
- Gastrointestinal: constipation, nausea, vomiting, anorexia, abdominal pain
- Renal: nephrocalcinosis, nephrolithiasis, polyuria, polydipsia
- Cardiovascular: bradycardia, short QT interval, hypertension

Management
- Attempt to identify and treat underlying etiology.
- For severe hypercalcemia, consider intravenous fluids (e.g., normal saline solution at two to three times maintenance) followed by furosemide every 6 to 8 hours.
- Consider bisphosphonates ± calcitonin in refractory hypercalcemia
- Steroids may be effective in specific cases (e.g., malignancy, sarcoidosis).

HYPOKALEMIA

Serum potassium concentration less than 3.5 mEq/L

Etiology
- Decreased intake: anorexia, low dietary intake, IVFs without potassium
- Renal losses: medications (diuretics, amphotericin B, penicillins), renal tubular acidosis, osmotic diuresis (e.g., diabetic ketoacidosis), mineralocorticoid excess (hyperaldosteronism, licorice abuse)
- Extrarenal losses: gastrointestinal losses (diarrhea, vomiting, fistulas), sweat losses (cystic fibrosis)
- Transcellular shift (into intracellular fluid): alkalosis, insulin, beta agonists, familial hypokalemic periodic paralysis

Clinical Manifestations
- Muscle: weakness, paresthesias, hyporeflexia, paralysis, rhabdomyolysis
- Renal: polyuria, polydipsia
- Cardiac: bradycardia, prolonged QT, flattened T-wave, appearance of U-wave, AV block, premature beats, paroxysmal atrial or junctional tachycardia, ventricular arrhythmias

Management
- Determine etiology: electrolytes, arterial blood gas, creatine phosphokinase, urinalysis, urine electrolytes (sodium, potassium, chloride)
- Obtain electrocardiogram; consider continuous ECG monitoring
- Replace potassium orally or in IVFs as potassium chloride or potassium bicarbonate (up to 40 mEq/L through peripheral IV and up to 80 mEq/L through central IV)
- For life-threatening hypokalemia, can give up to 1 mEq/kg per hour of IV potassium.
- Correct underlying acid/base disorder or other etiology.

HYPERKALEMIA

Serum potassium concentration greater than 5.5 mEq/L

Etiology
- Increased intake/production: excessive oral or intravenous administration, hemolysis, rhabdomyolysis
- Decreased excretion: renal failure, hypoaldosteronism, medications (potassium-sparing diuretics, beta-blockers)
- Acidosis causing transcellular shift
- "Pseudohyperkalemia": hemolyzed specimen, extreme leukocytosis or thrombocytosis

Clinical Manifestations
- Paresthesias, weakness, decreased reflexes, hyporeflexia
- Cardiac manifestations can be life-threatening:
  - ECG changes: peaked T-wave, depressed ST segment, widened P-R interval, loss of P-wave, wide QRS complex, sine wave pattern
  - Arrhythmias: ventricular fibrillation, asystole

Management
- Discontinue potassium intake; discontinue potassium-sparing diuretics
- Perform ECG
- Determine etiology: electrolytes, arterial blood gas, creatinine phosphokinase, urinalysis, urine electrolytes (potassium, sodium, chloride)
- If electrocardiogram changes other than peaked T-wave or serum potassium greater than 8 mEq/L, consider the following interventions:
  - Continuous ECG monitoring
  - Calcium (e.g., 10% calcium gluconate 0.5 mL/kg IV over 2 to 5 minutes)
  - Sodium bicarbonate (e.g., 2–3 mEq/kg IV over 30 to 60 minutes)
  - Insulin (0.1–0.3 U/kg) plus glucose (1 g/kg)
  - Beta-agonist (nebulized or IV): controversial because may cause arrhythmia
  - Kayexalate: decreases total body potassium
  - For renal failure or if refractory to treatment, consider dialysis.

HYPONATREMIA

Serum sodium concentration less than 130 mEq/L

Etiology
- Euvolemic: SIADH, hypothyroidism, adrenal insufficiency, stress, drugs, decreased solute intake ("tea-and-toast" diet)
- Hypervolemic: congestive heart failure, nephrotic syndrome, cirrhosis, renal failure, pregnancy
- Hypovolemic: vomiting, diarrhea, poor intake, third-space losses (burns, pancreatitis, trauma), renal losses (diuretics, osmotic diuresis, renal tubular acidosis, ketonuria)
- Excessive water intake: dilute infant formula, primary polydipsia
- Measurement artifact: hyperlipidemia, hyperproteinemia, hyperglycemia

Clinical Manifestations
- Anorexia, headache, nausea, vomiting, lethargy, muscle cramps
- Central nervous system: seizures, altered mental status, decreased reflexes
- Brain stem herniation and respiratory arrest are possible.

Management
- Rapid correction of hyponatremia (especially if chronic hyponatremia) can lead to pontine myelinolysis. In general, correct serum sodium at a rate 0.5 mEq/L/hour or less or 15 mEq/L in 24 hours.

- For hyponatremia with symptomatic hypovolemia: start with re-expansion of extracellular fluid volume with intravenous isotonic saline (e.g., NSS 20 mL/kg over 30 to 60 minutes; may repeat).
- If patient has symptomatic hyponatremia (e.g., seizures): consider IV hypertonic saline (e.g., 2–6 mL/kg of 3% NaCl over 1 hour).
- SIADH: water restriction (25% to 50% of daily maintenance requirement) with monitoring of serum sodium.
- Definitive management requires establishing the underlying etiology. Compare urine and serum osmolarity to differentiate between SIADH and water intoxication. Withhold offending medications.

HYPERNATREMIA

Serum sodium concentration greater than145 mEq/L

Etiology
- Euvolemic: diabetes insipidus (central or nephrogenic), insensible losses, decreased water intake
- Hypervolemic: sodium gain (sodium bicarbonate, NaCl tablets, seawater ingestion), hyperaldosteronism, Cushing syndrome
- Hypovolemic: extrarenal losses (diarrhea, emesis, burns), renal losses (diuretics, intrinsic renal disease, postobstructive diuresis)

Clinical Manifestations
- Irritability, muscle weakness, lethargy, restlessness, muscle twitching
- CNS: altered mental status, seizures, coma

Management
- Rapid correction of pronounced hypernatremia can result in life-threatening cerebral edema. In general, aim to lower serum sodium by 10 to 15 mEq/L per 24 hours.
- If patient is severely dehydrated, start with isotonic saline bolus (e.g., NSS 20 mL/kg over 1 hour; may repeat) to restore circulation.
- Free water deficits (FWD) should be corrected over 24 to 48 hours. FWD can be estimated by 4 mL FW/kg needed to reduce serum Na^+ by 1 mEq/L. Chose a solution that is hypotonic but that will not lower serum sodium too quickly. Remember to give maintenance fluid requirements as well.
- Follow serum Na^+ levels frequently (e.g., every 4 hours), until stable.
- Treat underlying cause of hypernatremia (e.g., discontinue osmotic diuretics)

Resources

Fluid Therapy
Behrman R, Kliegman R, Jenson H. Nelson Textbook of Pediatrics. 17th ed. Philadelphia: WB Saunders, 2004.

Hellerstein S. Fluid and electrolytes: clinical aspects. Pediatr Rev 1993;14:103–115.

Holliday MA, Segar WE. The maintenance need for water in parenteral fluid therapy. Pediatrics 1957;19:823–832.

Electrolyte Abnormalities
Adrogue HJ, Madias NE. Primary Care: hypernatremia. N Engl J Med 2000;342:1493–1499.

Adrogue HJ, Madias NE. Primary care: hyponatremia. N Engl J Med 2000;342:1581–1589.

Bushinsky DA, Monk RD. Calcium. Lancet 1998;352:306–311.

Halperin ML, Kamel KS. Potassium. Lancet 1998;352:135–140.

Kumar S, Berl T. Sodium. Lancet 1998;352:220–228.

Lteif AN, Zimmerman D. Bisphophonates for treatment of childhood hypercalcemia. Pediatrics 1998;102:990–993.

Singh J, Moghal N, Pearce SH, Cheetham T. The investigation of hypocalcemia and rickets. Arch Dis Child 2003;88:403–407.

Yeates KE, Singer M, Morton AR. Salt and water: a simple approach to hyponatremia. CMAJ 2004;170:365–369.

Rose C. Graham-Maar, MD, Heather Morein French, MD,
David A. Piccoli, MD

Esophagus and Stomach

GASTROESOPHAGEAL REFLUX DISEASE

Gastroesophageal reflux (GER) is the regurgitation of stomach contents into the esophagus. Gastroesophageal reflux disease (GERD) occurs when GER is accompanied by esophagitis, respiratory disease, failure to thrive, and/or neurobehavioral manifestations.

Epidemiology
- In infants, most GER is physiologic and benign.
- Functional GER occurs in more than half of all infants.
- Most common esophageal disorder

Pathophysiology
- Transient lower esophageal sphincter (LES) relaxation allows gastric contents to flow retrograde up the esophagus.
- Decreased gastric compliance in infants compared to adults

Clinical Manifestations
- *Functional/Simple GER:* silent oral regurgitation, effortless spitting, or forceful vomiting; symptoms peak at 1 to 4 months and resolve by 12 to 18 months of age; usually benign
- *Complicated GER (GERD):* significant complications develop in ~10% of untreated children:
  - Esophagitis: crying, irritability, food aversion, heartburn, epigastric or chest pain, odynophagia, hematemesis, anemia, and/or guaiac-positive stools
  - Respiratory: laryngospasm, bronchospasm, microaspiration pneumonia
  - Failure to thrive
  - Neurobehavioral manifestations: Sandifer syndrome (opisthotonic posturing, head tilting, seizure-like activity); arching; excessive irritability

Diagnostics
- With uncomplicated GER, no diagnostic tests are warranted. In infants or children with complicated GER, consider:
  - *Upper gastrointestinal (GI):* defines anatomy; useful to exclude malrotation, pyloric stenosis, webs, atresias, or other anatomic causes; not diagnostic for reflux
  - *Scintigraphy or "milk scan":* detects delayed gastric emptying and/or pulmonary aspiration; not diagnostic for reflux
  - *pH probe:* gold standard to quantify acid reflux; helps establish causal relationship between reflux and other symptoms
  - *Upper endoscopy:* allows direct visualization of the mucosa and the pathologic diagnosis of mucosal disease related to reflux; basal cell hyperplasia, papillary elongation, and an inflammatory cellular infiltrate seen in esophagitis

Management
- *Conservative therapy* is appropriate as a component of treatment for all GER, and may be sole therapy for uncomplicated GER: sit upright during and after feeds; small, frequent feeds; sleep with head elevated 30 degrees; prone position; thicken formula with cereal ($1/2$ to 1 tablespoon per ounce)

- *Medical Therapy:*
  - Antacid (e.g., Maalox, Mylanta): 0.5 mL/kg/dose (max 15 mL) three times daily 10 minutes before feedings; separate from other medications by 1 hour
  - Acid suppression (ranitidine, famotidine, omeprazole, lansoprazole); does not prevent GER but helps prevent complications
  - Prokinetics: metoclopramide (commonly used), low dose erythromycin (5 mg/kg/dose three times daily; rarely used)
- Post-pyloric feeds via feeding tube (naso-jejunal or gastro-jejunal)
- Fundoplication: indicated for severe complicated GERD with failure of maximal medical therapy; may result in other long-term complications such as gas-bloat syndrome, chronic retching, and dumping syndrome

PEPTIC ULCER DISEASE

Histologic inflammation and ulceration of the mucosa of the stomach and/or duodenum

Epidemiology
- During childhood typically occurs after age 8 years
- Accounts for 15% of abdominal pain seen in specialty practice

Etiology
- Primary peptic ulcer disease (PUD) (typically gastritis and duodenal ulcers) tends to have a chronic relapsing and remitting course. It may be *Helicobacter pylori*–associated, non–*H. pylori*–associated, or idiopathic.
- Secondary PUD (typically gastric ulcers) tends to be acute and, with therapy, recovery is usually complete. Etiologies include physiologic stress, illness, burns, sepsis, shock, head injury, trauma (i.e., retching, nasogastric tube), drugs (NSAIDs, alcohol, valproate, chemotherapy, KCl), allergic or eosinophilic gastritis, infectious, iron overdose, diabetes mellitus, Crohn disease, Zollinger-Ellison syndrome, hyperparathyroidism, cystic fibrosis, vascular insufficiency (sickle cell disease, HSP), radiation gastropathy

Pathophysiology
- Imbalance between cytotoxic factors (acid, pepsin, aspirin/NSAIDs, bile acids, *H. pylori* infection) and cytoprotective factors (mucous layer, local bicarbonate secretion, mucosal blood flow)
- Role of *H. pylori*: Gram-negative rod; causes chronic active gastritis and duodenal ulcers; spread by human to human transmission; *H. pylori* infection is often acquired during childhood but uncommonly leads to peptic ulcer disease (PUD).

Clinical Manifestations
- Abdominal pain: often epigastric but may not be localized in children; may be postprandial and nocturnal
- Anorexia, weight loss, early satiety, nausea, recurrent vomiting, upper GI bleeding, anemia
- On physical exam, may note oral ulcers (e.g., Crohn), wheezing (may imply GERD), abdominal tenderness
- Perform rectal exam to look for perianal disease (e.g., Crohn) and occult blood in stool

Diagnostics
- *Endoscopy* with biopsies of the upper intestinal tract
- *Blood antibody tests* for *H. pylori* are NOT recommended in pediatric patients due to low sensitivity and specificity
- *Stool antigen test* for *H. pylori* is available: studies have shown sensitivity 88%, specificity 95%
- *Blood and stool tests* do not allow diagnosis of PUD; current recommendations discourage noninvasive testing of patients without endoscopically diagnosed PUD.
- *Urea breath test:* useful for initial diagnosis of *H. pylori* and for follow-up after therapy but has limited availability

Management

Acid Suppression
- Use alone for non–*H. pylori* PUD or in conjunction with antibiotics for *H. pylori*–associated PUD
- H2 receptor antagonist: ranitidine, famotidine
- Proton pump inhibitor (PPI): omeprazole, esomeprazole, lansoprazole

H. pylori Therapy
- First-line options:
  1. PPI + amoxicillin + clarithromycin
  2. PPI + amoxicillin + metronidazole
  3. PPI + clarithromycin + metronidazole
- Second-line option: PPI + bismuth subsalicylate + metronidazole + (amoxicillin or tetracycline or clarithromycin)
- Doses:
  - omeprazole: 1 mg/kg/day up to 20 mg twice daily for 14 days
  - lansoprazole: 1 mg/kg/day up to 30 mg twice daily for 14 days

Hepatobiliary System

ALAGILLE SYNDROME

A genetic syndrome characterized by cholestatic liver disease from a paucity of bile ducts; cardiac defects; characteristic facies; vertebral, renal, and ocular anomalies

Epidemiology
- 1 in 70,000 affected
- Autosomal dominant inheritance with variable penetrance

Pathophysiology
- Mutations of *Jagged1* gene on chromosome 20p are identified in 70% of patients.

Clinical Manifestations
- Extremely variable clinical expression even within families
- *Diagnostic criteria:* intrahepatic bile duct paucity plus at least three of six major features: 1) cholestasis; 2) characteristic facies (frontal bossing, deep-set eyes, bulbous nose tip, pointed chin); 3) heart murmur (peripheral pulmonic stenosis, Tetralogy of Fallot); 4) butterfly vertebrae or other vertebral anomalies; 5) posterior embryotoxon or other eye anomalies; 6) renal anomalies
- Bile duct paucity may not be present before 6 months of age
- 10% to 50% progress to cirrhosis, portal hypertension, and liver failure.
- Also associated with vascular, bone, ear, intestinal disease
- Other features may include osteopenia; intracranial hemorrhage and stroke; growth retardation; pancreatic insufficiency
- On physical exam: poor growth, characteristic facies, jaundice, evidence of pruritus, xanthomata, heart murmur, hepatomegaly, splenomegaly (less common)

Diagnostics
- *Laboratory studies:* serum bilirubin (total and conjugated fractions), alkaline phosphatase, gamma-glutamyltransferase (GGT), alanine aminotransferase (ALT), aspartate aminotransferase (AST), albumin, PT, cholesterol level, electrolytes, BUN, creatinine, urinalysis
- Ultrasound: liver and kidney
- X-ray: spine and chest
- DISIDA scan
- Echocardiogram, ECG
- Liver biopsy
- Cholangiogram: intraoperative, percutaneous transhepatic, MRCP, or ERCP
- Ophthalmologic exam

Management
Medical
- *Cholestasis:* ursodeoxycholic acid (15–30 mg/kg/day divided two or three times daily); rifampin (5 mg/kg/day in one dose or divided twice daily)
- *Pruritus:* skin emollients, fingernail trimming, antihistamines
- *Growth failure:* vitamin supplements of A, D, E, K; nutritional supplements; possible magnesium supplements
- Manage cardiac and renal disease as necessary
- *Genetic evaluation and counseling:* test for Jagged1 gene

Surgical Management of Cholestasis
- Percutaneous biliary diversion: external biliary drainage
- Liver transplantation: 21% to 31% of Alagille syndrome (AGS) patients
- Cardiac repair may be needed
- Hepatoportoenterostomy (Kasai) is contraindicated

ALPHA 1-ANTITRYPSIN DEFICIENCY

An autosomal recessive disorder associated with chronic liver disease and premature pulmonary emphysema that is caused by a deficiency of the serine protease inhibitor, alpha1-antitrypsin

Epidemiology
- Most common inherited cause of liver disease in children
- Affects 1 in 2000 live births of white children in the United States

Pathophysiology
- Alpha-1 antitrypsin (Alpha1-AT) is predominantly produced in hepatocytes, released into the bloodstream, and functions in the lung to inhibit cleavage of connective tissue proteins.
- When Alpha1-AT is genetically mutated, it cannot be released from hepatocytes and becomes hepatotoxic
- Absence of Alpha1-AT or abnormal function allows uninhibited cleavage of connective tissue by elastase leading to lung injury.

Clinical Manifestations
- May present at any age from infancy to adulthood
- Variable presentation: some allele variants cause both liver and lung disease, while others cause only lung disease
- Liver disease (neonate to adult): prolonged conjugated hyperbilirubinemia in neonate, small for gestational age, acholic stools, elevated transaminases, severe bleeding episode (vitamin K deficiency from liver disease), severe liver failure, hepatomegaly, portal hypertension, varices, chronic hepatitis, cirrhosis, hepatocellular carcinoma
- Lung disease (adult): emphysema
- On physical exam: jaundice, hepatomegaly, splenomegaly, ascites, excoriations from pruritus

Diagnostics
- Serum Alpha1-AT level: normal is 150 to 350 mg/dL; may be misleading because it is an acute phase reactant and does not specify functionality
- Pi Typing (Pi = protease inhibitor): defines alleles present, which indicates a normal, dysfunctional, deficient, or absent Alpha1-AT protein
- Liver biopsy: necessity for diagnosis is controversial

Management
- Supportive care for liver dysfunction
- Counsel against cigarette smoking
- Protein replacement therapy (recombinant or purified): only for established emphysema; does not help liver disease
- Surgical options include: orthotopic liver transplantation, portocaval or splenorenal shunt, lung transplantation

AUTOIMMUNE HEPATITIS

A chronic inflammatory liver disease of unknown etiology characterized by hypergammaglobulinemia, autoantibodies, and clinical response to immunosuppressive therapy. There are three types of autoimmune hepatitis (AIH):

- Type I (classic AIH): antinuclear antibody (ANA)–, anti–smooth muscle antibody (SMA)– positive
- Type II: Liver-kidney-microsomal (LKM) antibody–positive; more common in pediatrics
- Type III: Soluble liver antigen (SLA)–antibody positive

Epidemiology
- Relatively uncommon; may present at any age
- Female predominance (4:1)
- 40% to 50% of patients have at least one other autoimmune disorder

Pathophysiology
- Likely autoimmune process in genetically susceptible persons
- Associated with certain HLA haplotypes (A1, B8, DR3, DR4)
- May overlap with autoimmune sclerosing cholangitis

Clinical Manifestations
- Extremely variable from asymptomatic to liver failure; may be acute or insidious and progressive
- Fatigue, malaise, nausea, anorexia, upper abdominal discomfort, arthralgia, myalgia, oligomenorrhea, skin rashes, mild pruritus, jaundice, dark urine, pale stools
- On physical exam: jaundice, cutaneous stigmata of liver disease, ascites, hepatomegaly, splenomegaly, rash, altered mental status

Diagnostics
- ALT, AST levels are increased. Alkaline phosphatase and GGT levels are normal or increased
- PT, albumin: to check liver synthetic function
- Gamma-globulin levels (high IgG, normal IgA)
- ANA; SMA; LKM-1; SLA and liver-pancreas antibody; perinuclear antineutrophil cytoplasmic antibody; 10% to 20% of patients with AIH are negative for traditional antibodies
- Liver biopsy: required to confirm diagnosis

Management
- Prednisone 2 mg/kg/day, maximum 60 mg/day; gradually decrease dose over 6 to 8 weeks to the minimal dose required to maintain normal ALT/AST
- Azathioprine (0.5 mg/kg/day, maximum 2 mg/kg/day): add if steroid alone not showing improvement
- Relapses require pulse steroids
- Continue therapy until laboratory results are normal for at least 1 year; do not wean just before or during puberty; many patients require lifelong immunosuppressive therapy
- Liver transplantation for initial presentation with severe liver failure or progressive disease unresponsive to medical therapy

BILIARY ATRESIA

A disease of unknown etiology in which there is progressive destruction of the extrahepatic biliary tree with variable involvement of the intrahepatic biliary system

Epidemiology
- Incidence: 1 in 10,000 to 20,000
- Females > males
- 10% to 25% of cases associated with other congenital anomalies

Pathophysiology
- Natural history is complete obliteration of bile ducts leading to biliary cirrhosis and liver failure
- Most cases affect the entire extrahepatic biliary tree

- 10% of cases affect only the distal biliary tree
- Untreated extrahepatic disease: life expectancy is 11 months

Clinical Manifestations
- Usually normal at birth
- Conjugated hyperbilirubinemia around 2 to 6 weeks of age
- Associated anomalies: polysplenia, abdominal heterotaxy, intestinal malrotation, cardiovascular malformations, and anomalies of hepatic arteries/portal vein
- On physical exam: jaundice/greenish hue to skin, hepatomegaly, splenomegaly, dark urine, acholic stools, ascites, edema

Diagnostics
- Bilirubin (total, conjugated, and unconjugated): conjugated fraction greater than 2 mg/dL or greater than 15% of total bilirubin
- ALT/AST (two to three times normal); GGT/ALP (markedly elevated); PT/PTT (elevated); albumin (low due to liver synthetic dysfunction)
- Thrombocytopenia/neutropenia: if there is hypersplenism
- Ultrasound: may not be diagnostic but important to rule out choledochal cyst and to detect polysplenia, heterotaxy
- DISIDA scan (diisopropyl iminodiacetic acid labeled with 99m-technetium): Normally, after injection this lipid-soluble, albumin-bound substance is depicted in the liver and followed by excretion into the small bowel. In biliary atresia, there is normal uptake by liver but excretion occurs into the urinary tract due to an absent/obstructed biliary tree.
- Liver biopsy: typically shows bile duct proliferation with cholestasis and fibrosis, but very early may not be diagnostic
- Surgical cholangiography: necessary if biopsy not diagnostic and clinical suspicion high

Management
Portoenterostomy (Kasai Procedure)
- Anastomosis of biliary tract directly to bowel
- 80% eventually require liver transplantation even if done early
- 70% to 80% success of palliation if done before 60 days of age; only 20% to 30% success if done after 90 days of age
- High morbidity and mortality
- Complications include cholangitis, portal hypertension/varices, malnutrition/fat-soluble vitamin deficiency

Liver Transplantation
- Indicated for extrahepatic biliary atresia when diagnosis is delayed past time window for Kasai
- Indicated after Kasai if: hepatic insufficiency, portal hypertension with recurrent variceal bleeding, irreversible failure to thrive, recurrent cholangitis, persistent cholestasis, hepatopulmonary syndrome

GALLBLADDER DISEASE

Cholelithiasis: gallstones

Choledocholithiasis: stones in common bile duct

Cholecystitis: infected or inflamed gallbladder

Calculous cholecystitis: infected or inflamed gallbladder that contains stones

Acalculous cholecystitis: infected or inflamed gallbladder that does not contain stones

Epidemiology
- Cholelithiasis and cholecystitis are uncommon in children and are often secondary to a predisposing condition
- More than 50% of cholecystitis in children is acalculous
- Biliary symptoms develop in only 20% of patients with gallstones

Etiology
• Conditions that predispose to cholelithiasis in children: prematurity, congenital anomaly of biliary tract, hemolytic disorders (e.g., sickle cell disease), ileal resection or disease, obesity, pregnancy, cystic fibrosis, furosemide, total parenteral nutrition (TPN), long-term ceftriaxone

Pathophysiology
Cholelithasis
• Due to alteration in relative proportions of bile components
• *Cholesterol gallstones* due to bile supersaturated with cholesterol
• *Pigment gallstones:* black pigment stones due to bile supersaturated with unconjugated bilirubin that complexes with free ionized calcium. Brown pigment stones involve biliary stasis and bacterial infection.

Choledocholithiasis
• *Primary:* stones formed in common bile duct (CBD)
• *Secondary:* stone migrates from gallbladder and lodges in CBD
• Causes obstructive cholestasis; may lead to pancreatitis, cholangitis

Cholecystitis
• *Calculous:* obstruction of cystic duct by stone leads to acute inflammatory response of gall-bladder mucosa; secondary bacterial infection may occur
• *Acalculous:* biliary stasis (e.g., post-surgery, TPN, infectious illness) causes acute symptoms whereas functional disorders (e.g., biliary dyskinesia) cause chronic symptoms

Clinical Manifestations
• *Cholelithiasis:* 80% asymptomatic; biliary colic
• *Choledocholithiasis:* biliary colic, obstructive jaundice, cholangitis, pancreatitis
• *Calculous cholecystitis:* acute presentation involves abdominal pain (right upper quadrant [RUQ] or diffuse), low-grade fever, nausea, vomiting, anorexia. Chronic presentation often includes history of biliary colic or history of acute cholecystitis episode that resolved. Symptoms may be minimal.
• *Acalculous cholecystitis:* acute presentation similar to acute calculous. Chronic presentation involves recurrent biliary type pain.
• May be ill-appearing with abdominal tenderness, rebound, guarding, palpable gallbladder, jaundice, splenomegaly
• *Murphy's sign:* on palpation of RUQ, pain worsens with inspiration, which leads to cessation of breath.

Diagnostics
• Bilirubin, aminotransferases, alkaline phosphatase: may be elevated or normal
• Leukocytosis: variable
• Amylase/lipase: may be elevated
• Abdominal x-ray: shows calcified stones
• Ultrasound: best to detect cholelithiasis, choledocholithiasis, and acute cholecystitis
• DISIDA scan: no filling of gallbladder in acute cholecystitis; delayed filling in chronic chole-cystitis (delayed ejection fraction with cholecystokinin [CCK] or pain with CCK stimulation suggests either chronic cholecystitis or biliary dyskinesia)
• ERCP: noninvasive cholangiogram, useful with common bile duct obstruction to find stones

Management
Cholelithiasis
• Observation in asymptomatic patients

Choledocholithiasis
• ERCP: both diagnostic and therapeutic, can remove stones
• Biliary stents
• Elective cholecystectomy
• Surgical correction of anatomic abnormality of biliary tree, such as choledochal cyst

Acute Cholecystitis
- Rehydration, analgesia, antibiotics, observation (usually resolves spontaneously in 2 to 3 days)
- Typical antibiotic regimens: ampicillin-sulbactam; ampicillin-sulbactam plus gentamicin; third-generation cephalosporin plus metronidazole; ticarcillin-clavulanate; piperacillin-tazobactam; imipenem (if life-threatening)
- Elective cholecystectomy after resolution of acute illness (early or up to 2 to 3 months later) in uncomplicated cases
- Emergent cholecystectomy is indicated if complicated by necrosis, perforation, or empyema.

Chronic Cholecystitis
- Cholecystectomy for chronic calculous cholecystitis (in general)
- For biliary dyskinesia, cholecystectomy has variable results

GLYCOGEN STORAGE DISEASE

A family of inherited disorders affecting glycogen metabolism. Glycogen is a highly branched polymer of glucose and is stored in liver and muscle. The glycogen found in these disorders is abnormal in quantity, quality, or both.

- Conversion of glycogen into pyruvate occurs in two parts: glycogenolysis from glycogen to glucose-6-phosphate and glycolysis from glucose-6-phosphate to pyruvate
- Some enzyme defects are localized in liver, others in muscles; a few are generalized

Epidemiology
- Frequency (all forms) ~1/20,000 live births
- Autosomal recessive inheritance
- Types I, II, III, and IX most commonly present in early childhood; type V (McArdle disease) most common in adults

Etiology
- More than 12 types; can be classified by organ involvement and clinical manifestations into liver and muscle glycogenoses (Table 10.1)
- *Hepatic Glycogen Storage Disease:* type I (von Gierke disease), type III, type IV, type VI, type IX, glycogen synthetase deficiency, and glucose transporter-2 defect; typically cause hepatomegaly and fasting hypoglycemia; types III and IV are also associated with hepatic cirrhosis.
- *Muscle Glycogen Storage Disease:* divided into two groups: progressive skeletal muscle weakness, cardiomyopathy or both (type II); muscle pain, exercise intolerance, myoglobinuria and fatigue (types V, VII)

Diagnostics
- Hepatic glycogen storage disease: enzyme defects can only be detected in a liver biopsy but preliminary screening can be performed with an oral glucose tolerance test or a glucagon test.
- Muscle glycogen storage disease: exercise test (semi-ischemic forearm test, bicycle ergometer test or treadmill test) used to demonstrate the failure of venous lactate and pyruvate to rise and the production of uric acid, inosine, hypoxanthine and ammonia to increase excessively; if exercise test is abnormal, myopathy should be verified by enzyme assay.

Management
- Prevention of hypoglycemia while avoiding storage of even more glycogen in the liver and muscle
- *Hepatic glycogen storage disease:*
  - Nasogastric tube feedings at night; frequent feedings every 2 to 3 hours during the day using a lactose-free and sucrose-free formula (e.g., Prosobee)
  - Uncooked cornstarch (1.75 to 2.5 g/kg) every 4 hours in infants and every 6 hours in older children
  - Restrict intake of fructose and galactose

Table 10.1: Classification of Glycogen Storage Diseases

Type	Deficient Enzyme	Tissue	Main Clinical Feature
Ia	Glucose-6-phosphatase "von Gierke disease"	Liver, kidney	Hypoglycemia, hepatomegaly, lactic acidosis, hyperlipidemia
Ib-d	Glucose-6-phosphatase–related transport	Liver	Above + neutropenia and infections (Ib)
II	Acid α-glucosidase "Pompe disease"	Generalized	Infant form: cardio-respiratory failure Later form: myopathy
III	Debranching enzyme	Liver, cardiac muscle	Hypoglycemia, hepatomegaly, myopathy
IV	Branching system	Liver	Hepatosplenomegaly, cirrhosis
V	Phosphorylase, "McArdle disease"	Muscle	Exercise intolerance
VI	Phosphorylase	Liver	Hepatomegaly
VII	Phosphofructokinase, phosphoglycerate kinase, phosphoglycerate mutase	Muscle	Exercise intolerance
IX	Phosphorylase b kinase	Liver	Hepatomegaly
O	Glycogen synthase	Liver	Hypoglycemia

- Supplementation with calcium and multivitamins
- Allopurinol is used to lower the concentration of uric acid.
- Liver transplantation has been successful.
• *Muscle glycogen storage disease:* muscle function may be influenced by diet (protein may compensate for increased muscle catabolism); glucose use depends on underlying condition

WILSON DISEASE

Autosomal recessive disease of copper metabolism that involves defective biliary copper excretion, which leads to abnormal copper accumulation in the liver, CNS, eyes, and kidneys.

Epidemiology
• Prevalence: 1:30,000

Pathophysiology
• Wilson disease gene on chromosome 13 encodes a transmembrane copper-transporting ATPase protein (ATPase 7B). Mutations result in an abnormal transporter protein, which prevents normal export of copper from hepatocytes.
• Copper accumulates first in the liver and then spills over to other tissues.

Clinical Manifestations
• Frequently presents in childhood but rarely before age 5 years
• Classic triad: hepatic disease, neurologic disease, Kayser-Fleischer rings
• In children, hepatic effects precede neurologic effects and typically present in the second decade of life.

- Liver: acute hepatitis, chronic active hepatitis, cirrhosis, fulminant hepatic failure
- CNS: basal ganglia involvement leads to dystonia, incoordination, tremor, fine motor skill difficulty, rigidity, dysarthria, and gait disturbances. Psychiatric manifestations include depression, aggressive behaviors, impulsivity, compulsivity, poor school performance, psychosis
- Ophthalmologic: Kayser-Fleischer rings, sunflower cataracts
- Other: hemolytic anemia, proximal renal tubular dysfunction, bone demineralization, osteoporosis, pathologic fractures, cardiac dysrhythmias, cholelithiasis

Diagnostics
- Laboratory tests: ceruloplasmin level less than 20 mg/dL; serum copper low or high; urine copper greater than 100 µg/day; CBC (hemolysis); LFTs (hepatitis, cholestasis)
- Liver biopsy: gold standard; quantitation of hepatic copper, typical findings of steatosis, inflammation, +/− fibrosis
- Head CT: ventricular dilatation, brain atrophy, basal ganglia abnormalities
- Head MRI: more sensitive than CT for specific changes

Management
- D-Penicillamine (20 mg/kg/day divided four times a day, maximum 1 g/day; start with reduced dose): copper chelator used as initial treatment in hepatic disease. Give 1 hour before or 2 hours after meals. Supplement with vitamin B6.
- Trientine: a copper chelator and alternative to D-penicillamine
- Zinc: antagonist of copper absorption used as adjunctive therapy or alternative maintenance therapy after chelation
- Ammonium tetrathiomolybdate: still experimental
- Restrict dietary sources of copper: animal liver and kidney, shellfish, chocolate, dried beans, peas, unprocessed wheat
- Liver transplantation: for severe disease with fulminant hepatic failure or worsening disease unresponsive to medical therapy
- Screening of asymptomatic relatives of patients with Wilson disease

Small and Large Intestine

CELIAC DISEASE

An autoimmune disorder of the small intestine characterized by a permanent intolerance to wheat gluten that results in mucosal damage and malabsorption.

Epidemiology
- Prevalence: 1 in 300 worldwide
- More common in persons of European descent
- Associated with juvenile-onset diabetes mellitus, IgA deficiency, dermatitis herpetiformis, autoimmune thyroid disease
- Increased risk of small bowel lymphoma

Pathophysiology
- Gut exposure to grain proteins in wheat, rye, barley, and oats results in an autoimmune reaction that is toxic to enterocytes and leads to a flattened mucosal lining and impaired small intestinal absorptive capacity.

Clinical Manifestations
- Symptoms are variable and can present at any age
- Classically presents around age 1 to 3 years
- Diarrhea, foul-smelling bulky greasy stools, abdominal distention and pain
- Poor growth, anorexia, malaise, muscle wasting, irritability
- Symptoms can be subtle with only mild diarrhea or abdominal complaints
- Physical exam: weight loss, short stature, edema, abdominal distention, rectal prolapse, muscle wasting, dental erosion, angular stomatitis, aphthous ulcers, osteopenia, rickets

Diagnostics

- *Antibody Tests:* antigliadin antibody (IgA and IgG; moderate sensitivity, low specificity), antiendomysial IgA (sensitivity = 90% to 95%, specificity = 98% to 100%; false-negative results more common in children younger than 2 years of age), anti-tissue transglutaminase antibody (IgA anti-tTG; sensitivity = 92% to 98%, specificity = 96% to 100%); antibody tests are good for initial screen but endoscopy currently required for definitive diagnosis.
- *Tests of Malabsorption:*
  - CBC: anemia due to iron, vitamin B_{12}, or folate deficiency
  - Calcium, magnesium, phosphorus, albumin, alkaline phosphatase: low
  - PT prolongation due to fat-soluble vitamin deficiency
  - D-xylose test: Evaluates carbohydrate malabsorption
    - Nothing by mouth starting 8 hours before test. Give 10% D-xylose orally (14.5 g/m^2; maximum dose = 25 g), and draw serum D-xylose level 1 hour after ingestion.
    - A level less than 30 mg/dL suggests decreased jejunal surface area. False-positive results can occur with delayed gastric emptying, rapid intestinal transit time, and small bowel bacterial overgrowth.
  - 72-hour fecal fat
- *Upper GI with small bowel follow-through*
- *Wrist x-ray:* evaluate for rickets
- *Endoscopy:* small bowel biopsies on a gluten-containing diet help make diagnosis; findings of villous atrophy, crypt hyperplasia, infiltration of lamina propria with inflammatory cells are consistent with celiac disease; resolution of abnormalities on gluten-free diet confirms diagnosis.

Management

- Permanent gluten-free diet leads to full clinical and histologic remission; gluten-free means no wheat, rye, barley, or oats; corn and rice are permitted.
- Dietary counseling and careful attention to ALL food and medicinal products that may contain traces of gluten
- Multivitamin/fat-soluble vitamins
- Medical therapy for iron-deficiency and rickets if present
- Very close follow-up of growth parameters and symptoms
- Periodic monitoring of dietary compliance with antibody profile; antibodies usually undetectable within 3 to 6 months after initiation of appropriate diet
- Screening of all family members

CONSTIPATION

A symptom of abnormal defecation characterized by infrequent stooling, incomplete evacuation of the rectum, passage of large painful stools, involuntary soiling, or the inability to pass stool.

Epidemiology

- Occurs in more than 10% of all children
- Majority of constipation in older children is functional.
- Encopresis occurs in 1% to 2% of all children.

Etiology

- Anatomic: Hirschsprung disease, imperforate anus, anal stenosis, malpositioned anus, ileal atresia, meconium ileus, colonic stricture, abdominal mass, hydrometrocolpos
- Physiologic: hypothyroid, spinal cord defect, infant botulism, muscular diseases, cystic fibrosis, diabetes, lead poisoning, post-viral "ileus," prune-belly syndrome, ascariasis, medications, excessive cow's milk ingestion, inadequate fluid intake, malnutrition, anorexia nervosa, functional constipation

Pathophysiology
- *Functional Constipation:* cycle begins with voluntary withholding of stool. Stool returns from anal canal to rectum. Sensation of urge to defecate is lost. Stool bolus becomes larger and harder, which perpetuates more withholding. Over time, rectal vault distends and normal sensation diminishes.
- *Retentive Encopresis:* involuntary soiling of liquid stool around solid stool, which results from chronic constipation
- *Grunting Baby Syndrome:* an infant with grunting, straining, and turning red while passing a *soft* stool has immature coordination of the stooling process and not true constipation.

Clinical Manifestations
- Signs of possible anatomic abnormalities: blood in stool, failure to thrive, emesis, abdominal distention
- Signs of functional constipation: retentive posturing; infrequent passage of large, hard bowel movements; involuntary soiling
- Complaints of abdominal pain
- Stool consistency may be hard, soft or even diarrheal.
- Stool frequency can be daily or infrequent.
- On physical exam, note abdominal tenderness/distention, anal wink, anal tone, stool in rectal vault, width of rectal vault, neurologic and back exams.

Diagnostics
- Consider laboratories depending on suspected cause.
- Abdominal x-ray
- Unprepped barium enema or rectal biopsy: to evaluate for Hirschsprung disease
- MRI: suspected spinal cord abnormality

Management
- Treat underlying medical disorders.
- Surgical correction of anatomic defects
- Treatment of functional constipation may take months to years:
  - Bowel clean-out: enemas, suppositories, lubricants, hyperosmolar agents
  - Maintenance: dietary fiber and fluids, hyperosmolar agents
  - Toilet sitting: twice-daily stooling attempts
  - Diary/journal: positive reinforcement
  - Educate patient and parents. Frequent follow-up is critical to success.
- Medications used to treat constipation:
  - *Enema:* mineral oil (rectally); sodium biphosphate (Fleets); or saline; all in children ≥ 2 years of age
  - *Suppositories:* glycerin, bisacodyl
  - *Lubricants:* mineral oil (orally)
  - *Osmotic laxatives:* PEG 3350 (Miralax), lactulose, PEG with lytes (GOLYTELY)
  - *Stimulant laxatives:* senna, bisacodyl, magnesium citrate, magnesium hydroxide
  - *Fiber/bulk forming agents:* Benefiber, Citrucel, Metamucil, Maltsupex
- Typical cleanout regimen:
  1. Enemas to clean out rectal vault
  2. Hyperosmotic and/or stimulant therapy: may require nasogastric tube for administration. Continue until clear effluent.

GASTROINTESTINAL BLEEDING

Loss of blood via the gastrointestinal tract:
- *Hematemesis:* bloody emesis due to active bleeding proximal to the ligament of Treitz
- *Hematochezia:* bright red or maroon stool due to active bleeding in the colon or brisk bleeding from a more proximal site
- *Melena:* dark, tarry stool due to bleeding proximal to the ileocecal valve.

Differential Diagnosis

- Upper intestinal bleeding
  - Infant: swallowed maternal blood, esophagitis, gastric ulcer
  - Older child: esophagitis, Mallory Weiss tear, varices, foreign body, duplication cyst, Dieulafoy disease, gastritis, gastric ulcer, vascular malformation, duodenitis, hemobilia, swallowed blood from oral/nasal pharynx, pulmonary bleeding
- Lower intestinal bleeding
  - Infant: anal fissure, swallowed maternal blood, milk protein intolerance, infectious enterocolitis, vascular lesion, necrotizing enterocolitis, Hirschprung disease, Meckel diverticulum (>2 months), intussusception, intestinal duplication
  - Older child: anal fissure, perianal strep cellulitis, solitary rectal ulcer, infection, infectious enterocolitis, intussusception, inflammatory bowel disease, vascular malformations, Meckel diverticulum, polyp, intestinal duplication, Henoch-Schönlein purpura, hemolytic uremic syndrome, hemorrhoids, rectal trauma, sexual abuse

Clinical Manifestations

- Variable presentation from hemodynamically stable to shock
- Note prior use of NSAIDs, steroids, indomethacin, antibiotics
- Note history of trauma, liver disease, umbilical vein catheterization
- May present with vomiting, retching, casual regurgitation of bloody fluid, abdominal pain, anorexia, fever, weight loss, sepsis, asphyxia, recent surgery, mental status changes
- Inspect mouth, nares, pharynx for trauma
- Abdomen: hepatomegaly, splenomegaly, prominent abdominal vessels, right lower quadrant mass or tenderness
- Rectal: blood, erythema, fissure, fistula, skin tag, polyp, hemorrhoid
- Stool: blood or mucous within or surrounding stool
- Extremities: capillary refill, digital clubbing, palmar erythema, purpura or petechiae
- Skin: pallor, jaundice, facial petechiae, pigmented freckles on lips/buccal mucosa, excoriations, hemangiomas
- For breastfeeding infant, inspect mother's nipples

Diagnostics

- *Stool guaiac:* false-positive results may be due to rare meat, horseradish, turnips, iron, tomatoes, fresh red cherries; false negatives may be due to vitamin C, outdated card or developing solution, storage of stool greater than 4 days
- *Nasogastric lavage:* use normal saline at room temperature; absent blood does not exclude an upper GI source; present blood does not identify the exact origin
- *Laboratory studies:* CBC, PT/PTT, LFTs, electrolytes, type and screen
- *Stool culture*
- *Abdominal x-ray:* free air, toxic megacolon, pneumatosis, small bowel dilation
- *Air or gastrograffin contrast enema:* for suspected intussusception
- *Meckel diverticulum scan*
- *Upper GI:* structural abnormality, tumor, polyp, signs of inflammatory bowel disease (IBD)
- *Red blood cell/bleeding scan:* localize an active slower bleed (<0.3 mL/min)
- *Angiography:* localize a brisk bleed (>0.5 mL/min)
- *Endoscopy or colonoscopy:* direct visual inspection, biopsy, culture

Management

- *Initial management of all GI bleeding:* identify and treat shock with IV access, isotonic fluids, oxygen, blood products (see Transfusion Medicine in Chapter 12)
- *Non-variceal upper GI bleed:* acid reduction (ranitidine); discontinue NSAIDs; endoscopic hemostasis therapy if bleed persists (bipolar electrocoagulation, heater probe, clips, injection therapy)
- *Variceal upper GI bleed:*
  - Fluid resuscitation; transfuse red cells to maintain hemoglobin near 10 g/dL; transfuse platelets to greater than 50,000/mm^3; FFP to correct coagulopathy

- Octreotide (bolus 1–2 μg/kg over 2 to 5 minutes, then 1–2 μg/kg/hour infusion): reduces splanchnic arterial blood flow to decrease portal pressure
- Endoscopic band ligation, sclerotherapy
- Emergent surgical therapy for unresponsive severe bleeding: portosystemic shunt, transjugular intrahepatic portal shunt (TIPS), Blakemore-Sengstaaken tube occlusive balloon therapy, liver transplantation
- *Lower GI bleed in an infant:*
  - Surgical evaluation for suspected intussusception, necrotizing enterocolitis, toxic megacolon, Hirschsprung disease
  - If otherwise healthy and has blood-streaked mucus in stool without evidence of fissure, send stool culture and consider changing to elemental formula for presumptive milk-protein allergy
  - Flexible sigmoidoscopy for persistent bloody stools despite elemental formula and negative stool culture
  - Anal fissures heal without intervention.
- *Lower GI bleed in an older child:*
  - Treat according to underlying cause if known.
  - Treat constipation if present.
  - Flexible sigmoidoscopy or colonoscopy for recurrent or persistent bleeding to detect colitis, polyps, IBD
  - Polyp removal by electrocautery
  - Meckel's scan if no source identified by endoscopy
  - Surgical evaluation if severe bleed of unidentified source

INFLAMMATORY BOWEL DISEASE

An idiopathic chronic disease of the GI tract resulting in inflammation, tissue destruction, diarrhea, protein-losing enteropathy, bleeding, abdominal pain, and many extraintestinal manifestations. IBD is divided into Crohn disease (CD), ulcerative colitis (UC), and indeterminate colitis (IC).

Epidemiology
- Family history is predisposing
- 20% to 30% of new IBD presents in persons younger than 20 years of age.
- 4% of pediatric IBD presents in children younger than 5 years of age.
- More common in developed countries

Etiology
- Interaction between environmental and genetic factors
- Dysregulation of mucosal immune system driven by normal intestinal flora

Pathophysiology
- Crohn disease:
  - May involve any segment of the GI tract, mouth to anus
  - Commonly involves small intestine and terminal ileum
  - Transmural disease with thickened nodular bowel, non-caseating granulomas, strictures, fistulas, abscesses, adhesions
  - Skip lesions, discontinuous disease
  - Perianal disease (15%)
  - Malabsorption of Fe, Zn, folate, vitamin B_{12}
  - Bacterial overgrowth
  - Carcinoma (increased risk over general population)
- Ulcerative colitis:
  - Limited to the colon; starts in rectum and ascends continuously
  - Diffuse mucosal involvement/submucosal sparing

- Crypt abscesses; toxic megacolon (<5%)
- Carcinoma (significant increased risk over general population)
- Indeterminate colitis: term used when disease is localized to colon but cannot be definitively said to be UC or CD

Clinical Manifestations
Intestinal Manifestations
- *Crohn disease:* abdominal pain, diarrhea, rectal bleeding, aphthous oral lesions, perianal fissures/tags/ fistulas, abdominal abscesses, anorexia, weight loss, linear growth deceleration
- *Ulcerative colitis:* bloody mucoid diarrhea, lower abdominal pain/tenderness, urgency to defecate, nausea/vomiting associated with defecation

Extraintestinal Manifestations:
- Systemic: fever, malaise, anorexia, weight loss, growth delay/linear growth deceleration, delayed puberty
- Skin: erythema nodosum, pyoderma gangrenosum, perianal disease
- Joints: arthritis, arthralgia, clubbing, ankylosing spondylitis, sacroileitis
- Eyes: uveitis, episcleritis, keratitis, retinal vasculitis
- Biliary: sclerosing cholangitis (UC > CD), chronic active hepatitis, fatty liver, cholelithiasis
- Bone: osteopenia
- Renal: stones, hydronephrosis, enterovesical fistula
- Vascular: thrombophlebitis, vasculitis
- Heme: anemia (Fe, vitamin B_{12}, folate deficiency, hemolysis, marrow suppression from medications, anemia of chronic disease), thrombocytosis, neutropenia
- Oncologic: lymphoma, acute myelogenous leukemia, colon cancer

Diagnostics
- CBC (low hemoglobin, low mean corpuscular volume, high platelets), ESR (high), C-reactive protein (high), albumin (low), alkaline phosphatase (low), iron studies, folate, vitamin B_{12} levels, electrolytes, calcium, magnesium, phosphorus
- Antineutrophil cytoplasmic antibody and anti-*Saccharomyces cerevisiae* antibody: can help support diagnosis of IBD; cannot differentiate CD from UC
- Stool guaiac: positive
- Stool for culture, *Clostridium difficile* toxins A and B, ova and parasites

Radiology
- Upper GI with small bowel follow-through
- Abdominal CT: assess complications of CD such as abscess or phlegmon
- Tagged white blood cell scan: may have role in finding inflammation in IBD
- MR-gadolinium: may have role in localizing disease in IBD
- Bone age: assess for delayed bone maturation
- Dexascan: follow effects of the disease and the medications on bone health

Endoscopy
- Gold standard for diagnosis
- Mucosa is erythematous, edematous, friable, ulcerated
- Loss of normal vascular pattern

Management
Medical
- Salicylates: first line
  - sulfasalazine, mesalamine (Pentasa, Asacol), balsalazide (Colazol)
- Antibiotics: often used in conjunction with salicylates and other therapies
  - metronidazole, ciprofloxacin
- Steroids: added for active flare
  - prednisone, methylprednisone, budesonide, hydrocortisone enema
- Immunomodulators: to reduce steroid dependency or as adjunct to infliximab
  - 6-mercaptopurine, azathioprine, methotrexate, cyclosporine, tacrolimus

- Biologic agents: fistulizing disease, refractory IBD, other indications
  - infliximab (Remicade)
- Other: omega-3 fatty acids (fish oil); probiotics (lactobacillus, VSL3)
  - high calorie foods, oral supplements, elemental formulas NG/GT
- Discharge criteria following acute flare depends on improvement of presenting symptoms (e.g., tolerating oral intake without severe pain, minimal gross blood in stool and maintaining stable hemoglobin level, fewer diarrheal stools, gaining weight if admitted with weight loss, resolution of emesis, resolution of obstruction)

Surgical
- Indicated in uncontrolled bleeding, bowel perforation, bowel obstruction, intractable disease, and intractable perianal disease
- CD: local resection, ostomy diversion, fistula management
- UC: total colectomy with ileo-anal anastomosis

MECKEL DIVERTICULUM

A true diverticulum that results from incomplete closure of the omphalomesenteric or vitelline duct. It may contain gastric or other mucosa, and occurs along the ileum usually within 100 cm of the ileocecal valve.

Epidemiology
- 2% of the population
- Has been associated with cleft palate, bicornuate uterus, and annular pancreas

Pathophysiology
- Persistence of vitelline duct; contains all three intestinal layers
- May contain ectopic tissue: gastric (50%), pancreatic (5%), other
- Bleeding occurs when acid secreted by ectopic gastric mucosa causes adjacent ileal ulceration or erodes into the vitelline artery

Clinical Manifestations
- Asymptomatic: 95% of cases
- Painless lower intestinal bleeding; most common symptom accounting for 50% of symptomatic presentations, generally in patients 2 months to 2 years
- Other manifestations: intestinal obstruction, intussusception, volvulus, herniation through mesenteric defect, severe right lower quadrant abdominal pain (Meckel diverticulitis), umbilical cysts/sinuses, palpable abdominal mass

Diagnostics
- Technetium-99m pertechnetate scintigraphic study
- Tagged red blood cell scan if active bleed
- Upper GI with small bowel follow through
- Barium enema (if intussusception suspected)
- Occasionally discovered as incidental finding at laparoscopy

Management
- Medically resuscitate the patient as with a lower GI bleed
- Symptomatic Meckel's should be surgically resected
- Meckel's found incidentally during surgery performed for another reason should be resected if: palpable heterotopic mucosa or mass, fibrous bands to umbilicus, surrounding inflammation

Pancreas

PANCREATITIS

Acute Pancreatitis: an acute inflammatory process of the pancreas characterized by abdominal pain, elevated pancreatic enzymes, and radiologic evidence of pancreatic inflammation

Chronic Pancreatitis: a condition of recurring or persisting abdominal pain, pancreatic inflammation, and progressive destruction of the pancreas that often leads to pancreatic insufficiency or failure

Epidemiology
- All ages; male – female
- Heritable forms of pancreatitis are the most common forms of chronic pancreatitis in children (cationic trypsinogen, SPINK1, CFTR gene mutations).

Etiology
- Acute Pancreatitis
  - *Systemic Disease*: infections; inflammatory/vascular (Henoch-Schönlein purpura, hemolytic-uremic syndrome, Kawasaki, IBD, collagen vascular); sepsis/shock; transplantation
  - *Mechanical/Structural*: trauma (blunt injury, child abuse, post-ERCP); anatomic (annular pancreas, pancreas divisum, choledochal cyst, stricture); obstruction (stones, tumor)
  - *Metabolic/Toxic*: hyperlipidemia, hypercalcemia, cystic fibrosis, severe malnutrition, refeeding, renal disease, organic acidemia, drugs/toxins
  - *Idiopathic*: up to 25% of cases
- Chronic Pancreatitis
  - Obstructive: congenital anomaly (choledochal cyst), ductal fibrosis or stricture, tumor, pseudocyst, sphincter of Oddi dysfunction, trauma, idiopathic fibrosing pancreatitis, autoimmune pancreatitis, sclerosing cholangitis
  - Calcific: heritable pancreatitis (cationic trypsinogen deficiency, SPINK1 and CFTR mutations), hypercalcemia, hyperlipidemia, juvenile tropical pancreatitis
  - Idiopathic (30%)

Pathophysiology
- Acute pancreatitis: inappropriate activation of enzymes within pancreatic parenchyma leads to inflammation and tissue destruction resulting in necrosis of peripancreatic fat, interstitial edema, and cytokine release. Complications include hypocalcemia, hyperglycemia, GI hemorrhage, severe necrosis, pseudocyst rupture, abscess, acute tubular necrosis, gastritis, duodenitis, and pleural effusion.
- Chronic pancreatitis: fibrotic parenchymal disease resulting from obstructive or calcific processes; exact mechanisms unknown. Complications include pancreatic exocrine and endocrine insufficiency or failure.
- Hereditary pancreatitis (cationic trypsinogen deficiency): autosomal dominant form of calcific chronic pancreatitis due to mutations of cationic trypsinogen, resulting in recurrent bouts of acute pancreatitis.
- Autoimmune pancreatitis: associated with increased IgG levels, presence of autoantibodies, diffuse enlargement of pancreas, narrowing of main pancreatic duct, and lymphocytic infiltration of the pancreas with fibrotic changes

Clinical Manifestations
- Acute pancreatitis: severe abdominal pain of acute onset; +/– epigastric location; nausea, vomiting, anorexia. Clinical course is highly variable and may progress to coma, hypotension, renal failure, pulmonary edema, hemorrhage, and shock.
- Chronic pancreatitis: recurring or persistent abdominal pain or painless; some patients have recurrent episodes of acute pancreatitis; pain diminishes as pancreas burns out (may take 10 to 20 years); other manifestations include pancreatic exocrine or endocrine insufficiency (end-stage), steatorrhea, excessive appetite, growth failure, obstructive jaundice

Diagnostics
- Amylase: level increases early; lasts 3 to 5 days
- Lipase: more specific than amylase; typically elevated longer
- In chronic pancreatitis, enzyme levels may not be increased
- C-reactive protein: peaks at 36 to 48 hours

- Markers of severe disease: hyperglycemia, hypocalcemia, hypoxemia, hypoproteinemia, high BUN, high white blood cells, low hematocrit
- Abdominal x-ray: to exclude other causes of abdominal pain
- Chest x-ray: evaluate for pleural effusion
- Ultrasound: pancreatic inflammation, calcification, ductular dilatation, stones, pseudocyst
- CT: only needed when ultrasound is technically unsatisfactory (sensitivity > 90% if necrosis involves > 30% of pancreas). Consider CT-guided fine-needle aspiration if diagnosis of necrosis/infection uncertain.

Management
- Supportive care, bed rest
- Nothing by mouth and nasogastric decompression
- Fluid and electrolyte replacement and maintenance
- Early nutrition, either total parenteral nutrition or jejunal enteral feeds
- Monitor acid/base status, electrolytes, renal function
- Analgesia: ibuprofen, tramadol, narcotics
- Adjuncts in chronic pancreatic pain: amitriptyline, nortriptyline, neurontin
- Antibiotics: for severe systemic illness or pancreatic necrosis (imipenem, ticarcillin-clavulanate, piperacillin-tazobactam, or ciprofloxacin + metronidazole)
- Repeat ultrasound every 3 to 4 days.
- Attempt to identify underlying cause to help prevent recurrence.
- ERCP to relieve stones or strictures
- Surgical management of complications such as symptomatic pseudocyst, abscess, necrosis, hemorrhage. Surgical correction of structural lesions is performed after acute illness resolves.
- Once symptoms resolve and able to tolerate oral feeds, maintain on low fat diet until complete recovery or indefinitely in chronic cases; consider pancreatic enzymes.

> * Medication recommendations in this chapter may be off label based on patient age or specific disease. Consult product insert for further information.

Resources

Esophagus and Stomach
Altschuler S, Liacouras C. Clinical Pediatric Gastroenterology. Philadelphia: Churchill Livingstone, 1998.

Faubion WA, Zein NN. Gastroesophageal reflux in infants and children. Mayo Clin Proc 1998;73:166–173.

Gold BD, Colletti RB, Abbott M, et al. *Helicobacter pylori* infection in children: recommendations for diagnosis and treatment. J Pediatr Gastroenterol Nutr 2000;31:490–497.

Gosciniak G, Przondo-Mordarska A, Iwanczak B, Blitek A. *Helicobacter pylori* antigens in stool specimens of gastritis children before and after treatment. J Pediatr Gastroenterol Nutr 2003;36:376–380.

Hassall E. Peptic ulcer disease and current approaches to *Helicobacter pylori*. J Pediatr 2001;138:462–468.

Orenstein SR, Izadnia F, Kahn S. Gastroesophageal reflux disease in children. Gastroenterol Clin North Am 1999;28:947–969.

Hepatobiliary System
Altschuler S, Liacouras C. Clinical Pediatric Gastroenterology. Philadelphia: Churchill Livingstone, 1998.

Baldassano R, Piccoli DA. Inflammatory bowel disease in pediatric and adolescent patients. Gastroenterol Clin 1999;28:445–458.

El-Youssef M. Wilson disease. Mayo Clin Proc 2003;78:1126–1136.

Feldman M, et al. Sleisenger & Fordtran's Gastrointestinal and Liver Disease. 7th ed. Philadelphia: WB Saunders, 2002.

Haber BA, Russo P. Biliary atresia. Gastroenterol Clin North Am 2003;32:891–911.

Indar AA, Beckingham IJ. Acute cholecystitis. BMJ 2002;325:639–643.

Lteif AN, Schwenk WF. Hypoglycemia in infants and children. Endocrinol Metab Clin North Am 1999;28:619–646.

Lykavieris P, Hadchouel M, Chardot C, Bernard O. Outcome of liver disease in children with Alagille syndrome: a study of 163 patients. Gut 2001;49:431–435.

McFarlane IG. Autoimmune hepatitis: diagnostic criteria, subclassifications, and clinical features. Clin Liver Dis 2002;6:317–333.

Mieli-Vergani G, Vergani D. Autoimmune hepatitis in children. Clin Liver Dis 2002;6:335–346.

Narkewicz MR. Biliary atresia: an update on our understanding of the disorder. Curr Opin Pediatr 2001;13:435–440.

Piccoli DA, Spinner NB. Alagille syndrome and the Jagged1 gene. Semin Liver Dis 2001;21:525–534.

Primhak RA, Tanner MS. Alpha-1 antitrypsin deficiency. Arch Dis Child 2001;85:2–5.

Suchy F, Sokol R, Balistreri W, eds. Liver Disease in Children. 2nd ed. Philadelphia: Lippincott, Williams, & Wilkins, 2001.

Walker, et al. Pediatric Gastrointestinal Disease: Pathophysiology, Diagnosis, Management. 3rd ed. Ontario: BC Decker, 2000.

Wolfsdorf JI, Weinstein DA. Glycogen storage diseases. Rev Endocr Metab Disord 2003;4:95–102.

Small and Large Intestine

Altschuler S, Liacouras C. Clinical Pediatric Gastroenterology. Philadelphia: Churchill Livingstone, 1998.

Baldassano R, Piccoli DA. Inflammatory bowel disease in pediatric and adolescent patients. Gastroenterol Clin 1999;28:445–458.

Baudon JJ, Johanet C, Absalon YB, et al. Diagnosing celiac disease: a comparison of human tissue transglutaminase antibodies with antigliadin and antiendomysium antibodies. Arch Pediatr Adolesc Med 2004;158:584–588.

Cuffari C, Darbari A. Inflammatory bowel disease in the pediatric and adolescent patient. Gastroenterol Clin 2002;31:275–291.

Fasano A. Celiac disease: the past, the present, the future. Pediatrics 2001;107:768–770.

Feldman M, et al. Sleisenger & Fordtran's Gastrointestinal and Liver Disease. 7th ed. Philadelphia: WB Saunders, 2002.

Fleisher G, Ludwig S, ed. et al. Textbook of Pediatric Emergency Medicine. 4th ed. Philadelphia: Lippincott, Williams & Wilkins, 2000.

Lawrence WW, Wright JL. Causes of rectal bleeding in children. Pediatr Rev 2001;22:384–385.

Mamula P, Mascarenhas MR, Baldassano RN. Biological and novel therapies for inflammatory bowel disease in children. Pediatr Clin 2002;49:1–25.

Olds G, McLoughlin R, O'Morian C, Sivak MV Jr. Celiac disease for the endoscopist. Gastrointest Endosc 2002;56:407–415.

Squires R. Gastrointestinal bleeding. Pediatr Rev 1999;20:95–101.

Walker WA, et al. Pediatric Gastrointestinal Disease: Pathophysiology, Diagnosis, Management. 3rd ed. Ontario: BC Decker, 2000.

Youssef NN, Peters JM, Henderson W, et al. Dose response of PEG 3350 for the treatment of childhood fecal impaction. J Pediatr 2002;141:410–414.

Pancreas

Morinville V, Perrault J. Genetic disorders of the pancreas. Gastroenterol Clin North Am 2003;32:763–787.

Okazaki K, Chiba T. Autoimmune related pancreatitis. Gut 2002;51:1–4.

Pietzak MM, Thomas DW. Pancreatitis in childhood. Pediatr Rev 2000;21:406–412.

Walker WA, et al. Pediatric Gastrointestinal Disease: Pathophysiology, Diagnosis, Management. 3rd ed. Ontario: BC Decker, 2000.

GENETICS

Trevor L. Hoffman, MD, PhD, Alix Seif, MD, MPH, Matthew Deardorff, MD, PhD, Paige B. Kaplan, MBBCh, Ian Krantz, MD

BECKWITH-WIEDEMANN SYNDROME

Overgrowth disorder characterized by macrosomia, macroglossia, visceromegaly, embryonal tumors, abdominal wall defects, characteristic linear creases on the ear lobe, and neonatal hypoglycemia

Epidemiology
- Approximately 1 in 10,000 births with 20% mortality rate in infancy
- 15% with family history consistent with autosomal dominant transmission
- Estimated risk of tumor development ~7.5%

Etiology
- Most cases involve genetic abnormalities in 11p15.5, which contains a number of genes implicated in this disorder.

Clinical Manifestations
- No consensus for diagnosis, but generally requires at least two major and one minor criteria.
- Major criteria: positive family history; macrosomia; linear ear lobe creases or posterior helical ear pits; macroglossia; omphalocele or umbilical hernia; visceromegaly of liver, kidneys, spleen, adrenal glands, and/or pancreas; embryonal tumor (Wilms, hepatoblastoma, rhabdomyosarcoma); hemihyperplasia; adrenocortical cytomegaly; renal structural abnormalities
- Minor criteria: polyhydramnios; prematurity; neonatal hypoglycemia; facial nevus flammeus; hemangioma; diastasis recti; advanced bone age; monozygotic twinning; cardiomyopathy and/or cardiomegaly; characteristic facies (infraorbital creases, midface hypoplasia)

Diagnostics
- Karyotype (normal in > 98%)
- UPD testing of 11p15.5
- Methylation testing in KCNQ1OT1 and H19 genes
- CDKN1C mutation testing
- False-negative test results may occur from somatic mosaicism in cases of UPD, so repeat testing may be indicated on second tissue type

Management
- Blood sugar monitoring to detect hypoglycemia (may require hydrocortisone analogue therapy during first 1 to 4 months of life)
- Consider electrocardiogram and/or echocardiogram given possible higher incidence of cardiomyopathy
- Renal ultrasound to screen for structural defects
- Surgery occasionally necessary to relieve airway obstruction from macroglossia
- Abdominal ultrasound monitoring every 3 months until 8 years of age to screen for embryonal tumors
- Serum alpha-fetoprotein every 3 months until 4 years of age to screen for hepatoblastoma

MARFAN SYNDROME

An autosomal dominant disorder of connective tissue, resulting in people who are tall and have long arms, long thin fingers, dislocated lenses, and aortic dilatation.

Epidemiology
- Prevalence: at least 3:10,000

Etiology
- Caused by mutation in the *fibrillin-1* gene (*FBN1*), which encodes a component of the extra-cellular matrix.

Pathophysiology
- *FBN1* is a large gene on chromosome 15q21
- Penetrance is high and most mutations are unique to a given family
- 25% of patients have new mutations (i.e., no family history)

Clinical Manifestations
- Skeletal system
  - *Major criteria* (four of the following): pectus carinatum; pectus excavatum requiring surgery; reduced upper/lower segment ratio, or arm span to height ratio greater than 1.05; positive "wrist" sign (thumb and fifth finger overlap appreciably when encircling the opposing wrist) or positive "thumb" sign (tip of the thumb protrudes beyond the border of the palm when the hand is clenched, enclosing the thumb); scoliosis (>20°) or spondylolisthesis; reduced extension of the elbows (<170°); medial displacement of the medial malleolus causing pes planus; protrusio acetabuli on pelvic x-ray (intrapelvic displacement of the medial wall of the acetabulum)
  - *Minor criteria*: pectus excavatum of moderate severity; joint hypermobility; highly arched palate with dental crowding; facial appearance (dolichocephaly, malar hypoplasia, enoph-thalmos, downslanting palpebral fissures, retrognathia)
- Ocular system
  - *Major criterion*: ectopia lentis
  - *Minor criteria*: abnormally flat cornea, increased axial length of globe, hypoplastic iris or hypoplastic ciliary muscle causing a decreased miosis
- Cardiovascular system
  - *Major criteria*: dilatation of the ascending aorta with or without aortic regurgitation and involving at least the sinuses of Valsalva; dissection of the ascending aorta
  - *Minor criteria*: mitral valve prolapse with or without regurgitation; dilatation of the main pul-monary artery; calcification of the mitral annulus; dilatation or dissection of descending thoracic or abdominal aorta
- Pulmonary system
  - *Major criteria*: none
  - *Minor criteria*: spontaneous pneumothorax; apical blebs
- Skin and integument
  - *Major criteria*: lumbosacral dural ectasia
  - *Minor criteria*: striae atrophica; recurrent or incisional hernias

Diagnositic Criteria
- *For the index case:* major criteria in two organ systems and involvement of a third system
- *For a patient with a positive family history:* one major criterion in one organ system and involvement of a second organ system

Management
- *Cardiovascular:*
  - Restrict physical activity to low impact activities
  - Beta blockers (propranolol) may slow progression of cardiovascular disease
  - May need mitral valve repair or replacement
  - Endocarditis prophylaxis prior to surgical procedures for those with cardiac disease (use American Heart Association criteria)
- *Ocular:* early ophthalmology evaluation; prevention of retinal detachment (avoid blows to head or globe)
- *Pectus excavatum:* if severe, repair as adolescent
- *Scoliosis:* bracing for scoliosis greater than 15° to 20°; surgery for pain, neurologic compro-mise, or curves greater than 45°

- *Integumentary:* surveillance for hernia; CT/MRI for dural ectasia in patients with neurologic symptoms
- *Respiratory:* smoking abstinence

NEUROFIBROMATOSIS TYPE 1

A genetic disorder characterized by the presence of café-au-lait spots, neurofibromas, axillary freckling, Lisch nodules, optic gliomas, and specific skeletal abnormalities

Epidemiology
- Occurs in approximately 1 in 4000 people
- 5% of affected individuals develop malignant tumors (neurofibrosarcomas, leukemia, brain tumors)
- 25% to 50% of individuals have associated learning disability

Etiology
- Caused by mutations in NF-1 gene
- 50% of cases inherited and 50% of cases from novel mutation

Pathophysiology
- NF-1 gene product acts as tumor suppressor. Mutations in the NF-1 gene predispose affected tissues toward neoplastic transformation.

Clinical Manifestations
- Diagnosis based on presence of two or more of the following diagnostic criteria:
  - Six or more café-au-lait spots greater than 5 mm in diameter before puberty or greater than 15 mm after puberty
  - Two or more neurofibromas or one plexiform neurofibroma
  - Axillary or inguinal freckling
  - Lisch nodules on iris
  - Optic glioma
  - Skeletal abnormality (sphenoid dysplasia, cortical thinning in long bones with or without pseudoarthrosis)
  - NF1 in parent, sibling, or offspring
- Short stature and macrocephaly common
- Café-au-lait spots and plexiform neurofibromas frequently present in first year of life. Isolated neurofibromas and intertriginal freckling usually develop near puberty.
- Progressive scoliosis may develop between ages 6 and 10.

Diagnostics
- Genetic testing rarely necessary as diagnosis often based on history and physical exam
- Ophthalmologic exam to evaluate for Lisch nodules and optic gliomas
- X-ray of lower extremity to screen for cortical thickening and pseudoarthroses

Management
- Annual ophthalmologic exam
- Regular developmental assessment
- Lower extremity x-ray in preambulatory children
- Removal of neurofibromas rarely necessary unless secondary complication occurs (e.g., hypertension from renal artery stenosis)
- Regular blood pressure monitoring
- In the absence of specific symptoms, brain MRI screening is controversial

TRISOMY 13

A genetic syndrome characterized by microcephaly, scalp defects, holoprosencephaly, micro-ophthalmia, cleft lip/palate, congenital heart disease, cryptorchidism, postaxial polydactyly, and severe developmental delay.

Epidemiology
- Occurs in approximately 1 in 5000 live births

Etiology
- Free trisomy 13 in 80% of cases; translocation in 20% of cases

Clinical Manifestations
- Intrauterine growth retardation
- Holoprosencephaly
- *Cardiac defects:* atrial septal defect (ASD), ventricular septal defect (VSD), dextrocardia, bicuspid aortic valve, coarctation of the aorta
- *Renal anomalies:* polycystic kidneys, horseshoe kidneys, hydronephrosis
- *Head and neck findings:* microcephaly, scalp defects at vertex, sloping forehead and hypotelorism, microphthalmia, cleft lip and palate, malformed ears, loose skin in posterior neck
- *Extremity findings:* postaxial polydactyly, hyperconvex nails, overlapping fingers and/or "fisting"
- Hypoplastic nipples
- Cryptorchidism (100%) and hypospadias in males
- Apnea

Diagnostics
- Karyotype analysis
- Segmented neutrophils on peripheral blood smears may have abnormal nuclear projections

Management
- Extremely poor prognosis with mean survival 130 days
- Generally, due to the poor prognosis, only supportive care is given

TRISOMY 18

A genetic syndrome characterized by growth deficiency, prominent occiput, micrognathia, low-set/malformed ears, fisting of hands, hypoplastic nails, cardiac anomalies, and severe mental retardation.

Epidemiology
- Occurs in approximately 1 of 5000 newborns; female predominance (4:1)
- Mean gestational age 42 weeks

Etiology
- Majority of cases from maternal nondisjunction of chromosome 18
- Small number of cases are familial secondary to robertsonian translocation

Clinical Manifestations
- Intrauterine growth retardation with polyhydramnios
- *Congenital heart disease:* VSD, ASD, bicuspid aortic valve, transposition, tetralogy of Fallot, dextrocardia
- *Renal anomalies:* cystic and horseshoe kidneys
- *Head and neck findings:* microcephaly, dolichocephaly with prominent occiput, short palpebral fissures, small mouth, micrognathia, low-set and/or malformed ears
- *Extremity findings:* overlapping fingers with "fisting," hypoplastic nails (especially on fifth digits), rocker-bottom or clubfoot with prominent calcaneus
- *Genitourinary findings:* cryptorchidism, prominent clitoris
- *Other findings:* failure to thrive; seizures; widely spaced nipples; hip dislocations; relative paucity of subcutaneous tissue, skeletal muscle, and adipose tissue; predominance of arches in dermatoglyphics

Diagnostics
- Karyotype analysis

Table 11.1: Risk of Trisomy 21 by Maternal Age	
Maternal Age (yr)	Incidence
15–29	1 in 1500
30–34	1 in 800
35–39	1 in 270
40–44	1 in 100
> 45	1 in 50

Management
- Extremely poor prognosis with mean survival of 48 days
- Generally, due to the poor prognosis, only supportive care is given
- Parental karyotype analysis necessary if robertsonian translocation identified

TRISOMY 21

Also known as Down syndrome (DS), a genetic syndrome characterized by dysmorphia, mental retardation, and hypotonia resulting from extra genetic material from chromosome 21.

Epidemiology
- 1/650–1000 newborns (Table 11.1)

Etiology
- Trisomy of all or of a large part of chromosome 21
- Typically due to maternal nondisjunction during meiosis
- Translocation in up to 6% of mothers under age 30

Clinical Manifestations
- *Principal findings in neonates:* hypotonia, poor Moro reflex, redundant skin at back of neck, flat facial profile, upslanted palpebral fissures, ears small, overfolding of angulated upper helix, ear lobes small or absent, clinodactyly (small middle phalanx of fifth finger), single palmar crease
- *Cardiovascular:* atrioventricular canal, ventricular septal defect, isolated secundum atrial septal defect, patent ductus arteriosus, tetralogy of Fallot, and other defects. Mitral valve prolapse or aortic regurgitation may develop in adolescents and young adults.
- *Other commonly associated findings:* protruding tongue (relative macroglossia), wide fontanelles ± third fontanelle, Brushfield spots in iris, inner epicanthal folds, wide gap between first and second toes ± deep plantar crease, cutis marmorata, hypogonadism, dental hypoplasia, mild-moderate short stature, mental retardation with IQ typically 25 to 50
- Conductive, sensorineural, or mixed hearing loss; risk for frequent otitis media
- *Ophthalmologic:* congenital cataracts, glaucoma refractive errors, strabismus, nystagmus
- *Gastrointestinal:* gastrointestinal atresia, Meckel diverticulum, tracheoesophageal fistula, celiac disease
- *Musculoskeletal:* juvenile rheumatoid arthritis-like arthropathy, joint subluxations, atlantoaxial instability
- *Endocrine:* diabetes mellitus, congenital hypothyroidism, hyperthyroidism
- *Hematologic:* acute lymphoblastic leukemia, acute myeloblastic leukemia, transient myeloproliferative disorder, myelodysplastic syndrome
- *Neurologic:* seizures, Alzheimer's disease
- *Dermatologic:* folliculitis, atopic and seborrheic dermatitis, fungal infections, xerosis, vitiligo, alopecia
- *Psychiatric:* attention deficit disorder, oppositional disorder, aggressive behavior, depression

- Other: obstructive sleep apnea; dental caries and orthodontic problems
- Women are typically fertile, while men have diminished fertility

Diagnostics
- Maternal triple screen (alpha-fetoprotein, human chorionic gonadotropin, unconjugated estriol) and prenatal ultrasound
- Prenatal diagnosis via amniocentesis or chorionic villus sampling if maternal risk factors or positive triple screen
- Karyotype of whole blood (or of tissue fibroblasts in cases of suspected mosaicism)

Management
Summary of recommendations by the American Association of Pediatrics and the Down Syndrome Medical Interest Group:
- *Assessment of newborns:* echocardiogram and cardiac evaluation; hearing assessment; ophthalmologic assessment by 6 months of age; parental karyotype analysis necessary if robertsonian translocation identified
- *Ongoing monitoring:*
  - Thyroxine and thyroid-stimulating hormone assays at birth, 6 months, and then yearly
  - Screening for celiac disease at 24 months of age (IgA anti-endomysial antibodies; see Celiac Disease in Gastroenterology chapter)
  - Atlantoaxial instability: screening with lateral neck films in flexion, extension, and neutral positions at 3 to 5 years.
  - Yearly audiologic and ophthalmologic evaluations
  - Frequent dental care
- *Obesity prevention:* dietary restriction beginning at 24 months of age; special attention to nutritional deficiencies, such as calcium and vitamin D

TURNER SYNDROME (TS)

A genetic syndrome characterized by females with short stature and gonadal dysgenesis resulting from a single, or abnormal, X chromosome.

Epidemiology
- 1/2000 newborn females

Etiology
- Absence of all or of a large part of chromosome X
- Typically due to paternal chromosome loss
- Not associated with maternal age
- Typically sporadic with minimal recurrence risk

Clinical Manifestations
- *Principal findings in neonates:* lymphedema, especially of hands and feet; low posterior hairline; redundant skin/webbing at back of neck; narrow palate; prominent ears; broad chest with wide-set nipples; short fifth metacarpal; narrow, hyperconvex fingernails
- *Cardiac anomalies:* usually bifid aortic valve or coarctation of the aorta
- *Other commonly associated findings:* short stature; cubitus valgus; medial tibial exostoses; bone dysplasia at metaphyses; multiple pigmented nevi; keloid formation; hypogonadism due to ovarian dysgenesis or agenesis; horseshoe kidney or other anomalies; mean IQ 90 with specific visuo-spatial, psychosocial, and psychomotor deficits; hearing loss; depression; Crohn disease; primary hypothyroidism; primary or secondary amenorrhea

Diagnostics
- Prenatal diagnosis via amniocentesis or chorionic villus sampling performed either for maternal risk factors for other chromosomal anomalies or for fetal anomalies; typically see nuchal thickening or fetal hydrops
- Karyotype of whole blood and of tissue fibroblasts to rule out mosaicism, especially in older children

Management

- *Short stature:* in consultation with a pediatric endocrinologist, growth hormone therapy may begin at age 2 if patient is less than fifth percentile.
- *Cardiovascular anomalies:* initial cardiac evaluation in the newborn period. Patients with bicuspid aortic valves, aortic stenosis, aortic coarctation or persistent hypertension require frequent imaging (echocardiography or cardiac MRI) to screen for aortic root dilatation. Patients with initial normal exams need close monitoring of blood pressure by primary pediatrician. Hypertension requires aggressive management. Subacute bacterial endocarditis prophylaxis may be indicated (as per American Heart Association)
- *Renal anomalies:* renal ultrasound in neonatal period. Follow closely for hypertension and evidence of urinary tract infection.
- *Hearing loss:* evaluate in newborn period and at every pediatric visit until age 1 year; then follow speech development. Evaluate for serous otitis media at well-child visits.
- *Obesity and glucose intolerance:* encourage appropriate diet and exercise. Screen for diabetes mellitus annually if patient is obese, has a strong family history of type 2 diabetes mellitus, or if she is Native American or African American.
- *Hypothyroidism:* annual or biannual evaluation of thyroxine and thyroid-stimulating hormone beginning at age 4 years
- *Orthopedic issues:* evaluate for congenital hip dysplasia; yearly evaluations for scoliosis beginning at age 5 years

Resources

American Academy of Pediatrics Committee on Genetics. Health Supervision for Children With Down Syndrome. Pediatrics 2001;107:442–449.

Delatycki M, Gardner RJ. Three cases of trisomy 13 mosaicism and a review of the literature. Clin Genet 1997;51:403–407.

De Paepe A, Devereux RB, Dietz HC, et al. Revised diagnostic criteria for Marfan syndrome. Am J Med Gen 1996;62:417–426.

Embleton ND, Wyllie JP, Wright MJ, et al. Natural history of trisomy 18. Arch Dis Child Fetal Neonatal Ed 1996;75:F38–41.

Frias JL, Davenport ML. Committee on Genetics and Section on Endocrinology. Health supervision for children with Turner syndrome. Pediatrics 2003;111:692–702.

Friedman JM. Neurofibromatosis 1. 1998. Available at: http://www.geneclinics.org. Accessed November 16, 2004.

Gorlin RJ, et al. Syndromes of the Head and Neck. Oxford: Oxford University Press, 2001.

Jones KL. Smith's Recognizable Patterns of Human Malformation. Philadelphia: WB Saunders, 1997:18–19.

Korf BR. The Child with Neurofibromatosis. New York: National Neurofibromatosis Foundation, 1993.

Online Mendelian Inheritance in Man, OMIM. Down syndrome. Available at: http://www.ncbi.nlm.nih.gov/entrez/dispomim.cgi?id=190685. Accessed November 16, 2004.

Pyeritz RE. The Marfan syndrome. Ann Rev Med 2000;51:481–510.

Roizen NJ, Patterson D. Down's syndrome. Lancet 2003;361:1281–1289.

Shuman C, Weksberg R. Beckwith-Wiedemann syndrome. 2000. Available at: http://www.geneclinics.org. Accessed November 16, 2004.

Char Witmer, MD, Leslie Raffini, MD

Anemia

Red Blood Cell Indices
- *Hematocrit (HCT)*: volume percentage of RBCs in the plasma. See Table 12.1 for age-related normal levels.
- *Mean corpuscular volume (MCV)*: average RBC volume
- *Mean corpuscular hemoglobin (MCH)*: average quantity of hemoglobin per RBC
- *Mean corpuscular hemoglobin concentration (MCHC)*: grams of hemoglobin per 100 mL of packed RBCs
- *Red cell distribution width (RDW)*: index of the variation in RBC size
- *Reticulocyte count*: percentage of young RBCs in the plasma

Differential Diagnosis Based on Mean Corpuscular Volume
Microcytic Anemia
- Iron deficiency, thalassemia, chronic inflammation, lead poisoning, sideroblastic anemia
- *Iron deficiency vs. thalassemia trait*: RBC count and RDW are often normal in thalassemia; in iron deficiency, low RBC count and elevated RDW; Mentzer index (MCV/RBC) serves as useful screen (<13 suggests thalassemia trait, >13 suggests iron deficiency)

Normocytic Anemia
- In normocytic anemia, assess the reticulocyte count. The reticulocyte index accurately reflects erythropoiesis by adjusting for the degree of anemia.
- Reticulocyte index (RI) = %Reticulocyte × Patient HCT/Normal HCT
  - RI is greater than 3% in compensated bleeding or hemolysis and less than 3% in anemia due to decreased RBC production. 1% is normal marrow activity.
- *Reticulocytes low*: pure RBC dysplasia (Diamond-Blackfan anemia), transient erythroblastopenia of childhood, aplastic crisis (parvovirus B19); renal disease; acute bleed; marrow infiltration (leukemia); erythroid aplasia; hormone deficiencies (e.g., hypothyroidism or growth hormone deficiency); anemia of chronic disease
- *Reticulocytes high*:
  - Chronic blood loss
  - Extrinsic hemolysis: antibody mediated hemolysis, disseminated intravascular coagulation (DIC), hemolytic-uremic syndrome, prosthetic heart valve, vitamin E deficiency, Wilson disease, liver disease, renal disease
  - Intrinsic hemolysis: membrane disorders (e.g., hereditary spherocytosis), enzyme deficiencies (e.g., G6PD), hemoglobin disorders (e.g., sickle cell disease)

Macrocytic Anemia
- Folic acid deficiency, vitamin B_{12} deficiency, normal newborn (MCV 100–125), Down syndrome, medications (e.g., valproate, Bactrim, hydroxyurea, azathioprine), aplastic anemia, dyserythropoietic anemia, hypothyroidism, liver disease.

GLUCOSE-6-PHOSPHATE DEHYDROGENASE DEFICIENCY

Deficiency in the major enzyme in the hexosemonophosphate shunt; results in a decrease in the oxidative protective mechanism of the RBC. An oxidative stress may cause RBC hemolysis.

Table 12.1: Normal Hemoglobin and Hematocrit Values by Age*		
Age	Hemoglobin (g/dL)	Hematocrit (%)
Newborn	16.8 (13.7–20.1)	55 (45–65)
2 wk	16.5 (13.0–20.0)	50 (42–66)
3 mo	12.0 (9.5–14.5)	36 (31–41)
6 mo–6 yr	12.0 (10.5–14.0)	37 (33–42)
7–12 yr	13.0 (11.0–16.0)	38 (34–40)
Women (adult)	14.0 (12.0–16.0)	42 (37–47)
Men (adult)	16.0 (14.0–18.0)	47 (42–52)

* Mean values with ranges in parentheses.

Adapted from Berman RE, et al., eds. Nelson Textbook of Pediatrics. 17th ed. Philadelphia: WB Saunders, 2004:1605.

Epidemiology
- X-linked inheritance; affects 10% of African-American males.
- African-American variant is less severe than Mediterranean variant

Clinical Manifestations
- Clinically and hematologically normal until "oxidative challenge"
- 6 to 24 hours after exposure to oxidative agent: dark urine, jaundice, pallor, tachycardia, nausea, abdominal pain
- 24 to 48 hours: low-grade fever, moderate splenomegaly and mild hepatomegaly

Diagnostics
- Glucose-6-phosphate dehydrogenase (G6PD) quantitation: G6PD concentration highest in young RBCs, so the presence of reticulocytosis leads to overestimation of true G6PD level.

During Hemolytic Episode:
- Normocytic, normochromic anemia with reticulocytosis
- Smear: anisocytosis (reflected by increased RDW), spherocytosis, blister cells, Heinz bodies on supravital staining with methyl violet (precipitates of denatured hemoglobin)
- Elevated unconjugated bilirubin
- Urine dipstick positive bilirubin
- Direct antiglobulin test negative (excludes autoimmune hemolysis)

Management
- Avoid oxidative stressors including sulfonamides, aspirin, fava beans, or antimalarial agents.
- Most episodes of acute hemolysis are self-limited with hemoglobin returning to normal within 3 to 6 weeks.
- If hemoglobin greater than 7 mg/dL but clinically stable and no hemoglobinuria, observe closely for 24 to 48 hours. If hemoglobin less than 7 mg/dL or between 7 and 9 mg/dL with continued brisk hemolysis (persistent hemoglobinuria), consider packed RBC transfusion (see Transfusion Medicine section).
- Management of neonatal jaundice associated with G6PD deficiency similar to approach for other causes of neonatal jaundice. Initiate prompt phototherapy if serum bilirubin greater than 15 mg/dL in first 2 days of life, or greater than 20 mg/dL during first week of life. Infants with the more severe type may require exchange transfusion to prevent kernicterus.

HEREDITARY SPHEROCYTOSIS

Disorder of the red blood cell membrane resulting in a decreased membrane surface area to intracellular volume ratio.

Epidemiology
- Most common in people of northern European heritage
- 75% inherited as autosomal dominant defects and 25% new mutations

Pathophysiology
- Defect or deficiency of red cell skeletal proteins (ankyrin, spectrin)
- Decreased deformability of the RBC results in sequestration in the spleen and depletion of membrane lipid results in spherocytes and premature destruction of RBCs

Clinical Manifestations
- Anemia: mild to severe; patients may have hyperhemolytic periods and are susceptible to an aplastic crisis from parvovirus.
- Jaundice, splenomegaly, gallstones
- 50% of patients present in the newborn period with jaundice.

Diagnostics
- Normocytic hemolytic anemia with increased reticulocyte count, high RDW and MCHC
- Smear: microspherocytes, hyperdense cells, polychromasia
- Increased red cell fragility on osmotic fragility test (may be normal in patients younger than 6 months of age)

Management
- Daily folic acid supplementation
- Splenectomy: for moderate to severe cases. This stops the hemolysis. If possible, delay splenectomy until the patient is 5 years of age or younger to decrease risk of infection.
- Transfusion support if needed

IRON DEFICIENCY ANEMIA

Microcytic anemia with a decreased reticulocyte count and increased RDW due to a deficiency of iron.

Etiology
- Dietary insufficiency, blood loss, or chronic intravascular hemolysis
- Most common etiology in children ages 1 to 3 years is dietary

Pathophysiology
- Iron is required for heme synthesis as well as other systemic enzymes (i.e., cytochromes).

Clinical Presentation
- Mild or moderate iron deficiency may have few overt symptoms
- Progressive pallor, irritability, fatigue, pica
- History of drinking greater than 24 ounces of cow's milk a day or transition to cow's milk before 12 months is common

Diagnostics
- CBC with reticulocyte count
- Iron studies: high TIBC, low transferrin, and low ferritin (first value to change with iron deficiency). Ferritin, an acute phase reactant, can be elevated in other conditions. The plasma iron level varies with recent consumption of iron and is not reliable.

Management
- Iron: 4–6 mg/kg/day of elemental iron in two to three divided doses
- Continue iron for 8 to 12 weeks after the Hb has normalized

- Dietary changes: limit milk intake; increase intake of iron-rich foods
- Response to therapy: reticulocyte count will start to increase in 72 hours

SICKLE CELL DISEASE

Normal adult hemoglobin is composed of four polypeptide chains ($2\alpha2\beta$). Sickle cell disease results from a genetic mutation in the β-globulin chain at the sixth position. Valine is substituted for glutamic acid. Sickle cell (HbS) trait is protective against malaria. 8% of African Americans are asymptomatic carriers.

- There are other genetic defects in the β-globulin chain resulting in abnormal hemoglobins (e.g., Hb C and Hb E). When these are combined with HbS, patients have a milder hemolytic anemia than sickle cell disease (SCD-SS).

Common Complications of Sickle Cell Disease

Painful Episode
- *Definition*: vaso-occlusive event resulting in an acute onset of pain; often involves hands and feet in infants.
- *Management*: some patients may be managed as outpatients with oral medications and hydration; for severe pain that requires hospitalization, appropriate pain control includes a combination of an anti-inflammatory agent such as ibuprofen or ketorolac (IV) with an opioid, and IV hydration.

Fever
- *Definition*: temperature > 38.5°C. Patients with SCD are more susceptible to bacterial infections because of splenic dysfunction. They are at highest risk for sepsis from encapsulated organisms, such as *Streptococcus pneumoniae*.
- *Management*: All fevers need to be urgently evaluated with a physical examination, blood culture, CBC with differential and a reticulocyte count; consider a urine culture, chest x-ray (dependent on age and symptoms); administration of antibiotics (ceftriaxone or high dose ampicillin) with observation
  - To prevent bacterial infections, patients with SCD should be vaccinated and take prophylactic penicillin VK (125 mg orally twice daily until age 3 years then 250 mg orally twice daily) from birth until at least the age of 5 years.

Splenic Sequestration
- *Definition*: intrasplenic trapping of red blood cells.
- *Clinical manifestations*: a decrease in hemoglobin with an acute enlargement of the spleen; in SCD-SS typical age of onset is 3 months to 5 years; often associated with acute viral/bacterial illnesses; in milder forms of SCD, SC or Sβ⁺ splenic sequestration can occur at an older age.
- *Management*: follow the hemoglobin and spleen size closely; if splenomegaly and anemia result in hypoxia, tachypnea, or significant tachycardia then transfuse with red blood cells (5 cc/kg), then reassess; transfusion causes remobilization of sequestered blood, resulting in a higher post transfusion hemoglobin than expected from the transfused blood alone.

Acute Chest Syndrome
- *Definition/Clinical manifestations*: clinical diagnosis based on the findings of fever, respiratory symptoms, and a new pulmonary infiltrate on chest x-ray (findings can lag behind the clinical symptoms). Multifactorial etiologies include bacteria (*Mycoplasma pneumoniae, Chlamydia pneumoniae, Staphylococcus aureus, S. pneumoniae*, or *Haemophilus influenzae*), viruses, or fat emboli.
- *Management*: antibiotics—macrolide (erythromycin, azithromycin, or clarithromycin) and ampicillin or a third-generation cephalosporin (cefotaxime or ceftriaxone); oxygen if hypoxic; pain control; incentive spirometry; red blood cell transfusion (simple or exchange) for respiratory or hemodynamic instability; may require intensive care monitoring

Aplastic Crisis
- *Definition:* marked anemia with reticulocytopenia, frequently secondary to Parvovirus infection. Patients with SCD are dependent upon their high reticulocyte count to maintain their hemoglobin secondary to their shortened RBC lifespan. During an acute infection with Parvovirus-B19 there is a temporary suppression of erythropoiesis.
- *Clinical manifestations:* increased fatigue, pallor, fever. Reticulocytopenia begins approximately 5 days after exposure and continues for 7 to 10 days.
- *Management:* packed RBC transfusion may be necessary if the patient is symptomatic.

THALASSEMIAS

Beta-thalassemia is usually the result of point mutations that result in impaired β-globulin production. There is only one gene on chromosome 11 for β-globulin.

- *β: thalassemia trait:* mild reduction in β-chain synthesis; heterozygous condition
- *β⁺:* markedly reduced β-chain synthesis (thalassemia intermedia when homozygous)
- *β⁰:* no detectable β-chains are made (thalassemia major or Cooley's anemia when homozygous)

Alpha-thalassemia is usually the result of large deletions that result in impaired α-globulin production. There are two genes on chromosome 16 for α-globulin, and four subsets of α-thalassemia:

- *Silent carrier:* deficient in one α gene
- *Alpha-thalassemia trait:* deficient in two α genes
- *Hemoglobin H (β4) disease:* deficient in three α genes
- *Hydrops fetalis:* deficient in all four α genes; not compatible with life; in utero the fetus develops hydrops fetalis

Clinical Manifestations
- *Alpha- and β-thalassemia trait:* mild microcytic anemia, asymptomatic
- *Hb H:* mild hemolytic anemia, jaundice, hepatosplenomegaly, gallstones
- *Homozygous β-thalassemia (β⁰ or β⁺):* massive hepatosplenomegaly, growth retardation, bony deformities including frontal bossing and maxillary prominence from extramedullary hematopoiesis (all preventable with aggressive transfusion therapy)
  - Precipitation of excess globulin chain on the red cell membrane causes a hemolytic anemia and hypersplenism.
  - Iron overload from chronic transfusions results in cirrhosis, endocrine abnormalities, cardiac dysfunction, and skin hyperpigmentation.

Diagnostics
- Hematologic parameters vary depending on severity of condition.
- *Alpha-thalassemia trait:* mild microcytic anemia, normal levels of HbA2 and HbF; Hb Barts on newborn screen
- *Beta-thalassemia trait:* mild microcytic, hypochromic anemia. HbA2 level 3.5% to 8%; HbF level 1% to 5% but significant variability depending on disease severity.
- *Hemoglobin H:* moderate hypochromic, microcytic anemia (Hb 7 to 10 g/dL); RBC fragmentation on peripheral smear and other findings of chronic hemolysis, reticulocytosis, Hb H (β4) on electrophoresis
- *Homozygous β-thalassemia (β⁰ or β⁺):* moderate to severe anemia (β⁰: Hb 3 to 7 g/dL; β⁺: 6 to 10 g/dL); reticulocytosis; HbF 20% to 100%; HbA2 2% to 7%; MCV 50 to 60 fL

Management
- No intervention for thalassemia trait
- Folic acid supplementation for those with Hb H
- Transfusion therapy for severe thalassemia; 10 to 15 mL/kg of pRBCs required every 3 to 4 weeks; keep pre-transfusion hemoglobin greater than 9.0 g/dL
- Chelation therapy for chronically transfused patients with iron overload; desferrioxamine, an iron chelator, is given SC/IV 5 to 7 days per week

TRANSIENT ERYTHROBLASTOPENIA OF CHILDHOOD (TEC)

An acquired, self-limited anemia in a previously healthy child characterized by bone marrow erythroblastopenia; can be severe

Etiology
- Unknown; often preceded by viral illness

Epidemiology
- Age of onset: 6 months to 4 years (80% are >1 year at diagnosis)

Clinical Manifestations
- Gradually progressive pallor in an otherwise healthy child
- No organomegaly, ecchymosis, petechiae, or jaundice
- Spontaneous recovery within 1 to 2 months

Diagnostics
- Hb level: 3 to 8 g/dL (normocytic and normochromic)
- Low reticulocyte count
- White blood cell and platelet counts are typically normal.
- Neutropenia (ANC < 1000/mm^3) in 10% of cases
- Bone marrow: decreased red blood cell precursors (not required for diagnosis)

Management
- Transfusions for symptomatic anemia (see Transfusion Medicine section)

Bleeding Disorders

COAGULATION STUDIES

Activated partial thromboplastin time (aPTT): measures the intrinsic clotting system, which includes factors V, VIII, IX, X, XI, XII, fibrinogen, prothrombin, and the other contact factors.

Prothrombin time (PT): measures the extrinsic clotting system which includes factor V, VII, X, fibrinogen and prothrombin (standardized with the International Normalized Ratio, INR).

Thrombin Time: measures the final step of the coagulation cascade with the conversion of fibrinogen to fibrin.

Bleeding Time: (poor test) evaluates platelet plug formation.

HEMOPHILIA

Bleeding disorder affecting primarily males that results from an inherited deficiency of either factor VIII (hemophilia A) or IX (hemophilia B).

Epidemiology
- Hemophilia A: 1 in 10,000 live male births (85%)
- Hemophilia B: 1 in 40,000 live male births (15%)
- Both are X-linked recessive; 70% inherited, 30% spontaneous mutation

Pathophysiology
- Factors VIII and IX participate in the activation of factor X
- Factor Xa converts prothrombin to thrombin, which can then cleave fibrinogen to fibrin leading to clot formation
- Deficiency of either factor VIII or IX results in impaired clot formation

Clinical Manifestations
- Hemophilia A and B are clinically indistinguishable
- Three major classifications (bleeding is related to factor levels): less than 1% = severe; 1% to 5% = moderate; 5% to 30% = mild

- Most common cause of morbidity is bleeding into joints (hemarthrosis), especially the knees, elbows, shoulders, ankles and hips.
- Life-threatening bleeding episodes may occur in the central nervous system or in the pharynx or retropharynx.
- Other bleeding sites include the urinary tract (with or without trauma), muscle bleeds, or excessive delayed postoperative bleeding. Post-circumcision bleeding is often the initial presentation in patients without a family history of hemophilia.

Diagnostics
- Prolonged PTT, normal PT
- Factor VIII or IX activity: decreased (factor IX levels are low in normal newborns making diagnosis difficult in the newborn period)
- Carrier testing and prenatal diagnosis are available.

Management
- Replace missing factor; in the past these factors were derived from pooled plasma, now there is recombinant therapy.
- Factor replacement therapy: determined by the type and severity of the bleed. Hemostatic levels are 35% to 40%. For life-threatening or major bleeds or head trauma, replace 100%. The initial half-life of factor VIII concentrate is 6 to 8 hours, with a subsequent half-life of 8 to 12 hours. The initial half-life of factor IX concentrate is 4 to 6 hours, with a subsequent half-life of 18 to 24 hours.
  - Dose of factor VIII (units) = % desired rise in plasma factor VIII × body weight (kg) × 0.5
  - Dose of factor IX (units) = % desired rise in plasma factor IX × body weight (may vary depending on product)
- Desmopressin (DDAVP): for mild hemophilia A only; causes the release of stored endogenously produced factor VIII and vWF
- Activated factor VII: directly activates the intrinsic pathway; can be used in patients with inhibitors.
- Aminocaproic acid: antifibrinolytic drug, good for oral bleeding; see formulary for dosing
- Avoid medicines that affect platelet function (e.g., aspirin, NSAIDs)
- Complications: chronic joint destruction causing pain and limiting mobility; transfusion transmitted diseases (not reported from recombinant products); inhibitor (neutralizing antibody) formation to factor VIII or factor IX.

VITAMIN K DEFICIENCY

Vitamin K is a fat-soluble vitamin found in green leafy vegetables, pork, soybeans, and liver. Vitamin K is required for the post-translational carboxylation of specific coagulation factors: II, VII, IX, X and protein C and S.

Pathophysiology
- Infants not supplemented with vitamin K after delivery may develop hemorrhagic disease of the newborn; infants born to mothers who were taking anticonvulsants, phenobarbital, and phenytoin are at high risk
- Insufficient dietary intake
- Altered gut colonization: vomiting, diarrhea, malabsorption (celiac disease, cystic fibrosis, biliary atresia, gastrointestinal tract obstruction), antibiotic use
- Drugs: warfarin

Diagnostics
- PT: prolonged
- PTT: prolonged
- Low vitamin K–dependent factors, normal factor V. Normal factor V helps distinguish from liver disease

Management
- Vitamin K may be given orally, SC, IM, or IV; see formulary for dosing; risk of anaphylaxis with IV administration.

VON WILLEBRAND DISEASE

Most common inherited bleeding disorder; caused by an abnormality of von Willebrand factor (vWF)

- Type 1: 70% to 80% of cases; decreased vWF levels (normal structure)
- Type 2A: 10% of cases; decreased intermediate and high molecular weight multimers; more severe than type 1
- Type 2B: 5% of cases; abnormal high molecular weight subunit; increased binding of vWF to normal platelets resulting in mild thrombocytopenia
- Type 2N: defect of the vWF factor VIII binding region; low factor VIII levels; mild hemophilia phenotype.
- Type 2M: functional defect of vWF; may be in the binding region; normal multimers.
- Type 3: homozygous deficiency; factor VIII is decreased and vWF levels are undetectable; severe disease; can present like hemophilia A

Epidemiology
- ~1% of the population
- Autosomal dominant inheritance is most common
- Acquired vWF deficiency may be due to Wilms tumor, hypothyroidism, SLE

Pathophysiology
- vWF is a large glycoprotein synthesized in megakaryocytes and endothelial cells.
- vWF has two roles in hemostasis: 1) allows platelets to adhere to damaged endothelium; 2) serves as a carrier protein for factor VIII.
- DDAVP can induce the release of stored vWF

Clinical Manifestations
- Mucocutaneous bleeding: easy bruising, recurrent epistaxis, menorrhagia
- Postsurgical or traumatic bleeding.

Diagnostics
Levels of vWF can fluctuate on a daily basis. Normal studies do not necessarily exclude vWD. When the diagnosis is strongly suspected, patients may require up to three sets of laboratory studies before excluding the diagnosis.

- Bleeding time (poor test): often prolonged (can be normal)
- PTT: often prolonged (can be normal)
- vWF antigen level (measures the total vWF plasma concentration)
- vWF activity (ristocetin cofactor): decreased in all types, except increased in type 2B. Ristocetin is an antibiotic that stimulates platelet aggregation in the presence of vWF.
- Factor VIII activity: decreased (can be normal)
- vW multimers: helps distinguish type of von Willebrand disease (vWD)

Management
- DDAVP: causes endothelial release of stored vWF with a two- to fivefold increase in plasma levels; most helpful for patients with type 1 vWD; side effects include hyponatremia, facial flushing, and headache; available in IV or intranasal formulations; see formulary for dosing
- Plasma-derived vWF concentrates (Humate P, Alphanate).
- Humate P—dosed in ristocetin units:

> 1 ristocetin U/kg = 2.4% increase in vWF antigen
> *no. ristocetin units = (weight in kg) × (% desired)/2.4*

- Cryoprecipitate: use if Alphanate and Humate P are not available; not detergent treated for viruses, but lower donor exposure than FFP
- Amicar: antifibrinolytic therapy; helpful in oral bleeding, see formulary for dosing

Thrombocytopenia

DIFFERENTIAL DIAGNOSIS

Increased Platelet Destruction
- Idiopathic thrombocytopenic purpura (ITP), disseminated intravascular coagulation (DIC), neonatal alloimmune thrombocytopenia (NAIT), hemolytic uremic syndrome, artificial heart valves or grafts, uremia, Kasabach-Merritt syndrome (see Dermatology chapter), thrombotic thrombocytopenic purpura (TTP), other immune-mediated thrombocytopenias (HIV, systemic lupus erythematosus)
- Medication-induced: aspirin, nitrofurantoin, heparin, sympathetic blockers, clofibrate, NSAIDs, sulfonamides, penicillin, quinidine, quinine, digoxin, procainamide, methyldopa, phenytoin, valproic acid, barbiturates, gold, cimetidine, ranitidine

Decreased Platelet Production
- Hereditary thrombocytopenias: thrombocytopenia-absent radii, amegakaryocytic thrombocytopenia, Wiskott-Aldrich syndrome, Fanconi anemia, trisomy 13, trisomy 18, inherited giant platelet disorders
- Marrow infiltration: acute lymphocytic leukemia, histiocytosis, lymphomas, neuroblastoma, storage diseases, marrow failure, aplastic anemia
- Medications: thiazide diuretics, chemotherapeutic agents, alcoholism, estrogen, furosemide, trimethoprim-sulfamethoxazole (Bactrim)
- Infection-induced: cytomegalovirus, Epstein-Barr virus, varicella, rubella, rubeola, mumps, parvovirus B19, tuberculosis, typhoid

Platelet Sequestration
- Splenomegaly

Other
- Pseudothrombocytopenia (clumped in collection tube); dilutional

IDIOPATHIC THROMBOCYTOPENIC PURPURA

An autoimmune disorder characterized by thrombocytopenia and mucocutaneous bleeding

Epidemiology
- Frequency: 4 to 8 cases per 100,000 children per year
- Peak age: 5 years; range, 2 to 6 years; male = female
- 80% resolve within 6 months.

Pathophysiology
- Autoantibodies (IgG) to glycoprotein IIb/IIIa complex and other platelet specific glycoproteins
- Autoantibody-coated platelets are cleared by macrophage Fcγ receptors in spleen and liver

Clinical Manifestations
- Sudden onset of petechiae, typically days or weeks after a viral illness
- Intracranial hemorrhage is rare; incidence is 0.1% to 0.5%

Diagnosistics
- CBC and peripheral smear with a direct antibody test
- Bone marrow aspirate may be helpful in atypical cases
- ITP is a diagnosis of exclusion. Other causes of thrombocytopenia need to be considered (see Differential Diagnosis of Thrombocytopenia).

Management
- There is little evidence that treatment changes the long-term outcome. Treatment should be strongly considered in patients with platelet counts less than 10,000/mm^3, "wet" mucosal bleeding or in toddlers with platelet counts less than 20,000/mm^3.

- *Immunoglobulin (IVIG):* 1 g/kg/day for 1 to 2 days; improves platelet count in 75% of patients within 48 hours; recommended for patients who are Rh negative; premedicate with acetaminophen and diphenhydramine hydrochloride (Benadryl) to decrease side effects
- *Anti-D (WinRho):* 50 to 75 µg/kg; patient must be Rh+; generally tolerated well; side effects include extravascular hemolysis (1 to 2 g/dL decrease in hemoglobin); rare intravascular hemolysis
- *Corticosteroids:* 1–4 mg/kg/day for 2 to 3 weeks. If the platelet count does not respond to IVIG or Anti-D, then bone marrow aspiration should be considered before starting steroids to rule out malignancy.
- *Chronic ITP (persistent thrombocytopenia for longer than 6 months):* splenectomy; prednisone; vincristine; azathioprine; cyclosporine; cyclophosphamide; rituximab

Thrombotic Disorders

MEDICATIONS FOR ANTICOAGULATION

Heparin
- *Mechanism of action:* complexes with natural anticoagulant antithrombin and accelerates activity; limits the expansion of thrombi by preventing fibrin formation; causes prolongation of aPTT (Table 12.2)
- *Dosage form:* parenteral
- *Dose:*
  - Initial bolus: 50–75 U/kg
  - Infusion: younger than 1 year = 28 U/kg/hour; older than 1 year = 20 U/kg/hour
- *Monitoring:* therapeutic aPTT is 60 to 85 seconds. Check first aPTT 4 hours after the loading dose and adjust according to Table 12.2.
- *Antidote:* protamine sulfate
- *Side effects:*
  - Bleeding
  - Heparin-induced thrombocytopenia (HIT): develops in 5% of adults taking more than 5 days of therapy; rare in children; 30% risk of thrombosis if HIT develops; immediately discontinue the heparin; consult hematology; consider direct thrombin inhibitor
  - Osteoporosis with long term use

Table 12.2: Unfractionated Heparin Dose Adjustment Based on Activated Partial Thromboplastin Time		
aPTT	Dose Adjustment	Time to Repeat aPTT
<50	50 U/kg bolus ↑ infusion rate by 10%	4 hr after rate change
50–59	↑ infusion rate by 10%	4 hr after rate change
60–85	Keep rate the same	Next day
86–95	↓ infusion rate by 10%	4 hr after rate change
96–120	Hold infusion for 30 min ↓ infusion rate by 10%	4 hr after rate change
>120	Hold infusion for 60 min ↓ infusion rate by 15%	4 hr after rate change

Adapted from Michelson AD, Bovill E, Andrew M. Antithrombotic therapy in children. Chest 1995;108(suppl):506–522s.

Low-Molecular-Weight Heparin

- *Mechanism of action:* accelerates antithrombin but inhibits factor Xa more than thrombin; long half life, good bioavailability; monitor with anti-factor Xa levels.
- *Dosage form:* subcutaneous
- *Dosing (enoxaparin):*

	Enoxaparin Treatment	Enoxaparin Prophylaxis
<2 months	1.5 mg/kg every 12 hours	0.75 mg/kg every 12 hours
>2 months	1 mg/kg every 12 hours	0.5 mg/kg every 12 hours

- *Monitoring:* therapeutic antifactor Xa level is 0.5 to 1 U/mL. Check anti-Xa level 4 hours after the second dose, and adjust as needed.
- *Antidote:* protamine causes partial reversal
- *Side effects:* bleeding; HIT
- Use with caution in patients with renal insufficiency; avoid in renal failure

Warfarin (Coumadin)

- *Mechanism of action:* inhibits vitamin K epoxide reductase, the vitamin K regenerative enzyme; decreases the plasma concentration of vitamin K dependent factors II, VII, IX, and X along with protein C and S; causes prolongation of PT.
- *Dosage form:* oral only (no solution formulations)
- *Dosing:* start while patient is therapeutic on Heparin or LMWH; initially reduces protein C (shortest half life) before other factors and has a prothrombotic effect. Prolongation of PT/INR begins at 24 to 48 hours but takes 5 to 7 days for full anticoagulant effect. See formulary for dosing.
- *Monitoring:* use the International Normalized Ratio (INR); therapeutic range depends on clinical scenario. For patients with deep venous thrombosis, therapeutic INR is 2 to 3.
- *Antidote:* Fresh frozen plasma, vitamin K
- *Side effects:* Bleeding; warfarin-related skin necrosis (result of starting warfarin without adequate anticoagulant coverage)
- Efficacy is affected by dietary intake of vitamin K

Thrombolytic Therapy

Necessary for life- or limb-threatening thrombosis; consider in patients with massive iliofemoral thrombosis; options include recombinant tissue plasminogen activator (r-tpa) or urokinase; local or systemic therapy.

- *Mechanism of action:* activates plasminogen to plasmin, which then degrades the fibrin clot
- *Dosing for systemic therapy:* urokinase 4400 U/kg bolus, followed by 4400 U/kg/hour; TPA (wide variation) 0.03–0.6 mg/kg/hour; duration depends on dose and clinical response.
- *Monitoring:* no specific test; fibrinogen should drop 25% to 50%; D-dimer and FDPs should increase; maintain platelet count over 50,000 and fibrinogen greater than 100 mg/dL; repeat imaging of thrombosis at 6 hours
- *Antidote:* none; if bleeding, stop drug; can give cryoprecipitate, red blood cells
- *Side effect:* bleeding
- *Precautions:* no IM injections; no urinary catheterization, rectal temperatures, or arterial puncture; patient should be in intensive care unit
- *Contraindications:* head trauma, CNS lesions, recent noncompressible hemorrhage, major surgical procedure

THROMBOSIS

Complete or partial occlusion of deep veins or arteries

Epidemiology
- Usually occurs in children with acquired and/or congenital risk factors for thrombosis

- *Congenital Risk Factors:* antithrombin deficiency; protein C deficiency; protein S deficiency; factor V Leiden (activated protein C resistance); prothrombin mutation; elevated lipoprotein(a); hyperhomocysteinemia; dysfibrinogenemia; heparin cofactor II deficiency
- *Acquired Risk Factors:* central venous catheter, antiphospholipid antibody syndrome, cancer, congenital heart disease, trauma, surgery, infection, severe dehydration, prematurity, pregnancy, nephrotic syndrome, inflammatory bowel disease, cystic fibrosis, sickle cell disease, estrogen, L-asparaginase

Pathophysiology
- Usually related to endothelial damage, venous stasis, or hypercoagulability; often in combination

Clinical Manifestations
- *Extremity deep vein thrombosis (DVT):* extremity pain, swelling, and discoloration. Consider this diagnosis in patients with a current or recent central venous catheter (CVC) in the affected extremity.
- *Superior vena cava syndrome:* swelling and plethora of the head and neck, and distended neck veins; caused by a large thrombus obstructing the superior vena cava (often associated with CVCs)
- *Pulmonary embolism (PE):* shortness of breath, pleuritic chest pain, cough, hemoptysis, fever and in the case of massive PE, hypotension and right heart failure.
- *Cerebral sinovenous thrombosis:* neonates often present with seizures, whereas older children often complain of headache, vomiting, seizures, and focal signs. They may also have papilledema and abducens palsy.
- *Renal vein thrombosis:* hematuria, abdominal mass, thrombocytopenia
- *Arterial thrombosis:* cold, pale, blue extremity with poor or absent pulses

Diagnostics
- *Laboratory studies:* see Box 12.1
- *Doppler ultrasound:* best for lower extremity DVT; may miss upper extremity DVT
- *Venography:* helpful for upper extremity DVT if ultrasound is negative and clinical suspicion is high; requires contrast
- *Ventilation-perfusion scan or spiral CT:* to evaluate for pulmonary embolism
- *Magnetic resonance venography of brain:* best test for sinovenous thrombosis (can be missed on CT)
- *CT venogram:* helpful for proximal thrombosis

Management
- *Anticoagulation:* patients with symptomatic deep venous thrombosis should receive anticoagulation with unfractionated heparin or low-molecular-weight heparin (LMWH). Unfractionated

---

Box 12.1: Recommended Laboratory Evaluation in Cases of Thrombosis

Complete blood cell count (CBC)
Prothrombin time (PT)
Activated partial thromboplastin time (aPTT)
Antithrombin activity
Protein C activity
Protein S, free and total
Factor V Leiden mutation
Prothrombin mutation
Fasting homocysteine
Lipoprotein (a)
Anticardiolipin antibody (IgG, IgM)
Dilute Russell viper venom time (test for lupus anticoagulant)

heparin can be immediately reversed and should be used in patients who may require urgent procedures. Maintaining a therapeutic effect is often easier with LMWH. Anticoagulation in neonates with cerebral sinovenous thrombosis is controversial.

Transfusion Medicine

CRYOPRECIPITATE TRANSFUSION

Product
• Contains fibrinogen, FVIII, vWF, and FXIII
• One unit is 5–15 mL; 150–250 mg/unit fibrinogen.

Indication
• Bleeding associated with hypofibrinogenemia.
• Bleeding in patients with factor VIII deficiency, vWD when other products are not available

Dosage
• Rule of thumb: 1 unit per 10 kg

FRESH-FROZEN PLASMA TRANSFUSION

Product
• Contains all of the clotting factors
• FFP 170–270 mL/unit; approximately 1 unit/mL all coagulation factors

Indication
• To correct a factor deficiency in a coagulopathic patient with bleeding or preoperatively (DIC, vitamin K deficiency, liver disease, congenital factor deficiency, warfarin overdose)

Dose
• 10–15 mL/kg
• Can follow response by measuring PT/PTT and/or monitoring clinical bleeding

PLATELET TRANSFUSION

Product
• Pooled concentrates vs. single donor product: single donor product decreases the risk of antiplatelet antibodies and is preferable for patients who require multiple platelet transfusions

Indication
• Thrombocytopenic patient who is bleeding, critically ill, or requires surgical intervention. Most procedures can be done if platelet count is maintained greater than 50,000/mm^3
• Given to prevent bleeding in patients with hypoproductive bone marrow when platelet count less than 10,000 to 20,000/mm^3 (chemotherapy, aplastic anemia)
• Patients with platelet function defects who require surgical procedures

Dose
• Children less than 30 kg: 10 mL/kg increases platelet count by ~50,000/mm^3
• Patients greater than 30 kg: one single donor unit; maximum volume of 15 mL/kg
• Platelets are stored at room temperature so there is a higher risk of bacterial contamination.

RED BLOOD CELL TRANSFUSION

Product
• Packed red blood cells (pRBCs); 180–350 mL/unit (Table 12.3)
• Should be typed and crossmatched prior to transfusion; can use O-negative or O-positive blood in emergent situation; O-negative is preferable, especially in females

Table 12.3: Risk of Viral Transmission with Red Blood Cell Transfusion in United States

Virus	Risk of Transmission
HIV I/II	1:2,135,000
Hepatitis C	1:1,935,000
Hepatitis B	1:205,000
HTLV	1:2,993,000

HIV, human immunodeficiency virus; HTLV, human T-cell leukemia virus. Data from Dodd RY, et al. Transfusion 2002;42:975–979.

- Hematocrit varies depending on the preservative solution: 55% to 65% in AS (adenine-saline) units to 70% to 75% in citrate-phosphate-dextrose-adenine (CPDA) units.
- Leuko-reduced product greatly reduces risk of cytomegalovirus transmission and febrile transfusion reactions
- Washed pRBCs: used for patients with IgA deficiency or a history of severe allergic transfusion reactions
- Irradiated pRBCs: prevents transfusion associated graft versus host disease; important for neonates and young infants, and immunocompromised patients

Indication
- Treatment of symptomatic anemia (tachycardia, hypotension, hypoxia) or acute blood loss greater than 15%

Dose
- Formula for RBC transfusion volume:

$$((TBV) \times (Desired\ HCT - Current\ HCT))/HCT\ of\ blood\ product$$

- Total blood volume (TBV) varies by age: 1) infants younger than 1 month. 85 mL/kg; 2) 1 month or older: 75 mL/kg; 3) adult: 4 to 5 L
- Rule of thumb: 5 cc/kg of RBCs increases hemoglobin 1 g/dL. In patients who weigh more than 70 kg: 1 unit of RBCs increases hemoglobin by 1g/dL
- For severe anemia in a hemodynamically compensated child, transfuse small volume, slowly (over approximately 4 hours) due to risk of precipitating heart failure; initial pRBC transfusion volume estimated as:

$$(1cc/kg\ of\ pRBC) \times (current\ hemoglobin)$$

TRANSFUSION COMPLICATIONS

Hemolytic Transfusion Reaction
- *Acute:* rapid destruction of red cells; usually due to blood type incompatibility (Table 12.4). Can result in fever, chills, hypotension shock, DIC, and renal failure; high mortality rate. If suspected, stop transfusion and institute supportive measures (fluids, pressors).
- *Delayed:* 3 to 10 days after transfusion, usually in patients who had previous transfusion as a result of an antibody that was present, but undetectable at the time of the transfusion. May result in fever, fatigue, jaundice, and dark urine
- *Evaluation:* check urine for hemoglobin, confirm patient blood type, screen for antibodies, repeat DAT on post-transfusion sera, culture donor blood for bacteria

Table 12.4: Risk of Adverse Transfusion Reactions

Hazard	Risk per Unit
Allergic transfusion reaction	1:50 to 1:100
Febrile transfusion reaction	1:100
Sepsis (bacterial contamination)	1:400 to 1:12,500
Anaphylaxis	1:20,000 to 1:50,000
Acute hemolysis (ABO mismatch)	1:6000 to 1:33,000
Death	1:500,000
Transfusion-related acute lung injury	1:5000

Data from AuBuchon JP, Kruskall MS. Transfusion safety: realigning efforts with risks. Transfusion 1997;37:1211–1216.

Febrile Nonhemolytic Transfusion Reaction
• Temperature increase of at least 1°C in association with transfusion, with or without chills; usually due to donor white cell antigens; uncommon with leuko-reduced products. Stop transfusion and evaluate (see previous section). Consider premedication with acetaminophen.

Allergic Transfusion Reaction
• Reaction to donor plasma proteins; ranges from minor urticaria to anaphylaxis. Stop transfusion, treat with antihistamines (epinephrine and steroids if respiratory compromise).

Infectious Disease Transmission
• See Table 12.3

Resources

AuBuchon JP, Kruskall MS. Transfusion safety: realigning efforts with risks. Transfusion 1997;37:1211–1216.

Behrman RE, Kliegman RM, Jenson HB: Nelson Textbook of Pediatrics. 16th ed. Philadelphia: WB Saunders, 2000.

Bolton-Maggs P, Tarantino MD, Buchanan GR, et al. The child with immune thrombocytopenic purpura: is pharmacotherapy or watchful waiting the best initial management? A panel discussion from the 2002 meeting of the American Society of Pediatric Hematology/Oncology. J Pediatr Hematol Oncol 2004;26:146–151.

Cines DB, Blanchette VS. Immune thrombocytopenic purpura. N Engl J Med 2002;346:995–1008.

Dodd RY, Notari EP IV, Stramer SL. Current prevalence and incidence of infectious disease markers and estimated window-period risk in the American Red Cross blood donor population. Transfusion 2002;42:975–979.

Hoyer LW. Hemophilia A. N Engl J Med 1994;330:38–47.

Iolascon A, Miraglia del Giudice E, Perrotta S, et al. Hereditary spherocytosis: from clinical to molecular defects. Haematologica 1998;83:240–257.

Jew R. The Children's Hospital of Philadelphia Pharmacy Handbook and Formulary. Huson, Ohio: Lexi-Comp, 2001.

Journeycake JM, Buchanan GR. Coagulation disorders. Pediatr Rev 2003;24:83–91.

Lanzkowsky P. Manual of Pediatric Hematology and Oncology. 3rd ed. San Diego: Academic Press, 2000.

Levine JS, Branch DW, Rauch J. The antiphospholipid syndrome. N Engl J Med 2002;346:752–763.

Manno CS. The promise of third-generation recombinant therapy and gene therapy. Semin Hematol 2003;40(suppl):s23–28.

Mannucci PM, Tuddenham E. The hemophilias—from royal genes to gene therapy. N Engl J Med 2001;44:1773–1779.

Michaels LA, Cohen AR, Zhao H, et al. Screening for hereditary spherocytosis by use of automated erythrocyte indexes. J Pediatr 1997;130:957–960.

Michelson AD, Bovill E, Andrew M. Antithrombotic therapy in children. Chest 1995;108:506–522s.

Miller DR, Baehner RL. Blood Diseases of Infancy and Childhood. 7th ed. St. Louis: CV Mosby, 1995.

Nathan DG, Orkin SH: Nathan and Oski's Hematology of Infancy and Childhood. 6th ed. Philadelphia: WB Saunders, 2003.

Olivieri NF, Brittenham GM. Iron-chelating therapy and the treatment of thalassemia. Blood 1997;89:739–761.

Olivieri NF. The beta-thalassemias. N Engl J Med 1999;341:99–109.

Revel-Vilk S, Schmugge M, Carcao MD, et al. Desmopressin (DDAVP) responsiveness in children with von Willebrand disease. J Pediatr Hematol Oncol 2003;25:874–879.

Roseff SD, Luban NL, Manno CS. Guidelines for assessing appropriateness of pediatric transfusion. Transfusion 2002;42:1398–1413.

Segel GB, Hirsh MG, Feig SA. Managing anemia in pediatric office practice: Part 1. Pediatr Rev 2002;23:75–84.

Segel GB, Hirsh MG, Feig SA. Managing anemia in pediatric office practice: Part 2. Pediatr Rev 2002;23:111–122.

Streif W, Andrew ME. Venous thromboembolic events in pediatric patients: diagnosis and management. Hematol Oncol Clin North Am 1998;12:1283–1312.

Weitz JI. Low-molecular-weight heparins. N Engl J Med 1997;337:688–698.

Deborah Palmer, MD, Richard M. Rutstein, MD, Theoklis E. Zaoutis, MD

Human Immunodeficiency Virus Infection

Chronic human immunodeficiency virus (HIV) infection leads ultimately to severe immuno-deficiency (acquired immunodeficiency syndrome [AIDS]). May be caused by HIV-1 or HIV-2. Centers for Disease Control (CDC) categories for HIV infection are based on clinical symptoms and immunologic status (CD4 lymphocyte count).

Epidemiology
- 90% of pediatric AIDS cases from perinatal transmission.
- In the United States, 0.15% to 0.2% of pregnant women are infected.
  - In untreated mothers, risk of transmission to infant is approximately 20% if not breastfeeding
- Risk factors for perinatal transmission: prolonged rupture of membranes, poor compliance with antiretroviral meds, untreated sexually transmitted disease, high viral load, low CD4, premature birth, chorioamnionitis, and advanced disease.

Differential Diagnosis
- Congenital immunodeficiency syndromes; congenital infections; other viral infections; malignancy; malnutrition or other causes of failure to thrive.

Pathophysiology
- Modes of HIV transmission in infants: 1) in utero (25%), 2) intrapartum (75% to 80%), 3) postnatal (breastfeeding increases risk by 14% to 29%)
- Modes of transmission in older children and adolescents: 1) sexual contact, 2) contaminated blood products, 3) perinatal

Clinical Manifestations
- Presentations vary but may include recurrent invasive bacterial or opportunistic infections and specific malignant neoplasms.
- Exam may be normal in first few months of life.
- 90% will have some physical exam abnormality by age 2 years.
- Most common findings: generalized lymphadenopathy, hepatomegaly, splenomegaly, recurrent thrush after 1 year of age, parotitis (recurrent or chronic); failure to thrive

Diagnostics
Concepts Related to Testing
- Nearly 100% of exposed infants have maternal HIV IgG antibodies. Exceptions: primary viremia and advanced disease.
- Maternal antibodies detectable in infant until age 15 to 18 months.
  - A positive HIV antibody test in an infant confirms maternal infection and infant exposure.

Testing the Infant with Known Maternal Infection
- HIV DNA polymerase chain reaction (PCR) and/or culture at birth, 1 to 2 month age, and 4 month age. Immediately repeat PCR/culture if any test is positive.
- Must have two positive virologic assays at two different times to be diagnosed with HIV infection (two cultures or two DNA PCR).
- Sensitivity of DNA PCR is 38% at 48 hours life, 93% by 2 weeks, and 96% by 4 weeks. Specificity = 96% to 98%.

- Considered HIV negative if PCR/culture persistently negative at greater than 4 months of age in the absence of breastfeeding, but must continue antibody testing until greater than18 months of age (enzyme-linked immunosorbent assay [ELISA]/Western Blot).
- Test for HIV IgG with ELISA every 3 months.
- HIV is ruled out if ELISA/Western Blot is negative at 18 months in absence of hypogamma-globulinemia and clinical symptoms, and with negative virologic assays.
- Recommend final HIV antibody test at 24 months of age for those with negative virologic assays and antibody tests.
- Test CD4 at 1 month and 3 months. If tests HIV positive, continue checking CD4 levels and viral loads every 3 months.

Testing the Infant with Unknown Maternal Status
- Test mother or baby for HIV IgG by ELISA/Western Blot after obtaining appropriate informed consent.
- Only do virologic tests if the screening antibody test is positive.

Testing in Older Children and Adolescents
- If greater than18 months old, perform screening antibody test with ELISA and confirmation with Western Blot. If positive results, repeat tests. HIV infection confirmed with two positive ELISA/Western blot assays.

Management
Laboratory Monitoring
- CD4 count: marker of immune function and risk of opportunistic infection
- HIV RNA quantification (viral load, VL): marker of viral burden
- Immune categories (Table 13.1)

Therapies
- Highly active anti-retroviral therapy (HAART): a combination drug approach to viral suppression.
- Who to treat: less than 1 yr age regardless of clinical, immune, or virologic status; older children with clinical symptoms of HIV; Evidence of immune suppression (low CD4 total or %); Asymptomatic child 1 year or older: may initiate therapy if falling CD4, increasing VL, or at any time; If social situation is supportive towards adherence.

Specific Agents
NUCLEOSIDE REVERSE TRANSCRIPTASE INHIBITORS (NRTIS)
- Common side effects: nausea, vomiting, diarrhea, abdominal pain, headache
- More severe side effects of this class include severe hypersensitivity reactions, peripheral neuropathy, pancreatitis, lactic acidosis, hyperuricemia, neutropenia, myositis, and liver toxicity.

Table 13.1: Category of Immune Suppression Based on CD4 Percentage and by Absolute CD4 Count		
Category of Suppression		
None (1)	Moderate (2)	Severe (2)
CD4%			

	None (1)	Moderate (2)	Severe (2)
CD4%	>25%	15–25%	<15%
Absolute CD4 count*			
Age < 12 mo	>1500	750–1499	<750
Age 1–5 yr	>1000	500–999	<500
Age 6–12 yr	>500	200–499	<200

*Per cubic millimeter.

- Specific NRTIs:
  - *Abacavir* (ABC, Ziagen)
  - *Didanosine* (ddl, Videx)
  - *Lamivudine* (3TC, Epivir)
  - *Stavudine* (d4T, Zerit)
  - *Tenofovir*
  - *Zalcitabine* (ddC, HIVID)
  - *Zidovudine* (ZDV, AZT, Retrovir)
  - *Trizivir* (ZDV + 3TC + ABC)
  - *Combivir* (ZDV + 3TC)

NON-NUCLEOSIDE REVERSE TRANSCRIPTASE INHIBITORS (NNRTIS)
- *Mechanism of action*: bind directly to enzymatic site of reverse transcriptase to inhibit without requiring metabolic activation by phosphorylation.
  - One point mutation may confer resistance to all NNRTIs.
- Common side effects: headache, fatigue, gastrointestinal complaints, rash, interact with P450
- *Delavirdine* (DLV, Rescriptor): Not recommended to be used with antihistamines, sedative-hypnotics, calcium channel blockers, amphetamines, cisapride or warfarin
- *Efavirenz* (EFV, Sustiva): central nervous system (CNS) effects (hallucinations, confusion, somnolence), teratogenic, mixed inducer/inhibitor of P450
- *Nevirapine* (NVP, Viramune): Stevens-Johnson, hepatitis, hypersensitivity reactions

PROTEASE INHIBITORS
- *Mechanism of action*: inhibit viral protease with little interaction with host proteases.
- Common side effects: interact with cytochrome P450, many drug interactions, hepatitis, hyperglycemia, spontaneous bleeding in hemophiliacs, pancreatitis, increased cholesterol/triglycerides
- Specific protease inhibitors:
  - *Amprenavir* (APV, Agenerase)
  - *Atazanavir* (Reyataz)
  - *Fosamprenavir* (Lexiva)
  - *Indinavir* (IDV, Crixivan)
  - *Lopinavir/Ritonair* (Kaletra)
  - *Nelfinavir* (NFV, Viracept)
  - *Ritonavir* (RTV, Norvir)
  - *Saquinavir* (SQV, Invirase)

Typical HAART Regimens
- 2 NRTIs + 1 PI (NFV, RTV, or lopinavir/ritonair)
- Efavirenz + 2NRTIs + PI (NFV)
- Other regimens also used

Prevention of Maternal Transmission
- ZDV (AZT) (300 mg two times per day) starting at 14 to 34 weeks' gestation.
- Maximize HAART therapy to lower viral load.
- Intrapartum ZDV treatment: 2 mg/kg IV over 1 hour followed by continuous infusion 1 mg/kg/hr
- Postnatal ZDV for infant beginning 8 to 12 hours after birth: 2 mg/kg every 6 hours (adjust for prematurity); continue until 6 weeks age.
- Regimens containing ZDV found to be most effective (decrease risk of MCT from 20% to less than 5%). In resource-poor countries, may use short course of Nevirapine (single dose to mother and infant).

Prophylaxis Against Opportunistic Infections
- *Pneumocystis carinii* pneumonia (PCP) prophylaxis in infants before diagnosis: discontinue AZT at 6 weeks age and start TMP-SMX prophylaxis (dosing based on trimethoprim component: 5–10 mg/kg/day divided twice daily or 150 mg/m^2/day divided twice daily for three consecutive days each week). Continue prophylaxis until two or more negative virologic test results (one at or after 4 months).
- PCP prophylaxis in greater than12 months if low CD4.
- *Mycobacterium avium* complex (MAC) prophylaxis if CD4 less than 100/mm^3. Azithromycin (20 mg/kg/dose given once each week, maximum 1200 mg/dose), clarithromycin (15 mg/kg/day divided twice daily, orally, maximum 1 g/day) or rifabutin (5 mg/kg/day given once daily, orally, maximum 300 mg/day).

FEVER IN HUMAN IMMUNODEFICIENCY VIRUS

Differential Diagnosis
- *First consider common viral and bacterial etiologies as in any pediatric patient* (e.g., otitis media, sinusitis, pneumonia, urinary tract infection). Pneumococcal bacteremia and pneumonia are the most common serious causes of fever.
- *Opportunistic infections:*
  - *PCP, Toxoplasma gondii*
  - *Bacterial:* MAC, *Mycobacterium tuberculosis, Cryptosporidium, Microsporidium*
  - *Fungal:* Candidiasis, *Cryptococcal neoformans, Aspergillus, Histoplasma capsulatum, Coccidioides immitis*
  - *Viral:* Cytomegalovirus (CMV), varicella-zoster virus, herpes simplex virus, Epstein-Barr virus (and related malignancies)

Clinical Manifestations of Opportunistic Infections
- Duration of illness greater than 7 days
- Chronic low grade fever
- Systemic complaints: weight loss, night sweats, malaise, fatigue
- Chronic cough or worsening shortness of breath
- Gastrointestinal complaints: abdominal pain, diarrhea
- Change in mental status or declining mental capacity
- *Risk factors:* Low CD4 ($<200/mm^3$), prior bacteremia, pneumonia, PCP, sinusitis, otitis, diarrheal disease, or other opportunistic infection; methoxasole-trimethoprim (Bactrim) prophylaxis (indicates PCP risk); clarithromycin or rifabutin prophylaxis (indicates MAC risk).

Diagnostics
Laboratory Studies
- CBC w/differential
- Blood culture with AFB smear, possible CMV antigenemia
- Urine culture, CMV rapid shell vial from urine
- Stool cultures, stool O/P, *Giardia, Cryptosporidium*, acid-fast bacteria (AFB), CMV culture
- *If respiratory symptoms:* lactate dehydrogenase; consider bronchoscopy: send silver stain, Gram stain, viral panel, AFB, bacterial, fungal, and CMV cultures
- *If abdominal complaints:* LFTs, amylase, lipase
- *If CNS symptoms (headache, neck pain) or ill-appearing:* send cerebrospinal fluid (CSF) for cell count, protein, glucose, gram stain, culture, herpes simplex virus (HSV) PCR, cryptococcal antigen. Save specimen for possible Lyme, varicella, CMV. Check for presence of antibodies to toxoplasmosis and cryptococcal antigen in serum.

Radiology
- Chest x-ray for respiratory symptoms
- If abdominal complaints or chronic fever: consider abdominal ultrasound or CT scan: large nodes indicate MAC or lymphoma.
- If suspicious of CNS process: obtain brain MRI with contrast

Ophthamology Consultation
- Consider to detect or manage CMV retinitis, herpes keratitis, papilledema (CNS mass lesion)

Common Opportunistic Infections: Diagnosis and Treatment
Recurrent Bacterial Infections (risk may be independent of CD4 count)
- Pneumococcal bacteremia (10% per year for first 3 years of life.)
- Pneumonia or sinusitis
- Likely due to defects in B-cell mediated immunity.
- Consider monthly IVIG or antibiotic prophylaxis.

Pneumocystis carinii *Pneumonia*
- Most common AIDS-defining illness in children
- Progressive dyspnea, tachypnea, hypoxemia, dry cough, fever

- May have more insidious onset
- Lactate dehydrogenase greater than 500 U/mL (indicates lung injury, not specific PCP)
- Chest x-ray: can be normal (~10% of cases). Classically: diffuse alveolar or interstitial infiltrates that spread from hilum to periphery
- Diagnosis: silver stain and immunofluorescent stains of respiratory specimens detects cyst forms
  - Children younger than 5 years of age should undergo bronchoalveolar lavage (BAL) initially
  - Diagnostic yield in children 5 years of age and older: Induced sputum, 20% to 40%; BAL, 75% to 95%; transbronchial biopsy, 75% to 95%; open lung biopsy, 90% to100%
- Empiric therapy: IV TMP-SMX 20 mg/kg/d divided every 6 hours. If diagnosis confirmed, treat for 21 days (oral therapy when stable)
- Adjunctive treatment with prednisone improves survival in those with severe illness: 2 mg/kg/d for 7 to 10 days followed by 10- to 14-day taper.

Mycobacterium avium *Complex*
- Disseminated disease, occurs in 5% to 10% of infected children
- CD4 less than 200/mm^3, usually less than 50/mm^3
- Indolent presentation: fever, weight loss, abdominal pain
- Diagnosis: culture from blood or tissue. Blood cultures may take 3 to 4 weeks to become positive. Use special collection tubes
- Abdominal ultrasound or CT scan usually reveals adenopathy
- Bone marrow and lymph node biopsies: acid-fast bacilli within macrophages
- Treat with clarithromycin or azithromycin plus ethambutol and/or rifabutin.
- Begin prophylaxis with clarithromycin or rifabutin if CD4 less than 100/mm^3 (see above in Prophylaxis against opportunistic infections for dosing for prophylaxis)

Mycobacterium tuberculosis
- Also refer to *Tuberculosis* within Infectious Diseases chapter
- Usually primary pulmonary infection but 10% to 50% have extrapulmonary disease: mastoid, bones, joints, skin, CNS
- A result of 5 mm on purified protein derivative test is positive
- Treatment with four drugs until susceptibilities return: isoniazid, rifampin, pyrazinamides, and ethambutol or streptomycin

| Table 13.2: Characteristics of the Exposure Source and Risk of HIV Transmission ||
HIV Infection Status of Exposure Source	Risk of HIV Transmission
Known not to be infected with HIV	No risk
HIV infection status unknown, HIV risk status unknown	Unquantified
HIV infection status unknown, but known not to have risk factors*	Low
HIV infection status unknown but known to have 1 or more risk factors*	Intermediate
Known to be infected with HIV	High

HIV, human immunodeficiency virus.

*Risk factors for HIV infection include male homosexual activity, injection drug use, blood transfusion or blood product infusion before 1985, or sexual activity with a member of a high-risk group. Some persons who have sex with members of a high-risk group do not identify themselves as at risk, because they are unaware of the risk history of their sexual partner. Their risk of HIV infection is related to the prevalence of HIV infection in their immediate community.

(Reprinted with permission from Havens PL, et al. Postexposure prophylaxis in children and adolescents for nonoccupational exposure to human immunodeficiency virus. Pediatrics 2003;111:1475–1489.)

Candidiasis
- Oral: thrush, hypertrophic candidiasis, atrophic candidiasis, or angular cheilitis. Treat with nystatin or oral azoles (e.g., fluconazole)
- Esophageal: substernal or abdominal pain, burning and dysphagia; barium swallow study shows distinctive pattern; endoscopy to exclude HSV or CMV; treat with fluconazole for 21 days.

Cryptococcus neoformans
- Much more common in adults than in children
- Chronic basilar meningitis and encephalitis
- Insidious onset; may be asymptomatic
- Headache, nausea/vomiting, cognitive dysfunction, psychosis

Table 13.3: Exposure Type and Exposure Risk Category for HIV

Exposure Type	Exposure Risk Category
Cutaneous exposure	
Fluid on intact skin or bite without skin break	No risk identified
Skin with compromised integrity (eczema, chapped skin, dermatitis, abrasion, laceration, open wound)	Low to intermediate
Traumatic skin wound with bleeding in donor and recipient*	High
Mucous membrane exposure	
Kissing	No risk identified
Oral sex, human milk (single ingestion), splash to eye or mouth	Low
Receptive vaginal sex without trauma	Intermediate
Receptive anal intercourse	High
Traumatic sex with blood (sexual assault)	High
Percutaneous exposure	
Superficial scratch with sharp object, including a needle found in the community	No risk identified
Puncture wound with *solid* needle	Low
Puncture wound with *hollow* needle *without* visible blood	Low
Body piercing or bite with break in skin	Low
Puncture wound with hollow needle with visible blood	Intermediate
Puncture wound with large-bore hollow needle with visible blood on needle, or needle recently used in source patient artery or vein	High

*For example, in a fight, a blow to the mouth might break a tooth that bleeds and lacerates the fist that also bleeds. If there was mixing of blood, both persons may be at risk.

(Reprinted with permission from Havens PL, et al. Postexposure prophylaxis in children and adolescents for nonoccupational exposure to human immunodeficiency virus. Pediatrics 2003;111:1475–1489.)

- Change in mental status on presentation is poor prognostic sign
- Diagnosis: CSF pressure increased in two thirds of patients; Cryptococcal antigen in CSF is positive in greater than 90%; gold standard is culture.
- Treatment: Amphotericin B with flucytosine

Cytomegalovirus

- Chorioretinitis: blurry vision, floaters; leads to retinal detachment and loss of vision; diagnosis based on typical retinal lesions
- Colitis: diarrhea, abdominal pain, weight loss, anorexia, and fever; must be diagnosed with mucosal biopsy
- Pneumonitis: cough, progressive dyspnea and hypoxemia; diffuse interstitial infiltrates; diagnosis based on intracellular inclusions in lung tissue or bronchoalveolar macrophages in absence of other pathogens
- CNS: encephalitis, radiculomyelitis, neuritis; mental status change, lethargy, cranial nerve findings, deafness, ataxia, vertigo; CD4 less than 50/mm^3; send CSF for CMV PCR.
- Treatment: ganciclovir, foscarnet, or cidofovir

Varicella Zoster

- Recurrent, persistent, and chronic skin infections
- Risk of life-threatening dissemination (especially liver, lungs, and CNS)
- Treatment: IV acyclovir (1500 mg/m^2/day divided every 8 hours) for 7 to 10 days; varicella immune globulin (VZIG) within 96 hours after close exposure to infected person.

POST-EXPOSURE PROPHYLAXIS

These recommendations for management of children with nonoccupational exposure to HIV are adapted from the American Academy of Pediatrics (Pediatrics 2003;111:1475–1489).

- Risk of transmission *per exposure event*: blood transfusion: 0.95; perinatal exposure: 0.13 to 0.45; needlestick in health care: 0.0032; ingestion of human milk: 0.00001 to 0.00004

Table 13.4: Suggested Approach* to PEP on the Basis of Exposure Risk Category and HIV Infection Status of the Source

Exposure Risk Category[†]	HIV Infection Status of Source[‡]	Suggested Approach
No risk identified	Any	No PEP
Any	Not HIV infected	No PEP
Low, intermediate, or high	Unknown	Consider PEP
Low or intermediate risk	HIV infected	Consider PEP
High risk	HIV infected	Recommend PEP

HIV, human immunodeficiency virus; PEP, post-exposure prophylaxis.

*PEP is not recommended if 1) exposure occurred > 72 hours previously, 2) exposed person refuses PEP, or 3) exposed person is unwilling or unable to commit to 28 days of therapy and appropriate follow-up. When considering PEP, the approach is suggested on the basis of type and severity of exposure, fluid involved, and HIV infection status of the exposure source. Characteristics of the exposed patient are also considered. Given the absence of compelling data on effectiveness of PEP, clinicians may make different, reasonable decisions in similar clinical circumstances.

[†]See Table 13.2.

[‡]See Table 13.1.

(Reprinted with permission from Havens PL, et al. Postexposure prophylaxis in children and adolescents for nonoccupational exposure to human immunodeficiency virus. Pediatrics 2003;111:1475–1489.)

- Steps in deciding whether to administer post-exposure prophylaxis (PEP): 1) identify HIV infection status of source (Table 13.2); 2) determine exposure risk category (Table 13.3); 3) combine results of steps 1 (HIV status of source) and 2 (exposure risk category) to identify suggested approach (Table 13.4)
- Optimal PEP regimen is not known, most clinicians use 2 NRTIs and 1 protease inhibitor. Additional information available at CDC Divisions of HIV/AIDS Prevention (www.cdc.gov.hiv/DHAP:htm).

Resources

Abrams EJ. Opportunistic and other clinical manifestations of HIV disease in children. Pediatr Clin North Am 2000;47:79–105.

AIDSinfo. Available at: http://aidsinfo.nih.gov/drugs/. Accessed November 16, 2004.

American Academy of Pediatrics. 2000 Red Book: Report of the Committee on Infectious Diseases. 25th ed. Elk Grove Village, IL: AAP, 2000.

Buckley MR, Gluckman ST, eds. HIV Infection in Primary Care. Philadelphia: WB Saunders, 2002.

Clifford DB. Opportunistic viral infections in the setting of human immunodeficiency virus. Semin Neurol 1999;19:185–192.

Committee on Pediatric AIDS. Evaluation and medical treatment of the HIV-exposed infant. Pediatrics 1997;99:909–917.

Marra CM. Bacterial and fungal brain infections in AIDS. Semin Neurol 1999;19:177–184.

Perez Mato S, Van Dyke RB. Pulmonary infections in children with HIV infection. Semin Respir Infect 2002;17:33–46.

Nielsen K, Bryson YJ. Diagnosis of HIV infection in children. Pediatr Clin North Am 2000;47:39–63.

Pickering LK, ed. 2000 Red Book: Report of the Committee on Infectious Diseases. 25th ed. Elk Grove Village, Ill: American Academy of Pediatrics, 2000.

Rutstein RM. Prevention of perinatal HIV infection. Curr Opin Pediatr 2001;13:408–416.

Working Group on Antiretroviral Therapy and Medical Management of HIV Infected Children. Guidelines for the Use of Antiretroviral Agents in Pediatric HIV Infection. Available at: http://aidsinfo.nih.gov/. Accessed December 7, 2004.

Approach to Primary Immunodeficiency

MAJOR CATEGORIES

The five major categories of primary immune deficiencies reflect the various arms of the immune system (Table 14.1):

T Cell Disorders ("cellular immunodeficiency")
- Present at birth or in early infancy
- Develop prolonged and severe respiratory viral infections
- Predisposition for fungal infections, mycobacterial infections, *Salmonella typhi,* and opportunistic infections such as *Pneumocystis jiroveci* (formerly *Pneumocystis carinii*)
- Association with autoimmune diseases

B Cell Disorders ("humoral immunodeficiency")
- Usually do not present until 3 to 6 months because of maternal antibodies; exception is common variable immunodeficiency (CVID), which presents in adolescence and early adulthood
- Predisposition for common infections: enteroviral infections (can be fatal in X-linked agammaglobulinemia [XLA] or CVID), bacterial infections (*Streptococcus pneumoniae, Haemophilus influenzae, Staphylococcus aureus, Pseudomonas aeruginosa, Neisseria meningitidis, Clostridium fetus, Mycoplasma hominis, Ureaplasm urealyticum*), and protozoal infections (*Giardia lamblia*)

Combined T Cell and B Cell Disorders
- Most present within the first year of life. One exception is the progressive presentation of ataxia-telangiectasia at ages 1 to 10 years
- Predisposed to common bacterial, viral and fungal diseases, and opportunistic and mycobacterial infections

Phagocyte Disorders
- Present in early childhood to adolescence
- Predisposition to catalase-positive organisms, *S. aureus, Burkholderia cepacia, S. typhi, Nocardia asteroides, Serratia marcescens, Candida* spp, *Aspergillus fumigatus*
- Poor wound healing, delayed separation of the umbilical cord, and umbilical granulomas
- Myobacterial infections

Complement Disorders
- Predisposition for common bacterial (*Neisseria* spp) and viral infections
- Associated with autoimmune disorders and immune complex disease (systemic lupus erythematosus)

WARNING SIGNS

- Recurrent otitis (>8 episodes), sinusitis (>2 episodes), or pneumonia (>2 episodes) in 1 year (from Jeffrey Modell Foundation)
- Failure to thrive
- Recurrent skin or organ abscesses

Table 14.1: Classification of Primary Immunodeficiencies

T Cell Disorders (Cellular)	22q deletion syndromes* Severe combined immune deficiency (T – B+)*
B Cell Disorders (Humoral)	Common variable immune deficiency* IgG subclass deficiency Selective IgA deficiency Transient hypogammaglobulinemia of infancy Agammaglobulinemia* Ataxia-telangiectasia*
Combined T and B Cell Disorders	Hyper IgM syndromes Severe combined immune deficiency* Wiskott-Aldrich syndrome* X-linked lymphoproliferative disease
Phagocyte Disorders	Chédiak-Higashi syndrome* Chronic granulomatous disease* Hyper IgE syndrome* Kostmann syndrome Leukocyte adhesion deficiency types I and II Macrophage activation defects Myeloperoxidase deficiency
Complement Disorders	Properdin deficiency Early component deficiencies (C1–C4) Terminal component deficiencies (C5–C9)

*Denotes topic discussed in detail in chapter.

- Persistent thrush in mouth or elsewhere on skin (after age 1 year)
- Need for intravenous antibiotics to clear common infections
- Family history of immunodeficiency

DIFFERENTIAL DIAGNOSIS OF NEUTROPENIA

- *Congenital:* congenital neutropenia with eosinophilia; Kostmann syndrome (severe congenital neutropenia); cyclic neutropenia; Barth syndrome (X-linked methylglutaconic aciduria type II); Fanconi anemia; trichothiodystrophy with chronic neutropenia; trimethylaminuria
- *Metabolic diseases associated with neutropenia:* Shwachman-Diamond syndrome; glycogen-storage disease type 1b; propionic acidemia; methylmalonic acidemia
- *Infection:* HIV, parvovirus, hepatitis viruses, malaria
- *Immune-mediated:* isoimmune neonatal neutropenia; autoimmune neutropenia of infancy; autoimmune neutropenia; Felty syndrome
- *Primary immunodeficiency:* X-linked agammaglobulinemia; common variable immune deficiency; hyper-IgM syndrome; cartilage-hair hypoplasia (CHH); reticular dysgenesis; Chédiak-Higashi syndrome (CHS)
- *Nutrition:* vitamin B_{12}, transcobalamin II, or folate deficiency; copper deficiency
- *Hematologic diseases:* aplastic anemia; myelodysplastic syndromes; WHIM syndrome (autosomal dominant, warts-hypogammaglobulinemia-infections-myelokathexis)

- *Drug-induced neutropenia*: chloramphenicol, penicillin, sulfonamides, aspirin, acetaminophen, phenylbutazone, barbiturates, benzodiazepines, chlorpromazine, phenothiazines, levamisole

DIAGNOSTIC APPROACH

- Serum immunoglobulin levels and IgG subclasses
- Response to vaccination: polyribose phosphate (PRP) antibodies after HiB vaccination, pneumococcal serotype-specific antibodies after pneumococcal conjugate (Prevnar) or polysaccharide (Pneumovax) vaccination, tetanus and diphtheria antibodies after DTaP vaccination
- IgM antibodies against ABO polysaccharides (called isohemagglutinins) are formed in the first 6 months. Normal values are available above age 2.
- Flow cytometry for T cell and B subsets
- Respiratory oxidative burst measurement for phagocytic defects
- Blood smear: for platelet size and morphology, cellular inclusions in neutrophils

Common Immunodeficiencies

22q DELETION SYNDROMES

A heterogeneous disorder of conotruncal cardiac defects, developmental delay, learning disorder, craniofacial dysmorphology, and T cell deficiency

- DiGeorge syndrome, velocardiofacial syndrome, and similar syndromes involve deletions within the 22q region, but wide heterogeneity of the phenotype results from differing amounts of chromosomal loss
- Fluorescent in situ hybridization shows monosomic loss of the 22q11.2 region; 5% of patients with DiGeorge syndrome do not have 22q11 deletion (10p14 region is implicated in some)

Epidemiology
- 1/3000 to 1/4000 live births
- Found in 8% of children with cleft palates and 1% with congenital heart disease

Etiology
- Deletion of a region in chromosome 22q11.2. Putative gene is *tbx1*

Differential Diagnosis
- HIV infection; T cell deficiencies

Pathophysiology
- Variably deficient embryonic development of the third and fourth pharyngeal pouches due to defective neural crest migration results in thymic hypoplasia, parathyroid dysfunction, and heart and facial defects
- Thymic hypoplasia: variable T cell deficiency in 80% and absent T cells in 0.5%
- Normal B cell count and function. Immunoglobulin levels are usually normal.

Clinical Manifestations
- Neonatal tetany and seizures from hypocalcemia (10% to 30%). The hypocalcemia is self-limiting; most children do not require calcium supplementation beyond 1 year.
- Congenital heart disease in 80% to 90%: Most common associated defects include interrupted aortic arch, right arch, ventricular septal defect, aberrancy of right subclavian and internal carotid arteries, tetralogy of Fallot, and truncus arteriosus.
- Recurrent otitis associated with decreased midface development and small eustachian tubes. Conductive hearing loss in 75%.
- Speech delay, non-verbal learning disorders, and mild mental retardation (40% to 50%)

- Paranoid schizophrenia and depression in adolescence
- Failure to thrive due to oromotor feeding difficulties
- Autoimmune diseases occur in 9%.
- Low set, cupped or folded ears; small mouth; short philtrum; hypertelorism, high-arched or cleft palate, micrognathia

Diagnostics
- Chromosome 22q11 FISH
- Serum calcium levels
- Echocardiography, ECG, chest x-ray
- Flow cytometry for T cell and B cell subsets and in vitro functional assays

Management
- Do not defer vaccination except with evidence of significant immune compromise
- All blood products must be CMV negative
- Thymic transplant under research for severe immunodeficiency
- Calcium supplementation if necessary

ATAXIA-TELANGIECTASIA

Combined T lymphocyte and immunoglobulin deficiency with neurocutaneous findings and a predisposition for malignancy

Epidemiology
- Incidence between 1/100,000 to 1/300,000, equal across races

Etiology
- Ataxia telangiectasia mutated (ATM) protein (gene on chromosome 11q22.3)
- Autosomal recessive inheritance

Pathophysiology
- ATM is involved with DNA breakpoint detection and cell cycle arrest

Differential Diagnosis
- DNA breakage defects: Nijmegen breakage syndrome, Berlin breakage syndrome, Fanconi pancytopenia, Bloom syndrome
- Early onset cerebellar ataxia: Pelizaeus-Merzbacher (X-linked leukodystrophy), Joubert syndrome (underdeveloped cerebellar vermis), Friedreich's ataxia (most prevalent inherited ataxia)

Clinical Manifestations
- Difficulty walking at the end of the first year of life; most are wheelchair bound by the teenage years. 70% of patients with ataxia telangiectasia have recurrent respiratory infections.
- Truncal ataxia by age 1 to 2, then appendicular ataxia, progressively worse
- Bulbar telangiectasias, at age 3 to 5. Other telangiectasias, on the face (ears, palate), extremities, and trunk, appear from ages 3 to 7.
- Deep tendon reflexes become diminished or absent by age 8.
- Leukemia (T cell) or lymphomas (B cell) occur in 10% to 15% and may rarely be the presenting finding.
- Immunoglobulin deficiencies develop in many patients, specifically IgG2 (80%) and IgA (60%).
- Ocular motor apraxia, impassive facies, and dysarthria
- Diminished large-fiber sensation

Diagnostics
- Most diagnoses made by clinical presentation and exam
- Elevated serum alpha-fetoprotein (>99%)
- Immunoglobulin levels and IgG subclasses to detect IgA and IgG2 deficiency, with normal total IgG and IgM levels

Management
- Supportive treatment and avoid live-virus vaccines
- IVIG supplementation for hypogammaglobulinemia

CHÉDIAK-HIGASHI SYNDROME (CHS)

Characterized by neutropenia, impaired neutrophil chemotaxis and phagocytosis, recurrent infections, pigmentary dilution, easy bruising, and abnormal natural killer (NK) cell function

Epidemiology
- Unknown, but extremely rare (<1/100,000)

Etiology
- *CHS1* (formerly *LYST*) gene on chromosome 1q42.1-q42.2; Autosomal recessive

Pathophysiology
- Defect is in lysosomal-trafficking regulator protein
- Defective membrane targeting of CTLA-4 negative co-stimulatory receptor in T cells
- Other cells, including NK cells and platelets, are defective because of similar trafficking defects affecting storage granules
- Neutropenia (which may be severe), defective chemotaxis, and defective phagocytosis result
- Pigmentary dilution results from autophagocytosis of melanosomes in melanocytes

Differential Diagnosis
- *Pigment:* Griscelli syndrome, types I and II (rare autosomal recessive immunodeficiency with partial albinism and neurologic impairment); Hermansky-Pudlak syndrome (autosomal recessive disorder characterized by albinism, visual impairment, platelet dysfunction, pulmonary fibrosis, inflammatory bowel disease, kidney disease)
- *Hemophagocytic episodes:* familial hemophagocytic lymphohistiocytosis; X-linked lymphoproliferative syndrome; herpes virus-associated hemophagocytic syndrome (EBV, CMV, HHV-6, HSV); Griscelli syndrome, type II; T cell lymphoma; fungal, parasitic, HIV, tuberculosis infection

Clinical Manifestations
- In infancy, recurrent skin and sinopulmonary infections, severe gingivitis and periodontal disease. Adenopathy is common.
- May present in late adolescence or early adulthood with parkinsonism, dementia, spinocerebellar degeneration, and peripheral neuropathy.
- Most (85% to 100%) patients enter an "accelerated phase" with hemophagocytosis, lymphohistiocytic infiltrates, fever, jaundice, hepatosplenomegaly, lymphadenopathy, pancytopenia, and bleeding, resembling T cell lymphoma.
- Pigmentary dilution: silvery hair, pale translucent irises, fair skin
- Gingivitis and periodontal disease
- Easy bruisability, atrophic scars from frequent skin infections

Diagnostics
- Blood smear: Characteristic giant granules in neutrophils, eosinophils, and granulocytes seen on light microscopy
- Bone marrow biopsy: Inclusions in leukocyte precursor cells

Management
- HLA-identical bone marrow transplant prevents "accelerated phase" of the disease.
- Survival is 3.1 years on average without transplantation

CHRONIC GRANULOMATOUS DISEASE

Recurrent bacterial infections due to failure of the neutrophil to deliver activated oxygen to phagocytic vacuoles

Epidemiology
Prevalence varies by mutation (e.g., Cybb 1/250,000; Cyba 1/2,000,000)

Etiology
- Mutations usually affect NADPH oxidase activation
- 67% X-linked inheritance; remainder autosomal recessive

Differential Diagnosis
- *Primary immunodeficiency:* hyperIgE syndrome, leukocyte adhesion deficiency, Rosai-Dorfman (sinus histiocytosis with lymphadenopathy), Chédiak-Higashi
- *Macrophage/monocytes disorders:* hemophagocytic syndromes, juvenile xanthogranuloma
- Other: inflammatory bowel disease, sarcoidosis

Pathophysiology
Oxygen and NADPH+H are reduced by NADPH oxidase to produce NADP+ and superoxide radical. An additional electron for the reaction comes from a transport apparatus including the four known proteins involved with CGD (cybb, cyba, ncf1, and ncf2).

Clinical Manifestations
- Patients with X-linked form present within the first 1 to 2 years (mean age at diagnosis 3.8 years, at first infection 4 months) of life with severe deep-seated infections: pneumonia (23% to 30%), lymphadenitis (18%), GI infections (18%; enteritis, colitis, intra-abdominal abscesses), skin infections (18%; impetigo, furuncles, and abscesses), and osteomyelitis (3%)
- Common infecting organisms include: *S. aureus, Serratia marcescens, Candida* spp, *Aspergillus fumigatus, Salmonella* spp, and *Burkholderia cepacia*
- Other features include failure to thrive, granulomas in the respiratory, gastrointestinal, or urogenital tracts (presenting with partial or total small bowel or urinary obstruction). May have granulomatous colitis and perirectal abscesses. Recurrent hepatic and splenic abscesses can lead to hepatosplenomegaly.
- Autosomal recessive form presents with similar infections, but often later in life (mean age at diagnosis 13.6 years, at first infection 1.1 years)
- The survival rate for 39 studied patients was 91% and 54% at 10 and 30 years of age.

Diagnostics
- Flow cytometry for dihydrorhodamine 123 (DHR) conversion to rhodamine 123 is more sensitive and specific and objective than the historically used nitroblue tetrazolium test. It can be used to detect carrier status and can identify X-linked CGD from other forms in a majority of cases.

Management
- Long-term prophylaxis with trimethoprim-sulfamethoxazole (TMP-SMX) and itraconazole to reduce severe bacterial and fungal infections
- HLA-identical bone marrow allograft transplant after myeloablative conditioning has been studied, with good engraftment and high cure rates. If an HLA-identical sibling exists, younger patients and those without concurrent severe infection do best.
- Interferon-gamma should be reserved for children with severe infections.

COMMON VARIABLE IMMUNODEFICIENCY

A heterogeneous group of disorders characterized by decreased antibody production and recurrent bacterial infections

Epidemiology
- 1/10,000 to 1/100,000 children affected

- More common in families with selective IgA deficiency (which may lie on one end of the common variable immunodeficiency [CVID] spectrum) and autoimmunity.
- Two distinct peaks of infection are seen (ages 1 to 5 and 16 to 20 years). The childhood CVID subgroup has more autoimmune disease and infections and a lower survival rate.

Etiology
- Multiple single genes and polygenic inheritance have been implicated

Differential Diagnosis of Hypogammaglobulinemia
- *Drug-induced:* antimalarial agents, captopril, carbamazepine, glucocorticoids, fenclofenac, gold salts, penicillamine, phenytoin, sulfasalazine
- *Genetic disorders:* Any combined immunodeficiency, transcobalamin II deficiency and hypogammaglobulinemia, X-linked agammaglobulinemia, X-linked lymphoproliferative disorder, some metabolic disorders
- *Chromosomal anomalies:* chromosome 18q- syndrome, monosomy 22, trisomy 8, trisomy 21
- *Infectious diseases:* HIV, Epstein-Barr virus, and congenital rubella, CMV, and *Toxoplasma gondii*
- *Malignancy:* chronic lymphocytic leukemia, thymoma, non-Hodgkin's lymphoma, B cell malignancy
- *Systemic disorders:* immunoglobulin hypercatabolism, immunoglobulin loss (nephrotic syndrome, severe burn, lymphangiectasia, severe diarrhea)
- *Prematurity:* most IgG is maternally transferred during third trimester.

Pathophysiology
- Defects in B cell maturation lead to insufficient development of plasma cells

Clinical Manifestations
- Recurrent infections, including sinusitis (>90%) and pneumonia (80%)
- Lymphoproliferative diseases are common: B cell non-Hodgkin's lymphoma (7.7%)
- Gastrointestinal diseases, including inflammatory bowel disease and malabsorption are common; chronic infectious diarrhea (often *Giardia lamblia* [3%] or *Campylobacter jejuni* [1%])
- Non-caseating granulomas of lungs, liver, and spleen
- Autoimmune disease is common (22%; especially in females): autoimmune hemolytic anemia (5%), immune thrombocytopenic purpura (8%), polyarticular arthritis (proximal > distal), and celiac disease
- 30% will have lymphadenopathy and/or splenomegaly
- Chronic, purulent cough from pneumonia and bronchiectasis

Diagnostics
- Two of three immunoglobulins (IgG, IgA, IgM) are 2 SD below age-appropriate normal levels
- Infrequently, B cell count can be lower as well.
- Isohemagglutinins: IgM antibodies to ABO blood group determinants often deficient
- Poor antibody response to vaccines
- Tetanus and pneumococcal antibody titers at least 4 weeks after immunization
- In vitro T cell and B cell functional studies

Management
- IVIG replacement every 3 to 4 weeks
- Prophylactic antibiotics are often required
- The 20-year survival rate after the diagnosis of CVID is made is 64% for male patients and 67% for female patients compared with 92% to 94% for the general population

HYPER-IgE RECURRENT INFECTION SYNDROME

A rare immunodeficiency characterized by high IgE levels and recurrent bacterial skin and pulmonary infections (Job syndrome)

Epidemiology
- Incidence unknown, but rare; equal incidence in males and females, and across races

Etiology
- Gene(s) unknown. Linkage studies suggest a region on 4q21
- Autosomal dominant inheritance with variable penetrance

Differential Diagnosis of Elevated IgE
- Antimalarial agents
- HIV, malaria, parasitic infections
- Atopy, allergic bronchopulmonary aspergillosis
- Eczema
- T cell leukemia, cutaneous T cell lymphoma
- Immunodeficiencies: Omenn syndrome (autosomal recessive form of SCID characterized by erythroderma, lymphadenopathy, and hepatosplenomegaly), Wiskott-Aldrich, DiGeorge syndrome, Netherton syndrome, IPEX
- Native Waorani tribe of Ecuador

Pathophysiology
- Defective neutrophil chemotaxis
- Normal numbers of T and B cells
- Other immunoglobulin levels normal
- Suggestion of non-lymphocyte defect because of failure to correct after bone marrow transplantation

Clinical Manifestations
- Typical eczematous rash in infancy or early childhood.
- Delayed eruption of secondary teeth due to failure of exfoliation of primary teeth (60% to 70%)
- Recurrent bacterial infections, including upper and lower respiratory tract infection (90%). Pneumatoceles following pneumonias are common. Organisms include *S. aureus*, *H. influenzae*, *P. aeruginosa*, and *A. fumigatus*.
- Fungal infections including thrush, esophageal candidiasis, and onychomycosis in 80%.
- Skin infections are common, including abscesses (hot and cold).
- Increased incidence of fractures with subsequent osteomyelitis, even with minor or incidental trauma (60% to 70%); scoliosis (70%)
- Facial asymmetry suggestive of hemihypertrophy, frontal bossing, wide alar base of nose with fleshy nasal tip (100%), high arched palate

Diagnostics
- Elevated IgE greater than 2000 IU/mL (100%), although this can fluctuate
- Elevated eosinophil count greater than 2 SD above normal (93%)
- Dental x-rays: Delayed development and retained primary teeth
- Abnormalities on neutrophil chemotaxis assays

Management
- Full evaluation after skeletal trauma
- Removal of primary teeth
- Monitor and treat scoliosis
- Some centers recommend anti-staphylococcal prophylaxis
- Anecdotal evidence of topical calcineurin inhibitors or cyclosporine A (5 mg/kg/day) improving dermatitis and infections
- Weak evidence of interferon-gamma improving IgE levels
- Anecdotal evidence of IVIG suppressing IgE levels and improving dermatitis
- Matched unrelated donor bone marrow transplantation after cytoreductive conditioning showed re-elevation of IgE levels and infections within 2 years of transplant.

SEVERE COMBINED IMMUNODEFICIENCY (SCID)

A group of disorders with severe T cell dysfunction causing recurrent infection and early death

Epidemiology
- Incidence between 1/75,000 to 1/1,000,000 liveborn children.
- Among Navajo Native Americans, SCID occurs with an incidence of 1/2000 live births.
- Increased incidence in males because of X-linked etiologies (see subsequent section), but equal across races

Etiology
- Deficient T cells and B cells (T – B–): Adenosine deaminase (*ADA*, 1q21.1)–autosomal recessive, 15% of SCID cases: Rag1/Rag2 (11p13)-autosomal recessive, 3% of SCID cases
- Deficient T cells, defective B cells (T – B+): Cytokine common gamma chain (Xq13) defects— X-linked inheritance, also *most common* cause of SCID (45%): Janus kinase 3 (Jak3, 19p13.1)–autosomal recessive, 6% of SCID cases; IL7-receptor alpha chain (5p13)-autosomal recessive, 9% of SCID cases
- Defective T and B cells (T+B+): Omenn syndrome, ADA, purine nucleoside phosphorylase deficiency

Differential Diagnosis
- HIV infection
- Primary immunodeficiencies: Wiskott-Aldrich syndrome, 22q deletion syndrome, autoimmune poly-endocrinopathy candidiasis ectodermal dystrophy (APECED) syndrome, lymphopenia from sepsis or severe illness

Pathophysiology
- In common receptor gamma chain SCID (T – B+), the gamma chain forms the functional signaling unit of the IL-2, IL-4, IL-7, IL-9, IL-15, and IL-21 receptors, thus affecting numerous cell types and functionality.

Clinical Manifestations
- Infants with SCID present early (diagnosis at mean age of 6 months) with pneumonia, diarrhea, otitis, sepsis, or skin infections. Opportunistic infections, including with *P. carinii*, are frequent and persistent. Fungal and viral infections also occur.
- Graft-versus-host (GVHD) reactions from engrafted maternal T cells can result in severe cutaneous, gastrointestinal, and hematologic disease and lymphadenopathy and hepatosplenomegaly.
- Failure to thrive because of recurrent infections
- Small or absent lymphoid tissues (lymph nodes, tonsils, and adenoids) despite infections
- With GVHD, a morbilliform erythroderma is frequently seen, and can progress to necrosis in severe cases.

Diagnostics
- Complete blood cell count to demonstrate lymphopenia (absolute lymphocyte count typically < 3000/mm^3)
- Flow cytometry with lymphocyte and NK cell markers to show decreased T cell (<20% CD3$^+$) populations
- Immunoglobulin levels to show low to absent IgG and IgM
- Abnormal T and B cell functional studies, including absent or near absent mitogen-driven proliferation of lymphocytes
- HIV DNA PCR to exclude other causes of lymphopenia

Management
- Avoid public exposure before transplantation
- SCID patients should never receive live-virus vaccines, nor should their housemates/siblings.
- All blood products must be irradiated, CMV-negative, and leuko-reduced.

- Myeloablative conditioning with matched bone marrow, cord blood, or stem cell transplant is the only successful therapy. Unconditioned transplantation with haploidentical donor stem cells is also highly successful in some centers. Transplantation before 3 months of age results in better survival.
- If transplantation is not acceptable, adenosine deaminase-deficient SCID patients can receive polyethylene glycol-modified bovine ADA to reduce infection and improve lymphocyte counts.
- Gene therapy has been successful in many forms of SCID.

WISKOTT-ALDRICH SYNDROME

T and B cell immunodeficiency disorder associated with thrombocytopenia (small platelets), eczema, susceptibility to opportunistic infections, and B cell lymphoma.

Epidemiology
- Wiskott-Aldrich syndrome (WAS) occurs in 1/250,000 live male births
- Case reports of heterozygotic females due to inactivation of the unaffected X-chromosome

Etiology
- Defect in the *WAS* gene (Xp11.23)

Differential Diagnosis
- Chronic immune thrombocytopenia purpura (ITP) but ITP has normal to large platelet size.
- HIV infection
- Combined immunodeficiencies with both T and B cells affected: SCID
- Most of the inherited thrombocytopenias (May-Hegglin, Fechter syndrome, Bernard-Soulier, Sebastian syndrome, gray platelet syndrome, Montreal platelet syndrome) have giant platelets.

Pathophysiology
- The WAS family of proteins (WASP) transduces signals from cell-surface receptors to the actin cytoskeleton.
- Aberrant WASP signaling results in defective antigen-receptor signaling, cell migration, and phagocytosis.
- Actin cytoskeletal defects lead to decrease in platelet size.

Clinical Manifestations
- Average age at diagnosis 8 months
- 30% have classic triad of thrombocytopenia, eczema, and chronic otitis media
- Recurrent otitis media, sinusitis, and pneumonia. Other infections include sepsis, meningitis, severe viral infections and opportunistic infections (including *P. jiroveci* infection)
- Infants often present with bleeding (e.g., bloody diarrhea or prolonged bleeding after circumcision) especially if platelet counts are less than 10,000/mm^3.
- Petechiae and purpura; epistaxis, bleeding from gums
- Eczema focused on the scalp and flexural areas (80%)
- Lymphoreticular malignancies (13% to 20%; e.g., B cell lymphoma)
- Autoimmune disease (40%; e.g., autoimmune anemia, vasculitis, colitis)
- Average age at death 8 years, usually from bleeding or infection

Diagnostics
- Thrombocytopenia (typically < 70,000/mm^3) with small platelets (MPV half normal) is required
- Lymphopenia (mostly T cells) is common
- Normal IgG, reduced IgM, and increased IgA and IgE levels
- Flow cytometry to evaluate T and B cells to rule out SCID

Management
- Splenectomy may improve thrombocytopenia, if severe.
- Peripheral blood stem cell or bone marrow transplantation after myeloablative conditioning has been successful. Non-myeloablative conditioning may be necessary in the context of

active infections. Overall 5-year survival post-transplant was 70%, and survival was improved in transplants from HLA-identical siblings.
- Experimental therapies include gene therapy and IL-11.

X-LINKED AGAMMAGLOBULINEMIA

A defect of B cell maturation, resulting in B cell and antibody deficiencies and recurrent bacterial infections

Epidemiology
- Approximately 1/200,000

Etiology
- *Btk* (Bruton tyrosine kinase) gene, on Xp22

Pathophysiology
- Btk interferes with B cell receptor signaling causing arrested development of pre-B lymphocytes, so B cells and plasma cells never develop. Thus all isotypes of antibodies are deficient.
- Btk is also expressed in myeloid stem cells so neutropenia can occur.

Differential Diagnosis
- Agammaglobulinemia: Fleisher syndrome, BLNK deficiency, Igα deficiency, μ heavy-chain deficiency, other defects in B cell development
- Common variable immunodeficiency
- Immunoglobulin hypercatabolism
- Immunoglobulin loss (nephrotic syndrome, severe burn, lymphangiectasia, severe diarrhea)
- Selective IgA deficiency
- Specific IgG subclass, IgM, IgE deficiencies

Clinical Manifestations
- Respiratory tract bacterial infections are very common (82%), including sinusitis, otitis, pneumonia, and bronchitis.
- Skin and joint infections are common (30%). Also, diarrhea from *Campylobacter* and *Salmonella* species is frequent (10%).
- Infections due to *S. pneumoniae, H. influenzae, S. aureus,* and *P. aeruginosa*
- Resistance to viral infections is generally intact, except to enteroviruses (echovirus, Coxsackie virus, polio), which can cause significant morbidity.
- Absence of lymphoid tissue (tonsils, adenoids, lymph nodes)

Diagnostics
- In children beyond the first 6 months of life, low levels of IgG (<200 mg/dL) and absent IgA and IgM
- Because of maternally acquired IgG and normally low IgA and IgM, testing levels in the newborn is not helpful. Instead, the peripheral B lymphocyte count can be used (<1% is typical).
- Neutropenia can be seen.

Management
- IVIG replacement (400–500 mg/kg every 3–4 weeks), started early in infancy, prevents many hospitalizations and pulmonary infections.
- Avoid live virus vaccines
- Because IVIG does not provide IgA or mucosal immunity, significant morbidity can occur.

Resources

Ballow M. Primary immunodeficiency disorders: antibody deficiency. J Allergy Clin Immunol 2002;109:581–591.

Bonilla FA, Geha RS. Primary immunodeficiency diseases. J Allergy Clin Immunol 2003;111(suppl):s571–581.

Buckley RH. Primary cellular immunodeficiencies. J Allergy Clin Immunol 2002;109:747–757.

Cunningham-Rundles C, Bodian C. Common variable immunodeficiency: clinical and immunological features of 248 patients. Clin Immunol 1999;92:34–48.

Emanuel BS, McDonald-McGinn D, Saitta SC, Zackai EH. The 22q11.2 deletion syndrome. Adv Pediatr 2001;48:39–73.

Filipovich AH, Stone JV, Tomany SC, et al. Impact of donor type on outcome of bone marrow transplantation for Wiskott-Aldrich syndrome: collaborative study of the International Bone Marrow Transplant Registry and the National Marrow Donor Program. Blood 2001;97:1598–1603.

Grimbacher B, Holland SM, Gallin JI, et al. Hyper-IgE syndrome with recurrent infections—an autosomal dominant multisystem disorder. N Engl J Med 1999;340:692–702.

Grimbacher B, Schaffer AA, Holland SM, et al. Genetic linkage of hyper-IgE syndrome to chromosome 4. Am J Hum Genet 1999;65:735–744.

Lekstrom-Himes JA, Gallin JI. Immunodeficiency diseases caused by defects in phagocytes. N Engl J Med 2000;343:1703–1714.

Liese J, Kloos S, Jendrossek V, et al. Long-term follow-up and outcome of 39 patients with chronic granulomatous disease. J Pediatr 2000;137:687–693.

Ochs HD, Smith CI. X-linked agammaglobulinemia. A clinical and molecular analysis. Medicine 1996;75:287–299.

Online Mendelian Inheritance in Man, OMIM. Ataxia-telangiectasia. Available at: http://www.ncbi.nlm.nih.gov/entrez/dispomim.cgi?id=208900. Accessed November 16, 2004.

Online Mendelian Inheritance in Man, OMIM. Bruton agammaglobulinemia tyrosine kinase. Available at: http://www.ncbi.nlm.nih.gov/entrez/dispomim.cgi?id=300300. Accessed November 16, 2004.

Online Mendelian Inheritance in Man, OMIM. Chédiak-Higashi syndrome. Available at: http://www.ncbi.nlm.nih.gov/entrez/dispomim.cgi?id=214500. Accessed November 16, 2004.

Online Mendelian Inheritance in Man, OMIM. Common variable immunodeficiency. Available at: http://www.ncbi.nlm.nih.gov/entrez/dispomim.cgi?id=240500. Accessed November 16, 2004.

Online Mendelian Inheritance in Man, OMIM. DiGeorge Syndrome. Available at: http://www.ncbi.nlm.nih.gov/entrez/dispomim.cgi?id=188400. Accessed November 16, 2004.

Online Mendelian Inheritance in Man, OMIM. Hyper IgE syndrome. Available at. http://www.ncbi.nlm.nih.gov/entrez/dispomim.cgi?id=147060. Accessed November 16, 2004.

Online Mendelian Inheritance in Man, OMIM. Wiskott-Aldrich syndrome. Available at: http://www.ncbi.nlm.nih.gov/entrez/dispomim.cgi?id=301000. Accessed November 16, 2004.

Perez E, Sullivan KE. Chromosome 22q11.2 deletion syndrome (DiGeorge and velocardiofacial syndromes). Curr Opin Pediatr 2002;14:678–683.

Seger RA, Gungor T, Belohradsky BH, et al. Treatment of chronic granulomatous disease with myeloablative conditioning and an unmodified hemopoietic allograft: a survey of the European experience, 1985–2000. Blood 2002;100:4344–4350.

Snapper SB, Rosen FS. A family of WASPs. N Engl J Med 2003;348:350–351.

Sullivan KM, Parkman R, Walters MC. Bone marrow transplantation for non-malignant disease. Hematology 2000:319–338.

The Immunodeficiency Resource. Available at: http://bioinf.uta.fi/idr/. Accessed November 16, 2004.

VCFS Educational Foundation, Inc. Available at: http://www.vcfsef.org/. Accessed November 16, 2004.

Snehal N. Shah, MD, Asim Aminsharif Ahmed, MD, Jason G. Newland, MD, Sarah Armstrong, MD, Louis M. Bell, MD, and Samir S. Shah, MD (with contributions from Michael F. Maraventano, MD, Rose C. Graham-Maar, MD, Heather Morein French, MD, Pamela G. Fitch, MD, Judit Saenz-Badillos, MD)

Syndromes and Complexes

BITE WOUND INFECTIONS

Infections usually localized to site of bite. Rare sequelae include meningitis, brain abscess, endocarditis, and septic arthritis.

Epidemiology
- Infection follows 3% to 18% of dog bites and 28% to 80% of cat bites.
- Greatest rate of infection after bites to the hands

Etiology
- Usually polymicrobial; derived from oral flora of biting animal
- Cat and dog bite infections: *Pasteurella canis* (dog), *Pasteurella multocida* (cat), Streptococci, *Staphylococcus aureus*, *Moraxella* spp, *Neisseria* spp, and anaerobes
- Human bites: *Staphylococcus aureus*, viridans group Streptococci, *Streptococcus pyogenes*, *Eikenella corrodens*, *Streptococcus intermedius*, *Capnocytophaga* spp, *Neisseria* spp
- Pig bite: *Chryseobacterium*
- Horse/sheep bite: *Actinobacillus* spp, *Streptococcus equisimilis*
- Marine settings/fish bite: *Halomonas venusta*, *Vibrio* spp, *Aeromonas hydrophila*, *Plesiomonas shigelloides*, *Pseudomonas* spp, *Mycobacterium marinum*

Pathophysiology
- Infection follows direct inoculation of bacteria into tissues.
- Hematogenous dissemination may occur.

Clinical Manifestations
- Note wound type (puncture, laceration, avulsion), edema, erythema, tenderness, drainage, depth of penetration, bruising, deformity, involvement of underlying structure, sensation, regional lymphadenopathy
- Look for signs of systemic infection (e.g., fever, hypotension)
- Animal: record type of animal, health of animal, provoked or unprovoked attack; observe for signs of rabies if applicable
- Patient: history of asplenia; immunosuppression or other illnesses; last tetanus immunization

Diagnostics
- Gram stain and culture of wound if time from injury greater than 8 hours or if signs and symptoms of infection exist. Send blood cultures if fever present.
- Radiographs indicated if: penetrating injuries overlying bones or joints, suspected foreign body or fracture

Management
Immediate Management
- Examine for foreign body, irrigate with copious amounts of normal saline; debride devitalized tissue
- Suturing is controversial: leave wound open if greater than 8 hours old or a puncture wound; primary wound closure for injuries to face and when cosmetic outcome is important

- Indications for operative exploration and debridement: extensive tissue damage; involvement of metacarpophalangeal joint from clenched fist injury; cranial bites by large animals

Tetanus Prophylaxis
- Tetanus toxoid and tetanus immune globulin to all patients with two or fewer primary immunizations
- Tetanus toxoid alone to those who have completed primary immunization series but have not had a booster in 5 or more years

Rabies Prophylaxis
1. Dogs, cats, ferrets: if animal is healthy and available for 10 days observation, prophylax patient only if animal develops signs of rabies. If animal is rabid or suspected, give patient immunization and rabies immune globulin (RIG). If unknown, consult public health officials.
2. Bats, skunks, raccoons, foxes, woodchucks, and most other carnivores: regarded as rabid unless geographic area is known to be free of rabies or proven negative via laboratory tests. Patients require rabies immunization and RIG.
3. Livestock, rodents, and lagomorphs: consider individually and consult public health officials.

Antibiotic Prophylaxis
- Prophylaxis is generally recommended for: moderate to severe bite wounds, especially if edema or crush injury; puncture wounds, especially if bone, tendon sheath, or joint penetration has occurred; facial bites; hand and foot bites; genital area bites; wounds in asplenic and immunocompromised persons
- Antibiotics for prophylaxis and treatment of infection:
  - *Dog/cat/human bites:* amoxicillin-clavulanate; if penicillin allergy: trimethoprim-sulfamethoxazole plus clindamycin or third-generation cephalorsporin plus clindamycin
- Duration of treatment: prophylaxis: 3 to 5 days; treatment of infection: 10 to 14 days

BRONCHIOLITIS

Acute lower respiratory tract infection that causes inflammation of the bronchioles and results in distal airway obstruction

Epidemiology
- Children usually younger than 2 years of age
- All geographic areas; winter to early spring
- Infectious agents: Respiratory syncytial virus (RSV; 60% to 90% of cases); parainfluenza viruses types 1,2, and 3; adenovirus; influenza; rhinovirus, *Mycoplasma pneumoniae*, human metapneumovirus
- Risk factors for severe illness: age less than 3 months, gestational age less than 34 weeks, ill or toxic appearance, respiratory rate greater than 70 per minute, pulse oximetry less than 94%, atelectasis on chest x-ray, cardiac or pulmonary disease, immunodeficiency

Pathophysiology
- Necrosis of airway epithelium and ciliated lining causes mucosal inflammation. Lymphocytic infiltration of peribronchial and peribronchiolar epithelium causes edema of submucosa and adventitia.
- Impaired mucociliary clearance leads to obstruction of smaller caliber distal airways without significant alveolar involvement.
- Epithelial regeneration lags behind clinical recovery
- May also cause uncomplicated upper respiratory tract infections

Clinical Manifestations
- Incubation period ranges from 2 to 8 days. Acute illness ranges from 3 to 7 days. Recovery is gradual over 1 to 3 weeks.
- Signs and symptoms: rhinorrhea (profuse), cough, low-grade fever, lethargy, increased work of breathing, tachypnea, wheezing, cyanosis, apnea (especially in age less than 3 months)
- Auscultation: prolonged expiratory phase, wheezing, rales, rhonchi

Diagnostics
- Chest x-ray: hyperinflation, patchy atelectasis, peribronchial cuffing
- Rapid viral identification of nasapharyngeal collection: immunofluorescence or enzyme immuno-assay; does not require viable virus; useful for cohorting hospitalized patients
- Viral culture: useful if rapid identification tests are negative
- Consider arterial blood gas and serum electrolytes if ill

Management
- Respiratory support: oxygen as needed; chest physiotherapy may improve clearance of secretions; consider noninvasive (continuous positive airway pressure) and invasive ventilation in those with severe respiratory distress.
- Infants with extreme tachypnea are at risk of aspiration. In these patients, consider nothing-by-mouth status and IV hydration.
- Nebulized beta-2 adrenergic agonists (albuterol, levalbuterol): insufficient evidence to support *routine* inpatient use. In moderately ill infants, consider trial doses with assessment of clinical response. May have more benefit in those with asthma history or ventilated patients. Potential exists for paradoxical effects and increased airway resistance.
- Nebulized alpha/beta adrenergic agonist (racemic epinephrine): insufficient evidence to support *routine* inpatient use. Studies show higher rate of clinical response than with beta-2 agonists but no difference in length of hospitalization. In moderately ill infants, consider trial doses with assessment of clinical response.
- Corticosteroids: studies do *not* show consistent clinical improvement with either systemic or inhaled form. Infants with strong family history of asthma *and* a previous episode of wheezing may benefit from early systemic steroid administration. Data remains controversial.
- Antivirals (Ribavarin): not routinely administered. Consider in high-risk patients (e.g., congenital heart disease)
- Infection control: transmitted primarily by direct contact with secretions and/or fomites. Use contact precautions, cohorting patients, and handwashing
- Passive immunization: either palivizumab (humanized monoclonal RSV antibody; preferred due to IM administration) or RSV-IGIV (immune globulin enriched for RSV-specific antibodies). The American Academy of Pediatrics (AAP) recommends monthly prophylaxis in following situations (see AAP policy statement for further guidance; Pediatrics 112:1442–1446):
  - Age younger than 24 months with chronic lung disease requiring medical therapy (e.g., supplemental O_2, diuretics, corticosteroids) within 6 months of RSV season
  - Infants younger than 6 months of age during start of RSV season and 1) born at younger than 32 weeks of gestation or 2) born between 32 and 35 weeks of gestation and have other risk factors (e.g., neurologic disease, daycare, exposure to tobacco smoke)
  - Patients younger than 24 months with cyanotic or hemodynamically significant acyanotic congenital heart disease (e.g., receiving medication to control congestive heart failure, moderate-severe pulmonary hypertension) (RSV-IGIV contraindicated in infants with cyanotic congenital heart disease)
  - Palivizumab does not interfere with response to vaccines. RSV-IGIV recipients should have MMR immunization deferred for 9 months after last dose of RSV-IGIV.

CELLULITIS

A primary, superficial skin infection

Etiology
- Immunocompetent children: *S. pyogenes, S. aureus, S. pneumoniae*
- Immunocompromised children: also *Pseudomonas* spp, enterobacteriaceae, *Cryptococcus neoformans*, anaerobes

Pathophysiology
- Most commonly follows local trauma (e.g., abrasions)
- Hematogenous dissemination is less common since introduction of *H. influenzae* type B vaccine.

Clinical Manifestations
- Constitutional symptoms including fever, chills, malaise
- Skin edema, warmth, erythema, and tenderness
- Red, lymphangitic streaks
- Regional lymphadenopathy
- Break in skin may be found on exam.

Diagnostics
- Culture of aspirate, skin biopsy, and blood cultures collectively yield causal organism in 25% of cases.
- Blood cultures have low yield in those treated as outpatients. Drain areas of fluctuance (especially in areas of high methicillin-resistant *S. aureus* [MRSA] prevalence).

Management
- Well-appearing children can be treated as outpatients: cephalexin or amoxicillin-clavulanate. Consider trimethoprim-sulfamethoxazole (TMP-SMX) or clindamycin in areas of high MRSA prevalence.
- Ill-appearing patients with high fever, rapid progression, or lymphangitis require hospitalization and IV antibiotics. Consider oxacillin, cefazolin, or clindamycin.
- Neonates should have gram-positive and gram-negative coverage.
- Typical duration of therapy is 7 to 10 days.

CROUP

Upper airway obstruction due to virus-induced inflammation may involve the larynx, infraglottic tissues, and trachea (laryngotracheitis).

Epidemiology
- Usually between ages 6 months and 3 years (peak at 18 months)
- Epidemics begin in late fall and peak in early winter.

Etiology
- Common: parainfluenza viruses (>65% of cases)
- Less common: respiratory syncytial virus, influenza virus A and B, adenovirus, coxsackieviruses, and measles

Pathophysiology
- Viral infection of the nasopharynx spreads to respiratory epithelium.
- Infection causes diffuse inflammation of the trachea and vocal cords.
- Inflammation of the subglottic trachea (narrowest part of child's upper airway) leads to dramatic airflow restriction.

Clinical Manifestations
- Initial rhinorrhea, pharyngitis, and low-grade fevers
- Upper airway obstruction 8 to 12 hours later
- Signs of obstruction include "barking" cough, hoarseness, inspiratory stridor, accessory muscle use, and hypoxia.
- Fever, tachypnea, restlessness, coryza

Diagnostics
- Diagnosis is made on clinical grounds.
- Neck x-rays are not required but can support the initial diagnosis.
- Only 50% of cases demonstrate abnormal neck x-ray findings. Antero-posterior view: narrowed air column in subglottic area (steeple sign). Lateral view: overdistention of the hypopharynx.

Management
- Cool mist tent or vaporizer: may reduce airway edema and facilitate clearing of secretions, but *benefits are unproven*. May increase patient anxiety leading to worsening respiratory distress.

- Corticosteriods: proven benefit for moderate to severe croup; decreases subglottic edema; improvement begins 6 to 8 hours after dose; consider dexamethasone (0.6 mg/kg orally or intramuscularly for one dose, maximum 10 mg), prednisone (1 mg/kg/day twice daily for 3 to 5 days, maximum dose 30 mg), or nebulized budesonide (2–4 mg) for one dose
- Nebulized racemic epinephrine (2.25%): consider for hypoxia or severe croup. Adrenergic effects induce vasoconstriction leading to decreased subglottic edema. Onset occurs in less than 10 minutes. Duration of effect is less than 2 hours and, therefore, requires 3- to 4-hour observation period before discharge.
- Criteria for discharge include: no stridor at rest; normal air entry, color, and level of consciousness
- Heliox therapy (70% helium, 30% oxygen mixture) for severe distress: helium improves laminar gas flow in edematous airway and decreases the mechanical work of respiratory muscles. Heliox may be effective only if the supplemental oxygen requirement is less than 30%.

ENCEPHALITIS

Inflammation of the brain

Epidemiology
- Most frequently observed in summer and early fall when enteroviruses and arboviruses are prevalent
- Commonly associated with meningitis

Differential Diagnosis
- Viruses (most common): arboviruses (West Nile, St. Louis, Eastern and Western equine, Venezuelan equine, Califonia, Powassan, and Colorado tick fever), enteroviruses, herpes simplex 1 and 2, human herpesvirus 6 and 7, varicella-zoster, influenza A and B, parainfluenza 1–3, mumps, measles, RSV, rotavirus, adenovirus, Epstein-Barr, rabies, Nipah virus
- Bacteria: *Haemophilus influenzae, Neisseria meningitidis, S. pneumoniae, Mycobacterium tuberculosis, Bartonella henselae*
- Other infections: *Mycoplasma pneumoniae*, Rocky Mountain spotted fever, ehrlichia, *Cryptococcus neoformans, Coccidioides immitis*, parasites, and helminths
- Postinfectious diseases: Guillain-Barré, Miller-Fisher, acute cerebellar ataxia
- Other: inborn error of metabolism, seizure disorder, toxin ingestion, mass lesion, subarachnoid hemorrhage, acute demyelinating disorder, acute confusional migraine

Pathophysiology
- Most commonly occurs by hematogenous spread to the brain following viremia or bacteremia
- May occur as a result of retrograde movement through the peripheral nerves (e.g., HSV and rabies)

Clinical Manifestations
- Common: fever, headache, altered mentation
- Other: behavioral or personality changes, generalized or focal seizures, hemiparesis, ataxia, movement disorders
- Neurologic abnormalities are based on areas of the brain affected: altered level of consciousness, cranial nerve palsies, ataxia, weakness
- If meningitis: nuchal rigidity, Kernig and Brudzinski signs (see Meningitis)

Diagnostics
- Clinical diagnosis is based on fever and altered mental status.
- Labs: CBC with differential, chemistry panel, liver function tests (especially if considering HSV), toxicology screen
- Lumbar puncture: Gram stain, bacterial and viral culture, protein, glucose, cell count and differential, opening pressure, polymerase chain reaction (PCR) for enterovirus and HSV
- Serologic titers and CSF PCR for arboviruses during the summer

- CT scan to exclude cerebral edema or mass that would put patient at risk for herniation during the lumbar puncture
- MRI of the brain with contrast to better delineate affected areas
- Electroencephalogram (EEG)

Management
- If associated with meningitis suggestive of bacterial disease then begin appropriate empiric antibiotics (see Meningitis section)
- HSV encephalitis: in neonates, acyclovir 60 mg/kg/day divided every 8 hours (older children, 1500 mg/m^2/day divided three times daily)
- Most patients with other viral encephalitides require only supportive care.
- Physical, occupational, and speech therapy are important in those children with severe disease and long-term complications.
- Complications: cerebral edema, long-term neurologic dysfunction, seizure disorder, death

GASTROENTERITIS

Infection of the gastrointestinal tract usually associated with vomiting and diarrhea

Epidemiology
- Infectious cases due to bacteria (25%) or viruses (35%); 35% undetermined etiology

Etiology
- *Viral:* rotavirus, adenovirus, calicivirus (Norwalk agent), astrovirus
- *Bacterial: Campylobacter, E. coli* (multiple species), *Salmonella, Shigella, Yersinia, Clostridium difficile, Vibrio, Aeromonas*
- *Parasitic/Protozoan: Giardia, Cryptosporidium, Entamoeba, Cyclospora, Isospora*

Pathophysiology
- *Osmotic/Malabsorptive:* intestinal epithelial damage leads to malabsorption and osmotic diarrhea.
- *Inflammation:* exudation of mucus, blood, and protein into the luminal space exacerbates water and electrolyte loss.
- *Secretory/Toxigenic:* toxin release results in active secretion of water into the luminal space (e.g., cholera toxin).

Clinical Manifestations
Rarely bloody (in order of frequency)
- *Rotavirus:* major cause of diarrhea in infants from late fall to early spring; may result in transient post-infectious carbohydrate intolerance
- *Caliciviruses (e.g., Norwalk agent):* can present with isolated vomiting; commonly accompanied by diarrhea, fever, headache, malaise, myalgia, and abdominal cramping; cause of outbreaks in closed populations (e.g., cruise ships, daycare)
- *Giardia lamblia:* non-bloody diarrhea with greasy, foul-smelling stools and excessive flatulence; associated with daycare and camping; can be chronic
- *Cryptosporidium:* non-bloody watery diarrhea, usually in immunocompromised hosts; outbreaks associated with contaminated city water supplies, swimming pools, and daycare
- *Clostridium difficile:* non-bloody diarrhea (enterotoxin effect) associated with recent antibiotic exposure (classically with ampicillin and clindamycin); can cause pseudomembranous colitis (cytotoxin effect)
- *Vibrio cholerae:* painless profuse and explosive rice-water diarrhea with significant fluid loss and dehydration. Most cases in the United States are due to consumption of raw or undercooked shellfish.

Often bloody (invasive or cytotoxin-producing; in order of frequency)
- *Salmonella paratyphi:* bloody diarrhea associated with raw eggs, undercooked poultry, and reptile exposure

- *Salmonella typhi:* bloody diarrhea and abdominal pain after recent foreign travel; "rose spots" on neck or torso during the second week of illness (can culture the organism from the rash in 50% of patients); leukopenia with normocytic, normochromic anemia (secondary to marrow infiltration)
- *Shigella:* neurologic signs or symptoms (e.g., seizures, encephalopathy) preceding bloody diarrhea; high peripheral band count
- *Campylobacter:* bloody diarrhea associated with painful or crampy abdominal pain; may be associated with new puppy or pet; also associated with development of post-infectious syndromes such as Guillain-Barré or Reiter's syndrome
- *Yersinia entercolitica:* severe pain mimics appendicitis; can cause bloody diarrhea, mesenteric adenitis, and reactive arthritis; associated with chitterlings exposure and iron overload
- *Escherichia coli:* five major pathogenic classes: *Enteropathogenic* strains cause fever and diarrhea primarily in infants. *Enterotoxigenic* strains elaborate enterotoxins that cause watery diarrhea, fever and crampy abdominal pain ("traveler's diarrhea"). *Enteroinvasive* strains may cause fever, watery diarrhea with or without blood, and occasionally foodborne outbreaks. *Enteroaggregative* strains produce a mild chronic watery diarrhea. *Enterohemorrhagic* strains (e.g., serotype O157:H7) produce toxins that can cause hemorrhagic colitis or hemolytic-uremic syndrome.
- *Entamoeba histolytica:* colicky abdominal pain and tenesmus; dysentery characterized by profuse bloody diarrhea, fever, and electrolyte alterations; hepatic amebiasis presents with fever, anorexia, tender hepatomegaly, and minimal GI symptoms

On physical exam
- *Mild dehydration:* increased thirst, dry mucous membranes
- *Moderate dehydration:* sunken eyes, decreased skin turgor, decreased urine output, delayed capillary refill, depressed fontanelle
- *Severe dehydration:* features of moderate dehydration PLUS rapid and weak pulse, cold extremities, depressed mental status/lethargy, and no urine output

Diagnostics (Tests to Consider)
- Hemoccult for presence of blood in the stools
- Fecal leukocytes: positive test suggests invasive or cytotoxin-producing bacteria (usually polymorphonuclear; if mononuclear, consider *S. typhi*); negative test less helpful
- Electrolytes, BUN, and creatinine
- CBC: excessive band forms (*Shigella*) or hemolysis (*E. coli* O157:H7)
- Rapid viral antigen tests on stool for rotavirus or adenovirus
- Stool viral culture
- Standard stool culture detects *E. coli, Salmonella, Shigella, Campylobacter*
- Special stool cultures required for *Yersinia enterocolitica, Vibrio cholerae, Vibrio parahaemolyticus, E. coli* O157:H7, *Listeria monocytogenes*
- Stool ova and parasite exam. Rapid immunoassays for *Giardia* and *Cryptosporidium* are often more sensitive than O&P. If *Cyclospora* is suspected, alert the microbiology laboratory.
- *C. difficile* toxin A&B detection in stool
- Culture for *E. coli* O157:H7 (MacConkey sorbitol agar) if hemolytic-uremic syndrome suspected.

Management
- See Table 15.1 for indications for antibiotic therapy.
- Oral rehydration is the preferred therapy in cases of mild to moderate dehydration. Small but frequent oral challenges can be given with assessments in response.
  - Consider commercial oral rehydration solutions (target osmolarity of 250, carbohydrates 25 g/L, sodium 45 mosm/L) or WHO oral rehydration solution (osmolarity of 310 with 90 mosm/L of sodium).
- For IV rehydration, replace up to 50% of the deficit over the first 8 hours in addition to one-third of the maintenance fluid requirements. Ongoing losses from vomiting and diarrhea can also be replaced with normal saline (10 mL/kg for each stool and 5 mL/kg for each episode of vomiting).
- Severe dehydration can be life-threatening. Isotonic IV fluids (0.9% saline or lactated Ringer's) are recommended. IV boluses (20 mL/kg) can be given initially (see Fluids and Electrolytes, Chapter 9). Treatment can be transitioned to oral rehydration solutions.

Table 15.1: Indications for Antibiotic Therapy with Diarrheal Illness

Bacteria	Indication	Antibiotic
Aeromonas spp	Prolonged disease	TMP/SMX, ciprofloxacin
Campylobacter jejuni	Severe or systemic infection or immunodeficiency	Azithromycin, fluoro-quinolones, erythromycin
Clostridium difficile	Symptomatic and not improving	Metronidazole (PO/IV) or oral vancomycin or cholestyramine
Traveler's diarrhea (*Escherichia coli*)	Severe or systemic infection	TMP/SMX, fluoroquinolones*
Salmonella spp	Age < 3 mo, immuno-deficiency, or disseminated disease	Ampicillin, cefotaxime, ciprofloxacin, azithromycin
Shigella spp	Dysentery or epidemic setting	Ceftriaxone, azithromycin, fluoroquinolones, TMP/SMX
Vibrio cholerae	Treatment decreases illness duration	Ciprofloxacin, TMP/SMX, tetracyclines
Yersinia enterocolitica	Sepsis, immunodeficiency	Cefotaxime, TMP/SMX, fluoroquinolones

TMP/SMX, trimethoprim-sulfamethoxazole; PO, orally; IV, intravenously.

*Antibiotic therapy in patients with *E. coli* O157:H7 increased risk of developing HUS in some studies but no increased risk or benefit found on meta-analysis of trials. Treatment not currently recommended for *E. coli* O157:H7.

INFECTIOUS MONONUCLEOSIS

Clinical syndrome characterized by fever, exudative pharyngitis, lymphadenopathy (LAD), and hepatosplenomegaly. Most (80% to 95%) cases are caused by Epstein-Barr virus (EBV), a B cell-lymphotropic member of the herpesvirus family. Infectious mononucleosis is occasionally caused by cytomegalovirus and rarely caused by *Toxoplasma gondii*, adenoviruses, rubella, and hepatitis A.

Epidemiology
- Spread by close personal contact usually via saliva; can also be transmitted through blood products; incubation period is 30 to 50 days.
- The majority of primary EBV infections are asymptomatic. Clinical disease develops in less than 10% of infected children, whereas clinical infection develops in 50% to 70% of infected adolescents and young adults.
- Virus can be excreted up to 18 months following infection.

Pathophysiology
- EBV infects B cells in oropharyngeal lymphoid tissues. These infected B lymphocytes disseminate the infection systemically through the reticuloendothelial system.

Clinical Manifestations
- Wide spectrum of disease
- A prodrome of malaise, fatigue, headache, and low-grade fevers may precede clinical infection.

- Classic presentation includes triad of high fever, exudative tonsillar pharyngitis, and lymphadenopathy, which is symmetric involving the posterior cervical chain more than the anterior cervical chain.
- Common findings: severe fatigue, malaise, splenomegaly, generalized maculopapular rash (associated with ampicillin and amoxicillin), and abdominal pain (especially in young children)
- Rare findings and complications include splenic rupture, pneumonia, myocarditis, hepatomegaly, pancreatitis, mesenteric adenitis, myositis, acute renal failure, glomerulonephritis, Guillain-Barré syndrome, meningoencephalitis, transverse myelitis, peripheral neuritis, optic neuritis, and hemophagocytic syndrome.
- In patients with cellular immune deficiencies, fatal dissemination or lymphoproliferative syndromes can occur.

Diagnostics
- Leukocytosis: peripheral white blood cell count often greater than 15,000/mm^3 with greater than 50% lymphocytes and greater than 10% atypical lymphocytes
- Hemolytic anemia in less than 1% of cases
- Mild thrombocytopenia but rarely less than 100,000/mm^3
- Mild elevation of hepatic transaminases
- Heterophile antibody analysis by Paul-Bunnell test (agglutination of sheep erythrocytes) or "Monospot" test (rapid slide agglutination reaction using horse erythrocytes) are often negative in children younger than 4 years of age.
  - In older children, specificity = 90% to 98%. Positive in approximately 40% during first week of illness and in two thirds during second week.
  - If detected initially, they become undetectable over 3 to 6 months.
- Specific EBV serologies for young children and when heterophile test result is negative:
  - Acute infection: elevated viral capsid antigen (VCA) IgM and IgG; early antigen (EA) IgG negative or low positive; EBV nuclear antigen (EBNA) IgG negative
  - Recent infection: VCA IgM negative (disappears 8 to 12 weeks after infection); VCA IgG and EA IgG positive; EBNA negative
  - Past infection: VCA IgM and EA IgG negative; VCA IgG and EBNA positive (appears more than 8 weeks after infection)

Management
- Supportive care for fever and pharyngitis
- Corticosteroids for patients with impending airway obstruction (e.g., prednisone 1 mg/kg/day for 7 days followed by a taper)
- Acyclovir, ganciclovir, and foscarnet demonstrate in vitro activity against EBV but have *not* been shown to improve clinical outcomes in previous healthy children.
- Avoid contact sports until full recovery and spleen is not palpable (generally 6 to 8 weeks)
- Reduction of immunosuppressive therapy for patients with EBV-associated posttransplant lymphoproliferative disorders

LYMPHADENITIS AND LYMPHADENOPATHY

Enlargement (>10 mm) of a lymph node (isolated) or a group of lymph nodes (regional) accompanied by inflammation or infection. The condition may be acute, subacute, or chronic.

Etiology
- Common: group A beta-hemolytic streptococci and *S. aureus*
- Less common: anaerobes (dental source), cat-scratch disease, non-tuberculous mycobacteria
- Rare: tularemia, *Yersinia pestis*, diphtheria, chancroid, rat bite fever, parasites (toxoplasmosis, leishmaniasis), fungal (histoplasmosis, coccidioimycosis, blastomycosis, cryptococcosis)
- Viral: EBV, CMV, adenovirus, HIV, rubella, measles, mumps, HSV, VZV, HHV6, HHV7, hepatitis B, parvovirus B19, dengue

Pathophysiology

- Local disease: organisms may enter lymph nodes and cause microabscesses and suppuration secondary to lymphatic drainage of a localized infected site.
- Generalized disease: organisms may enter lymphatics after hematogenous spread from a systemic infection.

Physical Exam

- Lymphadenitis: affected nodes are tender with overlying warmth or erythema. Fluctuance suggests abscess formation.
- Torticollis (cervical node involvement); dysphagia, drooling, and dyspnea (retropharyngeal node); cough, stridor, dyspnea (mediastinal node); abdominal pain (mesenteric adenitis); limp (inguinal node)
- Preauricular: Adenovirus, tularemia, *B. henselae* (causes Parinaud oculoglandular syndrome; see cat-scratch disease)
- Postauricular: scalp infections, HHV6, HHV7, rubella, parvovirus B19
- Occipital: tinia capitis (kerion), scalp infection (cellulitis), or superinfection of eczema or seborrheic dermatitis, rubella, toxoplasma
- Supraclavicular: left-sided "Virchow's node" associated with abdominal source (consider malignancy); right-sided associated with thoracic source (e.g., histoplasmosis, tuberculosis)
- Concerning for malignancy: very rapid increase in node size; confluent and matted shape; firm rubbery consistency; lack of tenderness; fixation to surrounding soft tissue structures
- Overlying violaceous discoloration of skin with draining sinus is characteristic of mycobacterial adenitis.

Diagnostics

- Radiologic evaluation is not necessary in most mild-moderate cases.
- Ultrasonography or CT to diagnose suppuration and assess extent of infection.
- Consider needle aspiration or incisional drainage of lymph node if 1) poor response to IV antibiotics; 2) fluctuance or evidence of extension into neck by radiologic studies. Send specimen for staining (Gram stain and acid-fast stain) and bacterial and mycobacterial culture. Also send for pathologic diagnosis.
- Cat-scratch serology or PCR of nodal aspirate
- PPD: 5 to 10 mm may be seen with non tuberculous mycobacteria; usually greater than 15 mm with tuberculosis

Management

- Optimal management depends on making an accurate diagnosis.
- Empiric antibiotics for suspected bacterial adenitis:
  - Oral: cephalexin or dicloxacillin (consider clindamycin in areas with high MRSA prevalence); alternate therapy: clindamycin, amoxicillin-clavulanate (trimethoprim-sulfamethoxazole does not have sufficient activity against *S. pyogenes*)
  - IV: oxacillin, cefazolin, clindamycin. Alternate: vancomycin, ampicillin-sulbactam
  - Average duration of therapy is 10 days. For suppuration requiring drainage, consider 14- to 21-day course of therapy.
- Special situations (also see Cat-Scratch Disease section)
  - Non-tuberculous mycobacteria: standard therapy requires surgical resection of all visibly affected nodes. Incisional drainage is not recommended since it may lead to a draining sinus tract. Medical management with clarithromycin, ethambutol, or rifampin is *rarely* successful.
  - *M. tuberculosis*: isoniazid, rifampin, and pyrazinamide + ethambutol or streptomycin

MASTOIDITIS

Acute mastoiditis: mastoid air cell infection resulting from an extension of acute otitis media (OM)

Chronic mastoiditis: low grade but persistent mastoid air cell infection resulting from chronic suppurative OM or, less commonly, inadequately treated acute mastoiditis

Etiology
- Acute mastoiditis:
  - Common: *S. pneumoniae, S. pyogenes, S. aureus*
  - Less common: *H. influenzae, P. aeruginosa,* other enteric gram-negative bacilli, anaerobes, *M. tuberculosis*
- Chronic mastoiditis: *P. aeruginosa, S. aureus, S. pneumoniae*

Pathophysiology
- Mastoid is located on posterior process of temporal bone.
- Series of interconnected air cells develop by 2 years of age and drain into the middle ear.
- Purulent material from middle ear is under pressure and invades mastoid air cells.
- Complications arise due to extension of infection into adjacent structures:
  - Anterior: facial nerve, auditory canal, jugular vein, internal carotid
  - Posterior: posterior cranial fossa, sigmoid sinus
  - Superior: middle cranial fossa
  - Medial: inner ear organs
  - Inferior: deep neck musculature

Clinical Manifestations
- Fever, ear pain, tinnitus, postauricular swelling, tenderness
- History of recent otitis media (days-weeks)
- Chronic mastoiditis presents with persistent posterior auricular swelling, history of multiple otitis media infections, hearing loss, and ear pain.
- Pinna deviated outward and downward (infant) or upward (older child)
- Posterior auricular swelling, erythema, tenderness
- Tympanic membrane bulging, immobile, opaque

Diagnostics
- Elevated peripheral white blood cell count
- Elevated ESR and C-reactive protein (may be normal in chronic mastoiditis)
- Lumbar puncture if intracranial complication suspected (after CT scan excludes mass effect)
- Tympanocentesis for bacterial, fungal, acid-fast stains and culture to guide therapy
- Head CT: shows destruction of mastoid air cells; 30% of bone must be demineralized for change to be visible on CT; fluid-filled air cells without bony destruction insufficient for diagnosis of mastoiditis; CT (or MRI) may reveal associated intracranial complications.

Management
Medical
- Acute: ampicillin-sulbactam OR cefotaxime for 3 to 4 weeks; may switch to oral antibiotics once patient improves (amoxicilln-clavulanate; levofloxacin; or clindamycin)
- Chronic: oxacillin (or vancomycin) + gentamicin (or ceftazidime) OR ticarcillin-clavulanate
- Alter antibiotics based on culture results

Surgical
- ENT consultation: myringotomy +/– tympanostomy tubes
- Mastoidectomy if 1) no improvement within 48 hours of myringotomy; 2) subperiosteal abscess, facial nerve palsy, brain abscess, meningitis

Follow-up
- Audiology exam

MENINGITIS

Inflammation of the meninges, which manifests as increased CSF white blood cells (WBCs)

Epidemiology
- Most common during late summer and early fall during enteroviral season
- Neonatal meningitis occurs in 2 to 10 cases per 10,000 live births

Etiology
- Bacteria
  - Neonates (0 to 1 month): group B *Streptococcus, E. coli, Listeria monocytogenes, S. pneumoniae,* other enteric gram-negative bacilli
  - Infants (1 month to 1 year): *S. pneumoniae,* group B *Streptococcus, Neisseria meningitidis, Haemophilus influenzae*
  - Children older than 1 year: *S. pneumoniae, Neisseria meningitidis, H. influenzae*
  - Other bacterial causes: *Borrelia burgdorferi, M. tuberculosis, S. aureus, Treponema pallidum*
- Viruses: Enteroviruses, herpes simplex virus 1 and 2, varicella-zoster, adenovirus, parainfluenza, mumps, measles, influenza A and B, lymphocytic choriomeningitis virus, arboviruses, HIV
- Fungi: *Blastomyces dermatitidis, Coccidioides immitis, Cryptococcus neoformans, Candida* species, *Histoplasma capsulatum*

Pathophysiology
- Bacteria and viruses gain entry into the bloodstream through mucosal surfaces. After entry into the blood, the organism invades the meninges and replicates, inducing an inflammatory response leading to the clinical manifestations.

Clinical Manifestations
- Neonates and infants: fever, lethargy, poor feeding, and/or irritability. On exam: bulging fontanelle, nuchal rigidity, inconsolable irritability. In neonates, fever alone should prompt an evaluation for meningitis.
- Toddlers and children: fever, severe headache, chills, photophobia, neck stiffness, seizures, and vomiting. On exam: nuchal rigidity, photophobia, presence of Kernig and/or Brudzinksi signs
- Kernig sign: while legs are flexed 90° at the hip, extension of the lower legs cannot be accomplished beyond 135°.
- Brudzinski sign: passive neck flexion elicits involuntary hip flexion.
- Complications: circulatory collapse, focal neurologic findings (paralysis, facial nerve palsy, visual field defects, hearing loss), seizures, hydrocephalus, brain abscess, subdural effusions, syndrome of inappropriate diuretic hormone release

Diagnostics
- Laboratory studies: blood culture, CBC with manual differential, chemistry panel, liver function test (especially if suspecting HSV)
- CSF studies (Table 15.2): cell count with differential, protein, glucose, Gram stain and culture, enterovirus PCR during summer and fall, HSV PCR if consistent with clinical picture
- Radiology: CT scan if evidence of increased intracranial pressure to identify masses and cerebral edema that may put patient at risk for cerebral herniation during lumbar puncture.

Management
- Empiric therapy in patients with suspected bacterial meningitis:
  - Neonate (0 to 1 month): ampicillin IV 300 mg/kg/day divided every 6 hours (max: 3 g every 6 hours) and cefotaxime IV 300 mg/kg/day divided every 6 hours. If suspicious for HSV, acyclovir 60 mg/kg/day divided every 8 hours in neonates.

Table 15.2: Normal CSF Values (by Age)			
Age	WBC (cells/mm³)	Protein (mg/dL)	Glucose (CSF/Serum)
Neonate (0–4 wk)	0–22	20–170	$\frac{1}{2}$–$\frac{2}{3}$ or > 40 mg/dL
Infant (4–8 wk)	0–15	35–85	$\frac{1}{2}$–$\frac{2}{3}$ or > 40 mg/dL
Children and adolescents	0–10	5–40	$\frac{1}{2}$–$\frac{2}{3}$ or > 40 mg/dL

WBC, white blood cell.

- All other children: vancomycin IV 60 mg/kg/day divided every 6 hours (maximum, 1 g per dose) and ceftriaxone 100 mg/kg/day divided every 12 hours (maximum, 1 g every 12 hours) or cefotaxime (max: 2 g every 6 hours)
- If CSF culture results remain negative for 48 hours, the antibiotics can be discontinued. However, if the patient received antibiotics before the lumbar puncture, 10 days of IV cefotaxime or ceftriaxone should be strongly considered because negative cultures in this circumstance do not reliably exclude a bacterial cause.
- Duration of therapy varies by organism and patient course. Typically: *N. meningitidis*, 5 to 7 days; *S. pneumoniae*, 10 days; GBS, 14 days
- Audiology exam indicated during follow-up

NEONATAL CONJUNCTIVITIS

Conjunctivitis occurring in infants less than 4 weeks of age

Epidemiology
- *Chlamydia trachomatis* acquisition in 50% of infants born vaginally to infected mothers; after acquisition, risk of conjunctivitis is 25% to 50% and risk of pneumonia is 5% to 20%.

Etiology
- Common (infectious): *C. trachomatis* and *N. gonorrhoeae*. Other organisms include *S. aureus*, *S. pneumoniae*, *H. influenzae* (nontypeable), *P. aeruginosa* (hospitalized preterm infants)
- Chemical: silver nitrate, erythromycin, foreign body

Pathophysiology
- Infection (bacterial or chlamydial) can be acquired in utero, transvaginally, or after birth.
- Incubation: *N. gonorrhoeae*, 2 to 7 days; *C. trachomatis*, 5 to 7 days
- *Chlamydia trachomatis* pneumonia develops at 4 to 12 weeks (afebrile, diffuse infiltrates, rales).
- *Neisseria gonorrhoeae* may rapidly progress to corneal ulceration and perforation resulting in blindness. *Pseudomonas aeruginosa* may cause systemic infection.

Clinical Manifestations
- Conjunctival injection, edema of eyelids, chemosis (swelling)
- Eye discharge may be serosanguineous or purulent.

Diagnostics
- Culture and Gram stain of the discharge; *N. gonorrhoeae* appears as intracellular gram-negative diplococci on Gram stain.
- *Chlamydia trachomatis* can be identified by direct fluorescent antibody test on conjunctival or nasopharyngeal (pneumonia) swab. Culture or (in past) detection of intracytoplasmic inclusions on Giemsa-stained conjunctival epithelial cells can also be used.

Management
- Perinatal ocular prophylaxis with topical 0.5% erythromycin, 1% silver nitrate, or 2.5% povidone-iodine reduces risk of conjunctivitis.
- *Chlamydia trachomatis* (conjunctivitis or pneumonia): oral erythromycin for 14 days (50 mg/kg/day in four doses) has 80% efficacy. Newborns of untreated mothers with chlamydia require close observation (without treatment) because efficacy of prophylactic oral erythromycin is unknown. An alternate regimen is oral sulfonamides.
- *Neisseria gonorrhoeae*
  - Hospitalization, consider evaluation (blood and CSF cultures) to exclude disseminated infection.
  - Ceftriaxone: 25–50 mg/kg single dose IV or IM (maximum 125 mg) for infected infants and for those born to an infected, untreated mother.
  - Saline eye irrigations every 10 to 30 minutes until discharge resolves.

OSTEOMYELITIS

Inflammation of bone, usually secondary to bacterial infection

Epidemiology
- 50% of all cases occur in children less than 5 years of age.
- Boys are affected more often than girls (except in first year of life).

Etiology
- *Staphylococcus aureus* is most common.
- Other organisms: *S. pneumoniae*; *S. pyogenes*; Enteric gram-negative rods and group B *Streptococcus* (neonates); *Kingella kingae*; *Neisseria gonorrhoeae* (adolescents); coagulase-negative staphylococci (prosthetic material-related); anaerobes (complicated sinusitis, super-infection of fracture site); *Salmonella* (sickle hemoglobinopathies); *P. aeruginosa* (puncture wound through sneaker)

Pathophysiology
- Hematogenous spread (most common) or extension of contiguous skin/muscle structure infection
- In neonates, infection often extends to the joint space via transphyseal capillaries which recede by 6 to 12 months of age.

Clinical Manifestations
- Most frequently occurs in long bones (in order of decreasing frequency): femur, tibia, hands and feet, humerus, pelvis, fibula
- 75% of cases have single bone involvement.
- Fever, occasionally anorexia, malaise, vomiting, irritability
- Pain and reluctance to use affected extremity ("pseudoparalysis")
- Focal swelling, point tenderness, warmth, and erythema (usually over metaphysis)
- Tenderness out of proportion to soft tissue findings
- Range of motion intact, limited only by pain/muscle spasm
- Neurologic deficits in vertebral osteomyelitis
- In neonates, the entire limb may have swelling, edema, and discoloration.

Diagnostics
- Leukocytosis (often but not always)
- C-reactive protein (CRP): elevated in more than 95% (may be normal in chronic osteomyelitis)
- Erythrocyte sedimentation rate (ESR): elevated in 90%
- Blood culture results: positive in 35% to 50%
- Bone aspirate: culture of bone, blood, and/or joint fluid positive in 50% to 80%
- Plain radiographs: low sensitivity for diagnosing osteomyelitis
  - Ten to 20 days after onset: may detect lytic lesions, periosteal elevation, and new bone formation
- Radionuclide bone scanning: useful in early diagnosis (sensitivity 80% to 100%)
  - Helpful if multiple sites suspected or poorly localizable pain
- MRI: differentiates cellulitis from osteomyelitis and is probably the best study if pain is localized. Sensitivity for detection of osteomyelitis is 92% to 100%.

Management
Medical
- Empiric therapy: Clindamycin or vancomycin is usually first choice due to increasing prevalence of MRSA. Trimethoprin-sulfamethoxazole is a reasonable alternative though experience with this drug in *S. aureus* infection is limited. May switch to oxacillin or ceftriaxone if methicillin-sensitive *S. aureus* is isolated.
- CRP typically begins to decline 2 to 3 days after initiation of antibiotics (normal by 10 days). ESR begins to decline approximately 5 to 7 days after initiation of antibiotics (normal in 3 to 4 weeks).

- Oral therapy (e.g., cephalexin, 150 mg/kg/day) may be considered in cases of *S. aureus* osteomyelitis. Discuss with infectious diseases specialist.
- Duration of therapy: normalization of CRP, resolution of signs/symptoms of infection, and minimum 3 weeks of therapy (typical duration 3 to 6 weeks)

Surgical
- Considerations for surgery: 1) subperiosteal abscess; 2) bacteremia persisting beyond 48 to 72 hours of treatment; 3) continued fever, pain, swelling after 72 hours of therapy; 4) development of sinus tract

Special Situations
- Nonhematogenous osteomyelitis: associated with open fractures, implanted devices, decubitus ulcers, mastoiditis, sinusitis
- Neonatal osteomyelitis: diagnosis often delayed because of nonspecific symptoms; 20% to 50% have multiple bones involved
- Vertebral osteomyelitis: 1% to 3 % of all cases of osteomyelitis; indolent, nonspecific initial symptoms, vertebral tenderness

OTITIS MEDIA

Classification of otitis media (inflammation of mucosal lining of middle ear):

Acute otitis media (AOM): purulent fluid in the middle ear with acute signs and symptoms of local or systemic illness

Otitis media with effusion (OME): asymptomatic middle ear effusion

Chronic suppurative otitis media (CSOM): purulent drainage through perforated tympanic membrane for more than 6 weeks

Epidemiology
- 90% of children have at least one episode of AOM by 2 years of age; 50% have three of more by age 3 years

Etiology
- AOM: *Streptococcus pneumoniae* (35% to 48%); Nontypeable *Haemophilus influenzae* (20% to 29%); *Moraxella catarrhalis* (12% to 23%)
  - Other pathogens include group A *Streptococcus* and *S. aureus*
- Viral pathogens responsible for 10% to 40% of middle ear effusions in AOM
- CSOM is usually polymicrobial: *Pseudomonas* spp; *S. aureus*

Pathophysiology
- For AOM: transient (e.g., upper respiratory tract infection) or chronic eustachian tube dysfunction causes negative middle ear pressure
- Middle ear fluid accumulates with subsequent bacterial superinfection

Clinical Manifestations
- Abrupt onset of crying, fever, or otorrhea
- Middle ear effusion: bulging tympanic membrane, impaired membrane mobility by pneumatic otoscopy, or air-fluid level behind membrane
- Middle ear inflammation: tympanic membrane with red or yellow color; otalgia

Diagnostics
- Diagnosis made by physical exam with pneumatic otoscopy
- Tympanocentesis to 1) relieve severe pain; 2) confirm pathogens in neonates and immunocompromised; 3) failed antibiotic therapy; 4) part of treatment for acute mastoiditis
- Tympanometry confirms middle ear effusion when pneumatic otoscopy cannot be performed

Management
Initial Management of Acute Otitis Media
- Pain control: acetaminophen or ibuprofen; in children older than 5 years, consider topical benzocaine (e.g., auralgan, americaine otic)

- For age 2 years or older, consider initial observation without antibiotics if nonsevere illness or uncertain diagnosis and then treat if no improvement within 48 to 72 hours. *If observation option exercised, must ensure mechanism for communication with physician, reevaluation, and obtaining medication if necessary.*
- For age less than 2 years and for severe illness (severe otalgia or fever 39°C or greater), treat with antibiotics (see below).

Antibiotic Options for Acute Otitis Media
- First-line, *non-severe* disease (if decision made to treat): high-dose amoxicillin, 80 to 90 mg/kg/day in three divided doses
  - Alternate agents for penicillin allergy: cefdinir, cefuroxime, cefpodoxime, azithromycin, clarithromycin, or clindamycin
- First-line, *severe* disease: amoxicillin-clavulanate using 90 mg/kg/day of amoxicillin component with 6.4 mg/kg/day of clavulanate
  - Alternate agents for penicillin allergy: ceftriaxone (1 to 3 days)
- Clinically defined treatment failure (no improvement within 48–72 hours): amoxicillin-clavulanate using 90 mg/kg/day of amoxicillin component (if previously on amoxicillin); otherwise use ceftriaxone (3 days) or clindamycin ± tympanocentesis
- Duration of therapy: 5 days if child older than 2 years of age with uncomplicated AOM; 10 days in child younger than 2 years of age or with underlying medical conditions, recurrent AOM, or tympanic membrane perforation

Additional Considerations
- Persistence of middle ear effusion after AOM: 40% at 1 month and 10% at 3 months
- Recurrent AOM (more than three episodes in 6 months or four or more episodes in 1 year) requires antibiotic prophylaxis after treatment course: consider sulfisoxazole or amoxicillin for 3 to 6 months
- Indications for tympanostomy tubes: 1) chronic otitis media with effusion and associated conductive hearing loss greater than 15 dB; 2) failed chemoprophylaxis for recurrent AOM; 3) tympanic membrane retraction with ossicular erosion or cholesteatoma formation
- OME: First 3 months, observe
  - After 3 months (chronic): tympanostomy tubes if bilateral effusions and hearing loss greater than 15 dB. Antibiotics and corticosteriods not indicated because effusion rapidly reaccumulates upon cessation.
- CSOM: Seven to 14 days of ototopical antibiotics (ciprofloxacin, ofloxacin, neomycin, polymyxin B)
  - Consider oral agents as for AOM
- Complications: middle ear (e.g., conductive hearing loss, cholesteatoma); temporal bone (e.g., mastoiditis, petrositis; see Mastoiditis topic); inner ear (e.g., labyrinthitis); intracranium (e.g., subdural abscess, lateral sinus thrombosis, meningitis)

PERIORBITAL/PRESEPTAL AND ORBITAL CELLULITIS

Periorbital or preseptal cellulitis: infections anterior to orbital septum

Orbital cellulitis: infections posterior to the orbital septum

Epidemiology
- Preseptal cellulitis: usually in children under 5 years of age
- Orbital cellulitis: mean age is 12 years; more common in boys

Etiology
Preseptal Cellulitis
- Infection after local trauma: *S. aureus, S. pneumoniae, S. pyogenes*
- Hematogenous seeding: usually *S. pneumoniae* (since introduction of *H. influenzae* type b vaccine)
- Soft tissue swelling in periorbital area due to compression of ophthalmic veins secondary to sinusitis (not true cellulitis): *S. pneumoniae, Moraxella catarrhalis,* Nontypeable *H. influenzae*

Orbital Cellulitis
- Usually extension of sinusitis into orbit
- Often polymicrobial; most commonly *S. pneumoniae*, group A *Streptococcus, S. aureus,* occasionally anaerobes

Clinical Manifestations
- Fever
- Eyelid edema and erythema (>95% unilateral)

Preseptal Cellulitis
- Evidence of local trauma
- Normal visual acuity, pupillary responses, intraocular pressure and extraocular movements
- No pain with eye movement

Orbital Cellulitis
- Proptosis
- Impaired or painful extraocular eye movements
- Loss of visual acuity or pupillary responses

Diagnostics
- Obtain CBC and blood culture if: suspected or confirmed orbital cellulitis, periorbital cellulitis with fever or toxic appearance.
- Perform a lumbar puncture if signs or symptoms of meningitis.
- CT scan of orbits and sinuses is recommended if: 1) orbital involvement confirmed by exam; 2) orbital involvement is suspected or cannot be excluded by exam; 3) progression of disease despite parenteral antibiotic treatment

Management
Preseptal Cellulitis
- Oral antibiotics if mild infection and child non-toxic
  - First-line: amoxicillin-clavulanate
  - Alternate: clindamycin, dicloxacillin
- Intravenous antibiotics if ill appearing or failed oral treatment
  - First-line: ampicillin-sulbactam; use clindamycin in areas of high MRSA prevalence.
  - Alternate: clindamycin, oxacillin, cefotaxime
  - Total duration: 10 days; may be completed orally if clinical improvement is documented.

Orbital Cellulitis
- Requires intravenous antibiotics initially:
  - First-line: ampicillin/sulbactam
  - Alternate: clindamycin, cefotaxime
  - Total duration of 10 to 14 days
- If no clinical improvement is noted in 24 to 36 hours or if symptoms progress: repeat CT scan and consider surgical drainage
- Surgical drainage if: large, well-defined abscess on initial or repeat CT scan; complete ophthalmoplegia; significant visual impairment

PNEUMONIA

Infection of lung parenchyma

Etiology
- Neonates: group B *Streptococcus*, enteric gram-negative rods, cytomegalovirus, *S. pneumoniae*, herpes simplex virus
- One to 3 months: respiratory syncytial virus (RSV); parainfluenza viruses; *S. pneumoniae; C. trachomatis; Bordetella pertussis; S. aureus*
- Three months to 5 years: RSV; parainfluenza viruses; influenza; adenovirus; *S. pneumoniae; Haemophilus influenzae; Mycoplasma pneumoniae*
- Five to 15 years: *M. pneumoniae, C. pneumoniae, S. pneumoniae*; influenza

- Aspiration: *P. aeruginosa, K. pneumoniae*, oral anaerobes
- Significant pleural effusions:
  - Common: *S. pneumoniae* and *S. aureus*
  - Less common: *S. pyogenes, M. tuberculosis*

Pathophysiology
- Absent systemic or secretory immunity to an organism
- Impaired lower respiratory tract defenses
- Direct inhalation or hematogenous seeding of organism

Clinical Manifestations
- Fever, cough, tachypnea
- Perhaps dyspnea, chest or abdominal pain, malaise
- Hypoxia, nasal flaring, grunting, retractions
- Crackles, egophony, bronchophony, whispered pectoriloquy
- Wheezing suggests a viral or atypical bacterial cause.

Diagnostics
- Chest x-ray findings suggest etiology but may lag behind clinical symptoms:
  - Hilar adenopathy: *M. tuberculosis*, endemic fungi (e.g., *Histoplasma capsulatum, Coccidioides immitis*), *M. pneumoniae*; Epstein-Barr virus
  - Pneumatocele: *S. aureus*, gram-negative rods

Laboratory Studies
- Leukocytosis with left shift with some bacterial infections
- Blood culture result positive in 10% to 25% with pleural effusion; 7% to 10% of hospitalized children with pneumonia; less than 2% of outpatients with pneumonia
- Pleural fluid:
  - Transudate: pH greater than 7.4; LDH less than 1000 U/L; white blood cell count less than 1000/mm^3; no bacteria on Gram stain; glucose greater than 60 mg/dL; pleural/serum LDH ratio less than 0.6
  - Exudate: pH less than 7.3; LDH greater than 1000 U/L; white blood cell count greater than 10,000/mm^3; bacteria present on Gram stain; glucose less than 40 mg/dL; pleural/serum LDH greater than 0.6
  - Send acid-fast culture and stains

Diagnosis of Specific Agents
- Viral pathogens: nasopharyngeal aspirate antigen detection or culture
- *M. pneumoniae* and *C. pneumoniae*: polymerase chain reaction (rapid, accurate); serology (time-consuming); cold agglutinins (too nonspecific)
- Tuberculosis: tuberculin skin test (PPD); culture and acid-fast smear of sputum, bronchoalveolar lavage, or gastric aspirates

Management
- Specific treatment ultimately depends on cause
- Empiric antibiotics depend on age and presentation:
  - Neonate: ampicillin + gentamicin (or cefotaxime) (IV)
  - One to 3 months: ampicillin or cefotaxime (IV); consider addition of macrolide if *C. trachomatis* is suspected.
  - Three months to 5 years: high-dose amoxicillin (oral) or ampicillin (IV); alternate: cefotaxime, ceftriaxone, clindamycin, macrolide
  - More than 5 years: same as 3 months to 5 years; consider using fluoroquinolone alone or adding macrolide to cover atypicals
  - Pleural effusion: clindamycin + cefotaxime. Alternate regimens: oxacillin + cefotaxime; clindamycin; vancomycin; ampicillin-sulbactam
  - Aspiration: amoxicillin-clavulanate (oral) or ampicillin-sulbactam (IV). Alternate: clindamycin, penicillin, levofloxacin, ticarcillin-clavulanate. Aspiration event *without* evidence of pneumonia does not require antibiotic treatment or prophylaxis.

- Pleural effusion:
  - If greater than 10 mm on decubitus CXR, sample pleural fluid by thoracentesis or chest tube
  - If exudative, requires chest tube
  - If loculated, requires open decortication or video-assisted thoracoscopy
- Complications: empyema, lung abscess, necrotizing pneumonia

RETROPHARYNGEAL AND PERITONSILLAR ABSCESS

Peritonsillar abscess: purulent collection in the tonsillar fossa

Retropharyngeal abscess: deep neck abscess involving the potential space between the posterior pharyngeal wall and the alar division of the deep cervical fascia

Epidemiology
- Peritonsillar abscess: typically occurs in older children (mean age 11 years) as a complication of streptococcal pharyngitis; 15% complicate EBV infection.
- Retropharyngeal abscess: typically occurs in young children (<5 years) and complicates pharyngitis. In older children and adolescents, it often complicates penetrating injury to the posterior pharynx.

Etiology
Peritonsillar Abscess
- Common: *S. pyogenes*
- Less common: *S. aureus*, anaerobes (*Fusobacterium, Peptostreptococcus, Bacteroides*), *H. influenzae*

Retropharyngeal Abscess (usually polymicrobial)
- Common: *S. pyogenes, S. aureus*, viridans group streptococci
- Less common: Anaerobes (*Fusobacterium, Peptostreptococcus, Bacteroides* spp), *Eikenella corrodens, H. influenzae, S. pneumoniae*

Pathophysiology
- Peritonsillar abscess begins with pharyngitis or cellulitis and progresses to abscess.
- Retropharyngeal space is limited posteriorly by the alar division of deep cervical fascia and anteriorly by the posterior pharyngeal wall.
- This space is divided by a midline raphe into two lateral compartments with each half containing lymph nodes.
- Infection of the nasopharynx spreads to retropharyngeal space by lymphatic routes. Lymph node inflammation followed by necrosis leads to abscess.
- Retropharyngeal abscess is unlikely in older children due to regression of lymph nodes.
- Complications: extension to carotid sheath (carotid artery, internal jugular vein, vagus nerve) or posteriorly (atlantoaxial dislocation); spontaneous rupture may cause aspiration, asphyxiation, empyema, or mediastinitis.

Clinical Manifestations
Peritonsillar Abscess
- Adolescent with fever, sore throat, unilateral pain, drooling, dysphagia, and "hot potato" (muffled) voice
- Trismus in two thirds
- Oropharynx: displacement of uvula away from affected side, palpable peritonsillar fluctuance, +/– tonsillar exudate
- Ipsilateral cervical adenopathy

Retropharyngeal Abscess
- Fever, decreased oral intake, sore throat
- Drooling, dysphagia, odynophagia
- Neck stiffness or pain with neck extension
- Torticollis, trismus, stridor, and dyspnea are less common (<5%)

Diagnostics
- Leukocytosis with neutrophil predominance
- Rapid streptococcal antigen test by throat swab
- Lateral neck x-ray in retropharyngeal abscess: 1) retropharyngeal space wider than one-half of the C2 vertebrae or greater than 7 mm; 2) retroflexion of cervical vertebrae from abscess pressure (obtain x-ray with neck hyperextended and during inspiration to minimize false positive results)
- Neck CT with contrast: in peritonsillar abscess, assesses extent of infection; in suspected retropharyngeal abscess, distinguishes cellulitis from abscess (false-negative rate of 10%)

Management

Peritonsillar Abscess
- Incision and drainage with 18-gauge needle confirms diagnosis and provides immediate relief
- Empiric therapy: penicillin or clindamycin. Alternate: ampicillin-sulbactam, amoxicillin-clavulanate, cefuroxime.
- Duration of therapy: 7 to 10 days

Retropharyngeal Abscess
- Emergency: secure airway (if necessary); obtain IV access; order nothing by mouth (NPO)
- Early detection (no mature abscess) may obviate surgery
- Most cases of mature abscess require surgical drainage: transoral approach limits exposure of vessels; external approach limits aspiration risk.
- Antibiotics: ampicillin-sulbactam. Alternate: cefotaxime + metronidazole; cefoxitin. Use IV antibiotics initially, and switch to oral antibiotics when symptoms have improved to complete 10- to 14-day course. Longer courses may be necessary for undrained collections.

SEPTIC ARTHRITIS

Microbial invasion of the joint space

Epidemiology
- Peak incidence under 3 years of age

Etiology
- Neonates: *S. aureus*, group B *Streptococcus*, enteric gram-negative rods
- School age: *S. aureus*, *Kingella kingae*, *S. pyogenes*, *S. pneumoniae*, *H. influenzae*
- Older children: *S. aureus*, *S. pyogenes*, *Borrelia burgdorferi*, *N. gonorrhoeae*
- Less common causes: *N. meningitidis*, *Pseudomonas* spp, *Candida* spp, tuberculous and nontuberculous mycobacteria, *Nocardia asteroides*

Pathophysiology
- Mechanism: 1) hematogenous dissemination; 2) contiguous extension (10% to 16% of cases); 3) direct inoculation
- Risk factors: joint instrumentation, urinary tract infection, skin or soft tissue infection, hemoglobinopathy, IV drug use

Clinical Manifestations
- Fever, malaise, poor appetite, irritability (infants)
- Frequency of joint involvement (in order of decreasing frequency): knee, hip, ankle, other
- Severe joint pain, decreased mobility, refusal to walk
- Joint swelling, erythema, warmth, exquisite tenderness, decreased range of motion
- Septic hip held flexed and externally rotated
- 90% of cases are monoarticular.
- Dermatitis-arthritis syndrome, sexually transmitted diseases (*N. gonorrhoeae*)
- History of erythema migrans rash, significant swelling, minimal pain (Lyme)

Diagnostics
- CBC: 70% with elevated WBC
- CRP: elevated at presentation in 95%

Table 15.3: Typical Synovial Fluid Findings

Diagnosis	Typical WBC per mm^3
Normal	<150
Bacterial arthritis	>50,000
Lyme arthritis	30,000–50,000
Reactive arthritis	<15,000

WBC, white blood cell.

- ESR: elevated at presentation in 90%
- Blood culture results: positive in 40%
- Joint fluid aspiration for cell count (Table 15.3)
- Joint fluid culture results: positive in 50% to 60%; yield increased if joint fluid inoculated directly into blood culture bottle
- Joint radiographs: important to exclude other causes of joint pain; not diagnostic for septic arthritis but may reveal distortion of fat pad, soft tissue swelling, and joint space widening
- Ultrasound: preferred initial study to identify excess joint space fluid
- MRI: highly sensitive in early detection of joint fluid; detects involvement of adjacent bone or soft tissue

Management (*This is a medical emergency*)
Surgical
- Hip or shoulder: prompt surgical drainage, joint space irrigation
- Knee, ankle, or wrist: needle aspiration; consider joint space irrigation if unable to perform adequate drainage
- Open surgical drainage of joints other than hip and shoulder is usually not required.

Medical
- Empiric antibiotic therapy
  - Neonate: intravenous oxacillin (or cefazolin) + gentamicin (or cefotaxime)
  - Older children: intravenous clindamycin or vancomycin, switch to oxacillin or cefazolin if methicillin-sensitive *S. aureus* is isolated.
  - Add cefotaxime if risk factors for gram-negative rods
  - Specific antibiotic therapy based on culture results (see also Lyme Disease)
- Oral versus intravenous antibiotics
  - Knee, wrist, or ankle: oral antibiotics once CRP improves
  - Hip or shoulder: IV antibiotics for entire course
- Duration:
  - Three to four weeks for *S. aureus* or enteric gram-negative rods
  - In general, 2 to 3 weeks is sufficient for most other organisms (must be individualized based on patient's course).
- Response to therapy: ESR peaks at end of first week and normalizes at 3 to 4 weeks. CRP peaks by day 2 to 3, and normalizes by day 7 to 9.

SINUSITIS

Inflammation of paranasal sinuses secondary to allergic, bacterial, fungal, or viral etiology. Bacterial sinusitis is classified clinically by the duration of symptoms:

- Acute bacterial sinusitis: symptoms for less than 30 days
- Subacute sinusitis: symptoms for 30 to 90 days
- Chronic sinusitis: symptoms for greater than 90 days

Epidemiology
- Complicates 5% to 10 % of upper respiratory infections

Etiology
- Acute and subacute bacterial sinusitis:
  - *S. pneumoniae*; *H. influenzae*; *Moraxella catarrhalis*
  - Less commonly: group A *Streptococcus*, group C *Streptococcus*, viridans group streptococci, anaerobes, *Eikenella* spp
- Chronic sinusitis: aerobic bacteria found in acute sinusitis, *S. aureus*, anaerobes

Pathophysiology
- Ciliary dysfunction and increased secretions lead to sinus obstruction.
- Contamination of usually sterile sinuses with nasopharyngeal bacteria
- Recurrent bacterial sinusitis should prompt investigation for underlying predisposition (e.g., allergic rhinitis, cystic fibrosis, dysmotile cilia, and HIV).

Clinical Manifestations
- Acute sinusitis:
  - Respiratory symptoms longer than 10 days and not improving. Findings include nasal discharge of any quality, daytime cough, facial pain, headache, painless eye swelling
  - Severe respiratory symptoms for longer than 3 days including purulent nasal discharge and high fever
- Chronic sinusitis: respiratory symptoms for longer than 90 days; nasal discharge of any quality; headache; fever uncommon
- On physical exam: periorbital edema; mucopurulent discharge in nose or posterior pharynx; nasal mucosa are erythematous or boggy and pale; tenderness to palpation and/or percussion over paranasal sinuses; asymmetric sinus transillumination; malodorous breath
- Orbital complications: orbital abscess, optic neuritis
- Intracranial complications require neurosurgical and infectious diseases consultation: epidural or subdural empyema, cavernous or sagittal sinus thrombosis, meningitis, brain abscess, osteomyelitis

Diagnostics
- Diagnosis is usually based on clinical findings.
- Plain radiograph (easy to obtain but poor sensitivity): findings include complete opacification, mucosal thickening greater than 4 mm, air-fluid levels
- CT scan (not routinely required): indications include: 1) complicated sinusitis; 2) numerous recurrences; 3) protracted or unresponsive course; 4) anticipated surgical drainage

Management
Medical
- First-line therapy in uncomplicated sinusitis: amoxicillin 45 mg/kg/day divided in two doses
- Consider alternate agent if 1) allergy to amoxicillin; 2) failure to improve on amoxicillin; 3) moderate to severe illness; 4) protracted symptoms (>30 days); 5) risk factors for amoxicillin resistance (e.g., recent antibiotics, daycare)
- Alternate agents: high-dose amoxicillin-clavulanate (80 mg/kg/day); cefdinir; cefuroxime; cefpodoxime; clarithromycin; azithromycin; clindamycin; levofloxacin
- Duration: treat until patient is symptom-free and then for an additional 7 days (usually total 10 to 14 days).
- Empiric therapy for complicated sinusitis (e.g., subdural extension): vancomcyin + third-generation cephalosporin + metronidazole

Sinus Aspiration
- Indications: 1) failure to respond to multiple course of antibiotics; 2) severe facial pain; 3) orbital or intracranial complications; 4) evaluation of an immunocompromised host

TOXIC SHOCK SYNDROME

An acute streptococcal or staphylococcal exotoxin-mediated infection resulting in fever, diffuse erythroderma, hypotension, and impairment of three or more organ systems

Epidemiology
- 90% of cases in 1980s occurred in context of superabsorbent tampon use. Now less than 50% of cases are associated with tampon use. Other associations include foreign body placement, primary *S. aureus* infection, postoperative wound infection, and mucous membrane or skin disruption.
- *Streptococcus pyogenes*–associated toxic shock syndrome (TSS) is associated with varicella infection, diabetes mellitus, and HIV infection.

Etiology
- *S. aureus* strains producing one or more of the following exotoxins: TSST-1, enterotoxin A, B, C, or D
- *S. pyogenes* strains producing streptococcal pyrogenic exotoxins A, B, or C, mitogenic factor, or streptococcal superantigen

Pathophysiology
- TSST-1 and other exotoxins act as superantigens by crosslinking MHC II and TCR, bypassing normal MHC-mediated antigen presentation. T cell activation causes massive cytokine release.
- Exotoxins cause perivascular infiltrates, decreased peripheral resistance, and interstitial edema resulting in intravascular volume depletion, hypotension, and shock.
- Activation of the coagulation cascade and thrombolytic enzymes induce microangiopathic hemolytic anemia and DIC.

Clinical Manifestations
- Fever, rash, hypotension, arthritis with multi-organ involvement and clinical course out of proportion to degree of local infection
- Diffuse erythroderma or blanching macular erythema that desquamates 1 to 2 weeks later

Diagnostics
- Elevated creatinine
- Platelets less than $100,000/mm^3$ or signs of DIC
- Elevated alanine aminotransferase, aspartate aminotransferase, or total bilirubin
- Blood, throat, and CSF cultures are usually negative; blood cultures may be positive in *S. aureus*–related TSS.

Management
- Anticipate shock and multisystem organ failure
- Remove or drain any loculated source of infection
- Empiric IV antibiotics: beta-lactamase resistant antistaphylococcal antibiotic (e.g., oxacillin, vancomycin) plus a protein-synthesis inhibitor (clindamycin). Consider adding aminoglycoside until diagnosis is more certain.
  - For *S. pyogenes* cases, switch to penicillin + clindamycin.
  - For *S. aureus* cases, continue with an appropriate beta-lactam antibiotic (based on susceptibility testing) and clindamycin.
  - Total antibiotic course of 10 to 14 days may include high-dose oral therapy when the patient is no longer critically ill.
- IVIG decreased mortality in animal models of TSS and in some anecdotal human reports. Early administration may predispose to recurrence by blunting initial immune response. Therefore, IVIG is only recommended for patients with an inaccessible focus of infection or those with continued deterioration following fluid and vasopressor support (dose: 400 mg/kg once).

URINARY TRACT INFECTION

Infection of lower (cystitis) or upper (pyelonephritis) urinary tract

Epidemiology
- 3% to 6% prevalence in young febrile children without a source
- Age and gender influence prevalence:
  - Incidence (in order of decreasing frequency): neonates, infants, school-aged
  - Neonates: boys affected more often than girls; uncircumcised boys at higher risk
  - Age older than 6 months: girls affected more often than boys

Etiology
- *E. coli* (70% to 90% of urinary tract infections [UTIs])
- Other organisms include: *Proteus* spp (boys >1 year); *P. aeruginosa; Enterococcus* spp; *Staphylococcus saprophyticus* (rare before puberty); group B streptococci (neonates); *S. aureus* (suggests additional site of infection, e.g., osteomyelitis, renal abscess)

Pathophysiology
- Host factors: inability to empty bladder completely (e.g., neurogenic bladder, posterior urethral valves, indwelling catheter); vesicoureteral reflux (20% to 30% of children with UTI)

Clinical Manifestations
- History of UTI, renal disease, undiagnosed febrile episodes, sexual activity, genitourinary trauma
- Neonates and Infants: fever or temperature instability; poor feeding; vomiting; jaundice; decreased activity
- Children 2 to 5 years of age: fever; abdominal pain; bedwetting or incontinence in previously toilet-trained child; foul-smelling urine
- Children older than 5 years: fever; vomiting; abdominal pain; dysuria; frequency; urgency; bedwetting or incontinence in previously toilet-trained child; suprapubic or costovertebral angle tenderness

Diagnostics
Laboratory Screening
- Positive urine dipstick ($\geq$ trace leukocyte esterase or nitrites) or urinalysis (on centrifuged urine) with 5 or more white blood cells (WBC) per high-power field has sensitivity of 79% and specificity of 97%. There are few false-positive results, so it can be used to guide decisions regarding initiation of empiric therapy in older children.
- Enhanced urinalysis: positive if greater than 10 WBC/mm^3 on unspun urine or bacteria detected on Gram stain (sensitivity = 94%; specificity = 84%)
  - Few false-negative results, so useful to evaluate infants younger than 8 weeks of age for UTI.

Laboratory Confirmation
- Midstream clean catch method preferred in toilet trained children (Table 15.4)
- Straight catherization recommended in children unable to provide clean catch specimen
- Suprapubic aspiration (see Procedures chapter) unsuccessful in 10% of attempts
- Urine bag specimens are *not* appropriate for culture.

Management
Medical
- Treatment of uncomplicated urinary tract infection: 5 to 7 days of treatment. Empiric therapy (oral): ceftibuten, trimethoprim-sulfamethoxazole (TMP-SMX), ciprofloxacin (adolescents)
- Febrile UTI or suspected pyelonephritis *outpatient* therapy: oral therapy acceptable for uncomplicated pyelonephritis
  - Children must be older than 1 month of age, well-hydrated, and tolerating oral medications; 10 to 14 days of treatment; empiric therapy (oral): ceftibuten, cefdinir, amoxicillin-clavulanate, TMP-SMX

Table 15.4: Interpretation of Urine Culture Results

Method	Probable	Possible
Suprapubic	≥ 100 CFU/mL One pathogen	Any growth One pathogen
Catheterization	≥ 10,000 CFU/mL One pathogen	≥ 1000 CFU/mL One pathogen
Clean catch	≥ 100,000 CFU/mL One pathogen Two cultures	≥ 100,000 CFU/mL One pathogen One culture

CFU, colony-forming unit.

- Febrile UTI or suspected pyelonephritis *inpatient* therapy:
  - Hospitalization and initial intravenous therapy for those with moderate dehydration, ill appearance, significant emesis, underlying urologic abnormalities, poor compliance, and failure of outpatient therapy.
  - Ten to 14 days of treatment; empiric therapy (intravenous): ampicillin + gentamicin, cefotaxime, or ceftriaxone; may switch to oral therapy when patient improved clinically
- No benefit to routine repeat urine cultures after initiation of therapy. Consider repeat cultures if fever or symptoms persist longer than 72 hours.

Imaging
- Ultrasound of urinary tract identifies: hydronephrosis, dilatation of distal ureters, hypertrophy of bladder wall, presence of ureteroceles
  - Recommended by AAP in: 1) all children younger than 2 years of age with first UTI; 2) males at any age; 3) if clinical improvement is slower than anticipated with appropriate treatment
- Voiding cystourethrogram identifies: vesicoureteral reflux (VUR), posterior urethral valves, bladder abnormalities
  - Recommended by AAP in: 1) all children with renal ultrasounds suggestive of VUR; 2) all males with UTI; 3) all girls younger than 5 years with UTI
- Consider VCUG before discharge. Early VCUG does *not* overestimate incidence of VUR.

Specific Pathogens

CAT-SCRATCH DISEASE

A subacute, self-limited regional lymphadenitis syndrome caused by cutaneous inoculation with *Bartonella henselae* (a fastidious pleomorphic gram-negative rod) through cat scratches or bites. Rarer causes include *Afipia felis* and *Bartonella clarridgeiae*.

Epidemiology
- Broad geographic distribution; peaks in fall and early winter
- 90% of cases have a history of recent contact with healthy cats, especially cats younger than 1 year of age or cats with fleas.

Clinical Manifestations
- Primary cutaneous inoculation lesion (papules at site of inoculation) often precedes lymphadenopathy by 1 to 2 weeks.
- Unilateral subacute tender lymphadenopathy in axillary, cervical, submandibular, periauricular, supraclavicular, epitrochlear, femoral, inguinal locations; 1 to 5 cm in size, 10% to 15% suppurate

- *Parinaud's oculoglandular syndrome:* conjunctival granuloma with ipsilateral preauricular lymphadenitis
- Encephalopathy may develop 1 to 6 weeks after primary disease and is associated with seizures and rarely coma with recovery in several weeks. Head CT is typically normal. CSF shows slight mononuclear pleocytosis. EEG is abnormal.
- Fever: up to 5% of cases of fever of unknown origin due to cat-scratch disease (CSD)
- Granulomatous hepatitis or splenitis
- Rare manifestations: osteomyelitis, endocarditis, thrombocytopenic purpura, bacillary angiomatosis in immunocompromised hosts

Diagnostics
- *Serology by indirect fluorescence assay:* IgG titers less than 1:64, no current infection; greater than 1:64 but less than 1:256 possible infection, repeat in 10 to 14 days; greater than 1:256, current or recent infection.
- *PCR* (blood or tissue biopsy specimens): useful to diagnose rare *B. henselae* manifestations
- *Histopathology:* Warthin-Starry silver stain may demonstrate pleomorphic bacilli in chains (not routinely necessary)
- *Culture:* difficult to isolate organism from tissue or blood
- *CT scan:* may reveal multiple hypodense liver or spleen lesions

Management
- Routine antibiotic use for cat-scratch adenitis is controversial because spontaneous resolution typically occurs within 1 to 4 months: azithromycin (10 mg/kg for 1 day, followed by 5 mg/kg for 4 days) may hasten initial decrease in lymph node volume. Antibiotics demonstrating in vitro susceptibility include clarithromycin, rifampin, and ciprofloxacin.
- Consider needle aspiration of painful suppurative nodes for symptomatic relief. Surgical excision is not typically required.
- No controlled trials of therapy exist for other infections (e.g., hepato-splenic CSD, osteomyelitis, bacillary angiomatosis). Consider parenteral gentamicin or azithromycin. Transition to oral therapy when patient is improved. Duration of therapy is unclear.

CLOSTRIDIUM DIFFICILE INFECTION

Clostridium difficile is an anaerobic spore-forming bacterium that causes diarrhea and colitis.

Epidemiology
- 30% to 70% of infants and 1% to 3% of adults are asymptomatic carriers.
- Predisposing factors: hospitalization, prolonged antibiotics, abdominal surgery, inflammatory bowel disease, immune deficiency

Pathophysiology
- Disturbance of normal colonic flora allows *C. difficile* to flourish.
- Spores produce toxins (A and B) that cause mucosal damage.

Clinical Manifestations
- Spectrum of mild diarrhea to severe colitis to toxic megacolon
- Fever and crampy abdominal pain may accompany foul-smelling, watery, often green stools.
- Colitis: stools often have blood or mucous.

Diagnostics
- Stool studies: *C. difficile* toxins A and B
- CBC: leukocytosis, possibly anemia if stool is bloody
- Endoscopy: classic pseudomembrane is a white or yellow plaque along hyperemic and inflamed colonic mucosa. Mucosa may be friable and erythematous without pseudomembrane.

Management
Initial Medical Management
- Contact precautions
- Discontinue offending antibiotics when possible
- Treat any dehydration, anemia
- Surgical consultation if toxic megacolon is present
- Metronidazole PO/IV (PO preferred) 20 mg/kg/day divided four times daily for 10 to 14 days, maximum 1 g/day

Management of Relapse
- 10% to 20% relapse within 4 weeks of stopping therapy due to re-infection, persistent spores, chronic antibiotics, or a pre-disposing underlying disease.
- Initial replase: repeat metronidazole course
- Further relapses: consider vancomycin 40 mg/kg/day PO divided four times daily for 10 to 14 days, maximum 1 g/day

Management of Chronic Relapsing C. difficile
- Prolonged oral vancomycin for 1 to 3 months plus one or several of the following: 1) cholestyramine 240 mg/kg/day PO divided three times daily for 2 to 4 weeks; 2) Lactobacillus; 3) *Saccharomyces boulardii*; 4) GOLYTELY whole bowel irrigation; 5) IVIG 400 mg/kg/dose every 3 weeks; or 6) rectal instillation of normal stool to repopulate the colonic flora ("fecal transplant"—rarely performed)

HEPATITIS A

Hepatitis A virus (HAV) is the predominant form of viral hepatitis and is an acute, self-limited illness.

Epidemiology
- Fecal-oral transmission: very rarely is virus bloodborne
- Humans are the reservoir for the virus; children are the most frequently infected group.
- Outbreaks occur in special living situations such as day care centers, summer camps, institutions, and boarding schools. Food and waterborne outbreaks occur less frequently.

Etiology
- HAV is a single-stranded RNA virus in the picornavirus family.
- No antigenic relationship to other hepatitis viruses

Pathophysiology
- HAV replicates in hepatocytes and is released into the bloodstream, causing viremia.
- Hepatocyte necrosis, especially in centrilobular areas, causes an increase in ALT and AST.
- Virus appears in feces approximately 3 weeks before onset of symptoms.

Clinical Manifestations
- Spectrum of disease varies greatly, ranging from silent infection to fulminant hepatitis. Infants and children are most often asymptomatic.
- Symptoms can include fever, malaise, nausea, emesis, anorexia, abdominal pain, and diarrhea during prodromal period.
- Jaundice, dark urine, acholic stool, hepatomegaly
- Less common: headache, chills, myalgia, arthralgia, pruritus, rash

Diagnostics
- Elevation of ALT, AST, GGT, bilirubin, and alkaline phosphatase
- Transaminitis is most prominent.
- IgM and IgG anti-HAV is detected by immunoassay.
- IgM may be detected for up to 4 months. IgG indicates convalescence and protection against reinfection.

Management
- Supportive: no specific antiviral therapy is available.
- Full recovery requires 2 to 3 months.
- Clinical symptoms can reappear 4 to 7 weeks later in conjunction with second peak of LFTs.
- Prevention: contact precautions; hepatitis A vaccine (not approved for children younger than 2 years); hepatitis A immune globulin given up to 2 weeks after exposure is more than 85% effective in preventing clinical illness.

HEPATITIS B

Hepatitis B virus (HBV) causes both acute and chronic liver disease, including cirrhosis and hepatocellular carcinoma.

Epidemiology
- Three modes of transmission: 1) horizontal transmission through exposure with infected blood products or body fluids; 2) vertical transmission from mother to child at childbirth; 3) sexual intercourse
- Risk of vertical transmission: 70% to 90% if mother is HBsAg and HBeAg positive; 5% to 20% if mother is HBsAg positive but HBeAg negative
- Risk of chronic infection is inversely related to the age at infection. Chronic infection occurs in 90% of infants infected perinatally and 30% of children aged 1 to 5 infected after birth.

Pathophysiology
- Cytotoxic T cells attack HBV-infected hepatocytes, causing inflammation and necrosis.
- Nonhepatic clinical conditions are thought to be mediated by circulating immune complexes composed of HBsAg and anti-HBs (e.g., membranous nephropathy, vasculitis, papular acrodermatitis).

Clinical Manifestations
- Spectrum of disease includes asymptomatic seroconversion (most common in children), acute hepatitis with jaundice and fulminant fatal hepatitis.
- Incubation period ranges from 50 to 180 days.
- Acute infection: 1 to 2 weeks of malaise and anorexia followed by nausea, vomiting, abdominal pain, jaundice, hepatomegaly, and splenomegaly
- Chronic infection: often asymptomatic but progression to cirrhosis and hepatocellular carcinoma varies by population.
- Extrahepatic manifestations:
  - Acute: arthritis, arthralgias, urticarial rash
  - Chronic: vasculitis, membranoproliferative glomerulonephritis
- Hepatocellular carcinoma is seen years after infection with HBV.
- Fulminant hepatic failure occurs in approximately 1 per 100 cases.

Diagnostics
- HBsAg and anti-HBc IgM are present when symptoms appear (Table 15.5). ALT and AST elevations persist for 1 to 2 months in acute infection.
- Chronic HBV: HBsAg present for longer than 6 months or HBsAg present concurrently with anti-HBc IgG. Anti-HBs does not develop. HBeAg is variably present.
- HBeAg indicates active viral replication. Upon conversion to anti-HBe antibody, HBV DNA disappears from serum.
- HBV DNA PCR test is not part of criteria for diagnosis but is useful to follow response to therapy.
- In immunized non-infected patients, only anti-HBs is detected.

Table 15.5: Serology During Four Stages of HBV Infection

Test	Acute Disease	Window Phase	Complete Recovery	Chronic Carrier
HBsAg	Positive	Negative	Negative	Positive
HBsAb	Negative	Negative	Positive	Negative
HBcAb	Positive (IgM)	Positive (IgG)	Positive (IgG)	Positive (IgG)

HB, hepatitis B; sAg, surface antigen; sAb, surface antibody; cAb, core antibody; Ig, immunoglobulin.

Management
Prevention
- Following perinatal exposure, administer hepatitis B immune globulin (HBIG) 0.5 cc IM to infant with the first dose of recombinant HBV vaccine (at different sites) within 12 hours of birth. This combination prevents perinatal transmission in 95% of exposed infants.
  - Second and third doses of HBV vaccine are repeated at 1 and 6 months of age.
  - Infants born to HBsAg-positive mothers should be tested for HBsAg and anti-HBs at 9 to 15 months of age. Testing before 9 months of age may reveal anti-HBs from HBIG administration.
- If mother not tested before delivery, administer first HBV vaccine to infant within 12 hours of birth. Test mother immediately. If she is HBsAg-positive, administer HBIG to infant as soon as possible and within 7 days of birth.

Medical
- Chronic HBV infection: Interferon alpha-2b (5 to 6 million IU/m^2, three times per week for 16–24 weeks) is approved in children > 1 year of age and leads to increased clearance of HBsAg compared to controls. Alternate: Lamivudine (3 mg/kg PO every day; maximum, 100 mg) for 52 weeks, is approved in children 2–17 years of age.
- Children with chronic HBV infection should be screened periodically for sequelae such as hepatocellular carcinoma by serum LFTs, alpha-fetoprotein, and abdominal ultrasound.

HEPATITIS C

Hepatitis C virus (HCV) causes acute and chronic liver disease.

Epidemiology
- Seroprevalence rate in children is 0.2% to 0.4%.
- Despite routine screening of blood products for HCV since 1989, infection is most frequently observed post-transfusion. Risk is estimated to be 0.001% per unit transfused.
- Common modes of infection: blood and blood product transfusions, hemodialysis, intravenous drug use, accidental needle stick injuries, sexually transmitted, vertical transmission from mother to infant (risk increased of perinatal transmission if mother is HIV positive)
- Incubation period: 6 to 7 weeks (range = 2 weeks to 6 months)

Pathophysiology
- Unclear whether direct cytopathic effect of HCV on hepatic parenchymal cells or immune attack by cytotoxic T cells leads to hepatocyte death

Clinical Manifestations
- Spectrum of disease varies greatly.
- Only 20% to 30% with acute infection develop symptoms. These symptoms are clinically indistinguishable from other viral causes of hepatitis and include anorexia, nausea, jaundice, dark urine, and right upper quadrant abdominal pain.
- Extrahepatic findings: arthralgias, palpable purpura, Raynaud phenomenon, peripheral neuropathy, glomerulonephritis

- Aminotransferase elevations are less pronounced than those with HBV.
- Two thirds of children with acute HCV infection progress to chronic disease. Cirrhosis develops in 10% to 20% of patients with chronic disease.
- Fulminant hepatic failure is exceedingly rare.
- Acholic stool, ascites, clubbing, palmar erythema, and spider angiomas are evidence of cirrhosis.

Diagnostics
- HCV RNA can be detected in plasma by reverse-transcriptase PCR within 1 to 2 weeks after infection. HCV RNA indicates current infection and risk of progression to chronic liver disease. A single negative test is not conclusive because viral RNA may be detected intermittently.
- Anti-HCV IgG appears 8 to 10 weeks after infection (no IgM assay available). Antibody detection does not distinguish between acute and chronic infection.

Management
- Data are sparse in children and no therapies are approved in children. In adults, interferon alfa-2b with or without ribavirin may prevent *acute* infection from progressing to *chronic* infection (successful in 98% of adults in one study) (Jaeckel et al., 2001). In children diagnosed with chronic HCV infection, up to 45% are HCV RNA seronegative after therapy.
- Pediatric studies are in development.

LYME DISEASE

Tickborne illness caused by the spirochete *Borrelia burgdorferi*

Epidemiology
- Geographic regions: Northeast, upper Midwest, West Coast
- In endemic areas: incidence of 20 to 100 cases/100,000
- Seasonal occurrence: April to October
- Incidence highest among children 5 to 10 years old

Etiology
- *Borrelia burgdorferi* is transmitted by the bite of infected tick vectors: *Ixodes pacificus* (West Coast), *Ixodes scapularis* (East and Midwest)
- Tick must stay on skin longer than 36 hours for transmission.

Pathophysiology
- Initial infection site: skin
- Once disseminated into bloodstream, *B. burgdorferi* adheres to multiple cell types and persists in tissue unless treated.
- Cytokines amplify inflammatory response and cause local tissue damage.

Clinical Manifestations
- Three stages: early localized, early disseminated, late disease
- *Early localized:* erythema migrans (EM; erythematous annular lesion with central clearing, usually > 5 cm); fever, malaise, headache, myalgias, and arthralgias
- *Early disseminated (3 to 5 weeks after tick bite):* multiple erythema migrans lesions, cranial nerve palsies (especially VII, usually last 2 to 8 weeks and then resolves), fatigue, myalgia, headache, occasionally meningitis or myocarditis
- *Late disease (months to years after tick bite):* mono-articular arthritis of a large joint (knee in > 90%); CNS involvement (chronic demyelinating encephalitis, polyneuritis, memory problems) rare in children
- Jarisch-Herxheimer reaction: transient fever, headache, myalgias after therapy is started

Diagnostics
- Two-test approach: ELISA and confirmatory Western blot
- IgM peaks at 3 to 6 weeks; IgG peaks weeks to months after the bite.

- Antibodies to *B. burgdorferi* usually are not detectable yet in patients with early localized EM rash, so at this stage empirically treat without testing.
- False-positive results to EIA tests may be secondary to other spirochetal infections (syphilis, leptospirosis), systemic lupus erythematosus, EBV, varicella.
- Lumbar puncture (if CNS involvement suspected): usually 10 to 150 WBC/mm^3 and less than 10% segmented neutrophils, elevated protein, normal glucose
- ECG: detect heart block in patients with disseminated Lyme
- Joint aspiration: WBC 25,000 to 125,000/mm^3 and positive Lyme PCR of joint fluid
- *No* proven utility of blood PCR or urine PCR or antigen tests

Management
- Early localized: 14 to 21 days of amoxicillin (<8 years) or doxycycline (≥8 years)
- Early disseminated (multiple EM lesions) and arthritis: oral amoxicillin or doxycycline (21 to 28 days); cefuroxime or erythromycin may be used in young children with penicillin allergy
- For arthritis unresponsive to oral therapy, meningitis, and carditis: IV ceftriaxone for 21 to 28 days. For carditis, if degree of heart block is mild (e.g., first-degree and asymptomatic) may switch to oral therapy.

MALARIA

Intraerythrocytic parasitic infection caused by *Plasmodium* spp (*P. vivax, P. ovale, P. malariae,* and *P. falciparum*)

Epidemiology
- View countries with malaria risk at CDC website (www.cdc.gov)

Pathophysiology
- Transmission is primarily through the bite of an infected *Anopheles* species mosquito. Other modes of transmission: transplacental; bloodborne (e.g., transfusion, needle stick); cryptic
- Sporozoites from mosquito infect hepatocytes, differentiate to merozoites, and infect RBCs.
- Periodic RBC lysis releases merozoites to infect other RBCs.
- *Plasmodium vivax* and *P. ovale* have a dormant hepatic phase that can cause late relapse if not properly treated.

Clinical Manifestations
- High fever: cyclical pattern (every 48 to 72 hours). Fevers may occur daily, especially with *P. falciparum.*
- Chills, rigors, headache, sweats
- Nausea, vomiting, diarrhea, arthralgias, abdominal or back pain
- Pallor, jaundice, signs of anemia and thrombocytopenia, hepatosplenomegaly
- *Plasmodium falciparum*: influenza-like illness. Other syndromes:
  - Severe hemolysis, acute tubular necrosis, adrenal insufficiency, hypoglycemia, shock ("Black water fever")
  - Cerebral malaria: altered mentation, seizures, increased ICP, and progression to coma and death
- *Plasmodium vivax* and *P. ovale*: relapse due to latent intra-hepatic stage
  - Hypersplenism with danger of late splenic rupture
- *Plasmodium malariae*: nephrotic syndrome; chronic asymptomatic parasitemia

Diagnostics
- Blood smears: microscopic exam of thick (detect organisms) and thin (identify species) Giemsa-stained peripheral blood smears. *Plasmodium* species can be distinguished based on morphology of their blood stages.
- Multiple smears (every 12 hours) over 48 to 72 hours may be necessary.
  - Parasitemia >2% suggests *P. falciparum*

- Other findings: anemia, leukopenia, thrombocytopenia, hypoglycemia, proteinuria, hematuria, elevated hepatic transaminases and indirect bilirubin (hemolysis)
- Other diagnostic tests are helpful but not yet widely available: malaria antigen detection, species specific PCR diagnosis of malaria, malaria antibody detection, *Plasmodium*-associated lactate dehydrogenase detection

Management
- Establish 1) malaria-specific immune status (nonimmune status if: age ≤ 5 years; not from an indigenous area; reside in an indigenous area for < 1 year); 2) Likelihood of *P. falciparum* infection; 3) Whether prophylaxis taken
- If *P. falciparum* infection is excluded, patient may be treated as outpatient with repeat smears in the first few days as well as day 7 and 28.
- If infecting species is *P. falciparum* or *P. falciparum* cannot be excluded, nonimmune individuals require hospitalization due to risk of rapid clinical deterioration.
- Supportive care includes monitoring for hypoglycemia, anemia (hemolysis), fluid and electrolyte disturbances, and renal failure.
- Consider exchange transfusion for parasitemia greater than 10% or severe complications at lower parasitemia (e.g., cerebral malaria).
- Parasitemia should decrease over first 48 to 72 hours to 25% of initial parasitemia.

Treatment
- Refer to 2003 Redbook or CDC (www.cdc.gov) for additional information.
- Chloroquine-resistant *P. falciparum*
  - Quinine sulfate (25 mg/kg/day divided three times daily; maximum, 650 mg three times daily) for 3 to 7 days plus doxycycline (2 mg/kg/day divided twice daily; maximum, 100 mg twice daily) for 7 days OR
  - Quinine sulfate (3 to 7 days) plus clindamycin (30 mg/kg/day divided three times daily; maximum, 900 mg three times daily) for 5 days OR
  - Atovaquone/proguanil for 3 days
- Chloroquine-resistant *P. vivax*
  - Quinine sulfate (3 to 7 days) plus doxycycline for 7 days OR
  - Mefloquine: 15 mg/kg followed by 10 mg/kg 8 to 12 hours later (maximum 750 mg followed by 500 mg 8 to 12 hours later)
- Any *Plasmodium* species not resistant to chloroquine
  - Chloroquine phosphate for 3 days OR
  - Quinidine gluconate (intravenous)
  - Prevention of relapse (*P. vivax* and *P. ovale*): Primaquine phosphate for 14 days; high risk of hemolysis in patients with glucose-6-phosphate deficiency

NEONATAL HERPES SIMPLEX VIRUS INFECTION

Three main manifestations of neonatal herpes simplex virus (HSV):
- Localized skin, eye, mouth (SEM) involvement (33% of cases)
- CNS involvement with or without SEM disease (33% of cases)
- Disseminated disease involving multiple organs with or without CNS involvement (33% of cases)
- Other TORCH infections discussed in Neonatology chapter

Epidemiology
- Incidence of 1 in 3500 live births
- Perinatal transmission rate is higher with maternal primary genital HSV infection (33% to 50%) than with recurrence (0% to 5%).
- Onset: 9% at less than 24 hours of life; 30% at 1 to 5 days; 60% at greater than 5 days of life; usual onset is at 11 to 17 days of life.
- Higher risk with history of maternal sexually transmitted diseases, scalp electrodes, prematurity, lethargy, seizures

Differential Diagnosis
- Non-infectious etiologies: erythema toxicum, miliaria, neonatal lupus, Langerhans cell histiocytosis, epidermolysis bullosa
- Infectious etiologies: *S. aureus, P. aeruginosa,* group B *Streptococcus,* cytomegalovirus, *Treponema pallidum,* varicella

Clinical Manifestations
- No single constellation of signs and symptoms identifies all infants with HSV infections. The presence of skin lesions and seizures is most suggestive.
- 17% to 39% do *not* have skin vesicles at time of presentation.
- Ill appearing, fever, lethargy
- Conjunctivitis, skin vesicles, seizures, hepatomegaly
- Respiratory distress, hypoxia, cough
- Disseminated intravascular coagulopathy

Diagnostics
- Send CSF cell count, glucose, protein, and bacterial culture/Gram stain. Also perform urine and blood cultures.
- CSF should also be sent for HSV PCR (gold standard).
  - PCR is reliable up to 7 days after initiation of acyclovir.
- Culture skin vesicles, conjunctiva, oropharynx, and rectum (specify HSV culture to laboratory).
- Direct fluorescent antibody (DFA) staining of vesicle scraping is rapid but less sensitive than cultures
- Elevated ALT and AST with disseminated disease
- Patients with proven HSV and possible CNS involvement should have an EEG and CT or MRI of head during the acute period.

Management
- High-dose intravenous acyclovir (60 mg/kg/day divided every 8 hours): treat 21 days for CNS or disseminated disease and 14 days for SEM disease
  - Some experts recommend repeating lumbar puncture before completion of therapy. If HSV PCR remains positive, they suggest treating for additional 1 to 2 weeks (limited data available).
- Side effects of acyclovir: neutropenia, renal failure
- Prognosis:
  - SEM: neurologic impairment only with recurrent skin lesions
  - CNS infection: low risk of death in those treated but greater than 60% of survivors have neurologic impairment
  - Disseminated infection: high risk of death despite treatment, but < 20% of survivors have neurologic impairment

PERTUSSIS

Respiratory disease caused by *B. pertussis*, a fastidious gram-negative rod

Epidemiology
- Humans are the only host for *B. pertussis*. Transmission occurs through respiratory droplets and direct or indirect contact with nasal secretions.
- One third of reported cases occur in infants less than 6 months of age (non-immunized or partially immunized infants).
- Most cases occur from July to October.
- Immunity is not permanent, and older individuals may be infected.

Pathophysiology
- Pertussis toxin is responsible for local epithelium damage, leading to peribronchial inflammation and necrotizing bronchopneumonia.

Clinical Manifestations

- Incubation period is 6 to 20 days
- Three stages of the disease:
  - *Catarrhal* (1 to 2 weeks): rhinorrhea, low-grade fevers, sneezing; most infectious stage
  - *Paroxysmal* (2 to 4 weeks): paroxysmal coughing after which the child may become flushed or cyanotic or have post-tussive emesis. "Whoop" occurs during sudden forceful inspiration. Infants may present with apnea or cyanosis and often lack the characteristic cough or whoop.
  - *Convalescent* (1 to 2 weeks): chronic cough can persist for weeks.
- Complications: superinfection (bacterial pneumonia causes 90% of morbidity), seizures, encephalopathy, and pulmonary hypertension

Diagnostics

- Chest x-ray: perihilar infiltrates, "shaggy right heart border"
- Typically, absolute lymphocytosis with WBC greater than 15,000/mm^3
- Risk of hyponatremia due to SIADH
- PCR of nasopharyngeal swab specimen is the preferred test at many institutions (high sensitivity). Direct immunofluorescence is less sensitive.
- Culture with Dacron swab; best in the catarrhal phase or early paroxysmal phase (60–70% sensitivity)

Management

- Therapy can curb symptoms if started in the catarrhal stage, but will not improve course of disease or symptoms if started later; however, all infants should be treated to prevent transmission to others. Erythromycin (40 to 50 mg/kg/day divided four times daily for 14 days) is the drug of choice.
- TMP-SMX, azithromycin, or clarithromycin are alternatives to erythromycin.
- Respiratory isolation for hospitalized patients until patient is no longer contagious (5 days of treatment; routine hospitalization to complete treatment is not warranted)
- Prophylaxis for close contacts with erythromycin, clarithromycin, or azithromycin
- Consider hospitalization of young infants at risk for apnea.

RICKETTSIAL DISEASES

Tickborne illnesses caused by obligate intracellular pathogens that share similar clinical and epidemiologic features and treatment: includes ehrlichiosis, Q fever, rickettsialpox, Rocky Mountain spotted fever (RMSF), and endemic typhus. RMSF and ehrlichiosis are most common and are discussed subsequently.

- RMSF is caused by *Rickettsia ricketsii*.
- Ehrlichiosis manifests as human monocytic ehrlichiosis (HME; *Erlichia chaffeensis*) and granulocytic ehrlichiosis (HGE; human granulocytic ehrlichia).

Epidemiology

- RMSF and HME are most prevalent in the southeastern, south central and northern Rocky Mountain states. HGE occurs in Wisconsin, Minnesota, Connecticut, New York, Massachusetts, and the West Coast.
- Highest prevalence in late spring, summer, and early fall
- Transmission:
  - RMSF: Dog tick (*Dermacentor variabilis*), Wood tick (*Dermacentor andersonii*), and Lone Star tick (*Amblyomma americanum*)
  - HME: Lone Star tick (*Amblyomma americanum*); animal resovoir is the white tail deer
  - HGE: *Ixodes scapularis*; animal resovoir is the white-footed mouse
- Incubation period: 2 to 14 days for RMSF (median 7 days); 7 to 14 days for HME and HGE (median 10 days)

Pathophysiology

- After inoculation, rickettsia multiply in small vessel endothelium leading to focal areas of small vessel inflammation, thrombus, and capillary leak.

Clinical Manifestations

- Early phases: fever, headache, rash, malaise, myalgia, nausea, vomiting, abdominal pain
- RMSF rash: typically begins on ankles and wrists spreading both centrally to the trunk (within hours) and to the palms and soles; initially blanching, erythematous, and macular but becomes petechial and then hemorrhagic; develops between third and fifth day of illness, but 10% of patients never develop rash
- Rash in 30% to 50% of HME; rash in less than 10% of HGE; rash can be macular, maculopapular, or petechial with variable distribution.
- Other organ systems may be involved:
  - GI: diarrhea, hepatomegaly, splenomegaly, jaundice
  - Renal: renal failure, acute tubular necrosis
  - Cardiac: congestive heart failure, arrhythmias, shock
  - Neurologic: meningitis, encephalopathy, seizures, ataxia, aphasia, cranial nerve palsies
  - Pulmonary and generalized edema, signs of capillary leak
- Duration of illness typically 1 to 2 weeks; 2% to 3% mortality

Diagnostics

- Thrombocytopenia, anemia, and leukopenia; PT and PTT prolongation; elevated bilirubin, ALT, AST, BUN and creatinine; low fibrinogen, albumin, and sodium.
  - Leukopenia, anemia, and hepatitis are more frequent in ehrlichiosis than in RMSF.
  - WBC and platelets nadir at 5 to 7 days of illness and then recover.
- CSF pleocytosis and elevated protein in a third of patients
- Rickettsia-specific serology: positive titers usually occur 6 to 10 days into illness. Fourfold increase in titer by indirect fluorescent antibody (IFA) between acute and convalescent sera (2 to 3 weeks later) confirms diagnosis.
- In RMSF, *R. rickettsii* can be identified by direct antibody staining of a rash biopsy specimen.
- In ehrlichiosis, 50% have intraleukocytoplasmic inclusions (morulae) in neutrophils (HGE) and monocytes (HME) on buffy coat or peripheral blood smear.
- Rickettsia-specific PCR of skin and blood is available at some reference laboratories but is limited by poor sensitivity.

Management

- Provide supportive management as indicated. Anticipate complications: hypotension, thrombocytopenia, DIC, hypoalbuminemia, and hyponatremia.
- Recommended antibiotic is doxycycline 2–4 mg/kg PO/IV divided twice daily. Alternatives for RMSF include chloramphenicol. Alternatives for ehrlichiosis include chloramphenicol or rifampin. Continue therapy until patient is afebrile for at least 2 days. The usual course is 7 to 10 days.
- Because delay of antibiotic treatment greater than 5 days after onset of symptoms is associated with greater mortality, treat suspected cases empirically.
- Expect clinical improvement in 24 to 36 hours and defervescence in 48 to 72 hours after initiation of therapy. Mildly ill patients can be treated as outpatients. Hospitalization is recommended for severely ill patients who have had systemic complications.

TUBERCULOSIS

Caused by *M. tuberculosis*, an acid-fast bacillus

Latent tuberculosis infection (LTBI): patient has positive tuberculin skin test (TST), no physical exam findings, and a chest x-ray that is either negative or reveals only calcifications or granulomas in lung, lymph nodes, or both.

Tuberculosis (TB) disease: patient with infection in whom symptoms, signs, and/or radiographic findings are apparent.

Epidemiology
- Increased risk of infection in certain populations: low income; urban; nonwhite racial groups; foreign born; residence in jails, nursing homes, or homeless shelters; injection drug use; HIV infection; emigration from developing country

Etiology
- Transmission is person to person usually via airborne droplets but can occur by direct contact with infected body fluids.
- Children rarely infect others because they have sparse bacilli in endobronchial secretions and diminished force of cough.
- Adolescents are potentially infectious.

Clinical Manifestations
Intrathoracic Disease (includes primary infection and reactivation)
- Most infected children have positive TST and no symptoms.
- Hilar adenopathy, focal infiltrate, and pleural effusion are common.
- Extensive pulmonary infiltrates and cavitation are rare.
- Symptoms of primary infection and reactivation may include nonproductive cough, hemoptysis, chest pain, dyspnea, fever, night sweats, anorexia, failure to thrive, weight loss

Miliary Tuberculosis
- Bacteremia leads to disease in two or more organ systems. TST is nonreactive in 30%.
- Usually early complication of primary pulmonary tuberculosis in infants
- Initially malaise, anorexia, weight loss, fever
- Progresses to high fever, respiratory distress, hypoxia, and symptoms of other organ system involvement (e.g., hepatomegaly, splenomegaly, diffuse adenopathy)

Central Nervous System Disease
- Most common in ages 6 months to 4 years
- Usually occurs 2 to 6 months after initial infection
- Clinical manifestations vary widely. Symptoms may be mild (e.g., fever, mild but persistent headache) or severe (e.g., cranial nerve abnormalities, seizures, and decorticate posturing).

Other Manifestations
- Pericarditis, lymphadenitis, bone or joint infections, abdominal infection (peritonitis, mesenteric adenitis), cutaneous lesions

Diagnostics
Tuberculous Skin Test
- Mantoux test containing 5 tuberculin units of purified protein derivative (PPD) administered intradermally
- Time from infection to development of positive TST is 2 to 12 weeks.
- Delayed hypersensitivity reaction to TST peaks at 48 to 72 hours.
- Nonreactive TST does not exclude infection or disease.
- Special situations warranting immediate TST include 1) radiographic or clinical findings suggesting TB; 2) vertebral osteomyelitis; 3) pericarditis; 4) prior to initiation of immunosuppressive therapy

Definition of Positive TST: based on diameter of induration
- *Induration 5 mm or greater in diameter*: 1) contact with infectious cases; 2) abnormal chest x-ray; 3) clinical evidence of tuberculosis disease; 4) HIV infection or other immunosuppressive conditions or therapy (e.g., corticosteroids, chemotherapy)
- *Induration 10 mm or greater in diameter*: 1) children at risk of disseminated disease (age < 4 years or compromising conditions such as diabetes mellitus, chronic renal failure, and

malnutrition); 2) birth in or travel to country with high TB prevalence; 3) frequently exposed to adults with TB risk factors

- *Induration 15 mm or greater in diameter:* children 4 years of age or older without risk factors

Laboratory Diagnosis

- Acid-fast smear and culture are most important tests for definitive diagnosis but organism may take 2 to 10 weeks to grow:
  - Early morning gastric aspirates (three specimens on consecutive days) are best for diagnosis of pulmonary TB in young children (positive in < 50% of children with pulmonary TB)
  - Cultures from sputum (in older children), CSF, pleural fluid, urine, or bone marrow biopsy specimen as indicated
- DNA probes and PCR are not widely available. PCR is approved only for smear-positive respiratory tract specimens due to poor sensitivity.
- Chest x-ray to distinguish LTBI from TB disease
- Head CT: in TB meningitis, detects basilar meningitis, increased intracranial pressure, and tuberculomas

Management

- Exposure to contagious household contact with TB disease
  - Treat with INH even if TST is negative (especially for immunocompromised and children younger than 4 years of age)
  - Repeat TST in 3 months: if still negative then discontinue INH. If TST becomes positive, continue INH for a total of 9 months.
- LTBI
  - Therapy prevents most cases of progression to TB disease.
  - Isoniazid (INH) for 9 months; consider 12 months of therapy for immunocompromised patients. Alternate regimen for adults: 2 months of rifampin + pyrazinamide
  - If contact has INH-resistant TB, use rifampin for 6 months
- Pulmonary TB
  - INH + rifampin + pyrazinamide for 2 months followed by INH + rifampin for 4 months. If drug resistance suspected, add either ethambutol or streptomycin to the three-drug regimen until susceptibility results are available.
  - For hilar adenopathy without other pulmonary disease, consider INH + rifampin for 9 months.
- Extrapulmonary TB (including meningitis and miliary TB)
  - INH + rifampin + pyrazinamide + streptomycin for 2 months followed by INH + rifampin for 10 months. Capreomycin or kanamycin can be substituted for streptomycin.
  - Corticosteriods (e.g., dexamethasone or prednisone) for 6 to 8 weeks in patients with TB meningitis; consider for TB pericarditis and pleural effusion to hasten fluid absorption
- Dosing
  - INH: 10 mg/kg every day (maximum, 300 mg); pyridoxine supplementation (with INH) is recommended for 1) milk- or meat-deficient diets; 2) HIV-infected children; 3) breastfeeding infants; 4) pregnant females
  - Rifampin: 10–20 mg/kg every day (maximum, 600 mg)
  - Pyrazinamide: 20–40 mg/kg every day (maximum, 2 g)
  - Ethambutol: 15–25 mg/kg every day (maximum, 2.5 g)
  - Streptomycin: 20–40 mg/kg every day (maximum, 1 g); IM administration only

VARICELLA ZOSTER INFECTIONS

Primary infection with varicella zoster virus (VZV) causes varicella (chickenpox). Reactivation of latent VZV causes herpes zoster (shingles).

Epidemiology

Varicella

- Transmission to 90% of unimmunized household contacts
- Transmission to 12% to 33% during less sustained exposures

Herpes Zoster
- Rare in immunocompetent children younger than 10 years of age
- Primary VZV infection acquired in utero or during first year of life is associated with increased risk of herpes zoster

Pathophysiology
Varicella
- Mucosal inoculation by respiratory droplets or by direct lesion contact
- Transmission to susceptible contacts exposed 24 to 48 hours before the appearance of skin lesions

Herpes Zoster
- Latent VZV infection in dorsal root ganglion
- Transmission by contact with lesions: VZV is present in skin lesions but is not released into respiratory secretions.

Clinical Manifestations
Varicella
- Incubation period of 10 to 21 days
- Prodrome 24 to 48 hours before rash appears (fever, malaise, anorexia, headache)
- Generalized pruritic rash begins on scalp, face or trunk and eventually involves the extremities (less intensely). Initial erythematous macules progress to clear fluid-filled vesicles with a surrounding erythematous irregular margin ("dew drops on a rose petal.") Lesions in multiple stages present on the same are of the body, especially on mucous membranes of the oropharynx, conjunctivae, and vagina.
- In 24 to 48 hours, lesions begin crusting.
- New lesions continue to appear for 1 to 7 days.

Herpes Zoster
- Vesicular lesions in dermatomal distribution of sensory nerve. Usually one to three dermatomal segments involved.
- Discrete vesicles appear first and then enlarge and coalesce.
- Rash is often preceded by pain, pruritis, or hyperesthesia.

Complications
- Complications of varicella: secondary bacterial infections with *S. aureus* or *S. pyogenes* (e.g., cellulitis, necrotizing fasciitis, pneumonia), meningoencephalitis, Reye syndrome, hepatitis, nephritis, post-infectious cerebellitis
- Complications of primary varicella in high-risk populations:
  - Fetus/newborn: congenital varicella syndrome if varicella is acquired in first 20 weeks of gestation; neonatal varicella if varicella develops in mother from 5 days before to 2 days after delivery; 30% fatality if untreated
  - Immunocompromised (lymphoproliferative malignancies, solid tumors, and solid organ transplantation): visceral dissemination and severe, progressive varicella
- Complications of herpes zoster:
  - Depends on distribution of involved nerve. Potential complications include conjunctivitis, keratitis, uveitis, iridocyclitis, and facial palsies.
  - Immunocompromised: visceral dissemination

Diagnostics
- Laboratory studies are not routinely indicated but a specific diagnosis of VZV guides treatment in immunocompromised children.
- Viral culture of lesion for definitive diagnosis (requires 3 to 7 days)
- Rapid diagnosis: direct fluorescent antibody (DFA) test performed on *epithelial cells* scraped from base of lesions is more rapid and sensitive than culture.
- PCR of body fluid/tissue is used to diagnose unusual VZV manifestations.
- VZV IgG is detectable within 3 days after onset and persists for life after primary infection.

Management

Varicella

- Varicella vaccination within 72 hours of exposure may prevent or significantly modify disease (administer if no contraindications to varicella vaccination)
- Indications for acyclovir: 1) Immunocompromised including malignancy, bone marrow or organ transplant, high-dose steroid therapy, HIV infection, and congenital T-lymphocyte deficiency; 2) neonatal varicella; 3) varicella-associated pneumonia or encephalitis
- IV dose:
  - If younger than 1 year old: 30 mg/kg divided every 8 hours given over 1 hour
  - If older than 1 year old: 1.5 g/m² divided into every 8 hours given over 1 hour
  - Duration: 7 days or until no new lesions have appeared
- Consider acyclovir for infection in the following situations: chronic cutaneous disorders, cystic fibrosis or other pulmonary disorders, diabetes mellitus, disorders requiring chronic salicylate therapy or intermittent corticosteroid therapy, children older than 12 years
  - Oral administration within 24 hours after initial lesions appear
  - Oral dose: 80 mg/kg/day divided every 6 hours (maximum, 800 mg/dose) for 5 days

Herpes Zoster

- Acyclovir reduces pain and duration of new lesion formation if initiated within 72 hours of infection onset and is recommended for patients at high risk for disseminated disease.
- Dose: same as that for primary infection for total of 7 days or for 2 days after last new lesion

Passive Antibody Prophylaxis with Varicella Zoster Immune Globulin Following Varicella Exposure

- Recommended for 1) immunocompromised children with no history of VZV; 2) pregnant women with no history of or antibodies to VZV; 3) infants born to mothers whose varicella began within 5 days before or 2 days after delivery; 4) premature infants less than 28 weeks, or less than 1000 g or hospitalized premature infant with no maternal history of varicella
- Ideally administer within 48 hours of exposure but acceptable if administered within 96 hours.
- Dose: 1 vial (125 U)/10 kg body weight (maximum 5 vials) IM

Fever and Bacteremia

CATHETER-RELATED BLOODSTREAM INFECTION

Bacteria or yeast cultured from a central venous or arterial catheter

Epidemiology

- Risk with nontunneled is greater than tunneled is greater than totally implantable catheter
  - Tunneled = Hickman, Broviac, Groshong, and Quinton catheters
  - Totally implantable = portacath, permacath (hemodialysis)
- Lower risk with silver chelated collagen cuff, antibiotic impregnated catheter (e.g., minocycline + rifampin, chlorhexidine + silver sulfadiazine), and chlorhexidine preparation compared to beta-dine preparation

Etiology

- Coagulase-negative staphylococci, *S. aureus*, *Enterococcus*, *P. aeruginosa*, and other gram-negative bacilli, *Candida* spp, rapid-growing Mycobacteria (e.g., *M. chelonae*, *M. fortuitum*, *M. abscessus*)

Pathophysiology

- Migration of skin organisms into catheter
- Hematogenous seeding of catheter from another focus of infection or translocated bacteria from the gastrointestinal tract

Clinical Manifestations
- Fever alone
- Fever, hypotension, tachycardia, tachypnea (septic shock)
- Abscess or cellulitis at catheter insertion site
- Complications warrant infectious diseases consult: sepsis, bacterial endocarditis, mycotic aneurysms, disseminated candidiasis (endophthalmitis, endocarditis, or hepatosplenic or renal candidiasis)

Diagnostics
- Blood cultures from the catheter *and* periphery are preferred. In children the difficulty in obtaining adequate volume from peripheral culture may limit results. Following criteria indicate CVC as source of infection:
  - *Quantitative blood cultures:* 1) CVC culture yields a colony count at least fivefold *higher* than peripheral blood culture; 2) 15 or more CFU from catheter tip by *semiquantitative* culture (colony counts directly from agar plate); or 3) 100 or more CFU from catheter tip by *quantitative* culture (serial dilutions of original specimen allows for more precise enumeration of colony count)
  - *Alternate (easier) method-differential time to positivity:* Positive result from CVC culture at least 2 hours earlier than from peripheral culture. Compared to quantitative blood culture methods, differential time to positivity has sensitivity = 80% to 90% and specificity = 75% to 94%
  - Culture and Gram stain of any insertion site exudate
  - CBC with differential
  - In severe illness: electrolytes, liver function tests, DIC panel
  - Echocardiogram if the blood culture remains positive despite appropriate therapy and/or a new murmur develops.
  - Rapid-growing mycobacteria grow in conventional blood culture bottles. Isolation of MAI requires special AFB isolator blood culture tubes (check with Infectious Diseases or with Microbiology Laboratory).
  - If culture grows *Candida* spp, obtain ophthalmologic exam to exclude ocular dissemination. Also consider CT of brain/abdomen and echocardiogram.

Management
- Empiric regimens may vary depending on regional antibiotic susceptibility patterns.
- Fever alone in presence of a central catheter:
  - Oxacillin 150 mg/kg/day divided every 6 hours
  - Gentamicin 3 mg/kg/day divided every 8 hours (peak/trough with third dose)
- Shock in presence of a central catheter:
  - Vancomycin 40 mg/kg/day divided every 6 hours (trough before third dose)
  - Ceftazidime 150 mg/kg/day divided every 8 hours
  - Gentamicin 3 mg/kg/day divided every 8 hours (peak/trough with third dose)
- Amphotericin B (AmB; 1 mg/kg every day) or Lipid-AmB (3–6 mg/kg QD) for *Candida* spp; may use fluconazole (6–12 mg/kg every day; maximum 400 mg every day) if *C. albicans* or *C. parapsilosis* is isolated. Pediatric data allumulating for caspofungin and voriconazole.
- Reasons to discontinue the central catheter: 1) rapid clinical deterioration; 2) cellulitis or abscess at or along catheter site; 3) persistently positive blood culture results despite appropriate therapy; 4) culture reveals *Candida* spp or is polymicrobial
- Treatment length is individualized for organism and clinical course. Typical regimens include:
  - Coagulase-negative staphylococci: 7 days
  - *S. aureus:* 10 to 14 days
  - Gram-negative rods: 10 to 14 days
  - *Candida* species: 14 days from first negative culture. Disseminated infection requires prolonged therapy.

FEVER IN NEONATES

Temperature 38.0°C or greater in neonate (age 0 to 28 days) or young infant (age 29 to 56 days).

Epidemiology
- Serious bacterial infection (SBI) occurs in 9% to 13% of febrile neonates, including urinary tract infections (4% to 8%), bloodstream infections (2%), pneumonia (1%), and meningitis (0.5% to 1%).

Etiology
- Urinary tract infections: *E. coli, Klebsiella,* and *Enterobacter* spp, group B *Streptococcus* (GBS)
- Bloodstream infections: GBS; *E. coli, Klebsiella,* and *Enterobacter* spp; *Listeria monocytogenes*; coagulase-negative staphylococci; *S. aureus*; Enteroviruses; HSV
- Pneumonia: GBS; *E. coli, Klebsiella,* and *Enterobacter* spp; *L. monocytogenes*; *Chlamydia trachomatis*; respiratory viruses; cytomegalovirus
- Meningitis: GBS; *E. coli, Klebsiella,* and *Enterobacter* spp; *L. monocytogenes*; Enteroviruses; HSV (see Neonatal HSV section)

Pathophysiology
- Degree of neonatal immune compromise is inversely related to gestational age and birth weight.
- High risk of systemic dissemination from any bacterial infection
- Labor and delivery expose neonates to unique pathogens.

Clinical Manifestations
- Important history: maternal fever or infection, birth history, ill contacts, level of activity, irritability, feeding, lethargy, vomiting, bowel habits, urine output, jaundice, respiratory distress, fever, or rashes
- Medical history should include immunization status, existing medical conditions (e.g., HIV, asplenia), prematurity
- Neurologic: bulging fontanelle, lethargy, irritability, hypotonia, hypertonia, weak suck or cry
- Respiratory: tachypnea, grunting, nasal flaring, retractions, hypoxemia, apnea, cyanosis
- Cardiovascular: tachycardia, bradycardia, hypotension, delayed capillary refill, diminished pulses
- Gastrointestinal: abdominal tenderness, distended or firm abdomen, diminished bowel sounds, periumbilical ecchymoses or erythema, discharge from umbilical stump
- Skin: jaundice, mottled skin, petechiae
- Skeletal: focal bone tenderness

Diagnostics and Management
- Specific protocol may vary by hospital. The Philadelphia protocol is described subsequently.
- All infants 56 days old or younger undergo complete evaluation: CBC with differential; blood culture; urinalysis with Gram stain and cell count; urine culture; CSF cell count, glucose, protein and culture; chest x-ray (if respiratory signs)
- Hospitalize all neonates (age 0 to 28 days) to administer empiric intravenous antibiotic therapy until either an organism is identified or all culture results are negative for 48 hours or longer: ampicillin + gentamicin OR ampicillin + cefotaxime
- In young infants (age 29 to 56 days), the Philadelphia protocol identifies those at low risk for bacterial disease who may not require empiric antibiotic therapy (Baker et al., 1993). Criteria to identify low risk infants (29 to 56 days) are:
  - Exam: well appearance and normal exam
  - CBC: less than 15,000 WBC/mm³; band to neutrophil ratio less than 0.2
  - Spun urinalysis: less than 10 WBC/hpf; no bacteria on Gram stain
  - CSF: less than 8 WBC/mm³; no bacteria on Gram stain
  - Chest x-ray (if performed): no evidence of discrete infiltrate

• If *ALL* results meet low-risk criteria and follow-up within 24 hours by a physician can be ensured, then consider outpatient management without antibiotics for those age 29 to 56 days. If any results are abnormal, admit to the hospital and treat empirically with intravenous antibiotics as for neonates (may use cefotaxime alone). If culture results are negative after 48 hours and suspicion for SBI no longer exists, then discharge. If any culture result is positive, alter therapy appropriately.

FEVER OF UNKNOWN ORIGIN

1) Fever 14 days or longer; 2) documented temperature 38.3°C or greater; 3) cause not apparent after physical exam and screening laboratory tests

Epidemiology
• Infection (28% to 52%), collagen vascular disease (6% to 20%), malignancy (3% to 16%)
• Resolution of fever without diagnosis in 20% to 40%

Differential Diagnosis
• Common infectious causes: systemic viral syndrome, upper or lower respiratory tract infection, osteomyelitis, urinary tract infection, CNS infection, bacterial enteritis
• Less common infectious causes: tuberculosis, cat-scratch disease, infectious mononucleosis, lyme disease, rickettsial diseases, malaria, periodontal abscess, endocarditis, HIV, viral hepatitis, acute rheumatic fever
• Other infectious causes: Q fever, brucellosis, tularemia, leptospirosis, intra-abdominal abscess, toxoplasmosis, syphilis, endemic fungi (e.g., histoplasmosis), psittacosis, chronic meningococcemia
• Non-infectious causes: collagen vascular diseases, juvenile rheumatoid arthritis, systemic lupus erythematosus, dermatomyositis, scleroderma, vasculitis, malignancy, Kawasaki syndrome, inflammatory bowel disease, Munchausen syndrome by proxy, factitious fever, periodic fever syndrome, central fever, dysautonomia, hyperthyroidism, drug fever

Clinical Manifestations
• Constitutional: fever onset and height, method used to take temperature, weight loss, night sweats, chills, anorexia
• History: travel, animal exposure, unpasteurized dairy products, tick bite, blood transfusion, trauma, fractures or puncture wounds, congenital or acquired heart disease, immune deficiency, foreign body ingestion, central venous catheter, medications
• Family stressor (Munchausen by proxy, pseudofevers)
• Perform repeated and thorough physical exams searching for findings that suggest specific cause.

Management
Initial Studies (select tests based on history and exam)
• Blood:
  - Blood culture, CBC, CRP, ESR, hepatic function panel
  - Serology for HIV, EBV, CMV, cat-scratch, lyme, and streptococcal enzyme titers (ASO, anti-Dnase B)
  - Antinuclear antibodies
• Urine: urinalysis and culture
• Stool: hemoccult testing, culture (bacterial/viral), ova and parasite exam
• Radiologic: chest radiograph
• Miscellaneous: tuberculin skin test, throat culture, rapid viral antigen testing of nasopharyngeal aspirate

Follow-up Studies to Consider
• Blood:
  - Repeat blood culture
  - Serology for toxoplasmosis, hepatitis A, B and C, tularemia, brucellosis, leptospirosis, Rocky Mountain spotted fever, ehrlichiosis, and Q fever.

- Stool: *C. difficile* toxins A and B
- Radiologic: radiographs of involved bones if tenderness or edema on exam, sinus CT, gastrointestinal barium study with small bowel follow-through (if symptoms suggest inflammatory bowel disease), abdominal ultrasound, bone scan, or gallium scan, MRI of pelvis, spine, or specific extremity, echocardiogram
- Miscellaneous: ophthalmologic exam, bone marrow biopsy (if abnormal CBC or suspected malignancy), lumbar puncture, evaluation for immune deficiency.

Resources

Syndromes and Complexes

Ambati BK, Ambati J, Azar N, et al. Periorbital and orbital cellulitis before and after the advent of *Haemophilus influenzae* type B vaccination. Ophthalmology 2000;107:1450–1453.

American Academy of Pediatrics. Management of sinusitis. Pediatrics 2001;108:798–808.

American Academy of Pediatrics. Revised indications for the use of palivizumab and respiratory syncytial virus immune globulin intravenous for the prevention of respiratory syncytial virus infections. Pediatrics 2003;112:1442–1446.

American Academy of Pediatrics. The diagnosis, treatment and evaluation of the initial urinary tract infection in febrile infants and young children. Pediatrics 1999;103:843–853.

American Academy of Pediatrics and American Academy of Family Physicians. Diagnosis and management of acute otitis media. Pediatrics 2004;113:1451–1465.

Asmar BI. Bacteriology of retropharyngeal abscess in children. Pediatr Infect Dis J 1990;9:595–597.

Bishai WR, Sears CL. Food poisoning syndromes. Gastroenterol Clin North Am 1993;22:579–608.

Bonadio WA, Stanco L, Bruce R, et al. Reference values of normal cerebrospinal fluid composition in infants ages 0 to 8 weeks. Pediatr Infect Dis J 1992;11:589–591.

Burnett MW, Bass JW, Cook BA. Etiology of osteomyelitis complicating sickle cell disease. Pediatrics 1998;101:296–297.

Craig FW, Schunk JE. Retropharyngeal abscess in children: clinical presentation, utility of imaging and current management. Pediatrics 2003;111:1394–1398.

Dagan R. Management of acute hematogenous osteomyelitis and septic arthritis in the pediatric patient. Pediatr Infect Dis J 1993;12:88–93.

Feigin RD, Cherry JD, Demmler GJ, Kaplan SL, eds. Textbook of Pediatric Infectious Diseases. 5th ed. Philadelphia: WB Saunders, 2004.

Flores G, Horwitz RI. Efficacy of beta 2-agonists in bronchiolitis: a reappraisal and meta-analysis. Pediatrics 1997;100:233–239.

Ghaffar FA, Wordemann M, McCracken GH Jr. Acute mastoiditis in children: a seventeen-year experience in Dallas, Texas. Pediatr Infect Dis J 2001;20:376–380.

Gross CW, et al. Infections of the deep fascial spaces of the neck. In: Jenson HB, Baltimore RS, eds. Pediatric Infectious Diseases: Principles and Practice. 2nd ed. Philadelphia: WB Saunders, 2002:721–727.

Guerrant RL, Van Gilder T, Steiner TS, et al. Practice guidelines for the management of infectious diarrhea. Clin Infect Dis 2001;32:331–350.

Hartling L, Wiebe N, Russell K, et al. A meta-analysis of randomized controlled trials evaluating the efficacy of epinephrine for the treatment of acute viral bronchiolitis. Arch Pediatr Adolesc Med 2003;158:957–964.

Hoberman A, Wald ER, Hickey RW, et al. Oral versus initial intravenous therapy for urinary tract infections in young febrile children. Pediatrics 1999;104:79–86.

Kairys SW, Olmstead EM, O'Connor GT. Steroid treatment of laryngotracheitis: a meta-analysis of the evidence from randomized trials. Pediatrics 1989;83:683–693.

Kallio MJ, Unkila-Kallio L, Aalto K, Peltola H. Serum C-reactive protein, erthyrocyte sedimentation rate and white blood cell count in septic arthritis of children. Pediatr Infect Dis J 1997;16:411–413.

Lee SS, Schwartz RH, Bahadori RS. Retropharyngeal abscess: epiglottitis of the new millennium. J Pediatr 2001;138:435–437.

Long SS, Pickering LK, Prober CG, eds. Principles and Practice of Pediatric Infectious Diseases. New York: Churchill Livingstone, 2003.

Margileth AM. Management of nontuberculous (atypical) mycobacterial infections in children and adolescents. Pediatr Infect Dis 1985;4:119–121.

McDonald A, Scranton M, Gillespie R, et al. Voiding cystourethrograms and urinary tract infections: how long to wait? Pediatrics 2000;105:e50.

McIntosh K. Community-acquired pneumonia in children. N Engl J Med 2002;346:429–437.

Pickering LK, ed. Red Book: 2003 Report of the Committee on Infectious Diseases. 26th ed. Elk Grove Village, IL: American Academy of Pediatrics, 2003.

Rittichier KK, Ledwith CA. Outpatient treatment of moderate croup with dexamethasone: intramuscular versus oral dosing. Pediatrics 2000;106:1344–1348.

Peltola H, Unkila-Kallio L, Kallio MJ. Simplified treatment of acute staphylococcal osteomyelitis of childhood. Pediatrics 1997;99:846–850.

Powell KR. Orbital and periorbital cellulitis. Pediatr Rev 1995;16:163–167.

Rich RR. Intravenous IgG: super therapy for superantigens. J Clin Invest 1993;91:378.

Romero JR, Newland JG. Viral meningitis and encephalitis: traditional and emerging viral agents. Semin Pediatr Infect Dis 2003;14:72–82.

Saez-Llorens X, McCracken GH Jr. Bacterial meningitis in children. Lancet 2003;361:2139–2148.

Schlievert PM, Kelly JA. Clindamycin-induced suppression of toxic-shock syndrome-associated exotoxin production. J Infect Dis 1984:149:471.

Shah SS, Alpern ER, Zwerling L, et al. Risk of bactermia in young children with pneumonia treated as outpatients. Arch Pediatr Adol Med 2003;157:389–392.

Shah SS, Gallagher PG. Complications of conjunctivitis caused by Pseudomonas aeruginosa in a newborn intensive care unit. Pediatr Infect Dis J 1990,17,97–102.

Shands KN, Schmid GP, Dan BB, et al. Toxic-shock syndrome in menstruating women: association with tampon use and Staphylococcus aureus and clinical features in 52 cases. N Engl J Med 1980;303:1436–1442.

Shaw KN, Bell LM, Sherman NH. Outpatient assessment of infants with bronchiolitis. Am J Dis Child 1991;145:151–155.

Shaw KN, McGowan KL, Gorelick MH, Schwartz JH. Screening for urinary tract infection in infants in the emergency department: which test is best? Pediatrics 1998;101:e1.

Slack CL, Dahn KA, Abzug MJ, ChanKH. Antibiotic-resistant bacteria in pediatric sinusitis. Pediatr Infect Dis J 2001;20:247–250.

Starkey CR, Steele RW. Medical management of orbital cellulitis. Pediatr Infect Dis J 2001;20:1002–1005.

Sumaya CV. Epstein-Barr virus serologic testing: diagnostic indications and interpretations. Pediatr Infect Dis 1986;5:337–342.

Sumaya CV, Ench Y. Epstein-Barr infectious mononucleosis in children: clinical and general laboratory findings. Pediatrics 1985;75:1003–1010.

Talan DA, Citron DM, Abrahamian FM, et al. Bacteriologic analysis of infected dog and cat bites. N Engl J Med 1999;340:85–92.

Venezio FR, Naidich TP, Shulman ST. Complications of mastoiditis with special emphasis on venous sinus thrombosis. J Pediatr 1982;101:509–513.

Whitley RJ, Gnann JW. Viral encephalitis: familiar infections and emerging pathogens. Lancet 2002; 359:507–513.

Williams JW Jr, Simel DL. Does this patient have sinusitis? Diagnosing acute sinusitis by history and physical examination. JAMA 1993;270:1242–1246.

Wohl DL, Isaacson JE. Airway obstruction in children with infectious mononucleosis. Ear Nose Throat J 1995;74:630–638.

Specific Pathogens

Altschuler S, Liacouras C. Clinical Pediatric Gastroenterology. Philadelphia: Churchill Livingstone, 1998.

Arisoy ES, Correa AG, Wagner ML, Kaplan SL. Hepatosplenic cat-scratch disease in children: selected features and treatment. Clin Infect Dis 1999;28:778–784.

Bakken JS, Aguero-Rosenfeld ME, Tilden RL, et al. Serial measurements of hematologic counts during the active phase of human granulocytic ehrlichiosis. Clin Infect Dis 2001;32:862–870.

Bakken JS, Dumler JS. Human granulocytic ehrlichiosis. Clin Infect Dis 2000;31:554–560.

Bass JW, Freitas BC, Freitas AD, et al. Prospective randomized double blind placebo-controlled evaluation of azithromycin for treatment of cat-scratch disease. Pediatr Infect Dis J 1998;17:447–452.

Feigin RD, Cherry JD, Demmler GJ, Kaplan SL, eds. Textbook of Pediatric Infectious Diseases. 5th ed. Philadelphia: Saunders, 2004.

Gerber MA, Zemel LS, Shapiro ED. Lyme arthritis in children: clinical epidemiology and long-term outcomes. Pediatrics 1998;102:905–908.

Halasa NB, Barr FE, Johnson JE, Edwards KM. Fatal pulmonary hypertension associated with pertussis in infants: does extracorporeal membrane oxygenation have a role? Pediatrics 2003;112:1274–1278.

Horsburgh CR Jr, Feldman S, Ridzon R, et al. Practice guidelines for the treatment of tuberculosis. Clin Infect Dis 2000;31:633–639.

Jacobs RF, Schutze GE. *Bartonella henselae* as a cause of prolonged fever and fever of unknown origin in children. Clin Infect Dis 1998;26:80–84.

Jaeckel E, Cornberg M, Wedemeyer H, et al. Treatment of acute hepatitis C with interferon alfa-2b. N Engl J Med 2001;345:1452–1457.

Kimberlin DW, Lin CY, Jacobs RF, et al. Natural history of neonatal herpes simplex virus infections in the acyclovir era. Pediatrics 2001;108:223–229.

Kimberlin DW, Lin CY, Jacobs RF, et al. Safety and efficacy of high dose intravenous acyclovir in the management of neonatal herpes simplex virus infection. Pediatrics 2001;108:230–238.

Leung DY, Kelly CP, Boguniewicz M, et al. Treatment with intravenously administered gamma globulin of chronic relapsing colitis induced by *Clostridium difficile* toxin. J Pediatr 1991;118:633–637.

Loeffelholz MJ, Thompson CJ, Long KS, Gilchrist MJ. Comparison of PCR, culture, and direct fluorescent-antibody testing for detection of Bordetella pertussis. J Clin Microbiol 1999;37:2872–2876.

Long SS, Pickering LK, Prober CG, eds. Principles and Practice of Pediatric Infectious Diseases. New York: Churchill Livingstone, 2003.

Margileth AM. Antibiotic therapy for cat scratch disease: clinical study of therapeutic outcome in 268 patients and a review of the literature. Pediatr Infect Dis J 1992;11:474–478.

Pickering LK, ed. Red Book: 2003 Report of the Committee on Infectious Diseases. 26th ed. Elk Grove Village, IL: American Academy of Pediatrics, 2003.

Ramrakhiani S, Bacon BR. Hepatology in the new millennium: advances in viral hepatitis, hepatic disorders and liver transplantation. Med Clin North Am 2000;84:1085–1105.

Senzilet LD, Halperin SA, Spika JS, et al. Pertussis is a frequent cause of prolonged cough illness in adults and adolescents. Clin Infect Dis 2001;32:1691–1697.

Small PM, Fujiwara PI. Management of tuberculosis in the United States. N Engl J Med 2001;345: 189–199.

Thorner AR, Walker DH, Petri WA Jr. Rocky Mountain spotted fever. Clin Infect Dis 1998;27:1353–1360.

Fever and Bacteremia

Baker MD, Bell LM, Avner JR. Outpatient management without antibiotics of fever in selected infants. N Engl J Med 1993;329:1437–1441.

Baker MD, Bell LM, Avner JR. The efficacy of routine outpatient management without antibiotics of fever in selected infants. Pediatrics 1999;103:627–631.

Callelo D, Shah SS. The child with fever of unknown origin. Pediatr Case Rev 2002;2:226–239.

Feigin RD, Cherry JD, Demmler GJ, Kaplan SL, eds. Textbook of Pediatric Infectious Diseases. 5th ed. Philadelphia: WB Saunders, 2004.

Long SS, Pickering LK, Prober CG, eds. Principles and Practice of Pediatric Infectious Diseases. New York: Churchill Livingstone, 2003.

Mermel LA, Farr BM, Sherertz RJ, et al. Guidelines for the management of intravascular catheter-related infections. Clin Infect Dis 2001;32:1249–1272.

Pappas PG, Rex JH, Sobel JD, et al. Guidelines for treatment of candidiasis. Clin Infect Dis 2004;38:161–189.

Steele RW, Jones SM, Lowe BA, Glasier CM. Usefulness or scanning procedures for diagnosis of fever of unknown origin. J Pediatr 1991;119:526–530.

Ralph J. DeBerardinis, MD, PhD, Irma Payan, RN, CRNP,
Neal Sondheimer, MD, PhD, Can Ficicioglu, MD, PhD

Fatty Acid Oxidation Disorders and Disorders of Ketone Metabolism

GENERAL PRINCIPLES

Class of metabolic diseases in which enzyme deficiencies in mitochondrial fatty acid import, β-oxidation, or ketone metabolism limit the ability of mitochondria to use fat as an energy source.

Epidemiology
- Overall incidence ~1:10,000; autosomal recessive inheritance
- Medium-chain acyl-CoA dehydrogenase (MCAD) deficiency is the most common single disease

Pathophysiology
Most significant danger is hypoketotic hypoglycemia, leading to failure of multiple organ systems. General considerations:
- Fatty acid oxidation (FAO) provides energy for heart and liver at baseline, and for skeletal muscle during prolonged exercise. FAO produces ketones used by brain as energy source during prolonged fast.
- FAO supports gluconeogenesis by providing ATP, acetyl CoA and reduced electron carriers
- Risk for hypoketotic hypoglycemia highest when relying on FAO for energy (e.g., prolonged fast, infection)

Clinical Manifestations
Varies with syndrome but initial presenting symptoms include hypoketotic hypoglycemia; neonatal neurologic symptoms; coma; Reye syndrome; cardiac arrhythmia; cardiomyopathy; sudden death, rhabdomyolysis.

Diagnostics
Decompensated Patient
- Dextrose stick; serum Na, K, Cl, HCO_3, hepatic function panel, ammonia, CPK, free fatty acids, plasma acylcarnitine profile, total and free carnitine
- Blood gas if concern for metabolic acidosis
- Urine for ketones, myoglobin (if blood in U/A), and organic acid profile
- Consider ECG, echocardiography

Other Studies
- Acylcarnitine profiles performed in newborn screening programs have identified FAO disorders (FAOD) in many presymptomatic patients
- Closely supervised fasting studies
- Enzyme assays on fibroblasts
- Mutation (DNA) diagnostics used in some disorders

Management
Acute
Goal is to reverse hypoglycemia immediately, to curtail lipolysis, and to treat associated morbidities:
- Place widest gauge IV catheter immediately. Some patients require central access to maintain high dextrose infusion rates.

- Dextrose bolus (2 cc/kg with D10 for neonates; larger boluses in older children), then start dextrose infusion with D10 at 1.5 × maintenance rate. Insulin surge after dextrose infusion inhibits further lipolysis
- Saline boluses if dehydrated
- Do not use intralipids
- Early consultation with biochemical geneticist or other specialist

Chronic
- Carnitine supplementation for primary carnitine deficiency (e.g., carnitine transporter defect [CTD]). Use in other FAODs is controversial
- Low fat, high carbohydrate diet
- Limit long-chain fatty acid intake
- For disorders affecting long-chain FAO, supplement diet with medium chain triglycerides (2–3 g/kg/day for infants; 1 g/kg/day in older children).
- Strategies to avoid hypoglycemia include frequent or continuous feeds, evening snacks with glucose polymers (e.g., corn starch) and close clinical evaluation during intercurrent illness.
- Immunizations are not contraindicated, but frequent feeds and prophylactic antipyretics can reduce catabolism associated with febrile reactions.
- Any procedure requiring sedation and nothing by mouth period requires admission for IV fluids before procedure.

SPECIFIC DISORDERS

Important diagnostic laboratory studies for each entity is provided in Table 16.1.

Carnitine/Acylcarnitine Translocase Deficiency
A mitochondrial FAO disorder affecting transport of acylcarnitines across the inner mitochondrial membrane, limiting ability to use fat as an energy source. Long-chain fatty acylcarnitine and free fatty acid accumulation may contribute to the clinical picture.
- Two clinical subtypes exist:
  - *Severe:* neonatal onset hypoketotic hypoglycemia, hypertrophic cardiomyopathy, ventricular arrhythmias, hyperammonemia, myoglobinuria
  - *Mild:* fasting- or stress-induced hypoketotic hypoglycemia

Carnitine Transporter Defect
The transporter defect impairs transport of carnitine across cytoplasmic membranes into the cell. This results in reduced renal conservation of carnitine (leading to reduced serum carnitine levels) and decreased intracellular carnitine levels (esp. muscle cells), both of which contribute to the impairment of FAO.
- Clinical manifestations include hypertrophic cardiomyopathy, progressive cardiac failure, skeletal muscle weakness, and hypoketotic hypoglycemia.

Carnitine Palmitoyltransferase I Deficiency
A mitochondrial FAOD affecting conversion of fatty acyl CoA esters to acylcarnitine. Defective mitochondrial fatty acid import reduces or abolishes ability to use fat as an energy source. The first episode of decompensation usually occurs in infancy or early childhood.
- Manifestations include hypoketotic hypoglycemia, hepatomegaly, and hepatic encephalopathy (Reye syndrome).

Carnitine Palmitoyltransferase II Deficiency
A mitochondrial FAOD affecting mitochondrial import of long-chain fatty acids, resulting in defective conversion of acylcarnitines to fatty acyl CoA.
- Three clinical subtypes are defined by age at onset of symptoms:
  - *Classical:* episodic muscle weakness and myoglobinuria after prolonged exercise or other stressors, starting in the second to third decade.
  - *Antenatal:* fatal multiorgan system disease including hypoglycemia, hepatic and renal insufficiency, congenital malformations, and death often in the neonatal period.

Table 16.1: Fatty Acid Oxidation Disorders and Disorder of Ketone Metabolism: Important Diagnostic Laboratory Values

Disorder	Acylcarnitine Profile	Urine Organic Acids	Plasma Free Carnitine	Method for Definitive Diagnosis
Carnitine/acylcarnitine translocase deficiency	↑ esters of 16–18 carbons	Normal or ↑ dicarboxylic acids	↓	Enzyme assay and mutation analysis
Carnitine transporter defect	↓ long-chain acylcarnitines	Dicarboxylic aciduria	↓	Carnitine uptake in skin fibroblasts
Carnitine palmitoyl-transferase I deficiency	↓ long-chain esters	Normal	Normal or ↑	Enzyme assay or mutation analysis
Carnitine palmitoyl-transferase II deficiency	↑ esters of 16-18 carbon length	Usually normal	↓	Enzyme assay or mutation analysis
Medium chain acyl CoA dehydrogenase deficiency	↑ C6:0, C8:0, 4-cis-C8:1, 5-cis-C8:1, 4cis-C10:1	Medium-chain dicarboxylic acids and acylglycines	Normal to ↓	Acylcarnitine panel
Mitochondrial trifunctional protein deficiency and long-chain-3-hydroxyacyl CoA dehydrogenase seficiency	↑ long-chain esters and long-chain 3-hydroxy esters	Dicarboxylic acids	Often ↓	Enzyme assay or mutation analysis
Multiple acyl CoA dehydrogenase deficiency*	Globally increased	Dicarboxylic, glutaric, ethylmalonic acids	↓	Enzyme assay or mutation analysis
Short-chain acyl CoA dehydrogenase deficiency	↑ butyrylcarnitine	Ethylmalonate, methylsuccinate, butyrylglycine	Normal or ↓	Enzyme assay

(Continued)

Disorder	Acylcarnitine Profile	Urine Organic Acids	Plasma Free Carnitine	Method for Definitive Diagnosis
Short chain L-3-hydroxyacyl-CoA dehydrogenase deficiency	3-hydroxy-C4 ester	Dicarboxylic acid (variable)	Variable	Enzyme assay
Beta-ketothiolase deficiency[†]	↑ C5:1 acylcarnitine	2-methylacetoacetate, 2-butanone, 2-methyl-3-hydroxybutyrate	Variable	Enzyme assay
Very-long-chain acyl CoA dehydrogenase deficiency	↑ very long-chain acylcarnitine	Dicarboxylic acid	Often ↓	Enzyme assay

*Also known as glutaricaciduria type II.

†Also known as methylacetoacetyl-CoA thiolase deficiency and T2 deficiency.

- *Infantile:* hypoglycemia, hypotonia, hepatic dysfunction, hepatomegaly, cardiomegaly, and seizures.

Medium Chain Acyl CoA Dehydrogenase Deficiency

A mitochondrial FAOD affecting β-oxidation of medium-chain (e.g., 4 to 12 carbon-length) fatty acids, causing fasting- or stress-induced episodes of hypoketotic hypoglycemia associated with emesis/lethargy.
• Hyperammonemia may lead to coma.
• Severe episodes can result in multi-organ system failure.
• Hepatic steatosis generally improves after resolution of decompensation, but acylcarnitine profile is abnormal between episodes in some patients.
• Long-term manifestations include developmental disabilities and seizure disorder, especially in patients with delayed diagnosis.
• Newborn screen acylcarnitine analyses detect MCAD deficiency in presymptomatic individuals.

Mitochondrial Trifunctional Protein Deficiency and Long-Chain-3-Hydroxyacyl CoA Dehydrogenase Deficiency

Mitochondrial FAOD affecting β-oxidation of long-chain fatty acids. For long chain (especially 12 to 16 carbon length) fatty acids, one enzyme (mitochondrial "trifunctional protein") carries out hydratase, 3-hydroxyacyl CoA dehydrogenase, and thiolase reactions. Some mutations affect all three activities, while others affect only the dehydrogenase. Impaired ability to oxidize long-chain fatty acids severely compromises use of fat as an energy source.
• Isolated long-chain 3-hydroxyacyl CoA dehydrogenase (LCHAD) deficiency is associated with hypoketotic hypoglycemia, fulminant hepatic disease, hypertrophic cardiomyopathy, episodic myoglobinuria, peripheral neuropathy, and pigmentary retinopathy.
• Mitochondrial trifunctional protein (MTP) deficiency manifests as hypoketotic hypoglycemia, dilated cardiomyopathy, episodic myoglobinuria, and hypotonia.
• MTP and LCHAD fetuses can cause acute fatty liver of pregnancy in mothers.

Multiple Acyl CoA Dehydrogenation Deficiency (Glutaric Aciduria Type II)

MADD affects transfer of electrons from fatty acyl CoA to the electron transport chain, resulting in FAOD. The block also affects oxidation of branched-chain amino acids (leucine, isoleucine, valine) and of glutaryl-CoA (an oxidation product of tryptophan, lysine, hydroxylysine).
• Three clinical subtypes exist:
  - Neonatal onset *with* congenital anomalies (prematurity, hypoglycemia, metabolic acidosis, hypotonia, hepatomegaly, cardiomegaly, polycystic kidneys, and genitourinary, skeletal and craniofacial abnormalities)
  - Neonatal onset *without* congenital anomalies (severe metabolic decompensation in first few days of life)
  - Later onset (variable phenotype including metabolic decompensations and myopathy)

Short Chain Acyl CoA Dehydrogenase Deficiency

A mitochondrial FAOD affecting β-oxidation of short-chain (e.g., 4 to 6 carbon-length) fatty acids. The clinical course is incompletely defined and seems to be variable.
• Newborn screen acylcarnitine analyses have detected SCAD deficiency in presymptomatic individuals

Short Chain L-3-Hydroxyacyl-CoA Dehydrogenase Deficiency

A mitochondrial FAOD affecting β-oxidation of short-chain (e.g., 4 to 6 carbon-length) fatty acids, involving dysfunctional production of energy from fat and accumulation of toxic metabolites.
• Causes cardiomyopathy, rhabdomyolysis, hypoglycemia, and hepatic steatosis.
• Ketosis may be present in sick patients.

β-Ketothiolase Deficiency (Methylacetoacetyl-CoA Thiolase deficiency, T2 Deficiency)
A ketone utilization defect affecting the interconversion of acetyl-CoA and acetoacetyl-CoA. Deficiency of T2 enzyme affects ketone utilization, so stresses associated with ketosis (fasting, infection, ketogenic diet, dehydration) cause severe ketoacidosis. Onset is typically in infancy or early childhood, but patients are asymptomatic between episodes.
• T2 deficiency is characterized by episodic ketoacidosis and headaches.
• Cardiomyopathy has been reported.

Very-Long-Chain Acyl CoA Dehydrogenase Deficiency
Very-long-chain acyl CoA Dehydrogenase (VLCAD) gene mutations result in an impaired ability to oxidize fatty acids longer than 14 carbons in mitochondria and severely compromises use of fat as an energy source. A "severe" phenotype involves neonatal- or infantile-onset hypertrophic cardiomyopathy and hypoketotic hypoglycemia/Reye syndrome. A "mild" phenotype involves episodic hypoketotic hypoglycemia during stress or fasting without cardiomyopathy.
• Newborn screen acylcarnitine analyses have detected VLCAD in presymptomatic individuals.

Urea Cycle Defects

GENERAL PRINCIPLES

Class of metabolic diseases in which an enzyme deficiency compromises activity of the urea cycle, which normally functions to remove waste nitrogen as urea

Etiology
• Mutations in urea cycle enzymes, including carbamyl phosphate synthetase (CPS), ornithine transcarbamylase (OTC), argininosuccinic acid synthetase (AS), argininosuccinic acid lyase (AL), and arginase
• N-acetyl glutamate synthetase deficiency has also been described
• OTC deficiency is an X-linked disease. Other urea cycle defects (UCDs) are autosomal recessive

Epidemiology
• Overall prevalence of UCDs: ~1:30,000
• Most common is OTC deficiency. ~1.40,000

Pathophysiology
• The urea cycle is a major mechanism for ammonia (NH_3) clearance by converting it to water-soluble urea.
• Decompensation states occur during "nitrogen imbalance," when the nitrogen load exceeds the excretion ability, resulting in hyperammonemia.
• Conditions of increased nitrogen load include high protein diets, muscle catabolism induced by fasting, stress or exercise, and medicines that increase protein turnover.
• Ammonia-stimulated hyperventilation causes respiratory alkalosis.
• Hyperammonemia increases tryptophan transport across blood-brain barrier, enhancing serotonin production. Intracerebral glutamine also accumulates, contributing to cerebral edema. The overall effect is an encephalopathy that can include somnolence and coma.

Clinical Manifestations
• Great variability in clinical spectrum
• Episodic decompensations with: hyperammonemia; encephalopathy (lethargy, seizures, coma); respiratory alkalosis; other acid/base disturbances
• Neonatal clinical presentation is very similar to sepsis
• Older patients: poor appetite, cyclical vomiting, psychosis
• On exam, focus on ABCs, hydration status, mental status, neurologic exam, and possible sources of infection.
• Unexplained tachypnea may be due to hyperammonemia.

Diagnostics

- Some newborn screening programs include an amino acid profile and detect UCDs in pre-symptomatic patients.

Decompensated Patient (initial hyperammonemic episode)

- Neonatal presentation is similar to that of sepsis. Send CBC and differential counts, blood culture, and inflammatory markers
- NH_3; ABG; dextrose stick; basic metabolic panel/anion gap; LFTs; PT/PTT; plasma amino acids; plasma lactate/pyruvate; plasma acylcarnitine profile, total and free carnitine. These studies help determine the cause of hyperammonemia.
- Urine for urinalysis, organic acids and orotic acid; urine amino acid analysis
- CSF lactate/pyruvate and amino acids if lumbar puncture performed; MR spectroscopy if brain MRI performed

Decompensated Patient (known urea cycle defect):

- NH_3, ABG, dextrose stick, basic metabolic panel/anion gap, plasma amino acids, urine for urinalysis

Definitive Diagnostics

- Amino acid profile is unequivocal in some UCDs (AL, AS deficiency); enzyme assays; mutation (DNA) analysis

Management (Decompensated Patient)

- *ABCs/fluid management:* Ventilatory and pressor support; wide gauge IV (consider central access); start infusion with 10% dextrose-based solution (D10W or D10 1/4 NS if using nitrogen scavenger sodium salts) at 6–8 mg glucose/kg/min; nasogastric tube
- *Bulk NH_3 removal:* Dialysis may be necessary; consider consults with nephrology and critical care; nitrogen scavenging agents (Table 16.2)
- *Reversal of catabolic state:* Stop protein feeds; D10 infusion as above; consider intralipids; amino acids must be provided within 24 to 48 hours or protein turnover will persist; for total parenteral nutrition, start with 1–1.5 g amino acids/kg/day; if tolerating enteral feeds, use protein-free formula with gradual reintroduction of protein
- *Laboratory monitoring during critical phase:* ABG every 4 hours or as indicated for intubated patients; basic metabolic panel every 4 hours; NH_3 every 1 hour until less than 300; plasma amino acids every day; other laboratory studies as indicated for dialysis patients
- *Transition/home management:* Enteral nitrogen scavengers include sodium phenylbutyrate and sodium benzoate/sodium phenylacetate; some patients require citrulline (OTC deficiency)

Table 16.2: Nitrogen Scavenging Agents						
	Children (mg/kg)			Adolescents/Adults (g/m²)		
Diagnosis	SPA	SB	Arg-HCl	SPA	SB	Arg-HCl
Presumed UCD	250	250	600			
CPS/OTC	250	250	210	5.5	5.5	4.0
AS/AL	250	250	660	5.5	5.5	12

Dose size is same for load and maintenance infusion. Deliver loading dose over 90 minutes, then start every 24-hour continuous infusion.

SPA, sodium phenylbutyrate; SB, sodium benzoate; Arg-HCl, arginine-HCl; CPS, carbamyl phosphate synthetase deficiency; OTC, ornithine transcarbamylase deficiency; AS, argininosuccinic acid synthetase deficiency; AL, argininosuccinic acid lyase deficiency.

(Adapted from Summar M. Current strategies for the management of neonatal urea cycle disorders. J Pediatr 2001;138:S30–39. And Batshaw ML, MacArthur RB, Tuchman M. Alternative pathway therapy for urea cycle disorders: twenty years later. J Pediatr 2001;138:S46–55.)

or arginine (AS, AL deficiency) therapy; routine monitoring of nutritional markers, plasma amino acids, NH_3; consider G-tube placement, especially for neurologically impaired patients; normal immunization schedule with prophylactic antipyretics; for procedures requiring sedation and nothing by mouth period, consider admission for IV fluids before procedure; liver transplantation is curative for some patients.

SPECIFIC UREA CYCLE DEFECTS

Arginase Deficiency (Argininemia)
Arginase catalyzes the cytoplasmic production of ornithine and urea from arginine. Arginase deficiency causes arginine elevation and increases risk for hyperammonemia as well as toxic effects of arginine and other guanidino compounds. Unlike other UCDs, arginase deficiency presents primarily as a chronic neurologic disorder with progressive spastic diplegia/quadriplegia, ataxia, and choreoathetosis.
- Episodic hyperammonemic episodes can occur, but are less prominent than those in other UCDs.
- Diagnosis is confirmed by plasma amino acid profile, which shows elevated arginine.
- Urinary orotic acid is also increased.

Argininosuccinic Acid Lyase Deficiency
Argininosuccinic acid lyase (AL) catalyzes the cytoplasmic production of arginine from argininosuccinic acid. In AL deficiency, citrulline accumulates and arginine becomes an essential amino acid.
- Diagnosis is confirmed by plasma amino acid profile, which shows elevated citrulline and argininosuccinate with decreased arginine.
- Urinary orotic acid is also increased.

Argininosuccinic Acid Synthetase Deficiency (Citrullinemia)
Argininosuccinic acid synthetase (AS) catalyzes the cytoplasmic production of argininosuccinic acid from citrulline and aspartic acid. In AS deficiency, citrulline accumulates and arginine becomes an essential amino acid.
- Plasma amino acids reveal elevated citrulline and decreased argininosuccinic acid and arginine.

Carbamoyl Phosphate Synthetase Deficiency
Carbamoyl phosphate synthetase (CPS) catalyzes production of carbamoyl phosphate from NH_4^+, HCO_3^-, and ATP. Citrulline and arginine, downstream urea cycle products, become essential amino acids.
- Diagnosis is confirmed by plasma amino acid profile, which shows elevated glutamine with decreased citrulline and arginine.
- Urinary orotic acid is normal.

Ornithine Transcarbamylase Deficiency (Ornithine Carbamoyltransferase Deficiency)
Ornithine transcarbamylase (OTC) deficiency is an X-linked disorder resulting from mutations in the gene encoding OTC, which catalyzes the entry step into the urea cycle. Citrulline and arginine, downstream urea cycle products, become essential amino acids. Classic presentation is a male neonate, well at birth, with progressive emesis, feed refusal, and encephalopathy within a few days. Seizures occur in approximately 50% of patients. Female OTC deficiency carriers may be symptomatic depending on X-inactivation pattern in hepatocytes. Older patients may present with cyclic vomiting or behavior disturbances rather than frank metabolic decompensation.
- Diagnosis is confirmed by plasma amino acid profile, which shows elevated glutamine and decreased citrulline and arginine; urinary orotic acid is also increased; enzyme assays can be performed on liver samples.

Defects of Amino Acid Metabolism

HEREDITARY TYROSINEMIA TYPE I

Hereditary tyrosinemia type I (HT1) is an inborn error of tyrosine metabolism causing progressive liver and renal failure. It is due to mutations in the gene encoding FAH, the terminal enzyme in tyrosine metabolism.

Epidemiology
- Incidence ~1:100,000; autosomal recessive inheritance
- Incidence much higher in the Lac-St. Jean region of Quebec

Pathophysiology
- Tyrosine metabolism is both ketogenic (producing acetoacetate) and gluconeogenic (producing fumarate). Tyrosine metabolism occurs in the hepatocyte and the proximal renal tubule.
- Elevated tyrosine is due to inhibition of upstream biochemical steps, and does not contribute to liver or renal injury.
- Blockade at the FAH step causes an accumulation of fumarylacetoacetate (FAA), an alkylating agent that promotes apoptosis and alters gene expression.
- Accumulation of succinylacetone, a byproduct of fumarylacetoacetate, contributes to renal Fanconi syndrome.
- Hypoglycemia may result from hepatic dysfunction, reduced availability of gluconeogenic precursors, and decreased expression of genes required for glucose production.
- Porphyria crises occur because succinylacetone inhibits δ-aminolevulinic acid dehydratase in the heme synthetic pathway.
- FAA's mutagenic activity may contribute to the development of hepatocellular carcinoma.

Clinical Manifestations
- Hepatic failure is progressive, usually beginning in the neonatal period or early infancy. Patients may present with acute hepatic crises, with hypoalbuminemia, ascites, and jaundice.
- High risk for cirrhosis and hepatocellular carcinoma if untreated.
- Coagulopathy due to compromised liver synthetic function may be the first symptom, sometimes manifested by gastrointestinal bleeding.
- Proximal renal tubular dysfunction often presents as a renal Fanconi syndrome.
- Neurologic symptoms due to attacks of porphyria include painful peripheral neuropathy, hypertonia, and autonomic instability.
- Causes of death include liver failure, hemorrhage, respiratory arrest (porphyria episodes), and hepatocellular carcinoma.

Diagnostics
- Plasma amino acids may reveal elevated tyrosine, phenylalanine, and methionine. Definitive diagnosis requires demonstration of succinylacetone on urine organic acid quantitation or on filter-blotted blood specimens. FAH enzyme activity and genetic testing can be used for confirmation.
- Elevation in alpha-fetoprotein (AFP) may predate elevated tyrosine levels.
- Tyrosine is often not severely elevated in affected 2-day-old infants, so newborn screening is difficult.
- Check coagulation studies and other markers of liver synthetic function. Hepatic transaminases may or may not be elevated.

Management
- 2-(2-nitro-4-trifluoromethyl-benzoyl)-1,3-cyclohexanedione (NTBC, nitisinone) inhibits 4-HPPD, an upstream step in tyrosine metabolism, reducing production of FAA and succinylacetone. NTBC decreases risk of liver failure and hepatocellular carcinoma. Starting dose is 1 mg/kg/day orally divided twice daily, adjusted for biochemical control.

- NTBC treatment increases blood tyrosine and phenylalanine levels, so treated patients require dietary modification.
- NTBC can cause corneal erosions and other ocular abnormalities, so baseline and routine ophthalmologic exams are indicated.
- Liver transplantation is an option for NTBC nonresponders.

PHENYLKETONURIA

PKU is an inborn error of phenylalanine (phe) metabolism associated with mental retardation. Mutations in the gene encoding phenylalanine hydroxylase (PAH) account for most cases. Inheritance is autosomal recessive.

Epidemiology
- Overall incidence in American children is 1:15,000

Pathophysiology
- Increased phe interferes with amino acid transport in both directions across the blood-brain barrier.
- Altered amino acid transport probably impacts CNS protein and neurotransmitter (especially dopamine, serotonin) synthesis.
- Phe is hydroxylated to form tyrosine (tyr), a precursor of melanin. Relative underpigmentation of PKU patients reflects decreased tyr availability.

Clinical Manifestations
Due to newborn screening, PKU patients are now diagnosed before symptoms develop. Historically, abnormalities included seizures, infantile spasms, increased tone/spasticity, and microcephaly.
- Tics, parkinsonism, and behavior abnormalities occur in poorly controlled patients.
- Light pigmentation of hair, skin, eyes
- Eczema in 20% to 40%
- Urinary phenylacetic acid causes the classic "mousy odor."

Diagnosis
- All U.S. neonates are now screened for elevated phe levels.
- Confirmatory testing requires plasma amino acid quantitation to verify elevated phe and to determine the phe:tyr ratio. A phe:tyr ratio greater than 3:1 reflects a state of hyperphenylalaninemia.

Management
- Consultation with a biochemical geneticist or other specialist
- Early treatment is associated with better neurodevelopmental outcomes. Dietary therapy should begin immediately after diagnosis, by the end of the first week of life if possible. Dietary management is recommended in patients with phe levels greater than 10 mg% (625 µM). Phe-reduced formulas and foods form the basis of dietary therapy. Patients also take a small amount of complete protein to provide requisite amounts of phe and tyr.
- Goal phe level is controversial, but many experts agree that 2 to 6 mg% until age 12 and less than 15 mg% after age 12 are acceptable levels.
- Mothers with PKU need strict dietary control before and during pregnancy. Poor first-trimester control increases fetal risk for microcephaly, mental retardation, and congenital heart disease.

Defects of Carbohydrate Metabolism

GALACTOSEMIA

Galactosemia is an inborn error of galactose metabolism resulting in toxicity after ingestion of lactose or galactose. Mutations may occur in any of three genes involved in galactose metabolism: galactokinase (GK), galactose-1-phosphate uridyltransferase (GALT), and uridine diphosphate-galactose 4' epimerase. GALT deficiency accounts for the majority of cases. "Classical" galactosemia is caused by severe GALT deficiency (<5% activity). "Partial" GALT deficiency (5% to 50%) is more common and is benign.

Epidemiology
- Prevalence of classical galactosemia is 1:30,000
- Inheritance is autosomal recessive

Pathophysiology
- Symptoms appear in neonates fed breast milk or cow's milk formulas, both of which contain lactose, a disaccharide of glucose and galactose.
- In patients with GALT deficiency, galactose-1-phosphate (gal1P) accumulates. Hypoglycemia occurs because: 1) galactose cannot be converted to glucose, and 2) gal1P inhibits phosphoglucomutase, an enzyme required for glycogenolysis.

Clinical Manifestations
- Affected children are well at birth with symptoms appearing in a few days
- In an American series (Waggoner et al., 1990) following galactosemic neonates: 89% had symptoms from hepatocellular damage (jaundice, hepatomegaly, ascites, transaminitis, hyperammonemia, and coagulopathy); 76% had food intolerance (poor feeding, emesis); 29% had failure to thrive; 16% had lethargy; 10% had sepsis (usually *Escherichia coli*); 1% had seizures.
- Other neonatal manifestations include hypoglycemia, renal Fanconi, and cataracts. Early death by sepsis, hepatic failure, or renal failure may occur unless patient is diagnosed and treated.
- Long-term sequelae include developmental delay, speech dyspraxia, cataracts, and ovarian failure.

Diagnostics
- In some states, newborn screening detects essentially 100% of affected neonates. Many programs assay GALT enzyme activity directly, allowing diagnosis to be made even in children on lactose-free formulas. However, not all states test for galactosemia, and many newborns become symptomatic before the diagnosis is reported by the laboratory, underscoring the need to recognize the clinical picture.
- *Evaluation of a sick neonate suspected of having galactosemia:* dextrose stick, basic metabolic panel, blood culture, liver function tests, PT/PTT, ammonia, urine for reducing substances, galactitol, amino acids, erythrocyte gal1P, GALT activity (whole blood or dried sample on filter paper).
- *Evaluation of an asymptomatic neonate referred because of a presumptive positive newborn screen result:* urine galactitol, erythrocyte gal1P, GALT activity
- *Interpretation of GALT activity:* less than 5%: classical galactosemia; 5% to 20%: Duarte/galactosemia (D/G); 50%: galactosemia carrier (benign); 75% to 90%: Duarte carrier (benign)

Management
- ABCs
- In sick neonates, discontinue feeds, reverse hypoglycemia if present, and begin dextrose infusion. If hyperammonemia is present, discontinue protein intake until resolved.
- In asymptomatic neonates with a positive galactosemia newborn screen, stop lactose/galactose-containing feeds, pending confirmation. Start non–lactose-containing formula (e.g., soy-based).
- Long-term management of classical galactosemia includes avoidance of dietary lactose and galactose (dairy products, some tomato products, canned foods, etc). Calcium supplementation is important. Consultation with a clinical nutritionist is helpful.
- In galactokinase deficiency, which causes isolated cataracts, elimination of dairy products alone is sufficient treatment.
- Severe epimerase-deficiency galactosemia is difficult to treat, because deficiency impairs not only production of glucose from galactose, but also galactose biosynthesis, which is necessary for processing of some proteins and lipids.

HEREDITARY FRUCTOSE INTOLERANCE

Hereditary fructose intolerance is an inborn error in metabolism resulting in toxicity after fructose ingestion. It is due to a mutation in the gene encoding aldolase B, an enzyme required for conversion of fructose to glucose. Exposure to fructose, sucrose (a glucose-fructose disaccharide), or sorbitol causes symptoms to occur.

Epidemiology
- In the United Kingdom, ~1% carry a common disease-causing allele and 1/20,000 are homozygous
- Inheritance is autosomal recessive.

Clinical Manifestations
- Most affected patients are asymptomatic until weaning, when they are exposed to sucrose or fructose.
- Symptoms include abdominal pain, vomiting, severe hypoglycemia (diaphoresis, lethargy, seizures, coma), hepatotoxicity (jaundice, coagulopathy, ascites), elevated uric acid, and renal Fanconi.
- Untreated patients progress to chronic hepatic and renal failure.

Pathophysiology
- Aldolase B deficiency primarily affects hepatocytes, mucosa of the small intestine, and the proximal renal tubules, major sites of aldolase B expression. Aldolase B cleaves fructose-1-phosphate (f1P) into 3-carbon products that can be used for glycolysis, glycogen synthesis, or gluconeogenesis.
- Aldolase B deficiency leads to accumulation of f1P and depletion of phosphate sources, especially inorganic phosphate (P_i) and ATP. P_i depletion activates purine degradation, resulting in hyperuricemia. f1P accumulation prevents glycogen breakdown and gluconeogenesis, contributing to hypoglycemia. Inhibition of gluconeogenesis causes precursors (e.g., lactate, pyruvate) to accumulate, resulting in metabolic acidosis, which is compounded by proximal renal tubular dysfunction.

Diagnostics
- Blood glucose; comprehensive metabolic panel including K, HCO_3, BUN, Cr, phosphate, liver function tests; PT/PTT; uric acid
- Urine for reducing substances, glucose, fructose and amino acids
- Plasma lactate/pyruvate and amino acids may also be helpful.
- Definitive diagnosis based on IV fructose challenge test under closely supervised conditions when patient is clinically well.

Management
- *Sick patient after fructose exposure:* ABCs; Establish intravenous access; Treat hypoglycemia, metabolic acidosis, and electrolyte abnormalities (especially hypophosphatemia)
- *Long-term management:* Avoid fructose and fructose-containing sugars, including sucrose and sorbitol. Consultation with a clinical nutritionist is helpful.
- *Sources of sucrose (table sugar) include:* candies/desserts, canned foods, soft drinks
- *Sources of fructose include* fresh fruits, raw vegetables, new potatoes, whole flour, brown rice
- *Sources of sorbitol include* some medications, diabetic products

Organic Acidemias

BRANCHED-CHAIN ORGANIC ACIDURIAS (Disorders of branched-chain organic acid metabolism; Branched-chain organic acidemias)

Branched-chain organic acidurias are a group of metabolic disorders due to inborn enzymes deficiencies in metabolism of branched-chain amino acids (leucine, isoleucine, valine), leading to accumulation of non-amino organic acids. Mutations in a variety of enzymes cause these disorders:

- Branched-chain oxo- (or keto-) acid dehydrogenase (Maple syrup urine disease, MSUD)
- Propionyl CoA carboxylase (propionic acidemia, PA)
- Methylmalonyl CoA mutase (methylmalonic acidemia, MMA)
- Isovaleryl CoA dehydrogenase (isovaleric acidemia, IVA)
- 3-methylcrotonyl-CoA carboxylase (3-methylcrotonyl-CoA carboxylase deficiency, 3MCCD)

Epidemiology
- *Incidence:* MSUD: 1:150,000 (1:1000 among Mennonites); PA: 1:150,000; MMA: 1:100,000; IVA: 1:150,000; 3-MCCD: 1:15,500
- Autosomal recessive inheritance

Differential Diagnosis
In patients with acidosis and neurologic dysfunction, consider:
- *Non-metabolic causes:* Sepsis, renal tubular acidosis, congenital cardiovascular or pulmonary malformation, hypocalcemia, other electrolyte abnormalities, toxins, intracranial bleed
- *Metabolic causes:* Biotinidase deficiency and holocarboxylase synthetase deficiency, cobalamin metabolism disorders, primary lactic acidosis syndromes

Pathophysiology
- Enzyme deficiency causes organic acid accumulation and consequently a variety of toxic effects on cellular function.
- Organic acid accumulation inhibits metabolic pathways including ketogenesis, gluconeogenesis, and ureagenesis.
- Organic acids also interfere with hematopoiesis.
- Decompensation occurs during states of catabolism (infection, fasting, exercise, other stress) or increased protein turnover (general anesthetics, steroids). Dietary protein overload can also promote decompensation.

Clinical Manifestations
Perform a comprehensive history and physical exam focusing on: ABCs; hydration status; tachypnea (may be due to acidosis or hyperammonemia); complete neurologic exam including mental status; cardiac exam; epigastric tenderness (vomiting may be due to pancreatitis); superficial skin desquamation; source of infection (if febrile); unusual odor in urine or breath

Neonatal Presentation
Similar to sepsis; typically a full-term baby, well for the first few days, then with dramatic decompensation:
- Lethargy and progressive neurologic dysfunction (seizures, abnormal tone, unusual movements, coma)
- Poor feeding, hypoglycemia, metabolic acidosis, ketonuria, hyperammonemia
- Stroke-like episodes, which may cause choreoathetoid or dystonic movements.
- Bone marrow suppression, cardiomyopathy, pancreatitis
- Unusual odor of body fluids

Later Presentation
- Poor appetite, failure to thrive, preference for non-protein foods
- Episodic vomiting, hypotonia, seizures
- Global developmental delay, especially with regression

Episodic Decompensation
- Catabolic states can cause appearance, recurrence, or exacerbation of any of the previous signs or symptoms.

Diagnostics
- Some newborn screening programs include an acylcarnitine profile, which detects organic acidemias.

Decompensated Patient (initial presentation)
- *General sepsis workup:* CBC count with differential, blood culture, inflammatory markers.
- NH_3, ABG with lactate, dextrose stick, basic metabolic panel/anion gap, LFTs, amylase/lipase in vomiting patient, plasma lactate/pyruvate
- *Metabolic tests:* plasma amino acids; plasma acylcarnitine profile and total/free carnitine; urine for urinalysis and organic acids; CSF for amino acids, lactate/pyruvate and organic acids if lumbar puncture is performed.
- Consider head CT if cerebral edema is suspected or brain MRI spectroscopy if persistent neurologic symptoms
- Perform ECG and echocardiography for signs of cardiac failure.

Decompensated Patient (known organic acidemia)
- ABG; Dextrose stick; Basic metabolic panel/anion gap; NH_3; CBC count and differential; LFTs and lipase/amylase for vomiting/abdominal pain; plasma amino acids; plasma total/free carnitine level; urine for urinalysis

Definitive Diagnostics
- Enzyme assays, usually on fibroblasts from skin biopsy

Management
- *ABCs/fluid management:* Ventilatory and pressor support as needed. Place widest gauge IV. Most patients will need multiple access sites and some will require central venous access; start infusion with D10-based solution at 6–8 mg glucose/kg/min; monitor urine output
- *Reverse acidosis:* Maintain HCO_3 at 22 to 25. If severely acidotic (pH < 7.22 or HCO_3 < 14 mEq/L), give $NaHCO_3$ bolus (1 meq/kg) followed by continuous infusion (2–4 meq/kg/day). If patient becomes hypernatremic, reduce rate of $NaHCO_3$ drip or replace with potassium acetate; THAM is contraindicated
- *Reverse catabolic state:* Stop protein feeds; In patients unable to tolerate enteral feeds, start total parenteral nutrition, with goal intake 20% above maintenance nutrition. Use dextrose (5–10 mg/kg/min) and intralipids (1–3 g/kg/day). Hold amino acids for 24 hours if severely ill, then start gradual reintroduction; if indicated (e.g., MSUD patients), use amino acid preparations lacking branched-chain amino acids; if tolerating enteral feeds, use protein-free formula with gradual reintroduction of protein to baseline.
- *Reverse hyperammoniemia:* Nitrogen scavenging agents (as in urea cycle defects) may be used; dialysis may be necessary. In severely ill patients, immediate consultations with nephrology and critical care are warranted.
- *Laboratory monitoring during critical phase:* ABG every 4 hours or as indicated for intubated patients; basic metabolic panel every 4 hours; NH_3 every 1 to 2 hours until less than 300; daily urine organic and plasma organic acids; daily plasma amino acids; daily CBC count with differential; plasma acylcarnitine profile every other day; other laboratory studies as indicated for dialysis patients
- *Medication Therapy:*
  - Carnitine: 50–200 mg/kg/day if carnitine deficient (MMA, PA)
  - Glycine: 10%: 250–600 mg/kg/day. Favors formation of rapidly excreted isovalerylglycine in IVA.
  - Thiamine: 25–100 mg/day. Co-factor for branch-chain ketoacid decarboxylase (MSUD).
  - Hydroxycobalamin: 1 mg intramuscular injection daily. Co-factor for methylmalonyl CoA mutase (MMA)
- *Transition/chronic care:* Choose appropriate home formula and daily protein allowance with metabolic dietitian; routine monitoring of nutritional markers, plasma and urine organic acids, acylcarnitine profile/carnitine levels, electrolytes, LFTs, CBC count with differential; may require long-term medication and alkalinization therapy; consider gastrostomy tube placement, especially for patients with failure to thrive; early intervention services; yearly developmental assessment; yearly bone density scans after age 4; normal immunization schedule with prophylactic antipyretics and protein-free diet; for procedures requiring sedation and nothing by mouth period, consider admission for IV fluids before procedure.

Primary Lactic Acidosis

RESPIRATORY CHAIN DEFECTS

Inborn errors in assembly, structure or function of the protein complexes necessary for oxidative phosphorylation. Respiratory chain defects (RCDs) are a large family of rare and incurable disorders, including clinical syndromes such as mitochondrial encephalomyelopathy with lactic acidosis and stroke (MELAS); myoclonic epilepsy with ragged red fibers (MERRF); neuropathy, ataxia, and retinitis pigmentosa (NARP); chronic progressive external ophthalmoplegia (CPEO); myoneurogastrointestinal disorder and encephalomyopathy (MNGIE); Barth syndrome; Pearson syndrome; Kearns-Sayre syndrome; many others.

Etiology
- The respiratory chain of the inner mitochondrial membrane contains five multi-subunit protein complexes.
- Complete assembly and maintenance of the electron transport chain requires the mitochondrial genome and hundreds of genes from the nuclear genome.
- Inborn errors in nuclear or mitochondrial genes can lead to RCD.
- Mitochondrial mutations are maternally inherited.
- RCDs resulting from errors in nuclear genes have been inherited in an autosomal recessive fashion.

Epidemiology
- Estimated prevalence of childhood RCD is 1:10,000

Pathophysiology
- Failure of the respiratory chain leads to inability to produce ATP from reduced electron carriers. This affects the efficiency of energy production from essentially all fuel sources.
- Decreased ATP production is associated with damage in tissues with high metabolic demand. Failure to re-oxidize electron carriers decreases TCA efficiency and leads to lactic acidosis.
- Ketosis results from shunting of acetyl CoA away from the TCA cycle and toward ketogenesis.
- Increased generation of toxic reactive oxygen species occurs.

Clinical Manifestations
Phenotypes in RCD are pleiotropic, even within a family. The presence of progressive dysfunction in seemingly unrelated organ systems should raise suspicion for an RCD. Tissues with high requirements for oxidative phosphorylation tend to be the most severely affected. These include:
- *Skeletal muscle:* weakness, myopathy, rhabdomyolysis, ophthalmoplegia
- *Central nervous system:* seizure, hearing loss, basal ganglia dysfunction, developmental delay, abnormal tone, retinopathy, stroke-like events
- *Liver:* steatosis, transaminitis, decreased synthetic function, hepatic failure
- *Bone marrow:* neutropenia, sideroblastic anemia
- *Pancreas:* diabetes mellitus, exocrine insufficiency
- *Heart:* arrhythmias, cardiomyopathy
- *Proximal renal tubule:* renal tubular acidosis, renal Fanconi

A wide range of findings are possible on physical exam:
- *Eyes:* Evaluate for ophthalmoplegia and retinal abnormalities
- *Respiratory:* Kussmaul respirations suggest metabolic acidosis, which can be due to lactemia or ketonemia
- *Cardiac:* Irregular rhythms, new murmurs/gallops, signs of congestive heart failure
- *Gastrointestinal:* Hepatomegaly
- *Neurologic:* Evaluate tone, mental status, and focal deficits

Diagnostics
In Patients Suspected of Having a Respiratory Chain Defect
- Basic metabolic panel, liver function tests, and creatine kinase
- Elevated lactate and lactate/pyruvate ratio may be present at baseline, or may be uncovered after glucose loading.
- Plasma ketones: Ketonemia may be present, even in fed state.
- Urine organic acids. May reveal elevated lactate, ketones, and TCA cycle intermediates (e.g., α-ketoglutarate).
- Urine amino acids: A generalized aminoaciduria reflecting proximal renal tubular dysfunction occurs in some patients.
- In patients with CNS disease, CSF lactate/pyruvate
- MRI of brain for structural or degenerative abnormalities
- MR spectroscopy to detect lactate, especially in basal ganglia

For Definitive Diagnosis
- Measurement of electron transport chain activity in tissue biopsy specimens, usually muscle, remains the gold standard.
- If the clinical presentation closely matches a particular syndrome (e.g., MELAS), then mutational analysis may be helpful.

Management
- There is no definitive management for RCDs. Supportive therapies vary according to organ system involvement.
- Consultation with a biochemical geneticist is recommended
- A variety of cofactors, antioxidants, and other agents have been attempted. These include CoQ10, vitamin C, vitamin E, thiamine, carnitine, and others. No therapy has been conclusively shown to be effective in improving outcome.

PYRUVATE DEHYDROGENASE DEFICIENCY

Pyruvate dehydrogenase (PDH) deficiency is an inborn error resulting in decreased activity of PDH, a mitochondrial enzyme complex that converts pyruvate to acetyl CoA. Inefficient oxidation of carbohydrates and a propensity for lactic acidosis occurs. Assembly and activity of PDH require products of at least nine genes, but the vast majority of patients have dysfunction of the E1α subunit.

Epidemiology
- Several hundred cases have been described; incidence unknown
- Despite its X-linked inheritance, PDH E1α deficiency has a similar incidence in males and females. The random nature of X-inactivation leads to a different phenotype in females.

Pathophysiology
- PDH, the biochemical step between glycolysis and the TCA cycle, is exclusively involved in carbohydrate metabolism.
- Inability to generate acetyl CoA from glucose severely limits the amount of energy (ATP) produced per mole of glucose.
- Involvement of the CNS reflects the exquisite dependence of the brain on aerobic glucose oxidation for cellular functions.
- Lactic acidosis results from the conversion of excess pyruvate to lactate by lactate dehydrogenase.

Clinical Manifestations
- Severity is variable, and is determined both by residual enzyme activity and, for females, the pattern of X-inactivation.
- Involvement of the central nervous system is universal and can cause poor feeding, hypotonia, lethargy, and coma in neonates.

- Two general phenotypes exist: a "metabolic" presentation of overwhelming, refractory neonatal lactic acidosis (especially in boys with profound E1α deficiency), and a chronic "neurologic" presentation causing developmental delay, seizures, and ataxia (typical in affected girls).
- Prenatal complications (low birth weight, decreased fetal movements, facial dysmorphisms) can occur in severely affected patients.
- Degenerative changes in the CNS, including subacute neurodegeneration of the brainstem and basal ganglia (Leigh disease) occur in some patients. Apnea and sudden death may occur as a result of brainstem dysfunction.
- Hepatomegaly is uncommon and suggests alternative diagnoses.

Diagnostics
- Plasma lactate and pyruvate. Elevations of both with a normal or near-normal ratio are strongly suggestive.
- Plasma amino acids often reveal an elevated alanine in PDH deficiency and other inborn forms of lactic acidosis.
- Lactate may also be elevated in other body fluids, including urine and cerebrospinal fluid. CSF lactate and pyruvate are helpful diagnostic aids in children with neurologic symptoms suspected to have a metabolic disease.
- Brain MRI to evaluate structural or degenerative CNS abnormalities. Concurrent MR spectroscopy to measure lactate peaks is very helpful.
- For definitive diagnosis, enzyme assays can be performed on a variety of tissues including skin fibroblasts, lymphocytes, and muscle. Various PDH components are examined separately in the assays, often allowing for precise biochemical diagnosis.

Management
- Consultation with biochemical geneticist
- Bicarbonate therapy to treat chronic acid load
- Use caution with dextrose-containing fluids, because glucose loads exacerbate lactic acidosis. Generally safe to start with D5-based solutions.
- A small minority of patients respond to thiamine (0.5–2 g/day).
- Dichloroacetate, which maintains the activated form of PDH, has improved lactic acidosis in some patients. Long-term benefits on development are unknown.
- Ketogenic (i.e., low carbohydrate) diets have in some cases been associated with improved development. They do not appear to reverse the ultimately fatal course of the disease.

Resources

Fatty Acid Oxidation Disorders and Disorders of Ketone Metabolism
al-Essa MA, Rashed MS, Bakheet SM, et al. Glutaric aciduria type II: observations in seven patients with neonatal- and late-onset disease. J Perinatol 2000;2:120–128.

Andersen BS, Olpin S, Poorthuis BJ, et al. Clear correlation of genotype with disease phenotype in very-long-chain acyl-CoA dehydrogenase deficiency. Am J Hum Genet 1999;64:479–494.

Mitchell GA, Fukao T. In: Scriver CR, Baudet AL, Sly WS, Valle D, eds. The Metabolic and Molecular Bases of Inherited Disease. 8th ed.. New York: McGraw-Hill, 2001.

Pollitt RJ, Leonard JV. Prospective surveillance study of medium chain acylCoA dehydrogenase deficiency in the UK. Arch Dis Child 1998;79:116–119.

Rinaldo P, Matern D, Bennett MJ. Fatty acid oxidation disorders. Ann Rev Physiol 2002;64:477–502.

Roe CR, Ding J. In: Scriver CR, Baudet AL, Sly WS, Valle D, eds. The Metabolic and Molecular Bases of Inherited Disease. 8th ed. New York: McGraw-Hill, 2001.

Saudubray JM, Martin D, de Lonlay P, et al. Recognition and management of fatty acid oxidation defects: a series of 107 patients. J Inhert Metab Dis 1999;22:488–502.

Stanley CA. In: Fernandes J, Saudubray J-M, Van den Berghe G, eds. Inborn Metabolic Diseases: Diagnosis and Treatment. 3rd ed. New York: Springer-Verlag, 2000.

Tyni T, Pihko H. Long-chain 3-hydroxyacyl-CoA dehydrogenase deficiency. Acta Paediatr 1999;88:237–245.

Vianey-Saban C, Divry P, Brivet M, et al. Mitochondrial very-long-chain acyl-coenzyme A dehydrogenase deficiency: clinical characteristics and diagnostic considerations in 30 patients. Clin Chim Acta 1998;269:43–62.

Urea Cycle Defects

Bachman C, Colombo JP. Increased tryptophan uptake in the brain in hyperammonemia. Life Sci 1983;33:2417–2424.

Batshaw ML, MacArthur RB, Tuchman M. Alternative pathway therapy for urea cycle disorders: twenty years later. J Pediatr 2001;138(suppl):S46–55.

Brusilow SW, Horwich AL. In Scriver CR, Baudet AL, Sly WS, Valle D, eds. The Molecular and Metabolic Bases of Inherited Disease. 8th ed. New York: McGraw-Hill, 2001.

Steiner RD, Cederbaum SD. Laboratory evaluation of urea cycle disorders. J Pediatr 2001;138(suppl):S21–29.

Summar M. Current strategies for the management of neonatal urea cycle disorders. J Pediatr 2001;138(suppl): S30–39.

Summar M, Tuchman M. Proceedings of a consensus conference for the management of patients with urea cycle disorders. J Pediatr 2001;138(suppl):S6–10.

Uchino T, Endo F, Matsuda I. Neurodevelopmental outcome of long-term therapy of urea cycle disorders in Japan. J Inherit Metab Dis 1998;21(suppl):S151–159.

Wyse AT, Bavaresco CS, Hagen ME, et al. In vitro stimulation of oxidative stress in cerebral cortex of rats by the guanidino compounds accumulating in hyperargininemia. Brain Res 2001;923:50–57.

Defects of Amino Acid Metabolism

Cederbaum S. Phenylketonuria: an update. Curr Opin Pediatr 2002;14:702–706.

De Braekeleer M, Larochelle J. Genetic epidemiology of hereditary tyrosinemia in Quebec and in Saguenay-Lac-St-Jean. Am J Hum Genet 1990;47:302–307.

Grompe M. The pathophysiology and treatment of hereditary tyrosinemia type 1. Semin Liver Dis 2001;21:563–571.

Halverson S. Screening for disorders of tyrosine metabolism. In Bickle H, Guthrie R, Hammerson G, eds. Neonatal Screenings for Inborn Errors of Metabolism. New York: Springer-Verlag, 1980.

Holme E, Lindstedt S. Tyrosinaemia type I and NTBC (2-(2-nitro-4-trifluoromethylbenzoyl)-1,3-cyclohexane-dione). J Inherit Metab Dis 1998;21:507–517.

Mitchell GA, et al. In: Scriver CR, Baudet AL, Sly WS, Valle D, eds. The Metabolic and Molecular Bases of Inherited Disease. 8th ed. New York: McGraw-Hill, 2001.

Phenylketonuria: Screening and Management. National Institutes of Health Consensus Statement 2000;17:1–27.

Scriver CR, Kaufman S. In: Scriver CR, Baudet AL, Sly WS, Valle D eds. The Metabolic and Molecular Bases of Inherited Disease. 8th ed. New York: McGraw-Hill, 2001.

Smith I, Lee P. In: Fernandes J, Saudubray J-M, Van den Berghe G, eds. Inborn Metabolic Diseases: Diagnosis and Treatment. 3rd ed. New York: Springer-Verlag, 2000.

van Spronsen FJ, Thomasse Y, Smit GP, et al. Hereditary tyrosinemia type 1: a new clinical classification with difference in prognosis on dietary treatment. Hepatology 1994;20:1187.

Defects of Carbohydrate Metabolism

Ali M, Rellos P, Cox TM. Hereditary fructose intolerance. J Med Genet 1998;35:353–365.

Gitzelmann R. In: Fernandes J, Saudubray J-M, Van den Berghe G, eds. Inborn Metabolic Diseases: Diagnosis and Treatment. 3rd ed. New York: Springer-Verlag, 2000.

Holton J, et al. In: Scriver CR, Baudet AL, Sly WS, Valle D eds. The Metabolic and Molecular Bases of Inherited Disease. 8th ed. New York: McGraw-Hill, 2001.

James CL, Rellos P, Ali M, et al. Neonatal screening for hereditary fructose intolerance: frequency of the most common mutant aldolase B allele (A149P) in the British population. J Med Genet 1996;33:837–841.

Schweitzer S, Shin Y, Jakobs C, Brodehl J. Long-term outcome in 134 patients with galactosemia. Eur J Pediatr 1993;152:36–43.

Shaw V, Lawson M. Clinical Paediatric Dietetics. London: Blackwell Science, 1994.

Van den Berghe G. In: Fernandes J, Saudubray J-M, Van den Berghe G, eds. Inborn Metabolic Diseases: Diagnosis and Treatment. 3rd ed. New York: Springer-Verlag, 2000.

Waggoner DD, Buist NR, Donnell GN. Long-term prognosis in galactosemia: results of a survey of 350 cases. J Inherit Metab Dis 1990;13:802–818.

Organic Acidemias

Berry GT, Heidenreich R, Kaplan P, et al. Branched-chain amino acid free parenteral nutrition in the treatment of acute metabolic decompensation in patients with maple syrup urine disease. N Engl J Med 1991;324:175–179.

Cohn RM, Roth K. Disorders of organic acid metabolism. In: Cohn RM, Roth KS, eds. Biochemistry and Disease. Baltimore: Williams & Wilkins, 1996.

de Baulny HO, Saudubray JM. Branched-chain organic acidurias. In: Fernandes J, Saudubray J-M, Van den Berghe G, eds. Inborn Metabolic Diseases. 6th ed. New York: Springer, 2000.

Morton DH, Strauss KA, Robinson DL, et al. Diagnosis and treatment of maple syrup disease: A study of 36 patients. Pediatrics 2002;109:999–1008.

Nyhan WL, Rice-Kelts M, Klein J, Barshop BA. Treatment of the acute crisis in maple syrup urine disease. Arch Pediatr Adolesc Med 1998;152:593–598.

Ozand PT, Generoso GG. Organic acidurias: A review. Part I. J Child Neurol 1991;6:195–219.

Ozand PT, Generoso GG. Organic acidurias: A review. Part 2. J Child Neurol 1991;6:228–295.

Sweetman L. Branched chain organic acidurias. In: Scriver CR, Baudet AL, Sly WS, Valle D, eds. The Metabolic Basis of Inherited Disease. 6th ed. New York: McGraw-Hill, 1989.

Primary Lactic Acidosis

Brown GK, Otero LJ, LeGris M, Brown RM. Pyruvate dehydrogenase deficiency. J Med Genet 1994;31:875–879.

Chinnery PF, Turnbull,DM. Epidemiology and treatment of mitochondrial disorders. Am J Med Genet 2001;106;94–101.

Kerr DS, et al. In: Fernandes J, Saudubray J-M, Van den Berghe G, eds. Inborn Metabolic Diseases: Diagnosis and Treatment. 3rd ed. New York: Springer-Verlag, 2000.

Munnich A. In: Fernandes J, Saudubray J-M, Van den Berghe G, eds. Inborn Metabolic Diseases: Diagnosis and Treatment. 3rd ed. New York: Springer-Verlag, 2000.

Robinson BH. In: Scriver CR, Baudet AL, Sly WS, Valle D, eds. The Metabolic and Molecular Bases of Inherited Disease. 8th ed. New York: McGraw-Hill, 2001.

Shoffner JM. In: Scriver CR, Baudet AL, Sly WS, Valle D, eds. The Metabolic and Molecular Bases of Inherited Disease. 8th ed. New York: McGraw-Hill, 2001.

Wexler ID, Hemalatha SG, McConnell J, et al. Outcome of pyruvate dehydrogenase deficiency treated with ketogenic diets. Studies in patients with identical mutations. Neurology 1997;49:1655–1661.

Laura A. Lawler, MD, Andrea A. Berry, MD, Snehal N. Shah MD,
Gary Frank, MD, MS, John Casey MD, CM, Mary Catherine Harris, MD

APGAR SCORES

APGAR scores are used to document the condition of a newborn infant on a scale of from 0 to 10. Newborns are given a score between 0 and 2 on each of five clinical categories. Scores are recorded at 1 and 5 minutes after birth. Thereafter, scores are recorded every 5 minutes until a score of 7 or more is achieved. Determination of an APGAR score should NOT delay resuscitation efforts. (Table 17.1)

APPARENT LIFE-THREATENING EVENT

Apparent life-threatening event (ALTE) is not a specific diagnosis but rather a general term used to describe an event. ALTE is defined by the National Institutes of Health as "an episode that is frightening to the observer and that is characterized by some combination of apnea (central or occasionally obstructive), color change (usually cyanotic or pallid but occasionally erythematous or plethoric), marked change in muscle tone (usually marked limpness), choking, or gagging. In some cases the observer fears that the infant has died."

- *Apnea:* absence of spontaneous ventilation for 20 seconds or of shorter duration if associated with cyanosis or bradycardia
- *Central apnea:* absence of respiratory effort
- *Obstructive apnea:* sustained respiratory effort without airflow
- *Mixed apnea:* a combination of central and obstructive apnea
- *Periodic breathing:* a pattern of breathing defined by three or more periods of apnea lasting at least 3 seconds and separated by less than 20 seconds of breathing

Epidemiology
- Incidence: 0.5% to 6%; peaks between 1 and 3 months

Differential Diagnosis
- Normal physiologic variation: normal infants may exhibit pauses in breathing of up to 10–20 seconds during sleep.
- Apnea of infancy: unexplained pauses in breathing that last longer than 20 seconds or accompanied by cyanosis, pallor, hypotonia, or bradycardia. These events usually cease by 43 weeks post-conception.
- Gastroesophageal reflux, seizure, anemia
- Infections: sepsis, pertussis, respiratory syncytial virus (RSV), meningitis
- Metabolic: inborn errors of metabolism, hypoglycemia, hypocalcemia
- Cardiovascular: conduction disorders (prolonged QT), congenital malformation, cardiomyopathy
- Respiratory disorders: airway anomalies, aspiration, reactive airway disease
- Child abuse: non-accidental head trauma, poisoning, suffocation, Munchausen's syndrome by proxy, factitious illness, drug effect

Clinical Manifestations
- Apnea, cyanosis, and difficulty breathing are most commonly reported
- Pallor, stiffness, floppiness, choking, red face, limb movements, vomiting
- Physical exam is often normal.

Table 17.1: APGAR Score

	0	1	2
Appearance (color)	Blue or pale	Pink body, blue extremities	Completely pink
Pulse (heart rate)	Absent	<100 bpm	>100 bpm
Grimace (reflex irritability)	No response	Grimace	Sneeze, cough
Activity (muscle tone)	Limp, flaccid	Some flexion	Active movements
Respiratory effort	Absent	Gasping; slow, irregular	Regular; good, lusty cry

bpm, beats per minute.

Diagnostics

- There is no standard ALTE workup. Decisions regarding what tests and studies to do are usually driven by the history and physical exam.
- *Thorough history:* determine the exact details of the event, including duration, preceding circumstances, relationship to feeding, location of the infant, and necessary intervention. Ask about the presence of respiratory effort, color change, choking, gasping, emesis, limpness, stiffness, rhythmic movements, eye movements, nasal congestion, and fever. Talk to all eyewitnesses. Try to determine the severity of the event.
- *Thorough physical exam:* focus on neurologic, respiratory, and cardiac exam; include pulse oximetry and funduscopy
- *Reasonable initial studies:* CBC with differential, serum electrolytes, glucose
- *Consider other initial studies:* serum lactate, chest radiograph, urinalysis, electrocardiogram, urine toxicology screen, nasal swab for RSV and pertussis
- *Full sepsis evaluation:* based on patient's age and severity of event, may need blood, urine, and cerebrospinal fluid cultures
- *Electroencephalogram (EEG):* if concerned about seizure
- *Head imaging:* if concerned about non-accidental head trauma
- *Metabolic workup:* blood and urine can be stored for future metabolic workup if indicated.
- *Upper gastrointestinal series:* evaluates for reflux and gastrointestinal anatomy
- *Four-channel pneumogram:* differentiates between central and obstructive apnea. The four channels include a nasal thermistor (detects airflow), pulse oximeter, chest leads to monitor heart rate, and chest leads to monitor chest wall movement. A pH probe (five-channel pneumogram) can also be included to define the relationship between reflux and apneic episodes.

Management

- Consider admission for period of observation and investigation. Place infants on continuous cardiorespiratory monitoring. Record further events in detail.
- Specific treatment should be directed towards results of the investigation.
- Antibiotics during a period of sepsis evaluation are often warranted based on the infant's age.
- Risk factors for significant disease include age above 2 months, abnormal findings on physical exam, lactate level greater than 2, and recurrent ALTE.
- ALTEs typically cause a high level of parental anxiety. Decisions regarding discharging an infant with a home apnea and bradycardia monitor can be difficult. The American Academy of Pediatrics (AAP) Policy Statement on Apnea, sudden infant death syndrome (SIDS), and Home Monitoring includes ALTE as an indication for home monitoring. However, parents must be informed that apnea is not predictive of or a precursor to SIDS, and that prevention of SIDS is not an indication for home cardiorespiratory monitoring. If a monitor is used, AAP

recommends discontinuing it by approximately 43 weeks post-conception or when extreme events cease to occur (whichever comes first).

HEMOLYTIC DISEASE: ABO INCOMPATIBILITY

Hemolysis caused by maternal-fetal ABO blood group incompatibility and resultant transplacental crossing of maternal IgG to the fetus is a major cause of neonatal hyperbilirubinemia. Usually, the mother is group O, and the newborn is group A or B.

Epidemiology
- Incidence of incompatibility: 1:5
- Incidence of mild disease (not requiring exchange transfusion): 1:150
- Incidence of severe disease: 1:3000
- More common in type B Asian and African newborns

Pathophysiology
- Mothers with type O blood do not have A or B antigens and therefore may produce anti-A and anti-B antibodies throughout life in response to gram-negative bacteria and other foreign antigens. Sensitization from a previous pregnancy is NOT required to cause disease.
- Maternal IgG crosses the placenta.
- IgG can attach to fetal red blood cells (RBCs), prompting hemolysis and removal.
- Disease is usually mild as compared to disease from Rh incompatibility because A and B antigens are expressed on tissues other than RBCs. Thus, maternal antibodies attach to the other sites, leaving less to attach to RBCs.

Clinical Manifestations
- Jaundice in the first 24 hours of life is a hallmark of hemolysis.

Diagnostics
- Type and screen reveal ABO incompatibility between mother and newborn.
- Direct Coombs test result is weakly positive or negative.
- Normal or mildly decreased hemoglobin
- Reticulocytes normal or increased
- Spherocytosis is characteristic.
- Total and fractionated bilirubin levels reveal an indirect hyperbilirubinemia.
- High reticulocyte count, positive Coombs, and presence of a sibling with neonatal jaundice are predictors for significant or severe disease.

Management
- Maintain adequate hydration
- Initiate phototherapy (see Hyperbilirubinemia)
- Exchange transfusion with type O blood of same Rh type as infant is occasionally required.
- Follow-up to detect late-onset hemolytic anemia occasionally requiring packed RBC transfusion.

HEMOLYTIC DISEASE: RH INCOMPATIBLITY

An often severe hemolytic anemia in the fetus and newborn caused by maternal-fetal blood group incompatibility of the Rhesus D antigen and resultant transplacental crossing of IgG antibodies from a previously sensitized mother to her fetus.

Epidemiology
- 15% prevalence of RhD(−) phenotype among whites in the United States; 9% incidence of incompatibility.
- Anti-D immunoglobulin for prevention of sensitization has reduced incidence of disease to approximately 10.6 cases per 10,000 live births

Pathophysiology
- Mothers who do not have D antigen are "RhD(−)" but can carry fetuses with paternally derived D antigen
- RhD(+) fetal RBCs cross into the maternal circulation during pregnancy or delivery with subsequent maternal antibody production against the foreign RhD antigen. More cells cross over with transplacental hemorrhage (e.g., cesarean section, toxemia, manual removal of the placenta).
- During the next pregnancy, the mother's IgG anti-RhD antibodies cross the placenta and attach to fetal RBCs, prompting hemolysis and removal.

Clinical Manifestations
- Fetal hydrops
- Anemia
- Hyperbilirubinemia
- Hypoglycemia due to islet cell hyperplasia of the pancreas
- Thrombocytopenia from liver dysfunction, disseminated intravascular coagulation, and/or repeated intrauterine transfusions
- Physical exam: signs of hydrops (ascites, pleural effusions, edema), pallor, jaundice, petechia/purpura, hepatosplenomegaly (due to extramedullary hematopoiesis and splenic sequestration)

Diagnostics
- Cord blood should be sent for laboratory tests, which reveal the following:
  - RhD(+) baby and RhD(−) mother
  - Decreased hemoglobin
  - Increased reticulocyte count
  - Increased nucleated RBCs
  - Positive direct Coombs test
  - Increased bilirubin

Management
Prevention
- Anti-D immunoglobulin prevents sensitization and should be given to RhD(−) mothers at 28 to 36 weeks' estimated gestational age and at delivery. More anti-D should be given when greater transplacental hemorrhage may have occurred.

In Utero Management
- Amniotic fluid bilirubin levels
- Umbilical vein blood sampling
- Intrauterine transfusions via umbilical vein
- Premature induction of labor. Consider glucocorticoids for lung maturation if premature delivery is anticipated.

Postnatal Management
- Phototherapy
- Exchange transfusion is sometimes required.
- Hydropic infants frequently require intensive care including: 1) therapeutic paracentesis or thoracentesis, 2) mechanical ventilation, 3) volume expanders (e.g., fresh-frozen plasma), 4) pressors, 5) diuretics, 6) isovolumetric partial exchange transfusion, among other therapies.
- Late anemia may develop following Rh isoimmunization.

INFANT OF A DIABETIC MOTHER

The infant of a diabetic mother (IDM) is distinguished because of increased risk of morbidity and mortality.

Epidemiology
- Pre-existing diabetes: 0.2% to 0.3% of pregnancies
- Gestational diabetes: 1% to 5% of pregnancies
- Perinatal mortality ranges from 2% to 4% in pregnancies complicated by insulin-dependent diabetes mellitus (IDDM). Mortality is three to six times higher than in the general population.

Pathophysiology
- Because glucose crosses the placenta in utero, maternal hyperglycemia leads to fetal hyperglycemia. Elevated fetal blood sugar results in increased insulin production. When the maternal glucose supply is interrupted at delivery, the elevated insulin levels lead to neonatal hypoglycemia.
- Because insulin is an anabolic hormone, elevated insulin levels lead to visceromegaly and macrosomia. Visceromegaly especially affects the heart, liver, and muscles. Increased insulin levels also delay lung maturation.
- Chronic fetal hyperinsulinism results in an increase in metabolic rate and oxygen consumption, leading to hypoxia in utero. Hypoxia increases erythropoietin production, leading to polycythemia. Hypoxia also contributes to the greater risk of fetal asphyxia and intrauterine fetal demise.
- Strict control of maternal blood sugar has resulted in improved morbidity and mortality.

Clinical Manifestations
- Hypoglycemia is often asymptomatic, but symptoms may include tachypnea, apnea, tremors, diaphoresis, irritability, and seizures.
- Risk of congenital malformations is significantly increased in infants born to mothers with IDDM. The most common malformations involve the heart, central nervous system, renal and urinary systems, limbs, ribs and spine, and caudal dysgenesis.
- Macrosomia and maternal diabetes are both independent risk factors for shoulder dystocia, with potential brachial plexus injury.
- Increased risk of respiratory distress syndrome
- Hypocalcemia and hypomagnesemia
- Polycythemia contributes to an increased risk of hyperbilirubinemia and venous thrombosis (especially renal).
- Hypertrophic cardiomyopathy with possible heart failure
- Research has raised concerns regarding the possibility of delayed growth and development, impaired psychosocial and intellectual capabilities, and future risk of developing diabetes.

Diagnostics
- The definition of neonatal hypoglycemia is controversial, and the level and duration of hypoglycemia that cause damage is unknown.
- Monitor glucose at delivery and frequently after birth (i.e., as soon as possible after birth, within 2 to 3 hours after birth, and before feeding). Confirm low values (<40 mg/dL) with a serum sample.
- Check glucose on any infant that is symptomatic and consider other etiologies if symptoms do not abate with therapy (e.g., sepsis, pneumonia).

Management
Management of Hypoglycemia
- Prevent hypoglycemia by testing blood sugars and initiating feeds early. Consider gavage feeds if infant will not easily take formula.
- Treat symptomatic hypoglycemia with 2 mL/kg of a 10% IV glucose solution. Then give continuous IV glucose at 5 to 6 mg/kg/min and increase or wean the rate as needed to maintain blood glucose greater than 50 mg/dL. Check blood sugars every 30 to 60 minutes until stable.

Other Management Issues
- Metabolic: may require calcium and magnesium therapy
- Cardiorespiratory: high risk for perinatal asphyxia, hyaline membrane disease, and hypertrophic cardiomyopathy. These infants may require management in an intensive care setting.

- Hematologic: manage hyperbilirubinemia and polycythemia as previously described in this chapter.
- Monitor for macrosomia, birth injury, and congenital malformations.

MECONIUM ASPIRATION SYNDROME

A common cause of neonatal respiratory distress, in which in utero or perinatal aspiration of meconium-stained amniotic fluid (MSAF) causes respiratory distress.

Epidemiology
- Approximately 14% of all deliveries are associated with MSAF.
- Approximately 5% to 12% of deliveries through MSAF develop MAS.

Pathophysiology
- Passage of meconium seldom occurs before 34 weeks' estimated gestational age, occurs more frequently with increasing gestational age, and is related to stress/asphyxia.
- Meconium is aspirated during gasping in utero, which is initiated by fetal distress. Airway obstruction by ball-valve mechanism causes simultaneous atelectasis and overexpansion, leading to air leaks.
- Chemical inflammation (pneumonitis) causes alveolar collapse and parenchymal damage. Inhibition of surfactant causes alveolar collapse and decreased lung compliance.
- Persistent pulmonary hypertension of the newborn (PPHN) can occur as a result of hypoxia-induced pulmonary artery vasoconstriction.

Clinical Manifestations
- Full-term or post-dates; often small for gestational age
- Infant born through MSAF (thick meconium more likely than thin meconium)
- Meconium staining of nails, skin, umbilical cord, placenta
- Respiratory exam: initial respiratory depression is quickly followed by tachypnea, retractions, grunting, flaring, prolonged expiratory phase, rales, rhonchi, barrel chest with increased antero-posterior diameter, cyanosis
- Neurologic depression

Diagnostics
- *Chest x-ray:* classic appearance is coarse, irregular pulmonary densities; may also see hyperinflation and flattening of the diaphragm. Other possible findings include pneumothorax, pneumomediastinum, pleural effusion, and cardiomegaly (secondary to hypoxia). X-rays can also look virtually normal.
- *Arterial blood gas:* hypoxemia; respiratory and metabolic acidosis from hypoxia, and poor perfusion/perinatal depression OR respiratory alkalosis from hyperventilation

Management
Prevention (perinatal resuscitation)
- Amnioinfusion: injection of normal saline into the amniotic sac to decrease cord compression and dilute meconium (efficacy unclear)
- Suctioning of the oropharynx by the obstetrician as soon as the head is visible
- Direct tracheal suctioning to remove meconium from the airway for "depressed" neonates (absent or depressed respirations, heart rate <100 beats per minute, poor muscle tone) before initiation of positive pressure

Postnatal Management
- Observation and monitoring in the neonatal intensive care unit: patients can rapidly decompensate
- Correction of acid-base status
- Chest physiotherapy and suctioning
- Oxygen and/or mechanical ventilation

- Minimal stimulation to prevent hypoxia
- Treatment of PPHN: liberal use of oxygen, hyperventilation, alkalinization, pressors
- Additional therapies: surfactant, nitric oxide, high frequency ventilation, extracorporeal membrane oxygenation

NEONATAL HYPERBILIRUBINEMIA

A common and often benign problem of newborns.

- *Unconjugated hyperbilirubinemia:* elevation of indirect serum bilirubin
- *Conjugated hyperbilirubinemia:* direct bilirubin level greater than 2.0 mg/dL and direct fraction greater than 10% of total serum bilirubin
- *Kernicterus:* pathologic findings of bilirubin toxicity in the brain, associated with staining and necrosis of neurons of the basal ganglia, hippocampus, subthalamic nuclei, and cerebellum. The clinical syndrome is characterized by cerebral palsy, mental retardation, uncoordinated movements, deafness, poor vision, and feeding and speech difficulties. Bilirubin levels greater than 25 mg/dL in otherwise healthy, term, or near-term infants are generally considered to be a risk factor for kernicterus.
- *Jaundice:* yellowing of skin, sclerae and mucous membranes due to high levels of serum bilirubin
- *Physiologic jaundice:* elevation of unconjugated bilirubin occurs in most infants during the first week of life and resolves spontaneously. Mean levels are ~5 to 6 mg/dL in bottle-fed white and African-American babies on the third day of life. Levels in breast-fed infants are higher (mean: 8 to 9 mg/dL) and peak later (fourth to fifth day).

Epidemiology
- Jaundice is observed in ~60% of term infants.

Etiology
Unconjugated Hyperbilirubinemia
- Functional: physiologic jaundice, breast-feeding
- Hemolytic anemia: ABO or Rh incompatibility, glucose-6-phosphate dehydrogenase (G6PD) deficiency, infection, drugs, hereditary spherocytosis or elliptocytosis, others
- Polycythemia: twin-twin transfusion, maternal-fetal transfusion, delayed cord clamping, small for gestational age, maternal diabetes, Down syndrome, Beckwith-Wiedemann syndrome, others
- Congenital: Crigler-Najjar syndrome, Gilbert syndrome, Lucey-Driscoll syndrome, congenital hypothyroidism
- Trauma: cephalohematoma, bruising

Conjugated Hyperbilirubinemia
- Anatomic: biliary atresia, Alagille syndrome, choledochal cyst, compression of the bile duct, other disorders of the biliary system
- Infectious: sepsis, intrauterine infection, urinary tract infection, other viral and bacterial etiologies
- Genetic/inborn errors: galactosemia, fructosemia, Niemann-Pick disease, cystic fibrosis, many others
- Other: total parenteral nutrition–induced cholestasis, medications, tumor, idiopathic neonatal hepatitis

Pathophysiology
- Physiologic jaundice is thought to be due to a combination of increased bilirubin load in neonates (larger RBC volume, shorter RBC life-span), decreased uptake of bilirubin by the liver, defective conjugation of bilirubin, and impaired excretion (bilirubin is excreted in stool and urine).

- Breast-fed infants are at higher risk of indirect hyperbilirubinemia in the first week of life than formula-fed infants due to relative dehydration and increased intestinal reabsorption of bilirubin. Additionally, ~2% of breast-fed infants develop indirect hyperbilirubinemia after the first week of life due to factors associated with human breast milk.
- Jaundice in the first 24 hours of life is generally pathologic.

Clinical Manifestations
- Jaundice: clinically visible at bilirubin levels ~5 to 7 mg/dL; apparent first in the face and then descends as levels increase.
- Early neurologic findings (bilirubin encephalopathy): lethargy, poor feeding, emesis, hypotonia
- Later neurologic findings: high-pitched cry, hypertonia, opisthotonus, seizures, fever
- Associated physical findings: cephalohematoma, petechiae, purpura, signs of prematurity or intrauterine growth retardation, plethora, hepatomegaly, splenomegaly, light-colored stools, dark urine

Diagnostics
- Serum bilirubin level: total, conjugated, unconjugated
- Initial laboratory tests: CBC and reticulocyte count, blood smear, blood type (mother and infant), Rh status (mother and infant), direct Coombs, electrolytes (to assess hydration), serum albumin
- Other laboratory tests to consider: urine for reducing substances, G6PD, hemoglobin electrophoresis, osmotic fragility, thyroid function, liver function, PT/PTT, blood and urine cultures, serum amino acids, urine organic acids
- Other studies to consider: liver ultrasound, hepatobiliary imaging (e.g., DISIDA scan), percutaneous liver biopsy
- See Figure 17.1 for bilirubin nomogram.

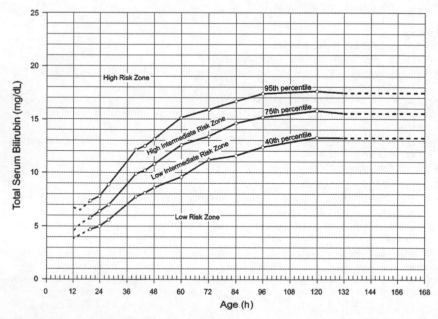

Figure 17.1 Bilirubin nomogram risk designation of term and near-term well newborns based on their hour-specific bilirubin values. (Reprinted with permission from Bhutani VK, Johnson L, Sivieri EM. Predictive ability of a predischarge hour-specific serum bilirubin for subsequent significant hyperbilirubinemia in healthy term and near-term newborns. Pediatrics 1999;103:6–14, figure 2.)

Management
Unconjugated Hyperbilirubinemia
- *Ensure adequate hydration:* consider supplementation of breast-fed babies with formula and/or intravenous fluids
- *Phototherapy:* light energy converts unconjugated bilirubin to a structural isomer, which can be excreted without conjugation. Blue lamps (420 to 480 nm) are most effective. The American Academy of Pediatrics recommends initiating phototherapy in *healthy, term, or near-term infants* with total serum bilirubin levels 15 mg/dL or greater at 25 to 48 hours, 18 mg/dL or greater at 49 to 72 hours, and 20 mg/dL or greater after 72 hours of age (see Figure 17.1). Phototherapy should be *considered* in healthy, term infants at total serum bilirubin levels 12 mg/dL or greater at 25 to 48 hours, 15 mg/dL or greater at 49 to 72 hours, and 17 mg/dL or greater after 72 hours of age based on clinical judgment. Phototherapy should be initiated at lower levels for premature infants.
- *Exchange transfusion:* double volume exchange transfusions are reserved for infants at high risk of kernicterus. Consider exchange transfusion in healthy, term infants with total bilirubin levels of 25 to 30 mg/dL.
- *Interruption of breast-feeding:* consider interrupting breast-feeding (and administering phototherapy) for 48 hours if bilirubin level is greater than 18 mg/dL.
- *Less common interventions:* albumin transfusion, phenobarbital, metalloporphyrins
- *Treat underlying disorder* if jaundice is non-physiologic.

Conjugated Hyperbilirubinemia
- Management is aimed at treatment of the underlying disorder.
- Phenobarbital, cholestyramine, and Actigall may promote bile flow and decrease serum bilirubin.
- Dietary management: formulas containing medium chain triglycerides are better absorbed; supplement vitamins A, D, E, and K.
- Kasai procedure (hepatoportoenterostomy) is used as bridge to transplantation in infants with biliary atresia.

POLYCYTHEMIA

A venous hematocrit (HCT) greater than 65%. Polycythemic neonates are at risk for hyperviscosity, which can compromise perfusion.

Epidemiology
- Incidence of polycythemia: 1% to 5%; highest at high altitudes
- Incidence of symptomatic polycythemia: 0.4% to 0.6%
- 10% to 15% of small for gestational age neonates are affected.

Pathophysiology
- A normal response to the relative hypoxic intrauterine environment is to increase RBC mass, causing a relative polycythemia.
- Polycythemia can occur because of increased red cell mass secondary to chronic intrauterine hypoxia (intrauterine growth retardation, maternal diabetes, maternal smoking) or erythrocyte transfusions. Factors that increase fetal blood volume, such as delayed cord clamping, positioning the infant below the introitus after delivery, maternal-fetal transfusion, and twin-twin transfusion, also increase risk for polycythemia.
- Viscosity is directly proportional to HCT but rises logarithmically above a HCT of 60%. When viscosity is increased, blood flow rate is decreased and tissue perfusion is poor.
- Fetal disorders that cause polycythemia include infants of diabetic mothers, congenital hypothyroidism, neonatal thyrotoxicosis, congenital adrenal hyperplasia, Beckwith-Wiedemann syndrome, and trisomies 13, 18, and 21.

Clinical Manifestations
- Most neonates with polycythemia are asymptomatic.
- Skin: plethoric, may have delayed capillary refill

- CNS symptoms: lethargy, apnea, tremors/jitteriness, poor feeding, hypotonia, and an exaggerated startle response. Strokes and seizures are rare.
- Cardiopulmonary symptoms: tachypnea, cyanosis, tachycardia, respiratory distress, and cardiomegaly. Prominent vascular markings on chest radiograph, elevated pulmonary vascular resistance and congestive heart failure are also possible.
- Hypoglycemia is the most common metabolic symptom. Hypocalcemia and hyperbilirubinemia are also possible.
- Renal dysfunction can present as oliguria, proteinuria, or hematuria. Renal vein thrombosis and renal failure are rare.
- Other rare complications: thrombus, thrombocytopenia, disseminated intravascular coagulation, necrotizing enterocolitis

Diagnostics
- HCT peaks at 2 hours of life and then progressively decreases, stabilizing by 6 to 24 hours of life. At 2 hours of life, it is common to use 70% as the upper limit of normal.
- Capillary HCT is significantly higher than venous values, and can only be used as a screening test. If the capillary value is above 65%, repeat with a venous stick. Blood obtained from arterial and umbilical vessels may yield a lower HCT.
- Other potential studies: serum glucose, serum calcium, serum bilirubin, serum electrolytes, urine specific gravity, blood gas, serum platelets

Management
- Partial exchange transfusion (PET): mainstay of therapy for symptomatic neonates with HCT greater than 65% or any neonate with a venous HCT greater than 70%.
  - The goal for PET is to decrease the HCT to 50% to 55%.
  - Volume to exchange (mL) is calculated by:

$$\frac{\text{Blood volume} \times (\text{Observed HCT} - \text{Desired HCT})}{\text{Observed HCT}}$$

  * Blood volume is estimated to be 90 to 100 mL/kg
  - Normal saline has become the replacement fluid of choice.
  - Blood should be removed using a central venous or arterial line and replacement fluid infused via a peripheral intravenous line.
  - Repeat HCT at end of procedure and 4 to 6 hours later.
- Asymptomatic neonates with HCT between 60% and 70% can be managed by liberalizing fluid intake and repeating HCT in 4 to 6 hours.
- Supportive care for metabolic abnormalities or hypoxia may be necessary.

TORCH INFECTIONS

A group of perinatally acquired infections with overlapping manifestations. Toxoplasmosis, syphilis, rubella, and CMV are discussed here. (See Infectious Diseases chapter for herpes simplex virus infection).

Epidemiology
- Congenital *Toxoplasma gondii* infection:
  - Maternal infection by ingesting cysts from infected meat or contact with cat excrement
  - Transmission if primary infection occurs during pregnancy
  - Maternal infection acquired in first trimester (rather than later) is associated with more severe fetal disease but fewer instances of fetal acquisition
- Congenital syphilis infection:
  - Fetal or perinatal death occurs in 40% to 50% of cases
  - Infection can be transmitted to fetus at any stage of disease but the rate is highest (60% to 90%) during primary and secondary stages.

- Congenital rubella infection:
  - 10% of young women are susceptible to rubella.
  - Congenital defects are more likely if infection occurs early in pregnancy.
- Congenital cytomegalovirus infection:
  - Most common human fetal infection
  - 1% of all liveborn infants are infected in utero but only 10% of those are symptomatic at birth.
  - Sequelae are more common in infants after maternal primary infection (25%) than after reactivation (8%).

Clinical Manifestations
Findings That Suggest TORCH Infection
- Intrauterine growth retardation, hydrops fetalis
- CNS abnormalities (microcephaly, hydrocephalus, intracranial calcifications), hepatospleno-megaly, bone abnormalities (osteochondritis, periostitis), myocarditis, ocular abnormalities (cataracts, chorioretinitis, glaucoma)
- Anemia and thrombocytopenia

Toxoplasmosis
- 70% to 90% are asymptomatic at birth
- Visual impairment, learning disabilities, or mental retardation become apparent several months to years later
- Hydrocephalus with *generalized* calcifications, seizures, opisthotonos, chorioretinitis, microph-thalmia, deafness, lymphadenopathy

Syphilis
- Two thirds of infected liveborn neonates are asymptomatic.
- Overt infection manifests in fetus, newborn, or later in childhood.
- Early congenital manifestations (detected before 2 years of age, typically before age 3 months): bullous lesions on palm and soles, copper color maculopapular rash, condyloma lata, snuffles (persistent, bloody nasal discharge), saddle nose deformity, osteochondritis and periostitis, parrot paralysis
- Late congenital manifestations (detected after 2 years of age): Hutchinson teeth, interstitial keratitis, eighth cranial nerve deafness, frontal bossing, rhagades (perioral fissuring), Clutton joints (chronic painless swelling of the knees), Saber shins

Rubella
- Blueberry muffin lesions (extramedullary dermal hematopoiesis), hemolytic anemia, cataracts, glaucoma, pigmented retinopathy, microphthalmia, cardiac malformations (patent ductus arte-riosus, pulmonary shunt, ventricular septal defect, atrial septal defect), deafness

Cytomegalovirus
- Microcephaly with *periventricular* calcifications, chorioretinitis, petechial rash, pneumonia, senso-rineural hearing impairment

Diagnostics
General Approach
- Blood: IgM (rubella, *Toxoplasma*), IgA and IgE (*Toxoplasma*), RPR (syphilis), hepatitis B surface antigen, polymerase chain reaction (PCR) (*Toxoplasma*)
- Cerebrospinal fluid: PCR (enterovirus, HSV, *Toxoplasma*), VDRL (syphilis)
- Skin lesion: direct fluorescent antibody (HSV, varicella), dark-field microscopy (syphilis)
- Viral culture: conjunctiva (HSV); mouth/throat (CMV, enterovirus, HSV, rubella); rectum (enterovirus, HSV); urine (CMV by rapid shell vial, rubella)
- Ophthalmology (CMV, HSV, rubella, syphilis, *Toxoplasma*, varicella)
- Hearing screen (CMV, rubella, *Toxoplasma*)
- Head CT (CMV, *Toxoplasma*)
- Additional studies: liver function tests, complete blood count
- Check the mother's prenatal laboratory results (including rubella, hepatitis B, and syphilis)

Toxoplasmosis
- Serologic diagnosis based on positive IgM or IgA assay within first 6 months of life or persistently positive IgG titers beyond 12 months

Syphilis
- Presumptive diagnosis: nontreponemal (VDRL or RPR) and treponemal (FTA-ABS or MHA-TP) tests on infant serum.
- Definitive diagnosis: identify spirochetes by dark-field microscopy or direct fluorescent antibody tests of lesions, exudate, or tissue
- Long bone radiographs for osteochondritis and periostitis

Rubella
- Diagnosis can also be made by demonstrating increasing serum rubella IgG over several months.

Cytomegalovirus
- Proof of congenital infection requires obtaining culture specimen within 3 weeks of birth
- Presumptive diagnosis can be made by fourfold antibody titer rise in paired serum samples (infrequently used method)

Management
- *Toxoplasmosis*: pyrimethamine combined with sulfadiazine for a prolonged (>1 year) course. Supplement with folinic acid
- *Syphilis*: aqueous crystalline penicillin G 50,000 U/kg per dose IV every 12 hours during first 7 days of life, and every 8 hours thereafter for a total of 10 days OR procaine penicillin G 50,000 U/kg IM once daily for 10 days
- *Rubella*: supportive care
- *CMV*: ganciclovir may decrease incidence of hearing loss. Consult with infectious diseases specialist.

Resources

American Academy of Pediatrics. Committee on Fetus and Newborn. Apnea, sudden infant death syndrome and home monitoring. Pediatrics. 2003;111:914–917.

American Academy of Pediatrics Provisional Committee for Quality Improvement and Subcommittee on Hyperbilirubinemia. Management of hyperbilirubinemia in the healthy term newborn: practice guideline. Pediatrics 1994;94:558–565.

Armentrout DC, Huseby V. Neonatal polycythemia. J Pediatr Health Care 2002;16:40–42.

Avery GB, et al., eds. Neonatology: Pathophysiology and Management of the Newborn. 5th ed. Philadelphia: Lippincott, Williams & Wilkins, 1999.

Beckerman RC, et al., eds. Respiratory Disorders in Infants and Children. Baltimore: Williams and Wilkins, 1992.

Bhutani VK, Johnson L, Sivieri EM. Predictive ability of a predischarge hour-specific serum bilirubin for subsequent significant hyperbilirubinemia in healthy term and near-term newborns. Pediatrics 1999;103:6–14.

Black VD, Lubchenco LO. Neonatal polycythemia and hyperviscosity. Pediatr Clin North Am 1982;29:1137–1147.

Cleary GM, Wiswell TE. Meconium-stained amniotic fluid and the meconium aspiration syndrome. An update. Pediatr Clin North Am 1998;45:511–529.

Cordero L, Landon MB. Infant of the diabetic mother. Clin Perinatol 1993;3:635–648.

Cornblath M, Hawdon JM, Williams AF, et al. Controversies regarding definition of neonatal hypoglycemia: suggested operation thresholds. Pediatrics 2000;105:1141–1145.

Davies F, Gupta R. Apparent life threatening event in infants presenting to an emergency department. Emerg Med J 2002;19:11–16.

Farrell PA, Weiner GM, Lemons JA. SIDS, ALTE, apnea, and the use of home monitors. Pediatr Rev 2002;23:3–8.

Feigin RD, Cherry JD, Demmler GJ, Kaplan SL, eds. Textbook of Pediatric Infectious Diseases. 5th ed. Philadelphia: WB Saunders, 2004.

Gomella TL, et al. Neonatology. 4th ed. Stamford, Conn: Appleton and Lange, 1999.

Greenough A. Rhesus disease: postnatal management and outcome. Eur J Pediatr 1999;158:689–693.

Kahn A. Recommended clinical evaluation of infants with an apparent life-threatening event. Consensus document of the European Society for the Study and Prevention of Infant Death, 2003. Eur J Pediatr 2004;164:108–115.

Long SS, Pickering LK, Prober CG, eds. Principles and Practice of Pediatric Infectious Diseases. New York: Churchill Livingstone, 2003.

AAP Subcommittee on Neonatal Hyperbilirubinemia. Neonatal jaundice and kernicterus. Pediatrics 2001;108:763–765.

Niermeyer S, Kattwinkel J, Van Reempts P, et al. International guidelines for neonatal resuscitation: an excerpt from the guidelines 2000 for cardiopulmonary resuscitation and emergency cardiovascular care: International Consensus on Science. Contributors and Reviewers for the Neonatal Resuscitation Guidelines. Pediatrics 2000;106:E29.

Pickering LK, ed. Red Book: 2003 Report of the Committee on Infectious Diseases. 26th ed. Elk Grove Village, Ill: American Academy of Pediatrics, 2003.

Rennie JM, Roberton NRC, eds. Textbook of Neonatology. 3rd ed. Edinburgh, New York: Churchill Livingstone; 1999.

Sarici SU, Yurdakok M, Serdar MA, et al. An early (sixth-hour) serum bilirubin measurement is useful in predicting the development of significant hyperbilirubinemia and severe ABO hemolytic disease in a selective high-risk population of newborns with ABO incompatibility. Pediatrics 2002;109:e53.

Schwartz R, Teramo K. Effects of diabetic pregnancy on the fetus and newborn. Semin Perinatol 2000;24:120–135.

Werner EJ. Neonatal polycythemia and hyperviscosity. Clin Perinatol 1995;22:693–710.

Wiswell TE, Gannon CM, Jacob J, et al. Delivery room management of the apparently vigorous meconium-stained neonate: results of the multicenter, international collaborative trial. Pediatrics 2000;105:1 7.

Christine T. Lauren, MD, Sarbattama Sen, MD, Kristen A. Feemster, MD, MPH, Joanne N. Wood, MD, Charles P. McKay, MD (with contributions from Ann E. Salerno, MD)

Glomerular Disease

HEMOLYTIC-UREMIC SYNDROME

Microangiopathic hemolytic anemia, thrombocytopenia, and acute renal injury following a prodromal illness of acute gastroenteritis.

Epidemiology
- Incidence in the United States: 1 to 3/100,000 population/year
- Peak age: 6 months to 4 years; seasonal peak during summer months

Etiology
- Caused by infection with Shiga toxin–producing *Escherichia coli* (STEC), especially O157:H7 (90% of cases), which can be found in undercooked hamburger meat, farm animals, alfalfa sprouts; may occur in outbreaks
- Other Shiga toxin–producing etiologies: non-O157 strains of *E. coli*, *Salmonella dysenteriae*, *Aeromonas*
- Other non–Shiga toxin infectious etiologies: *S. pneumoniae*, *C. canimorsus*, HIV
- Differential diagnosis includes atypical hemolytic-uremic syndrome (HUS); secondary HUS (bone marrow transplant, systemic lupus erythematosus [SLE], malignancy, post transplant); thrombotic thrombocytopenic purpura (TTP)

Pathophysiology
- Shiga toxin crosses gastrointestinal epithelium, enters bloodstream, and binds neutrophils, which carry the toxin to endothelial cells in other organs.
- Shiga toxin preferentially binds to endothelial cell receptors, causing a cascade of intracellular events leading to cell death, tissue ischemia, local activation of coagulation and fibrinolytic reactions and release of inflammatory cytokines and resulting in multiorgan injury.

Clinical Manifestations
- Fever, diarrhea, abdominal pain, vomiting 24 to 72 hours after inoculum
- Greater than 90% have bloody stools
- Two to 6 days after onset of gastrointestinal symptoms, HUS develops in 8%
- Pallor, petechiae, mild jaundice
- Oliguric or non-oliguric acute renal failure
- Volume overload, hypertension, hyperkalemia if oliguric or anuric
- Severe colitis; risk for bowel ischemia
- Other organs may be involved: e.g., pancreatitis
- Irritability, lethargy, restlessness
- Seizures, ataxia, tremors
- Cardiac failure from myocarditis, cardiomyopathy in rare cases

Diagnostics
- Culture stool for *E. coli* O157:H7
- Direct assay for Shiga toxin in stool
- Complete blood cell counts every 6 to 8 hours initially: thrombocytopenia often is first manifestation of HUS; hemolytic anemia with schistocytes on peripheral blood smear; leukocytosis in first week

- Serum chemistries and electrolyte panels every 6 to 8 hours initially
- Elevated amylase/lipase and glucose insensitivity if pancreas involved
- Hypoalbuminemia secondary to enteropathy

Management
- Intravenous fluid replacement of diarrheal losses during diarrheal prodrome
- Once HUS is diagnosed, fluids should be restricted to insensible losses + urine output + stool output + emesis.
- Meticulous management of electrolytes
- Provide sufficient calories with parenteral nutrition.
- Transfuse packed red blood cells only if hemoglobin less than 6 to 7 g/dL or cardiovascular compromise.
- Transfuse platelets only if active bleeding or before surgery.
- Avoid antibiotics, anti-motility medications
- May require dialysis
- Oral therapy with a Shiga-toxin binding agent does not appear to reduce the severity of diarrhea-associated HUS in children (Trachtman et al.).

IgA NEPHROPATHY

Immune complex–mediated glomerulonephritis characterized by microscopic or gross hematuria, IgA mesangial deposits, and mesangial proliferation.

Epidemiology
- Most common cause of primary glomerulonephritis worldwide
- 2% to 10% of cases of primary glomerulonephritis in the United States
- Prevalence: 25 to 50 per 100,000 individuals; male:female = 2-6:1
- Onset: usually 15 to 35 years of age; uncommon before 10 years

Etiology
- Etiology unknown. Genetic factors may lead to an increased susceptibility.
- Upper respiratory infection (URI) and other mucosal infections often precede onset by a few days.

Differential Diagnosis
- *Acute glomerulonephritis:* poststreptococcal glomerulonephritis, membranoproliferative glomerulonephritis, idiopathic rapidly progressive glomerulonephritis, Alport syndrome, Goodpasture syndrome, SLE
- *Other causes of hematuria:* stones, infection, trauma, exercise, anatomic anomalies, toxins, vascular

Pathophysiology
- Circulating IgA immune complexes and to a lesser extent other immune complexes are deposited in the glomerular mesangium
- C3 deposits are also found in the mesangium indicating that the alternative complement pathway may also be involved in the pathogenesis.
- Focal and sometimes generalized mesangial proliferation occurs

Clinical Manifestations
- Most children present with gross hematuria or with asymptomatic microscopic hematuria on screening urinalysis. Children with macroscopic hematuria often have a history of a URI or gastroenteritis 1 to 2 days before onset.
- Five clinical syndromes:
  1. Macroscopic hematuria: may be recurrent and associated with URI or other infection
  2. Asymptomatic microscopic hematuria and/or mild proteinuria
  3. Acute nephritic syndrome: hematuria with renal insufficiency and/or hypertension
  4. Nephrotic syndrome
  5. Mixed nephritic-nephrotic syndrome

- Renal function usually not significantly affected at initial presentation
- Proteinuria often minimal at time of initial presentation
- Generally has a benign course in children; however, up to 30% of patients may develop progressive renal failure.
- *Indicators of poor prognosis:* male gender; black race; older age at time of presentation; hypertension at time of presentation; renal insufficiency at time of presentation; lack of macroscopic hematuria; persistent proteinuria greater than 1 g/day; biopsy with crescents/large areas of fibrosis

Diagnostics
- Urinalysis: hematuria and or proteinuria (usually mild)
- Twenty-four–hour urine protein collection: usually less than 1 g of protein
- Serum creatinine and electrolytes: often normal
- Complement serum levels (C3 and C4): normal
- Serum IgA may be elevated in approximately 50% of patients but is not specific for IgA nephropathy.
- Skin biopsy if purpura: dermal capillary IgA deposits
- Renal biopsy required for definitive diagnosis:
  - Immunofluorescence: IgA deposits in glomerular mesangium
  - Light microscopy: mesangial proliferation usually focal but can be diffuse
  - Electron microscopy: electron dense mesangial deposits

Management
- Mainly supportive
- Consider steroids and immunosuppressants for patients with progressive disease or nephrotic features, but efficacy has not been proven.
- ACE inhibitors if hypertensive or proteinuric
- Fish oil if patient has large proteinuria
- Controversial/experimental: plasma exchange (removal of IgA antibodies); prophylactic antibiotics and/or tonsillectomy; phenytoin; danazol

NEPHROTIC SYNDROME

A composite of clinical findings (proteinuria, hypoalbuminemia, edema, hypercholesterolemia) which arises from a loss of glomerular membrane selectivity that leads to urinary protein loss.

Epidemiology
- Two to seven/100,000 in children younger than 16 years
- 50% are 1 to 4 years and 75% are younger than 10 years
- 75% of children with nephrotic syndrome have minimal change disease, 10% focal segmental glomerulosclerosis, 5% membranous glomerulopathy, 5% membranoproliferative glomerulonephritis (GN), 5% other causes

Differential Diagnosis
- *Minimal change disease:* normal glomerulus on light microscopy, loss of epithelial foot processes on electron microscopy; possibly related to allergic triggers, atopy
- *Focal segmental glomerulosclerosis:* segmental obliteration of capillary loops by increased collagen and the accumulation of lipid and proteinaceous material; thought to be idiopathic or secondary to urologic disease (unilateral renal agenesis or obstructive uropathy), sickle cell disease, glycogen storage disease, postinfectious GN, Alport syndrome, or obesity
- *Membranous glomerulopathy:* localization of immune complexes in the sub-epithelial zone. Etiologies include autoimmune disease (SLE, Hashimoto thyroiditis), infectious (hepatitis B/C, syphilis), therapeutic agents (penicillamine, captopril, NSAIDs), neoplastic disease (lung cancer), toxicity (heavy metal toxicity) or idiopathic. Immune complex stains for C3 and IgG are present.

- *Membranoproliferative GN:* localization of immune complexes to the mesangium and capillary walls; may be idiopathic or secondary to chronic bacterial/viral infection, bone marrow or renal transplant, autoimmune diseases or liver disease

Pathophysiology
- Nephrotic syndrome arises from a permeability defect in the glomerular capillaries that allows protein to be lost from the plasma into the urine.

Clinical Manifestations
- Facial, periorbital, and pretibial edema; anasarca or ascites
- Vomiting or diarrhea secondary to bowel wall edema
- Tachycardia if intravascularly depleted
- Foamy, frothy urine
- Abdominal pain due to reduced blood flow to the splanchnic bed
- Rales, dyspnea, and orthopnea in severe cases of fluid extravasation and pulmonary congestion/edema
- Urinary loss of antithrombin III, increased fibrinogen, and hemoconcentration predispose to hypercoagulability. Leg pain and Homan sign may signify a deep venous thrombosis (DVT).
- Urinary loss of IgG may predispose to infection. If fever is present, consider bacteremia and peritonitis.
- Occasionally, an acute flare may present with acute renal failure secondary to hypovolemia or infection.

Diagnostics
- Initial studies: urinalysis, serum chemistries, lipids, albumin, CBC
- Urinalysis: large protein, possible microscopic hematuria
- Twenty-four–hour urine collection: greater than 40 mg/m^2/day of protein
- Urine protein to creatinine ratio greater than 2 in first morning void
- Hypoproteinemia (<2 g/dL) and hypoalbuminemia (as low as 0.5 g/dL)
- Serum cholesterol greater than 200 mg/dL
- Hyponatremia, hypocalcemia
- Hemoconcentration causes elevated hemoglobin, platelets, hyperviscosity
- Consider renal biopsy if: 1) older than 10 years of age at presentation or disease has not responded to 4 to 6 weeks of treatment; 2) progressive renal insufficiency with persistently elevated BUN and creatinine; 3) younger than 1 year of age at diagnosis; 4) more than two relapses in a 6-month period; 5) steroid-resistant nephrotic syndrome

Management
- *Fluids:* due to low oncotic pressure, patients may appear to be fluid overloaded while they are actually intravascularly depleted. If vomiting, diarrhea, hypotensive, or tachycardic, give normal saline bolus IV and maintain on IV fluids to replace losses.
- *Albumin:* may be used to increase oncotic pressure in severe cases of edema or if hypotensive. Use with extreme caution if patient has respiratory compromise or elevated creatinine. Follow infusion with Lasix. Once intravascular volume is repleted, allow patient to drink to thirst.
- *Prednisone:* 60 mg/m^2 or 2 mg/kg daily for 4 to 6 weeks; proteinuria should clear within 3 weeks.
- Consider *loop diuretics* to increase urine output if patient is severly edematous.
- *Nutrition:* low sodium diet to reduce fluid retention.
- *ID:* blood culture and empiric antibiotic coverage for fever and/or severe abdominal pain.
- *Respiratory:* watch for signs of respiratory compromise secondary to pleural effusion, congestive heart failure (CHF)
- *Heme:* watch for clinical signs of DVT; discourage bed rest.
- Children with relapsing steroid-sensitive nephrotic syndrome may benefit from immunosuppressive therapy (e.g., cyclophosphamide, chlorambucil). Consult with pediatric nephrologist.

POST-INFECTIOUS GLOMERULONEPHRITIS

Immunologically mediated diffuse proliferative endocapillary inflammation of the glomerulus that results in damage to the basement membrane, mesangium, or capillary endothelium. The resulting syndrome is characterized by hematuria, proteinuria, hypertension, and renal insufficiency. The most common preceding infection is group A beta-hemolytic streptococci (pharyngitis or skin infection).

Epidemiology
- Affects children 2 to 12 years old; males more than females (2:1)
- May occur sporadically or as part of an epidemic
- Certain HLA haplotypes may be more susceptible
- Can occur in those with predisposition to endocarditis (anatomic abnormalities, IV drug users)

Etiology
- Streptococci (group A>group C>group G); staphylococci; gram-negative bacteria; intracellular bacteria

Differential Diagnosis
- Membranoproliferative glomerulonephritis, lupus nephritis, IgA nephropathy, Henoch-Schönlein purpura (HSP), Alport nephritis

Pathophysiology
- Deposition of circulating immune complexes
- Autoimmune response to a self antigen with molecular mimicry
- Microscopic changes:
  - Acute diffuse proliferative GN: infiltration of polymorphonuclear cells, influx of neutrophils, and endocapillary proliferation of mesangial cells and endothelial cells result in enlarged consolidated glomeruli.
  - Mesangioproliferative stage: begins several weeks after onset of illness. Neutrophils and endothelial hypercellularity resolve and leave only mesangial hypercellularity.

Clinical Manifestations
- Hematuria with RBC casts, dysmorphic RBCs, proteinuria, hypertension, and azotemia
- Latent period: 7 to 21 days after pharyngitis and 14 to 21 days after skin infection
- Hematuria: microscopic in two thirds of cases. Patient may have tea- or cola-colored gross hematuria. Patient may have transient oliguria. Anuria is rare and may indicate crescent formation.
- Hypertension: occurs in greater than 75%; usually secondary to fluid overload; can be treated with diuretics; 50% require antihypertensives.
- Edema: typically in the face and upper extremities; may present as anasarca or ascites; related to urinary sodium and fluid retention.
- Encephalopathy (headache, mental status change, seizure): may be related to a concomitant central nervous system (CNS) vasculitis or severe acute hypertension.
- Pallor
- Orthopnea, dyspnea, rales, and gallops may be associated with CHF.
- Pharyngeal erythema or impetigo have usually resolved.
- Resolution of disease: hypertension and edema typically resolve in 1 to 2 weeks. Hematuria and proteinuria may persist for months. Persistence of proteinuria longer than 1 year may indicate the persistence of proliferative glomerulonephritis and has a less favorable prognosis.

Diagnostics
- Urinalysis: urine may have rusty or tea color; presence of heme and protein. Microscopic evaluation reveals red cell casts or dysmorphic RBCs, occasional leukocytes and hyaline or granular casts.
- Electrolytes, BUN, creatinine
- Twenty-four–hour protein collection usually reveals sub-nephrotic range proteinuria (4 mg/m^2/day), but in 20% may be nephrotic range (40 mg/m^2/day).

- Throat/skin culture results positive in as few as 25% of patients
- ASO titer: doubling of this titer is highly indicative of recent streptococcal infection (70% sensitive). The peak value is found at 3 to 5 weeks.
- Streptozyme testing: 95% sensitive; does not correlate with severity of disease
- Blood culture: if clinical suspicion of subacute bacterial endocarditis
- Complement levels (particularly C3): reduced in the early acute phase and *usually return to normal in 8 weeks*
- Renal biopsy: if doubt as to diagnosis or prolonged or unusual course
- Renal ultrasound: if gross hematuria or azotemia
- Chest x-ray: to evaluate for pulmonary edema if severe fluid overload or CHF

Management
- Fluids: restrict fluids if patient has edema or hypertension; consider diuretics
- Electrolytes: replace electrolytes as needed; salt restriction if edema or hypertension; avoid potassium if renal failure present
- Treat hypertension due to fluid overload with loop diuretics. Calcium channel blockers can also be used.
- The presence of acute renal failure (ARF) is not associated with worse prognosis. Children rarely require dialysis for ARF associated with post-infectious GN.
- Steroids have not been shown to be associated with improved outcome.
- ID: if any evidence of a pharyngitis or skin infection persists, treat with a penicillin antibiotic or a macrolide if penicillin allergic.
- Long-term prognosis is generally good, with the main sequelae being hypertension. A small proportion have proteinuria, renal insufficiency, and hypertension 10 to 40 years after presentation.

Tubular/Interstitial Disease

RENAL TUBULAR ACIDOSIS

Failure of the kidney to maintain normal plasma concentration of bicarbonate due to impaired bicarbonate reabsorption or hydrogen ion (urinary acid) excretion resulting in a non–anion gap hyperchloremic metabolic acidosis.

Epidemiology
- Very rare; type 4 is most common followed by type 1 (type 3 doesn't exist)

Etiology
All forms may be either primary (sporadic or hereditary) or secondary to a wide range of conditions:
- *Type I: Distal RTA*
  - Inherited autosomal dominant or sporadic
  - Interstitial nephritis: obstructive uropathy, vesicoureteral reflux, sickle cell nephropathy, Ehlers-Danlos
  - Autoimmune: Sjögren syndrome, SLE, thyroiditis, chronic active hepatitis
  - Toxins/medications: amphotericin B, lithium, toluene, cisplatin
- *Type II: proximal renal tubular acidosis (RTA)*
  - Isolated: sporadic, hereditary (autosomal recessive), carbonic anhydrase deficiency
  - Fanconi syndrome: proximal tubular dysfunction with proteinuria, glycosuria, phosphaturia and amino aciduria; associated with a wide range of conditions including inborn errors of metabolism (cystinosis, Lowe syndrome, galactosemia, Wilson disease, glycogen storage disease, tyrosinemia), dysproteinemia (multiple myeloma, amyloidosis), toxins (heavy metals, gentamicin, cyclosporine/tacrolimus, outdated tetracycline), interstitial renal disease (Sjögren syndrome, renal transplant rejection)
  - Medications: acetazolamide, sulfonamide

- *Type IV: hyperkalemic RTA*
  - Hypoaldosteronism due to Addison disease, congenital adrenal hyperplasia or prolonged heparinization
  - Pseudohypoaldosteronism; obstructive uropathy; pyelonephritis, interstitial nephritis; diabetes mellitus; medications (trimethoprim-sulfamethoxazole [Bactrim], ACE inhibitors, cyclosporine)

Pathophysiology

- *Type I: Distal RTA:* impaired distal hydrogen ion secretion due to poor functioning of or damage to transporters or other proteins involved in the excretion of H^+ in the distal tubule. There is an inability to decrease urinary pH less than 5.5 even in setting of severe metabolic acidosis. Hypercalciuria results from the mobilization of calcium phosphate from bones. Increased citrate reabsorption decreases the solubility of calcium in the urine. Hypercalciuria and hypocitraturia promote nephrocalcinosis and nephrolithiasis.
- *Type II: Proximal RTA:* impaired proximal tubular reabsorption of bicarbonate due to defective sodium-hydrogen ion exchange. Decreased threshold for bicarbonate reabsorption causes increased bicarbonate excretion in urine. There is retained ability to acidify urine because distal tubule function is maintained. May be primary isolated form but is usually associated with more generalized proximal tubule dysfunction such as Fanconi syndrome. Not associated with hypercalciuria or hypocitraturia.
- *Type IV: Hyperkalemic RTA:* hypoaldosteronism or pseudohypoaldosteronism resulting in impaired hydrogen excretion and potassium secretion. Aldosterone acts directly on the H^+/ATPase responsible for acid excretion and promotes potassium secretion along the collecting tubule. Resultant hyperkalemia inhibits ammonia formation, which further inhibits hydrogen excretion. Poor response to aldosterone is most common mechanism in children.

Clinical Manifestations

All forms present with non-anion gap acidosis and growth failure within first few years of life. Distinguishing characteristics are:

- Type I: Distal RTA: bicarbonate levels may be more severe (<10), nephrocalcinosis and hypercalciuria (Urine Ca/Cr ratio); osteopenia; nephrolithiasis; alkaline urine with inability to bring pH lower than 5.5 even when severely acidotic; hypokalemia; hypocitraturia.
- Type II: Proximal RTA: severe sodium bicarbonate wasting resulting in polyuria and dehydration; anorexia, vomiting, and constipation; hypotonia; in Fanconi syndrome will see signs of phosphate wasting such as rickets; able to acidify urine (<5.5) in the face of acidosis because distal tubule function is intact. Hypokalemia is common secondary to hyperaldosteronism that results from decreased proximal reabsorption of Na^+.
- Type IV: Hyperkalemic RTA: polyuria and dehydration; hyperkalemia; elevated urine sodium and low urine potassium; pyelonephritis
- Signs of underlying etiology: bowing (rickets), Kayser-Fleischer rings (Wilson disease), hepatosplenomegaly, enlarged kidneys

Diagnostics

- Basic metabolic panel; pH via venipuncture, NOT heelstick; send sample STAT to prevent cell lysis and artificially low bicarbonate levels.
- Confirm type of metabolic acidosis (anion gap vs non-anion gap)

$$Anion\ gap = [Na^+] - [Cl^- + HCO_3^-]$$

- If anion gap greater than 20, acidosis is most likely NOT due to RTA.
- Urine anion gap (UAG):

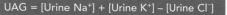

$$UAG = [Urine\ Na^+] + [Urine\ K^+] - [Urine\ Cl^-]$$

- Negative UAG: normal, GI bicarbonate losses, possible proximal RTA
- Positive UAG: suggests type I or IV RTA

- Urinalysis: metered urine pH (send STAT to lab); urine pH greater than 6 in face of acidosis suggests distal RTA. Urine pH cannot be interpreted in the presence of bicarbonate replacement, salicylates, penicillin, or ketoacids in urine.
- Detailed history: diarrhea; family history of renal disease, infant deaths, polyuria, polydipsia, failure to thrive, sensorineural deafness
- Renal ultrasound/abdominal x-ray: assess for anatomic abnormalities such as obstructive uropathy and nephrocalcinosis
- Bone radiographs: signs of rickets, failure to thrive, osteopenia

Management
- Bicarbonate replacement is the most important therapeutic step:
  - Usually as sodium bicarbonate, sodium citrate (Bicitra) or sodium/potassium citrate (Polycitra). Divide replacement into three to four doses per day. Titrate dose to maintain normal bicarbonate levels.
  - Type I (distal): Polycitra preferred because also have hypocitraturia and hypokalemia. Thiazide diuretics may aid in decreasing calcium excretion.
  - Type II (proximal): typically requires higher alkali doses (5–25 mEq/kg/day) than distal RTA (2–4 mEq/kg/day). Polycitra is recommended for hypokalemia. Consider dietary sodium restriction or thiazide diuretics.
  - Type II associated with Fanconi syndrome: consider phosphate replacement
  - Type IV: Bicitra or sodium bicarbonate 1–4 mEq/kg/day. Restrict potassium. If hyperkalemia does not improve, consider exchange resins such as Kayexalate. Give mineralocorticoids for hypoaldosteronemia.
- Treat underlying disease.
- In isolated RTA, normal growth is possible if steady bicarbonate levels are maintained.

RHABDOMYOLYSIS

Acute injury to skeletal muscle fibers, which results in the release of contents into the extracellular fluid and the circulation

Etiology
Physical
- *Compression and trauma:* crush injury, disasters, accidents, abuse, long-term positioning
- *Occlusion or hypoperfusion of vasculature:* thrombosis, embolism, surgical clamping, shock
- *Muscle overuse:* exercise, status epilepticus, status asthmaticus, tetanus
- *Electrical current:* injury, cardioversion
- *Hyperthermia:* malignant hyperthermia, neuroleptic malignant syndrome, sepsis, exercise

Non-physical
- *Infection:* influenza, coxsackievirus, HSV, herpes zoster, EBV, RSV, *Staphylococcus, Clostridium, Streptococcus, Leptospira, Legionella, Escherichia coli, Shigella*
- Drug-induced:
  - Direct: erythromycin, steroids, cyclosporine, itraconazole, colchicine, zidovudine, statins
  - Indirect: alcohol, central nervous system depressants, cocaine, amphetamine, ecstasy (MDMA), LSD, neuromuscular blocking agents
- Electrolyte abnormalities: hyperosmolarity, hyponatremia, hypocalcemia, hypokalemia, hypophosphatemia
- Metabolic myopathies: defects in carbohydrate metabolism and mitochondrial disorders
- Endocrinopathies: hypothyroid, diabetic coma/ketoacidosis
- Inflammatory myopathies: polymyositis, dermatomyositis, SLE, polyarteritis nodosum

Pathophysiology
- Regardless of etiology, muscle cell membrane integrity is compromised. There is a decrease in available intracellular ATP necessary for Na-K exchanger and calcium-exchanger, and calcium moves from the extracellular to intracellular space. This results in sustained contraction, energy depletion, and cell death as well as the release of enzymes and oxygen-free radicals.

- Myoglobin, released in large amounts, is unbound in serum and is filtered by the kidney. Myoglobin itself is not nephrotoxic; however, when urine flow is decreased (dehydration, hypotension) myoglobin can precipitate, leading to acute tubular necrosis, tubular obstruction and acute renal failure.
- Release of intracellular potassium and phosphorous
- Damage and cell death of muscle also results in large fluid shifts into the affected areas with ensuing hypernatremia, shock, and renal dysfunction.

Clinical Manifestations
Acute Rhabdomyolysis
- Evidence of primary etiology (i.e., abdominal trauma, viral prodrome)
- Myalgias, weakness, pain, muscle tenderness
- Dark/brown/red urine
- Edema of involved musculature
- Fluid shifts may result in hypotension, shock, tachycardia, hypernatremia
- Acute renal failure: oliguric or non-oliguric
- May progress to compartment syndrome
- Hypocalcemia initially; hypercalcemia during recovery phase
- Hyperkalemia, hyperphosphatemia
- Seizure, cardiac arrhythmia from electrolyte abnormalities

Chronic Rhabdomyolysis
- In metabolic myopathies: low grade chronic, episodic
- Muscle cramps precipitated by exercise, followed by weakness
- May be complicated by disseminated intravascular coagulation (DIC)

Diagnostics
- Elevated creatinine phosphokinase (MM fraction): from striated muscle breakdown; peak concentrations greater than 50,000 to 100,000 U/L
- Myoglobinuria and myoglobinemia
- Urinalysis, positive dipstick for blood, no or few RBCs, reddish-golden pigmented granular casts
- Elevated lactate dehydrogenase (LDH)
- Basic metabolic panel: multiple electrolyte abnormalities possible
- Elevated uric acid and other products of nucleic acid breakdown
- Initial hyperalbuminemia (dehydration phase) followed by hypoalbuminemia
- Anion gap acidosis due to organic acid release from necrotic cells
- Lactic acidosis
- Hematological parameters may reflect DIC
- ECG: changes consistent with electrolyte abnormalities

Management
- Strict monitoring of intake and output, daily weights, chemistries, urine pH with each void
- Half isotonic (0.45%) saline with sodium bicarbonate added to maintain circulatory volume and brisk urine flow; may require large volumes of fluid to replace fluid losses due to capillary leak in injured muscles. Avoid lactate and potassium-containing fluids.
- Sodium bicarbonate in fluid helps correct acidosis, prevents myoglobin precipitation by alkalinization of urine (goal urine pH>7) and reduces potassium levels; however, alkalinization will lower serum ionized calcium.
- Hyperkalemia: potassium binders, dialysis, bicarbonate, hypertonic glucose
- Hyperphosphatemia: non-calcium containing phosphate binders, dietary restriction
- Treatment of hypocalcemia is not recommended unless CaCl is necessary for arrhythmia, hypercalcemia, seizures, tetany. Treat severe hypercalcemia during recovery phase with forced diuresis, IV fluid, and furosemide (Lasix).
- Mannitol or furosemide if urine output is decreased
- Allopurinol for hyperuricemia

- Frequent neurovascular exams of affected muscle groups to detect signs of compartment syndrome
- Consider dialysis if severe renal failure.

UROLITHIASIS

Stones can be found in the lower (bladder, urethra) or upper (kidney, ureter) urinary tract.

Epidemiology
- In United States: less than 1% in children under 10 years and less than 3% in children under 19 years
- In children, most due to metabolic and genitourinary abnormalities or infection
- In children, 90% are found in the upper urinary tract

Etiology
- Calcium stones (calcium oxalate and calcium phosphate):
  - Most common stones in children
  - Normocalcemic hypercalciuria: distal RTA, loop diuretics, formulas high in calcium or parenteral calcium
  - Hypercalcemic hypercalciuria: increased absorption from bone (hyperparathyroidism, immobilization) or increased absorption of calcium from the gut (sarcoid granulomas)
  - Promoters of calcium stone formation: hypocitraturia, hyperuricuria, hyperoxaluria, hyperphosphaturia
- Uric acid stones:
  - Urinary pH less than 5.8 promotes uric acid crystal precipitation
  - Idiopathic: normal serum uric acid concentration
  - Inborn errors of metabolism that cause hyperuricemia (i.e., Lesch-Nyhan)
  - High cell turnover from myeloproliferative, lymphoproliferative, or chronic hemolytic disorders can cause high hyperuricemia
  - Ketogenic diet, inflammatory bowel disease, chronic diarrheal conditions
- Cystinuria:
  - Incompletely recessive autosomal disorder characterized by the failure of the renal tubules to reabsorb cystine, ornithine, lysine, and arginine
  - pH less than 7 precipitates cystine
- Struvite stones:
  - Related to urinary tract infection with organism that can split urea and increase NH_4, resulting in increased urinary pH
  - *Proteus* (70%), *Pseudomonas, Klebsiella, Streptococcus, Serratia* species
  - Tend to grow rapidly and form staghorn calculi
  - More common in children with anatomic abnormalities of the urinary tract

Clinical Manifestations
- Sudden onset of severe, crampy abdominal or flank pain that radiates anteriorly to scrotum or labia
- May have nausea, vomiting, dysuria, frequency, restlessness
- Hematuria (microscopic or gross) in 90%
- With urethral stones may be unable to void
- May have fever if associated with UTI

Diagnostics
- Urinalysis: hematuria, signs of concomitant urinary tract infection
- Urine microscopy: may reveal crystals; normal RBC morphology
- If febrile, send blood and urine cultures
- Urine calcium/creatinine ratio

- Serum electrolytes and creatinine
- Abdominal film may pick up radio-opaque stones.
- Renal and bladder ultrasound will reveal shadowing of stones, nephrocalcinosis, and obstruction.
- Gold standard for diagnosis is spiral CT without IV contrast.
- Attempt to obtain stone by straining urine stream.
- If first episode, every child should have a complete evaluation as to etiology: chemical analysis of stone/gravel; serum electrolytes; serum calcium, phosphorus and parathyroid hormone level if calcium is elevated; 24-hour urine collection after stone has passed to evaluate for metabolic abnormalities.

Management
- Intravenous fluids at 1.5 to 2 times maintenance
- Narcotic pain medication if needed
- *Uric acid stones:* increase fluid intake, alkalinization, allopurinol
- *Hypercalciuria:* increase fluid intake, dietary sodium restriction. Dietary calcium restriction is NOT recommended. Thiazide diuretics will decrease urinary calcium excretion. Potassium citrate will inhibit stone formation.
- *Cystinuria:* urinary alkalinization with potassium citrate; low methionine and sodium diet. If this fails, consider penicillamine and Thiola, but these have serious side effects and patients should be monitored closely.
- *Struvite stones:* antibiotic treatment; however, the stones harbor the bacteria and thus the UTI will recur when the antibiotics are stopped. Most require surgical intervention; may benefit from hemiacidrin irrigation or a urease inhibitor; GU evaluation to rule out anatomic abnormality.
- Approximately 36% of patients with a structural abnormality also have a metabolic abnormality so both possibilities should be fully evaluated.
- Stone removal may be needed if stone is obstructing the urethra and causing hydronephrosis, is causing a chronic UTI, or is a struvite stone:
  - Stones below the pelvic brim: ureteroscopy with direct stone removal or lithotripsy
  - Upper tract stones: extra corporeal shock wave lithotripsy
  - Large burden of upper urinary tract stones: percutaneous nephrolithotripsy
  - Open surgical stone removal is rarely needed.

Other Renal Diseases

ACUTE RENAL FAILURE

Acute renal failure (ARF) is a decrease in renal function over hours to days, resulting in the failure to excrete nitrogenous wastes and regulate electrolyte and water homeostasis.

- Anuria: complete cessation of urine output.
- Oliguria: excretion of less than 1 cc/kg/hour in infants, less than 0.5 cc/kg/hour in children and less than 400 mL/day in adults.

Etiology
- Prerenal: decrease in effective blood volume (dehydration, bleeding, shock, hypoalbuminemia, burns, postoperative); heart failure; drug-induced disruption of renal autoregulation; renal artery or venous occlusion
- Intrarenal: post-infectious glomerulonephritis (post-streptococcal glomerulonephritis [PSGN]); small vessel vasculitis; interstitial nephritis; acute tubular necrosis (ATN); pyelonephritis; HUS; medications (aminoglycosides, macrolides, IV contrast material, IVIG, acyclovir, amphotericin, NSAIDs, ACE inhibitors, cyclosporin, and tacrolimus); toxins (carbon tetrachloride, diethylene glycol, arsenic, mercury, lead, gold, and other heavy metals); toxic metabolites (myoglobin, hemoglobin deposits); organ/bone marrow transplantation

- Postrenal: bladder outlet obstruction (posterior urethral valves, occluded catheter); upper bilateral ureteral obstruction; intra-abdominal tumor obstructing urinary flow

Clinical Manifestations
- Cardiovascular: hypertension, peripheral edema, CHF, pulmonary edema, hypotension, tachycardia, arrhythmias
- Neurologic: mental status changes, seizures
- Gastrointestinal: nausea, vomiting, ileus
- Signs of urinary tract obstruction: suprapubic tenderness, palpable bladder
- Signs of chronic renal failure: edema, hypertension, poor growth parameters
- Signs of underlying disease process: e.g., rash of HSP, SLE

Diagnostics
Urinary Sediment and Indexes
- Obtain urine before fluid resuscitation or diuretic administration
- Calculate the fractional excretion of sodium (FENa):

$$FENa = ([Na_{urine}]/[Na_{plasma}]) \times 100/([Creatinine_{urine}]/[Creatinine_{plasma}])$$

  - Can only be interpreted in the presence of oliguria
- Prerenal etiologies: high specific gravity; hyaline and fine granular casts; cellular casts unusual; urine [Na] less than 20 mmol/L; FENa less than 1%
- Renal etiologies: may see brown granular casts and tubular epithelial cells; FENa greater than 1% (<1% in pigment nephropathy)

Laboratory Studies
- Elevated BUN and creatinine, decreased glomerular filtration rate (GFR)
- Schwartz formula for estimation of GFR

$$GFR\ (mL/min/1.73\ m^2) = K \times Ht\ (cm)/SCr\ (mg/dL)$$

  Where K = 0.35 (preterm infants), 0.45 (term infants), 0.55 (girls and prepubertal boys), 0.70 (postpubertal boys); SCr = Serum Creatinine
- Dilutional hyponatremia; hyperkalemia; hyperphosphatemia; hypocalcemia
- Anion gap acidosis
- Hematologic changes: anemia (dilutional, decreased production, hemolytic); neutropenia (SLE), thrombocytopenia (HUS, SLE), eosinophilia (allergic interstitial nephritis), leukocytosis (acute pyelonephritis)
- C3, C4: low in post-streptococcal GN (PSGN), SLE, and membranoproliferative GN
- Streptococcal specific studies in PSGN (ASO and anti-DNase B titers)

Imaging/Other Studies
- Ultrasound for intrinsic and post renal causes
- ECG: for changes due to hyperkalemia, hypocalcemia
- Radionuclide scanning may be clinically indicated

Management
Fluid Management
- Daily weights, strict input and output
- If volume depleted/pre-renal or toxin mediated: fluid replacement with isotonic fluid (normal saline 20 cc/kg IV, may repeat if clinically warranted)
- Fluid overload states require fluid restriction and a trial of furosemide. Restrict fluids to insensible losses (300 to 400 cc/m²/day) + urine output + GI losses (cc for cc)
- Bladder catheterization may be indicated if there is outlet obstruction.

Electrolyte Management
- Metabolic acidosis should be treated judiciously with sodium bicarbonate; correction of acidosis with bicarbonate can further lower the ionized calcium and precipitate tetany
- Hyperkalemia: no potassium in fluids; consider the following interventions:
  - ECG (also see Hyperkalemia in Fluids and Electrolytes chapter)
  - Kayexalate 1g/kg rectally or orally
  - 10% calcium gluconate 0.5 mL/kg over 2 to 4 minutes with continuous heart monitoring
  - Insulin 1 U intravenously with 5 g dextrose; check D-sticks frequently
  - Sodium bicarbonate infusion
- Hypocalcemia: in hyperphosphatemic patients, calcium may precipitate $CaPO_4$ deposition in tissues.
- Hyponatremia: will improve with fluid restriction

Other Management Issues
- Nutrition: give at least 25% of daily calorie requirements; consider parenteral dextrose; limit protein; low potassium, low phosphorous diet
- Cardiovascular: anti-hypertensive medications may be indicated
- Renal: avoid nephrotoxic medications. *Adjust dosing/schedule of medications for level of renal impairment.*
- Indications for dialysis (failure of conservative management of fluid and electrolyte imbalance or cardiopulmonary compromise): hyperkalemia (K^+ > 6.5 or peaked T-waves); acidosis (HCO_3^- <10); uremia (BUN > 150 or symptoms such as seizure, altered mental status, pericarditis); volume overload (congestive heart failure, pulmonary edema); dialyzable toxins (isopropyl alcohol, methanol, ethylene glycol, salicylates, lithium, theophylline)
- Post-renal failure secondary to obstruction: place bladder catheter, may require surgical intervention

HEMATURIA

Greater than five to ten RBCs per high-powered-field in a urine sample
- 3 to 10 RBCs per microliter can be detected by a standard dipstick

Epidemiology
- Microscopic hematuria is more common among children than gross hematuria
- Microscopic hematuria: 4% to 6% incidence on single urine sample; fewer than half remain positive when repeated in 7 days

Differential Diagnosis
Red Urine with a Negative Dipstick for Blood
- *Medications:* ibuprofen, chloroquine, deferoxamine, metronidazole, nitrofurantoin, Pyridium, rifampin, salicylates, doxorubicin
- *Dyes:* fruits/vegetables (i.e., beets, blackberries, food coloring)
- *Metabolites:* melanin, methemoglobin, porphyrin, urates, tyrosinosis
- *Bacteria: Serratia* urinary tract infection

Positive Urine Dipstick for Blood, but Absence of Red Blood Cells
- *Hemoglobin:* suggests a hemolytic process
- *Myoglobin:* associated with rhabdomyolysis from trauma, infection, prolonged seizures, or severe electrolyte abnormalities

Repeatedly Positive Urine Dipstick for Blood and Presence of Red Blood Cells
- *Common:* menstruation, bladder catheterization, perineal irritation, cystitis
- *Glomeruli:* glomerulonephritides, IgA nephropathy, Alport syndrome, postinfectious glomerulonephritis, membranous nephropathy, membranoproliferative glomerulonephritis, focal segmental glomerulosclerosis, thin basement membrane disease, systemic illnesses, SLE nephritis, HSP, Goodpasture syndrome, hemolytic-uremic syndrome, microscopic polyarteritis nodosa, Wegener granulomatosis

- *Interstitial:* acute tubular necrosis, papillary necrosis, interstitial nephritis, pyelonephritis, nephrocalcinosis
- *Vascular:* arterial or venous thrombosis, arteriovenous malformations, nutcracker syndrome
- *Interstitial and vascular:* hemoglobinopathies, sickle cell trait or SC hemoglobin, anatomic anomalies, polycystic kidneys, hydronephrosis, tumors (i.e., Wilms'), trauma
- *Urinary tract:* cystitis/urethritis, hypercalciuria, urolithiasis, trauma, coagulopathy, urethral prolapse, sports hematuria

Pathophysiology
- Lesions in the glomerulus, renal interstitium, renal vascular supply, or urinary tract result in bleeding or leakage of red blood cells into urinary tract.
- *Glomeruli:* disruption of the glomerular basement membrane due to immune mediated inflammatory damage. Acidic urine changes hemoglobin to hematin resulting in brown or tea-colored urine.
- *Renal papillae/tubules:* microthrombi or anoxia secondary to hemoglobinopathies. Antibiotics and other medications (i.e., NSAIDs) can cause inflammation of tubules and the interstitium.
- *Lower urinary tract:* trauma to kidney/bladder results in contusions, hematomas or lacerations. Increased vascularity from infection results in RBCs leaking into urine.

Clinical Manifestations
- Glomerular lesions present with brown or cola-colored urine with red cell casts and proteinuria.
- Presence of leukocytes or tubular epithelial cells suggests an interstitial or renal tubular etiology.
- Urinary tract or vascular causes present with gross hematuria occasionally with blood clots, normal RBCs, and absent or minimal proteinuria.
- Hypertension, edema, or azotemia suggested acute glomerulonephritis.
- Abdominal mass suggests tumor, hydronephrosis, polycystic kidney disease, or urinary obstruction.
- Skin lesions suggest tuberous sclerosis, HSP, or SLE.
- Fever and dysuria suggest a UTI.
- Preceding respiratory or gastrointestinal illness suggests IgA or HSP.
- Headaches and vision changes suggest severe hypertension.

Diagnostics
The diagnostic pathway depends upon whether there is gross or microscopic hematuria as well as other abnormal findings. Begin with a urinalysis with microscopy as well as a thorough history and physical exam.

- *Positive urine dipstick in the absence of macroscopic hematuria:* confirm with a microscopic evaluation. In the absence of RBC casts, proteinuria, hypertension, azotemia, or other concerning clinical signs, further evaluation should not be initiated until at least three urine specimens collected over 2 to 3 weeks show an abnormal number of RBCs.
- *Gross or microscopic hematuria with tea- or cola-colored urine, proteinuria, dysmorphic RBCs in urine, or RBC casts* indicates glomerular origin: CBC with differential; serum electrolytes, BUN, creatinine to assess renal function; blood pressure; cholesterol, C3, C4, albumin; ASO and Anti-DNase B (elevated in PSGN), ANA, antineutrophil antibody if complement levels are low (elevated in SLE); throat culture if history suggests possibility of group A streptococcal infection; check parents for hematuria to help identify benign familial hematuria
- *Gross or microscopic hematuria without proteinuria or RBC casts* suggests an extraglomerular origin:
  - Urine culture to rule out infection
  - Renal/bladder ultrasound: if hydronephrosis, renal scarring, or pyelocaliectasis, then follow-up with a renal scan
  - Urine calcium/creatinine ratio: collect 24-hour urine if nephrocalcinosis, urolithiasis, crystalluria

- Sickle cell preparation (in African-American children and in those with family history of sickle cell disease)
- *Macroscopic hematuria*: renal ultrasound to rule out malignancy

Management
- Consider a renal ultrasound to rule out tumor.
- Patients with gross hematuria, persistent microscopic hematuria, or microscopic hematuria associated with azotemia, proteinuria, hypertension, or hypocomplementemia should be referred to a pediatric nephrologist.
- Further management depends on etiology.

HYPERTENSION

Systolic blood pressure (SBP) or diastolic blood pressure (DBP) at 95th percentile or greater for height, age, and gender measured on at least three separate occasions. For children younger than 1 year, systolic BP defines hypertension.

- Normotensive: SBP and DBP less than 90th percentile for age, height, and gender
- High-normal blood pressure: SBP and DBP between 90th and 95th percentiles (see Appendix B for normal BP values)

Epidemiology
- Primary hypertension is more common in adolescents and adults.
- Secondary hypertension (caused by an underlying disease process) is more common in young children.
- Overall prevalence: 1% to 3% but as high as 15% among adolescents

Differential Diagnosis
- Inaccurate measurement due to improper technique or cuff size
- Anxiety, white coat hypertension, pain
- Primary (essential) hypertension: genetics, diet, stress, obesity, etc.
- Secondary hypertension:
  - *Renal:* acute glomerulonephritis, HSP, HUS, ATN, acute nephritis, chronic and acute renal failure, reflux nephropathy, polycystic kidney disease, post transplant or renal surgery
  - *Renovascular:* renal artery thrombosis or stenosis, vasculitides, fibromuscular dysplasia
  - *Cardiac:* coarctation of the aorta
  - *Endocrine:* pheochromocytoma, adrenocortical disorders, hypercalcemia, neuroblastoma
  - *Drugs/Medications:* cocaine, oral contraceptives, corticosteroids, amphetamines, sympathomimetics, cyclosporine, tacrolimus, heavy metals
  - *Central/Autonomic Nervous System:* increased intracranial pressure, Stevens-Johnson syndrome, Guillain-Barré syndrome, encephalitis, posterior fossa lesions
  - *Other:* withdrawal from antihypertensives, vitamin D intoxication, burns, extracorporeal oxygenation

Pathophysiology
- Blood pressure is determined by cardiac output and peripheral vascular resistance. Hypertension is caused by dysregulation of one or more of the mechanisms of blood pressure regulation: sodium and water balance, renin-aldosterone-angiotensin system, sympathetic nervous system, vascular tone.
- Severe blood pressure causes vascular damage, such as proliferation of the intimal layer and fibrinoid necrosis.
- Essential hypertension may be due to poor ability of the renal system to maintain appropriate sodium balance, reduced glomerular filtration, insulin resistance, or increased sympathetic nervous system activity.

Clinical Manifestations

- In children, hypertension is often asymptomatic.
- If there has been a prolonged and persistent increase in blood pressure or there is an acute onset of severe hypertension, patients may develop headache, vision changes, nosebleeds, nausea, epistaxis, and seizures.
- *Hypertensive emergency/malignant hypertension:* severe hypertension associated with a life-threatening complication or end-organ damage; may present with encephalopathy (stroke, focal deficits), acute heart failure or myocardial infarction, pulmonary edema, aortic aneurysm, or acute renal failure.
- *Hypertensive urgency:* symptoms may include headache, blurred vision, or nausea; may progress to hypertensive emergency.
- Signs of underlying etiology: gross hematuria, diarrhea, vomiting, rash
- Potential physical exam findings:
  - *General:* growth failure, obesity
  - *Skin:* café-au-lait spots or neurofibromas, rashes or flushing
  - *HEENT:* moon facies, blurred disk margins on funduscopic exam, proptosis indicating hyperthyroidism
  - *Chest/CV:* rales; hyperdynamic chest; rub, gallop, or murmur; decreased lower extremity pulses
  - *Abdomen:* hepatosplenomegaly, renal bruit, abdominal mass
  - *Neurologic:* focal deficits such as Bell's palsy

Diagnostics

Because hypertension is often asymptomatic, blood pressure screening is an important part of the well visit. If the blood pressure is greater than the 90th percentile, follow with two to three readings over at least 6 weeks to document a sustained elevation and to rule out anxiety or issues with technique. If persistently above the 95th percentile:

- Basic metabolic panel including BUN and creatinine
- Lipid profile, especially if patient is obese
- Urinalysis to screen for proteinuria/hematuria and urine culture
- CBC
- Renal ultrasound
- Echocardiogram to assess for end-organ damage

If indicated by initial studies or concern for specific etiology, consider:

- DMSA renal scan
- VCUG
- Urine for catecholamines and metanephrines; can be followed by MIBG scan to localize pheochromocytoma tumors
- Plasma renin activity and aldosterone levels
- Thyroid function, cortisol levels
- Renal angiogram with sampling for renal vein concentrations

If the blood pressure remains between the 90th and 95th percentiles:

- Monitor every 6 months before initiating an extensive evaluation.
- If the child is obese, institute a weight control plan.
- If no improvement, additional evaluation may be warranted.

Management

General Management Issues

Management depends on the severity of the blood pressure and the underlying etiology. The overall goal is to decrease the risk of cardiovascular disease and to prevent the sequelae of severe hypertension.

- *Nonpharmacologic:* for management of mild essential hypertension and for prevention, encourage weight reduction, sodium restriction in diet, exercise, and smoking cessation.

- *Pharmacologic*: initiate when nonpharmacologic efforts fail or if severe elevation of blood pressure or signs of end organ damage.
  - *ACE inhibitors* (e.g., captopril, enalapril, lisinopril): block conversion of angiotensin I to angiotensin II; increase in vasodilatory kinins; first line in patients with proteinuria; renoprotective effects; side effects include ARF, hyperkalemia, angioedema, cough, neutropenia, anemia, and birth defects.
  - *Angiotensin receptor blockers* (e.g., losartan): renoprotective and anti-proteinuric; limited data in pediatrics; fewer side effects than ACE inhibitors; also contraindicated in pregnancy
  - *Calcium channel blockers* (e.g., amlodipine, nifedipine): inhibit calcium movement into vascular smooth muscle cells, inhibiting vasoconstriction; side effects include sodium and water retention, peripheral edema, flushing, tachycardia, nausea, headache, postural hypotension
  - *Beta-blockers* (e.g., propranolol, atenolol, labetalol, esmolol): decrease cardiac output, peripheral vascular resistance, renin secretion and CNS sympathetic activity by blocking beta receptors; side effects include bronchoconstriction, insulin resistance, altered lipid profiles, bradycardia, syncope, CNS depression
  - *Diuretics*: promote salt and water excretion
    - *Loop diuretics* (e.g., furosemide): rapid diuresis; side effects include hypokalemia, alkalosis, hypercalciuria, nephrocalcinosis, ototoxicity
    - *Thiazide diuretics* (e.g., hydrochlorothiazide): more sustained but less vigorous diuresis; side effects include hypokalemia, alkalosis, hypercalcemia, glucose intolerance
    - *Potassium-sparing diuretics* (e.g., spironolactone): block aldosterone effect; weak diuretic; side effects include hyperkalemia.
  - *Central alpha-2-adrenergic blockers* (e.g., clonidine): stimulation of alpha-2 adrenergic receptors in CNS; side effects include sedation, depression, sleep disturbances, impotence, rebound hypertension
  - *Peripheral alpha-1-adrenergic blockers* (e.g., terazosin): peripheral vasodilation by antagonizing vascular alpha-1 sympathetic receptors; side effects include orthostatic hypotension, salt and fluid retention
  - *Direct vasodilators*: direct vascular smooth muscle relaxation
    - Hydralazine: side effects include hypotension, salt and water retention, headache, tachycardia, flushing
    - Minoxidil: side effects include hirsutism, salt and water retention
    - Nitroprusside: vasodilator via nitric oxide donation; side effects include cyanide toxicity

Hypertensive Emergency
- Intravenous access, monitor
- Goal is to lower BP promptly (within 1 hour) to prevent a life- or organ-threatening injury, but also gradually to preserve cerebral perfusion.
- Reduce mean arterial pressure by one third of planned reduction over 6 hours, additional third over next 24 to 36 hours and final third over next 48 hours.
- After elevated intracranial pressure is ruled out, do not delay treatment.
- Medications: IV labetalol, esmolol, nitroprusside, nicardipine

Hypertensive Urgency
- Requires prompt but gradual and controlled reduction in blood pressure over 24 hours.
- Medications: hydralazine PO/IV/IM, nifedipine PO, labetalol IV, clonidine PO, enalaprilat IV

Maintenance Therapy
- ACE inhibitors for renovascular, renoparenchymal disease, proteinuria
- Diuretics for volume-dependent hypertension and steroid-induced hypertension.
- Often, long-term management involves a combination of medications that act via different mechanisms
- For essential hypertension, initial therapy is often a diuretic and beta-blocker or calcium-channel blocker.
- *Invasive*: Surgery is required for coarctation of the aorta. Angioplasty can be used for renal artery stenosis. Consider dialysis if hypertension is secondary to volume overload from acute or chronic renal failure.

Resources

Glomerular Disease

Andreoli SP, Trachtman H, Acheson DW, et al. Hemolytic uremic syndrome: epidemiology, pathophysiology and therapy. Pediatr Nephrol 2002;17:293–298.

Brenner BM, Rector FC, eds. The Kidney. 6th ed. Philadelphia: WB Saunders, 2000.

D'Amico G. Natural history of idiopathic IgA nephropathy: role of clinical and histological prognostic factors. Am J Kidney Dis 2000;36:227–237.

Donadio J, Grande J. Medical progress: IgA nephropathy. N Engl J Med 2002;347:738–748.

Durkan AM, Hodson EM, Willis NS, Craig JC. Immunosuppressive agents in childhood nephrotic syndrome: a meta-analysis of randomized controlled trials. Kidney Int 2001;59:1919–1927.

Kaplan BS, Meyers KE, Schulman SL. The pathogenesis and treatment of hemolytic uremic syndrome. J Am Soc Nephrol 1998;9:1126–1133.

Mitsioni A. IgA nephropathy in children. Nephrol Dial Transplant 2001;16(suppl):123–125.

Patel HP, Bissler JJ. Hematuria in children. Pediatr Clin North Am 2001;48:1519–1537.

Roth K, Amaker BH, Chan JC. Nephrotic syndrome: pathogenesis and management. Pediatr Rev 2002;23:237–247.

Rubin E, Farber JL, eds. Pathology. Philadelphia: Lippincott-Raven, 1999.

Slutsker L, Ries AA, Maloney K, et al. A nationwide case-control study of Escherichia coli O157:H7 infection in the United States. J Infect Dis 1998;177:962–966.

Trachtman H, Christen C. Hemolytic uremic syndrome: current understanding of the pathogenesis and therapeutic trials and interventions. Curr Opin Pediatr 1999;11:162–168.

Trachtman H, Cnaan A, Christen E, et al. Effect of an oral Shiga toxin-binding agent on diarrhea-associated hemolytic uremic syndrome in children: a randomized clinical trial. JAMA 2003;290:1337–1344.

Wong CS, Jelacic S, Habeeb RL, et al. The risk of hemolytic-uremic syndrome after antibiotic treatment of Escherichia coli O157:H7 infections. N Engl J Med 2000;342:1930–1936.

Yoshikawa N, Tanaka R, Iijima K. Pathophysiology and treatment of IgA nephropathy in children. Pediatr Nephrol 2001;16:446–457.

Tubular/Interstitial Disease

Battino BS, DeFoor W, Coe F, et al. Metabolic evaluation of children with urolithiasis: are adult references for supersaturation appropriate? J Urol 2002;168:2568–2571.

Behrman R, Kliegman R, Jenson H. Nelson Textbook of Pediatrics. 17th ed. Philadelphia: WB Saunders, 2004.

Chan JC, Scheinman JI, Roth KS. Renal tubular acidosis. Pediatr Rev 2001;22:277–287.

Trachtman H, Gauthier B, eds. Pediatric Nephrology. The Netherlands: Harwood Academic, 1998.

Minevich E. Pediatric urolithiasis. Pediatr Clin North Am 2001;48:1571–1585.

Vanholder R, Sever MS, Erek E, Lameire N. Rhabdomyolysis. J Am Soc Nephrol 2000;11:1553–1561.

Other Renal Diseases

Behrman R, Kliegman R, Jenson H. Nelson Textbook of Pediatrics. 17th ed. Philadelphia: WB Saunders, 2004.

Chan JC, Williams DM, Roth KS. Kidney failure in infants and children. Pediatr Rev 2002;23:47–58.

Feld LG, Meyers KE, Kaplan BS, Stapleton FB. Limited evaluation of microscopic hematuria in pediatrics. Pediatrics 1998;102:E42.

Fleisher GR, Ludwig S. Textbook of Pediatric Emergency Medicine. 4th ed. Philadelphia: Lippincott Williams & Wilkins, 2000.

Klahr S, Miller SB. Acute oliguria. N Engl J Med 1998;338:671–675.

Patel HP, Bissler JJ. Hematuria in children. Pediatr Clin North Am 2001;48:1519–1537.

Rakel. Conn's Current Therapy. 55th ed. Philadelphia: Elsevier, 2003.

Thadhani, R, Pascual M, Bonventre JV. Acute renal failure. N Engl J Med 1996;344:1448–1460.

Update on the 1987 Task Force Report on High Blood Pressure in Children and Adolescent: A Working Group Report from the National High Blood Pressure Education Program. Pediatrics 1996;98:649–658.

Annapurna Poduri, MD, Renée A. Shellhaas, MD, Dennis J.
Dlugos, MD, Peter H. Berman, MD, Gihan I. Tennekoon, MD

General Principles

ACUTE WEAKNESS

Acute weakness is the acute loss of strength.
- *Bulk:* assess symmetry of muscle bulk
- *Tone:* assess by passive movement of limbs with patient relaxed; may be normal, increased (spastic or rigid), decreased
- See Table 19.1: Scales for strength and deep tendon reflexes

Etiology (by localization)
- *Central Nervous System (CNS)-Brain:* acute stroke, unilateral or bilateral
- *CNS–Spinal cord (anterior horn cell body):* cord infarction, cord compression, trauma, contusion, infection (e.g., enterovirus), transverse myelitis, spinal epidural abscess, syringomyelia
- *Spinal root of peripheral nerve:* acute inflammatory demyelinating polyneuropathy (Guillain-Barré)
- *Peripheral nerve (axon):* intensive care unit (ICU) neuropathy, HIV or zidovudine therapy, hereditary tyrosinemia, acute intermittent porphyria, medication-related (e.g., phenytoin, vincristine, nitrofurantoin, INH), toxins (heavy metals, glue), metabolic (uremia-mixed sensory and motor, or pure motor after dialysis), autoimmune (lupus), other vasculitis, chronic juvenile rheumatoid arthritis
- *Neuromuscular junction:* myasthenia gravis, botulism, tic paralysis, pharmacologic blockade, aminoglycoside toxicity
- *Muscle:* myositis (infectious, dermatomyositis, polymyositis), metabolic (hypocalcemia, hypokalemia, hypothyroid state), medication-related (especially steroids), ICU myopathy, familial periodic paralysis (hypo/hyperkalemic)

Clinical Manifestations
- *Central nervous system:* stroke; typically unilateral weakness in a cerebrovascular distribution; expected concomitant language, cranial nerve, or sensory changes; initial low tone then spastic; extensor plantar response ("upgoing toe") on affected side (Table 19.2)
- *Spinal cord:* acute flaccid paraparesis ("spinal shock") then spastic, bowel or bladder symptoms, incontinence, evolving spasticity, sensory level, back pain or trauma, fasciculation, fever (epidural abscess), hypotension (infarction), decreased rectal tone, extensor plantar responses ("upgoing toes")
- *Spinal root of peripheral nerve:* symmetric length-dependent weakness, often concomitant sensory disturbance, distal more than proximal weakness, areflexia, possible back pain, normal to decreased tone
- *Peripheral nerve:* weakness and sensory loss in distribution of specific nerve, in several discrete nerve distributions (mononeuritis multiplex), or diffusely in polyneuropathy (may be painful); may have decreased deep tendon reflexes (DTRs)
- *Neuromuscular junction:* hypotonia; DTRs present; no sensory loss (see Myasthenia Gravis and Botulism sections)
- *Muscle:* proximal more than distal weakness; normal tone; myalgias; normal to decreased DTRs

Table 19.1: Scales for Strength and Deep Tendon Reflexes

	Strength		Deep Tendon Reflexes
5	Full, normal strength	4+	Increased with clonus
5–	Nearly full strength	3+	Increased without clonus
4	Able to meet some resistance	2+	Normal
3	Able to overcome gravity but not resistance	1+	Diminished
2	Able to move in space but not overcome gravity	0	Absent
1	Flicker of movement but no movement in space		
0	No movement		

Table 19.2: Summary of Examination for Weakness by Localization

Examination Summary	Strength	Tone	DTRs	Sensory Loss	Fasciculations
Spinal cord	↓	↓ then ↑	↓ then ↑	+	+/–
Anterior horn cell	↓	↓	—	—	+
Spinal root	↓	↓	—	—	—
Peripheral nerve	↓	↓	↓/–	+	—
Neuromuscular junction	↓	↓	+(nl)	—	—
Muscle	↓	↓	+(nl)	—	—

DTRs, deep tendon reflexes.

Diagnostics
Imaging
- CT of head if stroke or hemorrhage is suspected
- MRI of brain if stroke is suspected
- MRI of spine if spinal cord compression, infarction, or transverse myelitis is suspected; can confirm diagnosis of Guillain-Barré syndrome

Electrophysiology (Electromyography and Nerve Conduction Velocities)
- May show evidence of anterior horn, peripheral nerve axon, neuromuscular junction, or muscle process; may show evidence of demyelination
- Remains normal until at least 1 week from onset of symptoms

Laboratory Studies
- Creatine phosphokinase (CPK) if myopathy is suspected
- Lumbar puncture if Guillain-Barré is suspected
- Lyme titers for mononeuritis multiplex
- Amino-levulinic acid for porphyria
- Muscle biopsy: as warranted based on previous workup

Management
Management will depend on clinical setting.
- *Stroke:* prompt recognition and management are important.

- *Spinal cord emergencies:* early steroids may stem evolution to compression; neurosurgical intervention may be needed; antibiotics if suspect abscess
- *Uremic neuropathy:* may respond to dialysis early in course
- *Neuromuscular weakness:* close monitoring of respiratory status; specific treatments for Guillain-Barré, botulism, myasthenia
- *With elevated CPK:* monitor for rhabdomyolysis, monitor renal function, and maintain hydration

ALTERED MENTAL STATUS

Decreased alertness or consciousness resulting from a pathologic process affecting the brain, whether an intrinsic central nervous process or diffuse metabolic derangement.

Normal: awake, easy to arouse and maintain alertness

Lethargic: difficult to maintain alertness

Obtunded: decreased alertness, responsive to pain, other stimuli

Stuporous: decreased alertness, responsive only to pain

Comatose: unresponsive even to pain

Orientation to person, place, time, and medical situation

Language: fluency, comprehension, naming, and repetition

Etiology
- Metabolic derangement: low or high glucose, Na^+ or Ca^{2+}, low Mg^{2+}, thyroid dysfunction, hypoparathyroidism, hepatic or renal encephalopathy, hypotension, hypertensive encephalopathy, hyperammonemia, sepsis, hypoxemia, hypercarbia, adrenal insufficiency, inborn error of metabolism
- Toxin or overdose (e.g., CO, cyanide, acetaminophen, narcotics, benzodiazepines, barbiturates)
- Seizure: nonconvulsive seizures or post-ictal state
- Infection: meningitis, encephalitis, CNS abscess
- Increased ICP: space-occupying lesion, obstructed VP shunt, cerebral edema
- Vascular: subarachnoid, subdural, intracerebral hemorrhage; stroke; migraine
- Trauma: concussion, contusion, hemorrhage

Pathophysiology
- Dysfunction in both cerebral hemispheres, and/or the ascending reticular activating system

Clinical Manifestations
- Abnormal mental status exam, change in breathing pattern
- Possible loss of brainstem reflexes, including pupillary, corneal, vestibulo-ocular
- Vesicular lesions suggest herpes simplex virus.
- Evaluate on coma scale

Diagnostics
- Glucose, electrolytes, liver function tests, ammonia, arterial blood gas, complete blood count, thyroid function tests, toxin screen, blood culture, urine culture
- Lumbar puncture unless obvious cause identified; avoid lumbar puncture if concern for herniation (clinically or radiologically)
- Head CT, ECG, and EEG

Management
Treatment of reversible causes:
- Correct electrolyte, acid-base, ABCs, glucose disturbances
- Antibiotics; consider acyclovir
- Anticonvulsants
- Maintain normal body temperature
- Consider naloxone
- Consider specific antidotes

ATAXIA

Impaired control of coordination, movement, and balance

Etiology
- Intrinsic cerebellar disturbance
- Disturbance of input to cerebellum (from frontal lobes, posterior columns, and/or spinocerebellar tracts)
- Vestibular dysfunction

Differential Diagnosis
- Acute ataxia
  - Post-infectious cerebellitis
  - Infectious cerebellitis: usually viral
  - Drug ingestion: alcohol, phenytoin, carbamazepine, sedatives, hypnotics, phencyclidine, thallium
  - Other: head trauma, cerebellar hemorrhage, neuroblastoma (opsoclonus-myoclonus-ataxia), acute disseminated encephalomyelitis (ADEM), hydrocephalus, Miller-Fisher variant of Guillain-Barré syndrome, meningitis, labyrinthitis, seizure or post-ictal state, basilar migraine, posterior circulation stroke, conversion
- Intermittent ataxia: metabolic disorder (e.g., pyruvate dehydrogenase deficiency), acute paroxysmal vertigo
- Subacute, chronic, or progressive ataxia: brain tumor, congenital anomaly, degenerative spinocerebellar diseases (e.g., Friedreich ataxia, ataxia-telangiectasia)

Clinical Manifestations
Manifestations depend on location of the lesion:

- Cerebellar vermis: truncal ataxia
- Cerebellar hemispheres: gait veers toward involved side, dysmetria of ipsilateral extremity
- Sensory ataxia (peripheral nerve or posterior columns): abnormal sensation of light touch, proprioception, vibration, high-stepping gait, + Romberg, difficulties with fine motor movements, no dysmetria when eyes open, + dysmetria when eyes closed

Physical Exam
- *Cerebellar exam:* coordination, truncal ataxia, limb ataxia
- *Cranial nerves:* lower brainstem abnormalities raise concern for tumor or vascular insufficiency; vermis lesions cause direction-changing nystagmus; opsoclonus (concern for neuroblastoma)
- *Motor:* unilateral weakness is concerning for posterior-fossa lesions; loss of DTRs suggests sensory ataxia
- *Sensory:* afferent sensory input abnormalities are exacerbated by eye closure (not true of cerebellar ataxia).
- *Mental Status:* consider encephalitis if abnormal

Diagnostics
Radiology
- Brain imaging: CT acutely to rule out hemorrhage or space-occupying lesion; MRI best for posterior fossa and for leptomeningeal enhancement
- Body CT if concern for neuroblastoma

Laboratory
- CBC, electrolytes, toxin screen
- Lumbar puncture
- Urine VMA/HVA (if opsoclonus-myoclonus)
- Consider metabolic/genetic evaluation (especially if intermittent or progressive ataxia)

Management
- Treat underlying etiology.
- Post-infectious cerebellitis is self-limited (begins to resolve in 1 to 4 weeks). Steroids are not indicated.
- Physical and occupational therapy

BRAIN DEATH

Irreversible loss of cortical and brainstem function, including respiratory drive

- Death by Neurological Criteria protocols differs, and physicians must act in accordance with their own institution's policies.
- Does NOT apply to children younger than 7 days (41 weeks conceptional age)
- A comatose patient with intact circulatory function must be declared dead by neurologic criteria before organ donation can be pursued.

Guidelines for the Determination of Brain Death in Children
- Eliminate reversible causes of coma (e.g., opiates)
- Physical exam criteria (see below): coma, absent brainstem reflexes, apnea
- In some institutions, at least one exam must be performed by a neurology or neurosurgery attending physician.
- A second exam consistent with death by neurologic criteria at a specified time, depending on age
- Apnea test (to be performed as part of the last exam)
- Ancillary testing may be required (see below).
- Age-specific requirements:
  - *7 days to 2 months:* two exams and EEGs 48 hours apart
  - *2 months to 1 year:* two exams and EEGs 24 hours apart OR one exam and initial EEG demonstrating electrocerebral silence plus no cerebral blood flow on a radionuclide angiogram
  - *More than 1 year:* two exams 12 to 24 hours apart with other studies optional

Physical Exam
- Normal temperature and blood pressure
- Mental status = coma (unresponsive to any stimulus)
- Absent brainstem function: midposition or fully dilated pupils; no oculocephalic (doll's eye) response; no vestibulo-ocular response to (cold) caloric testing; no corneal, gag, or cough reflexes; no suck or root reflex
- Flaccid tone, no spontaneous or induced movements (except spinally mediated reflex movements)
- Persistence of this exam consistent with death by neurological criteria for appropriate length of time, as above.
- Apnea test (performed as part of the second or last exam): give 100% O_2 for 10 minutes before test. Allow hypercapnia (maximal respiratory stimulus) to develop by holding assisted ventilation. Monitor for spontaneous respirations. Monitor CO_2 level every 5 minutes, and continue to observe until pCO_2 is 60 torr or greater. Stop test if pO_2 less than 50 torr.

Diagnostics
- Workup for reversible causes of coma should be negative.
- Drug levels should not be in toxic range.
- If required, EEG must be done using special protocol and must determine electrocerebral silence to be consistent with death according to neurologic criteria.
- Radionuclide angiogram must demonstrate lack of cerebral blood flow to be consistent with death according to neurologic criteria.

Management
- If patient satisfies definition for death by neurologic causes, physician should explain to family that patient is dead.
- Consider organ donation, depending on wishes of family.

COMA

A state of profound unconsciousness from which one cannot be aroused
Glasgow Coma Score less than 8 (Table 19.3)

Etiology
- Trauma, infection, vascular, metabolic, increased intracranial pressure (ICP), seizure, toxin, or overdose

Differential Diagnosis
- Profound neuromuscular disease, severe akinetic mutism, locked-in state, catatonia

Physical Exam
- ABCs, vital signs, primary survey
- Normal aggregate Glasgow Coma Score, based on age: Birth to 6 months: 9; older than 6 to 12 months: 11; older than 1 to 2 years: 12; older than 2 to 5 years: 13; older than 5 years: 14
- Focused neurologic exam

Management
Resuscitation
- ABCs, correct glucose, electrolytes
- Control seizures, consider Naloxone and mannitol

Table 19.3: The Glasgow Coma Scale

Response	Score	Infants	Children
Ocular	4	Open spontaneously	Open spontaneously
	3	To sound	To sound
	2	To pain	To pain
	1	Not at all	Not at all
Verbal	5	Coos, babbles	Oriented
	4	Cries but consolable	Confused
	3	Cries to pain, irritable	Inappropriate words
	2	Moans to pain, inconsolable	Nonspecific sounds
	1	None	None
Motor	6	Normal spontaneous movement	Follows commands
	5	Withdraws to touch	Localizes pain
	4	Withdraws to pain	Withdraws to pain
	3	Decorticates (abnl flexion) to pain	Decorticates (abnl flexion) to pain
	2	Decerebrates (abnl extension) to pain	Decerebrates (abnl extension) to pain
	1	Flaccid	Flaccid

abnl, abnormal.

- IV fluids: normal saline at maintenance unless fluid-electrolyte disturbances
- There is no evidence to support expectant hyperventilation.

Medical Management
- Empiric broad-spectrum antibiotics (e.g., third-generation cephalosporin + acyclovir). Do not wait for neuroimaging and lumbar puncture if suspicion for infection is high.

Surgical Management
- Neurosurgical consultation
- Decompression of space-occupying lesion (hemorrhage or tumor) or shunt for acute hydrocephalus
- Ventriculostomy to monitor ICP, if indicated

CRANIAL NERVES

Problems with cranial nerve (CN) function suggest brainstem abnormalities. For localization, consider the *Rule of Fours*: CN I to IV arise at midbrain level; CN V to VIII arise at pons level; CN IX to XII arise at medulla level.

- CN I: Olfactory: smell of non-noxious scents (e.g., coffee)
- CN II: Optic: pupillary response, visual acuity, visual fields, fundus exam
- CN III: Oculomotor: eye movements: vertical and horizontal adduction
- CN IV: Trochlear: eye movements: intorsion with adduction (down and in)
- CN V: Trigeminal: facial sensation (three distributions)
- CN VI: Abducens: eye movements: abduction
- CN VII: Facial: closure of muscles of facial expression
- CN VII: Auditory: cochlear-hearing; vestibular-balance
- CN IX: Glossopharyngeal: palate elevation, phonation
- CN X: Vagus: palate elevation, phonation
- CN XI: Spinal accessory: trapezius and sternocleidomastoid strength
- CN XII: Hypoglossal: tongue symmetry, strength

Acquired Neurologic Disease

ACUTE DISSEMINATED ENCEPHALOMYELITIS

Monophasic inflammatory demyelinating condition of the CNS resulting in scattered focal white matter greater than deep gray matter lesions

Typically occurs after viral illness and *very rarely* after vaccination (rabies, hepatitis, measles vaccines)

Epidemiology
- 70% have prodromal illness: usually upper respiratory infection or nonspecific febrile illness.
- ~90% of children recover completely.

Differential Diagnosis
- Meningitis, cerebellitis, sarcoidosis, CNS vasculitis, embolic events, acute hemorrhagic leukoencephalitis, multiple sclerosis (Table 19.4)

Pathophysiology
- Vasculitis: probably complement-mediated, with antigen-antibody complexes causing endothelial damage
- Demyelination: immune-mediated destruction of myelin

Table 19.4: Distinguishing Acute Disseminated Encephalomyelitis from Multiple Sclerosis

ADEM	Multiple Sclerosis
Monophasic	Multiple episodes
Lesions throughout (white and gray)	Peri-ventricular white matter lesions
Viral prodrome	Viral prodrome unusual
Ataxia common	Ataxia uncommon
Thalamic involvement common	Thalamic involvement very rare
Lesions may resolve on subsequent MRI	May find new lesions on subsequent MRI
More often in children	More often in adults

ADEM, acute disseminated encephalomyelitis; MRI, magnetic resonance imaging.

Clinical Manifestations
- Multifocal neurologic deficits (ataxia, hemiparesis, optic neuritis, cranial nerve palsies)
- Impaired consciousness (~65%), ataxia (~60%), meningismus (~25%), fever (~50%), headache (~45%), seizures
- Perform general exam to evaluate for infection
- Detailed neurologic exam reveals multifocal deficits

Diagnostics
Laboratory Studies
- Lumbar puncture (LP): increased protein, increased WBCs (usually <50, lymphocyte-predominant), culture negative, glucose normal. LP entirely normal in ~25%.
- If history or distribution of lesions is suspicious for multiple sclerosis, send for myelin basic protein and oligoclonal bands.
- Other laboratory studies as indicated by clinical situation

Radiology
- Early imaging may be normal.
- Enhanced head CT may not demonstrate abnormalities.
- T2-weighted MRI: scattered increase signal white greater than gray matter lesions. Lesions are typically bilateral, asymmetric, and variable in size.

Management
- Often resolves over 2 to 4 weeks without treatment
- Pulse methylprednisolone: dose varies but some use 15–30 mg/kg/dose given once daily for 3 days
- IVIG may also be useful (consult Neurology service)
- Physical and occupational therapy

ACUTE MYOPATHY

Motor dysfunction at the level of muscle

Acute weakness, typically proximal, may be painful or painless.

Etiology
- *Myositis:* infectious (e.g., influenza), benign acute childhood myositis, idiopathic inflammatory progressive myopathies (dermatomyositis, polymyositis)

- *Metabolic myopathy:* hypocalcemia, hypokalemia, inherited disorder of carbohydrate metabolism, critical illness myopathy

Differential Diagnosis
- Joint disease, peripheral neuropathy (Guillain-Barré, axonal neuropathy), neuromuscular junction disorder (neuromuscular blockade, botulism, myasthenia gravis)

Diagnostics
- Laboratory studies: CPK, BUN, and creatinine (if CPK is elevated), erythrocyte sedimentation rate (ESR) (may be elevated), Mi-2 antibodies (+ in 25% of dermatomyositis patients)
- Nerve conduction studies and electromyography (EMG): normal conduction velocities, myopathic features can be seen from 1 week after onset, EMG reveals small and polyphasic motor unit potentials
- Muscle biopsy: inflammatory changes, fiber necrosis replaces muscle by fat, dermatomyositis leads to perifascicular atrophy, polymyositis leads to endomysial inflammation, lipid myopathy
- Muscle MRI: can help define extent of edema or fatty infiltration

Management
- Analgesia, steroids
- Immunosuppression: methotrexate, azathioprine, or cyclophosphamide (consult with neurology service for indications and dosing)
- IVIG for refractory inflammatory myopathies (2 g/kg acutely then monthly)
- Monitor for rhabdomyolysis and hydrate if CPK is elevated (see Rhabdomyolysis, in Nephrology chapter)
- Physical therapy to avoid contractures from inactivity
- Dermatomyositis: screen for neoplasm (e.g., testicular cancer)

BOTULISM

Neuroparalytic illness caused by neurotoxins produced by *Clostridium botulinum* (anaerobic, spore-forming, bacillus)

Epidemiology
- *Clostridium botulinum* is found in soil, honey, and home-canned foods.
- Four types: foodborne, wound, infant, adult
- Seventy to 100 cases of infant botulism are reported annually to Centers for Disease Control.
- 70% to 90% of cases occur in breast-fed infants.
- Typical age: 6 weeks to 9 months (90% younger than 6 months)

Differential Diagnosis
- Sepsis, toxin ingestion (e.g., organophosphates), Guillain-Barré, myasthenia gravis, stroke

Pathophysiology
- *Infant botulism:* ingested spores germinate and colonize GI tract (infection) then release toxin.
- *Children and adults:* ingested toxin from contaminated food
- Neurotoxin binds irreversibly to presynaptic nerve endings, inhibiting acetylcholine release. Toxin does not cross the blood-brain barrier.

Clinical Manifestations
- Symmetric, descending flaccid paralysis
- Infants may present with constipation, poor feeding, and weak cry, followed by respiratory compromise.

- Cranial nerves (ophthalmoparesis, ptosis, disconjugate gaze, diminished gag, difficulty swallowing, weak suck) involved initially and then descends to upper extremities and respiratory muscles.
- Neurologic sequelae are rare.
- Progressive weakness and hypotonia with bulbar and spinal nerve abnormalities; hyporeflexia develops later in course.
- Autonomic dysfunction is common including decreased tearing and salivation.
- Normal pupillary light reflex fatigues with repeated stimulation over 1 to 2 minutes.

Diagnostics
Laboratory
- Stool for *C. botulinum* toxin assay
- Rule-out sepsis workup in infants
- Serum toxic screen
- EMG reveals: incremental response in muscle action potential with high-frequency stimulation; normal nerve conduction velocity
- Brain and/or spine imaging if diagnosis unclear

Management
- Human-derived botulinum immune globulin for infants
- Trivalent equine antitoxin for adults (risk of anaphylaxis)
- To obtain antitoxin or immune globulin (in any state), call California Department of Health Services: 510-540-2646.
- Supportive care: may require mechanical ventilation, nasogastric feeds, suppositories for constipation
- Avoid aminoglycosides because they can causes lysis of the bacteria.
- Contact state/local public health authorities for suspected or documented cases of botulism (except infant botulism).

GUILLAIN-BARRÉ SYNDROME

Acute inflammatory demyelinating polyradiculoneuropathy

Affects spinal nerve roots and peripheral nerves

May affect axons in acute motor axonal neuropathy

Classic Guillain-Barré syndrome: progressive often ascending weakness in more than one limb, areflexia

Miller-Fisher variant: ataxia, ophthalmoparesis, areflexia

Classic CSF finding: albumino-cytologic dissociation (markedly elevated protein level with normal or trivially elevated CSF WBCs)

Epidemiology
- Incidence: 0.6 to 1.9 cases per 100,000 children/year
- Slight male predominance
- Most common paralytic illness in children in developed countries

Etiology
- Follows viral infection in over 50% of cases
- May follow bacterial infection (e.g., *Campylobacter jejuni*), surgery, vaccination
- Seen in a higher-than-expected rate in patients with sarcoidosis, SLE, lymphoma, HIV infection, Lyme disease, and solid tumors
- Often no clear trigger

Differential Diagnosis
- Transverse myelitis, spinal cord compression, myositis, myopathy, posterior fossa lesion, acute cerebellar ataxia, bilateral strokes
- Infections: poliomyelitis (LP with elevated WBCs), HIV seroconversion (LP with elevated WBCs), diphtheria
- Tick paralysis, porphyria
- Drugs: INH, vincristine, amitriptyline, hydralazine, nitric oxide
- Toxins: lead, mercury, arsenic, thallium, organophosphates, glue, acrylamide
- Neuromuscular blockade: botulism, myasthenia gravis

Pathophysiology
- Immune-mediated inflammation and demyelination of spinal nerve roots and peripheral nerves
- Likely molecular mimicry
- Anti-GM1 Ab and *C. jejuni*
- Anti-GQ1B Ab in Miller-Fisher variant

Clinical Manifestations
- Progressive, often ascending weakness in the limbs: 50% plateau by 2 weeks, 80% by 3 weeks
- Numbness or paresthesias in the extremities in a classic stocking-glove distribution. Children *often* complain of pain.
- Facial weakness in 50%, weakness of respiratory muscles
- Ataxia, ophthalmoparesis, may have autonomic instability
- Back pain from spinal nerve root inflammation
- Constipation or bowel/bladder incontinence
- Clinical recovery is the rule with good supportive care: may take weeks to months; complete recovery in 80%
- Acute relapses occur in 1% to 5% of patients in large series.
- Chronic inflammatory demyelinating polyradiculoneuropathy (CIDP) can begin with a rapid onset of weakness indistinguishable from Guillain-Barré syndrome.
- Vital signs: may have instability
- Preserved mental status
- Cranial nerves: facial weakness, may have ophthalmoparesis
- Motor: weakness, usually distal greater than proximal, loss of DTRs
- Sensory: length-dependent loss of sensation
- Check gait for degree of weakness and for ataxia

Diagnostics
- *Lumbar puncture required:* albumino-cytologic dissociation = elevated CSF protein (typically 80–200 mg/dl); normal or mildly elevated CSF WBC (<10 mononuclear cells/mm^3); may be normal in first week of disease
- *Electromyography:* for confirmation of diagnosis; abnormal in 50% of patients in the first 2 weeks and in 85% of patients afterwards; evidence of segmental demyelination
- *MRI:* if suspicion for spinal cord compression; Guillain-Barré syndrome pattern: enhancing nerve roots

Management
- Admit patient for observation
- Supportive therapy: monitor respiratory status with serial negative inspiratory force (NIF); intubation if necessary
- Hastening of recovery: *IVIG* 2 g/kg divided into five daily doses OR *plasmapheresis:* plasma exchange volume 200 to 250 mL/kg divided in three to five treatments over 7 to 14 days
- Pain control (mostly back, limb; pain control often achieved with gabapentin and sometimes with opioids or NSAIDs), bowel regimen, Foley catheter if voiding limited, deep venous thrombosis prophylaxis if immobile

INCREASED INTRACRANIAL PRESSURE

Abnormal elevation of pressure inside the skull, caused by an increase in brain volume, intracranial blood, CSF, and/or mass. Normal ICP varies with age: neonate: less than 2 cm H_2O; younger than 12 months: 1.5 to 6 cm H_2O; child: 3 to 7 cm H_2O; adolescent: less than 15 cm H_2O; adult: less than 20 cm H_2O

Differential Diagnosis
- Brain tumor, meningitis, pseudotumor cerebri, hydrocephalus due to ventriculo-peritoneal shunt malfunction, intracranial hemorrhage, metabolic derangement, seizure

Pathophysiology (of edema)
- *Vasogenic edema*: impaired blood-brain barrier; increased capillary permeability; increased capillary transmural pressure; retention of extravasated fluid in interstitial space; occurs near tumors, hemorrhages, inflammatory foci
- *Cytotoxic edema*: impaired Na^+-K^+-ATPase pump due to decreased cerebral blood flow; causes increased extracellular K^+ and increased intracellular Ca^{2+}, leading to cell death secondary to membrane dysfunction; occurs near areas of ischemia and hypoxemia
- *Interstitial edema*: high pressure obstructive hydrocephalus leading to ischemia
- *Hydrostatic edema*: increased transmural vascular pressure resulting in increased extracellular fluid; may result from abrupt loss of cerebral autoregulation
- *Osmotic edema*: decreased serum osmolality and hyponatremia ($Na^+ < 125$ mEq/L)

Clinical Manifestations
- Mental status changes: may progress to coma
- Headache: especially early morning and positional
- Irritability, nausea, vomiting, diplopia
- Focal neurologic findings depending on etiology
- Glasgow Coma Scale score (see Table 19.3)
- Cushing's triad: bradycardia, hypertension, irregular respirations
- Acutely increasing head circumference; full or bulging fontanel or increased separation of sutures
- Detailed cranial nerve, motor, sensory, and cerebellar exam
- Infants rarely have papilledema

Diagnostics
Radiology
- Ventriculo-peritoneal (VP) shunt series in patients with ventricular shunt
- Emergent head CT or brain MRI with and without contrast: can have normal head CT with increased ICP; ultrasound usually sufficient for diagnosis in infants with open fontanel

Laboratory Studies
- If clinically indicated, LP only if neuroimaging excludes mass lesion or effaced ventricles
- Serum electrolytes and osmolarity
- Ammonia level if diffuse cerebral edema

Intracranial Pressure Monitoring (intensive care unit setting)
- Indicated if: Glasgow Coma Scale score less than 8; rapidly deteriorating neurologic status; pharmacologic paralysis; mechanical ventilation with increased mean airway pressures or increased pulmonary end-expiratory pressure

Management
Resuscitation
- ABCs, control seizures
- Maintain adequate mean arterial pressure (MAP) because:
  - Cerebral perfusion pressure: $CPP = MAP - ICP$
- Low CPP results in ischemia (aim for CPP greater than 50 mm Hg).

- Goal cerebral perfusion pressure: greater than 60 mm Hg in adolescents; greater than 50 mm Hg in infants and children

Reduce Cerebral Blood Volume
- Elevate head of bed
- Hyperventilation to $PaCO_2$ 25 to 30 mm Hg recommended in acute setting, but avoid chronic hyperventilation
- Cerebral vasoconstricting sedation (thiopental, pentobarbital)
- Avoid hyperthermia

Reduce Brain and Cerebrospinal Fluid Volume
- Mannitol: 0.25–1.0 mg/kg IV (effect seen in 10 to 15 minutes and lasts up to 8 hours); must monitor blood pressure, electrolytes, serum osmolarity
- Furosemide: 0.5–1.0mg/kg IV (or 0.15–0.3 mg/kg IV when used along with mannitol)
- Acetazolamide: 30 mg/kg/day IV/PO in four to six divided doses, maximum 1 g/day (may cause transient increased ICP due to CO_2 release, but then decreases CSF production significantly).
- Dexamethasone: 1–2 mg/kg IV/PO loading dose (maximum 10 mg) followed by 1 mg/kg/day in four divided doses (maximum 16 mg/day) to decrease vasogenic edema
- Ventriculostomy drain or ventriculo-peritoneal shunt (Neurosurgery consultation)
- Consider decreasing fluid infusion to two thirds of maintenance requirements using 0.9% normal saline rather than 0.45% normal saline

Reduce Intracranial Volume
- Surgical decompression, VP shunt

For Suspected Shunt Malfunction
- Head CT, shunt series, sterile shunt tap to assess proximal and distal flow; emergent shunt revision

MULTIPLE SCLEROSIS

Multiple demyelinating episodes in time and space. Multiple sclerosis (MS) is a lifelong disease with variable course.

- *Clinically Definite MS:* Two clinical attacks at least 24 hours long and separated by 1 month AND clinical evidence (on neurological exam) of two lesions OR clinical evidence of one lesion AND paraclinical evidence of a second lesion (see subsequent section)
- *Laboratory Supported Definite MS:* Two attacks AND clinical or paraclinical evidence of one lesion AND lumbar puncture evidence of MS

Epidemiology
- Geographic variation in prevalence. Northern United States, greater than 30/100,000; Southern United States, 5 to 30/100,000; children who move before age 15 acquire risk of new environment.
- Pediatric cases are 1.8% to 5% of all cases.
- Female:male ratio: 1:1 before puberty; 2.2–3:1 after puberty
- Youngest reported case: 10 months

Etiology
- Likely multifactorial; genetic component
- Possible viral or environmental trigger
- 25% risk of developing MS if monozygotic twin has MS
- In patients with MS, family history is positive in 10% to 26%.

Differential Diagnosis
- Systemic lupus erythematosus, Sjögren, neurosarcoidosis, HIV, syphilis, CNS infection, Lyme, vitamin B_{12} deficiency, CNS vasculitis, autoimmune disease, Behçet, recurrent ADEM, antiphospholipid antibody syndrome

Pathophysiology
- Immune-mediated inflammation and demyelination of central white matter
- Lesions are plaques: 1 mm to 4 cm in diameter; loss of myelin, sparing of axons; T cells, macrophages; evolution to gliosis
- Likely molecular mimicry and attack of myelin basic protein

Clinical Manifestations
- Attacks tend to last days to weeks and may be precipitated by acute infection or metabolic derangement
- Loss of sensation, coordination, or gait; nystagmus
- Motor: weakness (acute or chronic), spasticity
- Frequent brainstem involvement; sensory greater than motor dysfunction
- Optic neuritis: painful; usually unilateral loss of vision; on exam may see swollen disc, decreased color saturation, and decreased acuity with acute optic neuritis; a pale disc is seen with previous optic neuritis.
- Transverse myelitis or spinal cord syndrome
- Ataxia, other cerebellar dysfunction, bladder dysfunction
- Seizures: 10% to 22% of children with MS, more with younger age of onset
- Mental status: usually normal at disease onset, possible cognitive difficulties
- L'Hermitte's phenomenon: neck flexion yields electrical sensation down arms
- Uhtoff's phenomenon: symptoms worsen or brought on by heat
- Progression of disease: two thirds of children with MS have relapsing-remitting form; other forms: primary or secondary progressive, progressive relapsing

Diagnostics
- *Magnetic resonance imaging of brain and spinal cord with gadolinium:* classic periventricular white matter lesions; in isolated optic neuritis, helps predict progression to MS; active lesions enhance; old lesions do not enhance
- Lumbar puncture: oligoclonal bands, elevated IgG index
- Paraclinical evidence (extensions of the neurological exam): MRI, brainstem auditory evoked responses, visual-evoked response, documented urologic dysfunction
- Laboratory studies to rule out other processes. Antibodies: anti-nuclear antibody (ANA), anti-neutrophil cytoplasmic antibodies, anti-ssA, anti-ssB, ACE, anti-scl70, anticardiolipin antibody. Inflammatory markers: ESR, CRP. Infectious: RPR, HIV, Lyme; vitamin B_{12} level
- If history of oral and genital ulcers: skin pathergy test for Behçet

Management
Acute Management of an Attack
- Evaluate and treat precipitating infection, (temp, urinalysis, chest x-ray, etc).
- If symptoms are severe and progressive (e.g., non-ambulatory), consider pulse steroids (methylprednisolone 15–30 mg/kg/dose given once daily for 3 days; maximum 1 g/day) and taper to hasten recovery from attack.
- Optic neuritis: IV steroids hasten recovery (no effect on final vision) and may slow progression of MS (IV only)

Prevention of Disease Progression
- IFN1α weekly injections: first-line as it has been evaluated as safe and tolerable in children
- Other agents studied in adults: glatiramer acetate, IFN1β

MYASTHENIA GRAVIS

An antibody-mediated autoimmune disease resulting in depletion of nicotinic acetylcholine (ACh) receptors at the neuromuscular junction and subsequent fatigable weakness

- Myasthenic crisis: life-threatening respiratory weakness

Epidemiology
- Fifty to 125 cases per million population (approximately 10% are children)
- Can develop at any age
- Girls affected more often than boys post-pubertally
- 15% of adults with MG will have thymomas but rare in children; 85% of adults have thymic lymphofollicular hyperplasia.
- 10% of children will have associated autoimmune disease

Differential Diagnosis
- Congenital myasthenic syndrome, transient neonatal myasthenia, drug-induced myasthenia, hyperthyroidism, Lambert-Eaton syndrome, botulism

Pathophysiology
- Auto-antibodies cause deficit of ACh receptors at neuromuscular junctions leading to accelerated degradation, functional blockade of the binding sites, and complement-mediated damage to the receptors.
- Abnormal ACh receptors (simplified membrane folds) and wide synaptic space also contribute.
- Resulting decreased amplitude of end-plate potentials causes failure to trigger action potentials, reducing muscle power.

Clinical Manifestations
- Weakness and fatigability of skeletal muscles, ptosis, dysphagia, shortness of breath, blurred vision
- Muscles usually strongest early in the morning. Symptoms improve with rest.
- Diplopia, ptosis most often: 50% at presentation, 80% to 90% later
- Generalized weakness in 2/3 of children: bulbar, truncal, limb
- Intact deep tendon reflexes, sensation, and coordination
- "Closed eye rest test": rest with eyes closed for 15 minutes. Observe degree of ptosis before and after test.

Diagnostics
Anticholinesterase Test (Edrophonium, Tensilon)
- Tensilon, 0.1–0.2 mg/kg (maximum 10 mg) IV; start with 20% as test dose and wait 2 minutes, then 30% and wait 2 minutes, then 50%
- Positive if unequivocal improvement in objectively weak muscle
- Monitor for bradycardia, hypotension, respiratory compromise
- Have atropine ready STAT if patient becomes bradycardic

Radioimmunoassay for ACh-receptor Antibodies
- Positive in 50% to 90% of pediatric patients

Other
- Thyroid function studies: 3% to 8% will have hyperthyroidism
- Consider screening for other autoimmune disorders.
- Purified protein derivative test before immune therapy
- Serum vitamin B_{12} level
- Electromyography: repetitive nerve stimulation, single fiber EMG if unclear
- Consider chest CT to evaluate thymus
- If isolated CN weakness, consider brain imaging to rule out mass.

Management
Chronic Medical Management
- Anticholinesterase agents: Pyridostigmine (Mestinon) is first line therapy:
  - Initial dosing in children is every 4 to 6 hours. In adults, usually given three times a day but sustained release formulations permit every day to twice-daily dosing
  - Titrate dose to effect.

- Immunosuppression: prednisone, azathioprine, others
- Other immunotherapy: plasmapheresis, IVIG; used for myasthenic crisis, preparation for thymectomy, or failure to respond to medications

Crisis
- Criteria to consider mechanical ventilation include forced vital capacity less than 15 mL/kg, less than 30% predicted for age, severe aspiration, or labored breathing; consider plasmapheresis or IVIG

Surgical Management
- Thymectomy has a therapeutic effect in childhood generalized myasthenia gravis; prevention of spread of thymoma in adults (rare in childhood).

PSEUDOTUMOR CEREBRI

Syndrome characterized by increased ICP, normal CSF, normal/small ventricles, no intracranial mass
- ICP greater than 200 mm H_2O if non-obese, greater than 250 mm H_2O if obese patient
- Also known as idiopathic intracranial hypertension

Epidemiology
- Classically, obese women of child-bearing age
- Pre-puberty: no gender difference, less commonly associated with obesity, less often chronic

Etiology
Associated conditions and possible risk factors include:
- *Neurologic:* venous sinus thrombosis, meningitis (including Lyme)
- *Systemic:* malnutrition, re-feeding, SLE, hypertension, vitamin B_{12} or iron deficiency, hypervitaminosis A, renal failure, significant weight change
- *Medications:* steroid withdrawal, tetracycline, doxycycline, minocycline, vitamin A, isotretinoin, ciprofloxacin, lithium, thyroxine, nalidixic acid, oral contraceptive pills
- *Endocrine:* obesity, hyper/hypothyroid, hypoparathyroidism, Addison, pregnancy

Pathophysiology
Theories include decreased CSF absorption by arachnoid granulation tissue versus CSF over-production.

Clinical Manifestations
- Headache worse in morning or lying flat, +/- nausea, vomiting, and photophobia
- Diplopia, blurry vision (common in children), loss of central vision (central scotoma), may progress to blindness
- Transient visual obscurations likely due to optic nerve ischemia
- May have normal level of consciousness and intellectual functioning
- Strabismus, pulsatile tinnitus, neck/back pain, irritability, somnolence
- Papilledema (not universal); visual field loss (central scotoma)
- Visual acuity and color vision spared initially
- CN VI palsy (resolves when ICP normalized)
- Symptoms may improve immediately post-lumbar puncture

Diagnostics
Pseudotumor cerebri is a diagnosis of exclusion:
- *Neuroimaging:* emergent imaging to evaluate for mass or hydrocephalus; MRI/MRV best for venous sinus thrombosis.
- *Laboratory Studies:*
  - LP with opening pressure, cell count, glucose, protein, cultures (should be normal except pressure; protein can be low).

- Specific laboratory tests to evaluate for specific etiologies (e.g., vitamin A)
- Consider electrolytes, BUN, creatinine, ANA, urinalysis, hypercoagulability tests
- *Vision Testing:* visual acuity and quantitative perimetry testing at diagnosis and at regular intervals thereafter

Management
Medical
- If substantial visual field loss: admit, administer steroids such as dexamethasone (see Increased Intracranial Pressure) or prednisone (1–2 mg/kg/day up to 60–100 mg/day with a gradual taper over 2 weeks), follow serial visual field exams.
- Stop any precipitating agents.
- No specific treatment if headache resolves in 24 to 48 hours
- Acetazolamide (Diamox) for symptomatic children (see Increased Intracranial Pressure topic for dosing guidelines). Watch for dose-dependent paresthesias.
- Furosemide if patient cannot tolerate acetazolamide
- Consider steroids as last resort or if rapid vision loss

Surgical
- For patients who fail medications and are symptomatic
- Optic nerve sheath fenestration
- Lumbar peritoneal shunt

Other
- Weight loss in obese patients
- Serial LPs are NOT effective long-term

SPINAL CORD EMERGENCY

Etiology
- *Trauma:* breech or traumatic delivery; in older children, mostly cervical spine in order of decreasing frequency: motor vehicle accidents, diving, falls; may occur in setting of head injury or other trauma
- *Infection:* epidural abscess, tuberculosis, HIV, often after trauma or vertebral osteomyelitis
- *Infarction:* hypotension (e.g., after arrest), aortic dissection, anterior spinal artery occlusion
- *Hemorrhage:* arteriovenous malformation, intramedullary tumor
- *Inflammation:* demyelinating spinal cord process (e.g., transverse myelitis), vasculitis

Clinical Manifestations
- Sudden flaccid paraparesis (spinal shock)
- Evolution to spastic paresis or plegia
- Neck or back pain, fever if abscess
- Bowel and bladder compromise
- History of trauma
- A fall may occur as a result of the spinal cord process and resultant weakness and may not be the inciting factor.
- Vital signs: may have diaphragm paralysis if C3-C5 are involved
- Femoral pulses
- Preserved mental status unless there is concurrent head injury
- Cranial nerve function should be preserved.
- Motor: weakness with a spinal level; initial low tone, then increased; initial loss of deep tendon reflexes, then increased
- Sensory: spinal level

Diagnostics
- MRI of the spine
- Depending on clinical suspicion: electrolytes, CBC, ESR, CRP, ANA, bone radiographs, LP

Management
- Immobilization of the spine
- ABCs (minimal neck extension if cervical trauma)
- Emergent neurosurgical consultation
- Steroids within 8 hours of injury: methylprednisone 30 mg/kg IV bolus, then 5.4 mg/kg/hour for 23 hours
- Monitor respiratory status with serial measurements of NIF (negative inspiratory force)
- Other: supportive therapy, pain control, bowel regimen, Foley catheter, DVT prophylaxis, intubation if necessary

STROKE

Stroke: **prolonged or permanent dysfunction of brain due to interruption of blood flow**

Transient Ischemic Attack (TIA): **symptoms last less than 24 hours**

Epidemiology
- Two to 3 cases/100,000 children/year
- Neonatal stroke (infants < 30 days old): 1/4000 live births
- Approximately 50% have persistent neurologic abnormality or seizure disorder after stroke; 5% to 10% of affected children die, ~30% have a recurrence, ~30% have no sequelae
- Incidence of ischemic stroke is similar to hemorrhagic stroke, but mortality rate is 41% in hemorrhagic and 5% in ischemic.

Etiology
- Thrombosis, embolism, hemorrhage, hypoperfusion
- No cause detected in 20%
- *Risk factors for arterial ischemic stroke:* congenital heart disease, sickle cell disease, coagulation disorders, infection (e.g., endocarditis, varicella), moyamoya, arterial dissection
- *Risk factors for hemorrhagic stroke:* arteriovenous malformation, cerebral aneurysm, cavernous malformations, head trauma, bleeding diathesis
- *Risk factors for venous sinus thrombosis:* severe dehydration, sepsis, hypercoagulability

Pathophysiology
- *Arterial ischemic stroke:* decreased cerebral blood flow causes ischemia. Cell death causes edema and surrounding damage. Patients may have hemorrhage into stroke territory.
- *Hemorrhagic stroke:* mass effect causes local damage and may result in midline shift or herniation.
- *Venous sinus thrombosis:* venous hypertension, venous infarction with hemorrhages
- Maximal edema occurs 2 to 3 days after stroke.

Clinical Manifestations
- *Ischemic stroke:* focal neurologic deficit
- *Hemorrhagic stroke:* headache, mental status change, focal neurologic deficit
- Children often present hours or days after symptoms begin.
- Vital signs: watch for signs of herniation including Cushing's triad of hypertension, bradycardia, and abnormal respirations.
- Perform detailed neurologic exam to identify focality and evaluate level of consciousness.
- May have papilledema
- Evidence of trauma or predisposing disease
- Serial exams are required

Diagnostics
Radiology
- Non-contrast head CT
- Brain MRI better for early infarcts (diffusion-weighted MRI)

- MR Angiography/Venography to evaluate vascular abnormalities: include MRA of neck if suspect arterial dissection and MRV if suspect venous sinus thrombosis
- Cerebral angiography if further information required after MRA
- Transcranial Doppler ultrasound can predict increased risk in patients with sickle cell disease.

Laboratory Studies
- CBC, PT/PTT/INR, lipid profile, HIV, RPR
- Hypercoagulability workup (see Box 12.1): protein C and protein S levels, AT-III, factor V Leiden, homocystine level and MTHFR gene, antiphospholipid, prothrombin 20210 gene mutation, lipoprotein a, β-2 glycoprotein 1
- Screen for vasculitis: ESR, C3, C4, ANA
- Toxicology screen: cocaine
- Hemoglobin electrophoresis: sickle cell disease
- Blood culture if suspect endocarditis
- If infarct not in typical vascular distribution: plasma ammonia, lactate, pyruvate, amino acids, urine organic acids, CSF lactate
- Also consider ECG and echocardiography

Management

For initial resuscitation: ABCs, treat hypoglycemia, treat seizures, maintain temperature 36.5°C to 37°C

Acute Medical Management
1. *Arterial ischemic stroke:* lay flat (maximize cerebral perfusion); liberal IV normal saline (avoid dextrose to minimize edema); correct electrolyte abnormalities (avoid hyperosmolality); maintain normotension; monitor ICP; if arterial dissection or cardiac clot, consider heparin
2. *Hemorrhagic stroke:* monitor vital signs, ICP; elevate head 45 degrees; maintain normotension; correct electrolyte imbalances; *avoid* anticoagulation
3. *Venous sinus thrombosis:* monitor ICP; liberal IV normal saline; if not contraindicated, start heparin (*no bolus*)

Anticoagulation
- *Aspirin (ASA)* (acute and chronic therapy): 2–3 mg/kg/day causes antiplatelet effect ("low-dose" = 1 mg/kg/day).
- *Heparin* (risk of recurrence or extension versus risk of bleed): do NOT bolus; younger than 12 months: 28 U/kg/hr; older than 12 months: 20 U/kg/hr; target aPTT: 60 to 85 seconds
- *Low-molecular-weight heparin (Enoxaparin):* children and adults use 1 mg/kg/dose every 12 hours; neonates use 1.5 mg/kg/dose every 12 hours
- *Warfarin* is most effective long-term anticoagulant in children: avoid contact sports; target International Normalized Ratio (INR) is 2.0 to 3.0
- *Thrombolytics* have not been well studied in children with stroke and are not recommended at this time.

Surgical
- Emergent evacuation of large hemorrhage and/or increased ICP
- May require ventriculostomy to monitor ICP
- Consider surgery for vascular malformations, large middle cerebral artery infarcts, and hydrocephalus.

TRANSVERSE MYELITIS

Acute or subacute inflammatory process involving both gray and white matter of the spinal cord, resulting in bilateral motor, sensory, and autonomic dysfunction

Epidemiology
- One to four new cases/million/year; seasonal clustering (winter)
- Peak incidence at ages 10 to 19 and 30 to 39 years

- No gender or familial predisposition
- One third recover completely, one third moderate permanent disability, one third severe persistent disability

Differential Diagnosis
- Guillain-Barré syndrome, ADEM, multiple sclerosis, compressive lesions of spinal cord, fibrocartilaginous emboli
- Ischemia; if symptom nadir occurs in less than 4 hours: arteriovenous malformation, vasculitis

Pathophysiology
- *Anatomic changes:* edema, demyelination, necrosis of spinal cord
- *Post-infectious:* associated with numerous infections, including viral URI, herpes zoster, HIV, EBV, influenza, *Mycoplasma,* and mumps
- *Post-vaccination:* polio, cholera, typhoid, rabies
- *Autoimmune:* abnormal cell-mediated response to myelin sheath component

Clinical Manifestations
- Back pain, then weakness and sensory changes develop over days
- Usually legs more than arms
- Voiding dysfunction common
- Often fever, nuchal rigidity
- Deficits progress quickly, usually reaching maximum in 2 days
- May see signs of recovery after 6 days: full in 50%, partial in 40%, and none in 10%
- On physical exam: flaccid (early) or spastic (late) paraplegia or quadriplegia; sensory level (often mid-thoracic); sphincter abnormalities; abnormal deep tendon reflexes (decreased early, increased late); perform ophthalmologic exam for optic nerve involvement.

Diagnostics
Laboratory Studies
- LP: increased WBC (lymphocytic predominance), normal or increased protein, normal glucose. Send bacterial and viral cultures, oligoclonal bands, IgG index. Consider cytology, specific viral studies (e.g., VZV, EBV, Lyme titer, *Mycoplasma*)
- Serum/CSF viral titers if clinically indicated
- Screening for autoimmune disease
- HIV, HTLV-1, RPR tests
- U/A and culture if urinary retention

Other Studies
- *Gadolinium-enhanced MRI of spine:* fusiform swelling of spinal cord
- *Gadolinium-enhanced MRI of brain:* to evaluate for multifocal disease
- *Electromyography:* denervation associated with poor prognosis

Management
- High-dose IV methylprednisolone (15–30 mg/kg/dose, maximum 1 g/day) for 5 days is standard of care.
- *Sphincter dysfunction:* intermittent catheterization; treat constipation (see Constipation in Gastroenterology chapter)
- *Supportive:* physical and occupational therapy

Seizures and Epilepsy

GENERAL PRINCIPLES

Seizure: paroxysmal event caused by abnormal electrical discharges in the brain

Epilepsy: recurrent unprovoked seizures, usually stereotyped

Simple partial: motor signs, sensory or psychic experience with preserved awareness

Complex partial: partial seizure with impairment of awareness (often staring)

Generalized seizures: tonic-clonic, tonic, clonic, atonic, myoclonic, or absence

Simple seizures may evolve to complex partial seizures, and either may evolve to a generalized seizure.

Epidemiology
- 1% of children will have an afebrile seizure by age 14 years.
- 2% to 4% of American children will have a febrile seizure.
- Active epilepsy: 0.4% to 0.9% of children, 1% overall population

Etiology
- Fever, hypoxia, ischemia, head trauma, hemorrhage, CNS infection, hyperammonemia, toxin, medication, medication withdrawal, inborn error of metabolism
- Structural abnormality (tumor or malformation)
- Electrolyte disturbance: low or high glucose, Na or Ca, low Mg
- Idiopathic: presumed genetic
- Symptomatic: following hypoxic-ischemic injury, trauma, hemorrhage, stroke, CNS infection; associated with brain tumor, neurological syndrome
- Cryptogenic

Differential Diagnosis
- Syncope: anoxia may precipitate a provoked seizure
- Breath-holding spell, tic, cardiac dysrhythmia with collapse, myoclonus, behavioral event (e.g., staring), parasomnia, conversion disorder (nonepileptic), gastroesophageal reflux (GERD)

Physical Exam
- During a seizure, the following are possible: impaired awareness, change in vital signs, focal seizure activity.
- After a seizure, the following are possible: decreased awareness and responsiveness, Todd's paresis (transient postictal paresis that resolves within 24 to 48 hours), eye deviation toward the side of seizure focus

Management
Acute management focuses on maintaining control of ABCs and, when appropriate, cessation of seizures with benzodiazepines, e.g., Lorazepam (0.05–0.1 mg/kg IV); maximum dose is 4 mg for children and 8 mg for adults. Chronic management consists of raising the seizure threshold and should be initiated after a second seizure

- Medications that can be loaded by IV route:
  - *Phenytoin* 20 mg/kg IV SLOWLY (no faster than 1mg/kg/minute, usually over 1 hour) in non–dextrose-containing solution; monitor for cardiac arrhythmia. Fosphenytoin: same dose given as "phenytoin equivalents," but can be administered either IM or as a faster IV infusion compared to phenytoin.
  - *Phenobarbital* 20 mg/kg IV; monitor for hypotension and respiratory suppression
  - *Valproic acid* 15 mg/kg IV above 2 years old and if no suspicion for metabolic disease
- Outpatient anticonvulsant can be chosen based on seizure type, EEG, and side effect profile. If one of the above medications has been loaded, continue orally and check a level in one week:
  - *Phenytoin* 5 mg/kg/day divided three times a day
  - *Phenobarbital* 5 mg/kg/day divided twice daily (8 mg/kg/day for neonates)
  - *Valproic acid* 20 mg/kg/day divided three times daily
  - *Carbamazepine* or oxcarbazepine for partial epilepsy

FEBRILE SEIZURES

Simple febrile seizure: a brief (<15 minute), generalized seizure in a 6-month to 5-year-old child who has a fever (>38.4°C). To classify as simple, there can only be one seizure in 24 hours, and there can be no intracranial infection or significant metabolic abnormality.

Complex febrile seizure: prolonged (>20 minutes), focal, or recurrent (greater than one in 24 hours) seizure in 6-month to 5-year-old child with fever

Epidemiology
- 2% to 5% of all children have a febrile seizure.
- Peak age of onset is 18 to 22 months
- Recurrence risk: age younger than 12 months: 50%; age older than 12 months: 30%; second febrile seizure: 50% have at least one additional recurrence
- Overall risk of epilepsy in children with simple febrile seizures is similar to 1% risk in general population. Children with multiple febrile seizures and the first seizure at younger than 12 months of age have an ~2% risk.

Diagnostics
- *Lumbar puncture:* should always be performed if age less than 12 months; often, if age 12 to 18 months; only if clinical suspicion of intracranial infection if age greater than 18 months; if risk factors: complex febrile seizure, suspicious findings on exam, lethargy, concurrent antibiotic treatment
- *Laboratory studies:* electrolytes, Mg^{2+}, Ca^{2+}, CBC count, glucose: only if age less than 6 months, suspicious history, or abnormal findings on physical exam
- *CT/MRI:* not indicated for simple febrile seizure if recovery is complete and exam is normal
- *EEG:* not indicated for simple febrile seizure in a normal child

Management
- Antipyretic medications do *not* prevent recurrent febrile seizures.
- Daily *phenobarbital* and *valproate* can reduce the risk of recurrence, but they have significant side effects (especially sedation) and are *rarely* used as prophylaxis against febrile seizures.
- *Continuous or intermittent anticonvulsant medications are not recommended for prevention of simple febrile seizures.*
- In cases of prolonged febrile seizures, it may be appropriate to prescribe rectal diazepam (for age less than 5 years, 0.5 mg/kg; for 5 years or older, 0.25 mg/kg, maximum 10 mg) for use as abortive therapy.

INFANTILE SPASMS

Generalized epilepsy characterized by seizures with brief bilateral contractions of neck, trunk, and extremities, often occurring in clusters (flexor, extensor, or mixed). Seizures often occur on awakening or falling asleep:
- *Idiopathic/Cryptogenic* (10% to 45%): normal prenatal and postnatal history before onset of seizures, normal brain imaging
- *Symptomatic* (50% to 90%): directly related to risk factors (e.g., periventricular leukomalacia, congenital infections, brain malformations, head trauma, hypoxic-ischemic encephalopathy); associated with 80% to 90% risk of mental retardation.
- *West syndrome:* infantile spasms, developmental plateau/regression, and hypsarrhythmia on EEG

Epidemiology
- One in 4000 to 6000 live births
- 85% begin before age 1 year (peak age of onset 3 to 5 months).
- Normal development occurs in ~25% of patients with idiopathic infantile spasms (fewer if symptomatic).

Clinical Manifestations
- Brief symmetric contractions of head, neck, and extremities
- Often occur in clusters on falling asleep or awakening
- Often associated with loss of developmental milestones

Diagnostics
- *EEG:* hypsarrhythmia (disorganized, high-amplitude multifocal epileptiform pattern); electrodecremental seizures
- *Brain MRI:* evaluates for malformations, bleeds, etc.

Management
- Goals include disappearance of hypsarrhythmia, reduction in seizures, and stabilization of development:
  - *ACTH:* suppresses CRH synthesis; must be given IM; 70% to 80% will respond; adverse effects include hypertension, irritability, weight gain, hyperkalemia, hyperglycemia, risk of sepsis, risk of infection at injection sites.
  - *Vigabatrin:* first line in many countries because of good response and fewer side effects, but not available in United States due to retinal toxicity and peripheral vision loss.
  - *Topiramate, pyridoxine, valproate,* and *benzodiazepines* have all been used to treat infantile spasms.
  - Excision of focal lesion can occasionally be curative.

NEONATAL SEIZURES

Seizure that occurs in the first month of life

Epidemiology
- Occurs in 4.4/1000 live births; incidence increases with earlier gestational age
- Approximately 50% of infants with seizures due to hypoxic-ischemic encephalopathy have moderate to severe neurologic abnormalities at follow-up.

Etiology
- Most common cause in first 24 hours of life is hypoxic-ischemic encephalopathy.
- Other causes: metabolic abnormality, infection (TORCH, meningitis), trauma, structural abnormality, hemorrhage, pyridoxine dependency, inadvertent local anesthetic injection during delivery, familial neonatal convulsions

Pathophysiology
- Electric discharges in the neonatal brain are regional and rarely spread to contralateral hemisphere; therefore, generalized tonic-clonic seizures are rare in neonates.

Diagnosis
History
- Family history of neonatal seizures, metabolic disorders
- Maternal drug use
- Apgar less than 5 at 5 minutes, base deficit greater than 10 at birth

EEG
- Normal EEG in term infant or mildly abnormal EEG = good prognosis
- Flat or burst-suppression pattern on EEG = poor prognosis
- EEG abnormal for greater than 2 weeks in newborn with asphyxia = always poor prognosis
- If EEG positive for subclinical seizures, consider continuous EEG during medication loading until subclinical seizures cease.

Laboratory Studies
- Glucose, electrolytes, BUN, creatinine, Ca^{2+}, Mg^{2+}, PO_4, bilirubin, ammonia
- Blood gas (rule out acidosis)
- If metabolic acidosis and increased ammonia, send urine organic acids
- Check state newborn metabolic screening results.
- Consider serum amino acids, lactate, pyruvate, long-chain fatty acids.
- Consider karyotype.

- TORCH titers
- LP: cell count, protein, glucose, culture, HSV, metabolic laboratory studies
- Serum/urine toxicology screen from mother and/or neonate

Radiology
- Head ultrasound to evaluate for intraventricular hemorrhage; brain MRI with and without contrast to evaluate structural lesions

Evaluate for Pyridoxine Dependency
- Give 100 mg IV pyridoxine during EEG monitoring, then continue 100 mg orally every day for 1 week. Positive if all clinical seizures stop (minutes) and EEG normalizes (hours)

Management
- If identifiable, treat underlying disorder
- Seizures due to hypoxic-ischemic encephalopathy subside after 72 hours, regardless of therapy.
- Anti-epileptic drugs:
  - *Phenobarbital* is first-line therapy. Load 15–20 mg/kg IV, then maintenance 5–8 mg/kg/day.
  - *Phenytoin* is second-line therapy. Load 20 mg/kg IV to achieve level 15–20 µg/mL, then maintenance 4–6 mg/kg/day. *Fosphenytoin*: same dose given as phenytoin equivalents, but can be administered either IM or as a faster IV infusion compared to phenytoin.
  - *Benzodiazepines* are useful to acutely stop seizures while loading other medications, and for breakthrough seizures.
  - Check levels after loading and follow levels regularly if seizures continue or if subclinical seizures are noted on EEG.

STATUS EPILEPTICUS

A seizure lasting more than 20 minutes or multiple seizures without return to baseline

Epidemiology
- Greater than 50% in patients not previously known to have seizures
- 10% of epilepsy presents with status epilepticus
- Occurs in approximately 25% of children with epilepsy, most within the first 5 years of diagnosis
- Most common pediatric neurology emergency

Diagnostics
- After stabilizing the patient (ABCs), check STAT glucose.
- Electrolytes, BUN, Cr, LFTs, ABG, anticonvulsant levels, urine toxin screen
- In a patient without known epilepsy: NH_3, metabolic screens
- CT head once patient is stable
- Lumbar puncture when patient is stable; blood and urine cultures (especially if fever); also consider CSF HSV, enteroviral, or arboviral PCR testing

Management
Acute management focuses on maintaining control of ABCs and cessation of seizures. Successive doses of anticonvulsants may suppress respiration and necessitate intubation.

Convulsive Status Epilepticus
- ABCs
- Check glucose and give 50% glucose solution 1 mg/kg
- Anticonvulsants to be loaded parenterally:
  1. *Ativan (lorazepam)* 0.05–0.1 mg/kg IV or IM (maximum dose 8 mg) or *Versed* 0.2 mg/kg IV or 0.2–0.5 mg/kg PR. Doses may be repeated every 5 to 10 minutes, but if seizures persist after approximately three doses, proceed to:
  2. *Phenytoin* 20 mg/kg IV SLOWLY (no faster than 1 mg/kg/minute, usually over 1 hour) in non–dextrose-containing solution; monitor for cardiac arrhythmia or *Fosphenytoin* (same dose but can be given either IM or as a faster IV infusion compared to phenytoin)
  3. *Phenobarbital* 20 mg/kg IV; monitor for hypotension and respiratory suppression
  4. *Valproic acid* 15 mg/kg IV if patient is above 2 years old and no suspicion for metabolic disease

- If these are ineffective, *pentobarbital* can be loaded with concurrent EEG monitoring. Dose with 10 mg/kg boluses and titrate to EEG burst suppression.
- If there is concern for ongoing subclinical seizures after convulsive seizures have stopped, an EEG should be obtained.
- Consider empiric antibiotics and acyclovir if concern for CNS infection.

Nonconvulsive Status Epilepticus
- ABCs, check glucose
- Anticonvulsants should be given judiciously. The longer the seizures continue, the harder it may be to stop them. However, these seizures do not pose the same immediate danger as convulsive status epilepticus.
- Consider *Ativan* or *Versed*, *valproic acid*, *phenobarbital*, or *phenytoin* as described above.

UNPROVOKED SEIZURE, FIRST

A seizure for which no specific trigger is identified

Epidemiology
- In the United States, 25,000 to 40,000 children have a first unprovoked afebrile seizure each year.
- Overall recurrence risk ~1/2; remote symptomatic seizure recurrence greater than 2/3; cryptogenic seizure recurrence ~1/3
- If unexplained seizure, normal physical exam, and normal EEG, recurrence risk is 15% to 20%.

Diagnostics
Laboratory Studies
- Selection of laboratory studies based on clinical circumstances (e.g., vomiting, dehydration, mental status)
- Electrolytes, BUN, creatinine, Ca^{2+}, Mg^{2+}
- Urine toxicology screen if prolonged post-ictal state or high suspicion
- CBC if infection suspected
- Lumbar puncture: required in infants younger than 6 months, for failure to return to mental status baseline, or for meningeal signs.
- If increased ICP suspected, obtain head CT before LP.

Neuroimaging
- *Indications for emergent head CT*: focal deficit on exam; patient does not return to baseline within several hours of the seizure
- *Indications for outpatient brain MRI*: age younger than 1 year; unexplained cognitive or motor deficits; abnormal neurologic exam; partial onset seizure; focality on EEG

EEG
- *Urgent/Inpatient*: if patient does not return to baseline
- *Outpatient (within 1 to 2 weeks)*: indicated for all children with first unprovoked seizure

Management
- Outpatient neurologic consultation within 1 to 2 weeks
- No evidence that antiepileptic drugs (AEDs) change natural history of seizure disorders. Usually, AEDs are not indicated after a first unprovoked seizure

UNPROVOKED SEIZURE, SECOND

Epilepsy: recurrent unprovoked seizures, usually stereotyped

Epidemiology
- Affects 0.4% to 0.9% of children, 1% of overall population
- Occurs in 40% of those who had a first unprovoked seizure

Diagnostics

- *Neuro-imaging:* CT only if patient looks ill or has new focal neurologic exam. Obtain MRI with gadolinium to evaluate for seizure focus.
- *EEG:* to identify features of generalized epilepsy or focality; if there is doubt as to the nature of the paroxysmal events, consider prolonged monitoring with ambulatory EEG or in-patient video EEG.
- *Laboratory studies:* if patient is unstable and/or is in the emergency department, check glucose, electrolytes, and calcium. Consider a metabolic screening workup if suspicion is raised by developmental regression or other worrisome features in the history (see Metabolism chapter).

Resources

General Principles

Behrman R, Kliegman R, Jenson H. Nelson Textbook of Pediatrics. 16th ed. Philadelphia: WB Saunders, 2000.

Dinolfo EA, Adam HM. Evaluation of ataxia. Pediatr Rev 2001;22:177–178.

Fenichel, G.M. Clinical Pediatric Neurology: A Signs and Symptoms Approach. 4th ed. Philadelphia: WB Saunders, 2001.

Guidelines for the Determination of Brain Death in Children. Pediatrics 1987;80:298.

Kirkham FJ. Non-traumatic coma in children. Arch Dis Childhood 2001;85:303–312.

Maria B. Current Management in Child Neurology. 2nd ed. Hamilton: BC Decker, 2002.

Reilly PL, Simpson DA, Sprod R, Thomas L. Assessing the conscious level in infants and young children: a paediatric version of the Glasgow Coma Scale. Childs Nerv Syst 1988;4:30–33.

Swaiman KF, Ashwal S, eds. Pediatric Neurology, Principles and Practice. 3rd ed. St. Louis: Mosby, 1999.

Acquired Neurologic Disease

Abd-Allah SA, Jansen PW, Ashwal S, Perkin RM. Intravenous immunoglobulin as therapy for pediatric Guillain-Barré syndrome. J Child Neurol 1997;12:376–380.

Albers JW, Kelly JJ Jr. Acquired inflammatory demyelinating polyneuropathies: clinical and electrodiagnostic features. Muscle Nerve 1989;12:435–451.

Behrman R, Kliegman R, Jenson H. Nelson Textbook of Pediatrics. 16th ed. Philadelphia: WB Saunders, 2000.

Bracken MB, Shepard MJ, Collins WF, et al. A randomized, controlled trial of methylprednisolone or naloxone in the treatment of acute spinal cord injury. N Engl J Med 1990;322:1405–1411.

Callen JP. Dermatomyositis. Lancet 2000;355:53–57.

Carlin TM, Chanmugam A. Stroke in children. Emerg Med Clin North Am 2002;20:671–685.

Drachman DB. Mysathenia gravis. N Engl J Med 1994;330:1797–1810.

Duquette P, Murray TJ, Pleines J, et al. Multiple sclerosis in childhood: clinical profile in 125 patients. J Pediatr 1987;111:359–363.

Evans OB, Vedanarayanan V. Guillain-Barre syndrome. Pediatr Rev 1997;18:10–16.

Farber JM, Buckwalter KA. MR imaging in nonneoplastic muscle disorders of the lower extremity. Radiol Clin North Am 2002; 40:1013–1031.

Fenichel GM. Clinical Pediatric Neurology: A Signs and Symptoms Approach. 4th ed. Philadelphia: WB Saunders, 2001.

Ghezzi A, Deplano V, Faroni J, et al. Multiple sclerosis in childhood: clinical features of 149 cases. Multiple Sclerosis 1997;3:43–46.

Hynson JL, Kornberg AJ, Coleman LT, et al. Clinical and neuroradiologic features of acute disseminated encephalomyelitis in children. Neurology 2001;56:1308–1312.

Jones HR Jr. Guillain-Barre syndrome in children. Curr Opin Pediatr 1995;7:663–668.

Jones JS, Nevai J, Freeman MP, McNinch DE. Emergency department presentation of idiopathic intracranial hypertension. Am J Emerg Med 1999;17:517–521.

Lahat E, Pillar G, Ravid S, et al. Rapid recovery from transverse myelopathy in children treated with methylprednisolone. Pediatr Neurol 1998;19:279–282.

Larsen GY. Increased intracranial pressure. Pediatr Rev 1999;20:234–239.

Lynch JK, Hirtz DG, DeVeber G, Nelson KB. Report of the National Institute of Neurological Disorders and Stroke workshop on perinatal and childhood stroke. Pediatrics 2002;109:116–123.

Mackay MT, Kornberg AJ, Shield LK, Dennett X. Benign acute childhood myositis. Laboratory and clinical features. Neurology 1999;53:2127–2131.

Maria B. Current Management in Child Neurology. 2nd ed. Hamilton: BC Decker, 2002.

Mastaglia FL, Phillips BA, Zilko PJ. Immunoglobulin therapy in inflammatory myopathies. J Neurol Neurosurg Psychiatry 1998;65:107–110.

O'Riordan JI, Thompson AJ, Kingsley DP, et al. The prognostic value of brain MRI in clinically isolated syndromes of the CNS. A 10-year follow-up. Brain 1998;121:495–503.

Poser CM, Paty DW, Scheinberg L, et al. New diagnostic criteria for multiple sclerosis: guidelines for research protocols. Ann Neurol 1983;13:227–231.

Roach ES, deVeber G, Riela A, et al. Recognition and treatment of stroke in children. The Child Neurology Society Ad Hoc Committee on Stroke in Children. Available at: http://www.ninds.nih.gov/news_and_events/proceedings/stroke_proceedings/childneurology.htm. Accessed December 28, 2004.

Ruggieri M, Polizzi A, Pavone L, Grimaldi LM. Multiple sclerosis in children under 6 years of age. Neurology 1999;53:478–484.

Shapiro RL, Hatheway C, Swerdlow DL. Botulism in the United States: A Clinical and Epidemiologic Review. Ann Intern Med 1998;129:221–228.

Sindern E, Haas J, Stark E, et al. Early onset MS under the age of 16: clinical and paraclinical features. Acta Neurol Scand 1992;86:280–284.

Soler D, Cox T, Bullock P, et al. Diagnosis and management of benign intracranial hypertension. Arch Dis Childhood 1998;78:89–94.

Swaiman KF, Ashwal S, eds. Pediatric Neurology, Principles and Practice. 3rd ed. St. Louis: Mosby, 1999.

Tenembaum S, Chamoles N, Fejerman N. Acute disseminated encephalomyelitis: a long-term follow-up study of 84 pediatric patients. Neurology 2001;59:1224–1231.

Transverse Myelitis Consortium Working Group. Proposed diagnostic criteria and nosology of acute transverse myelitis. Neurology 2002;59:499–505.

Zochodne DW. Autonomic involvement in Guillain-Barré syndrome: a review. Muscle Nerve 1994:17: 1145–1155.

Seizures and Epilepsy

Behrman R, Kliegman R, Jenson H. Nelson Textbook of Pediatrics. 16th ed. Philadelphia: WB Saunders, 2000.

Brunquell PJ, Glennon CM, DiMario FJ Jr, et al. Prediction of outcome based on clinical seizure type in newborn infants. J Pediatr 2002;140:707–712.

Committee on Quality Improvement, Subcommittee on Febrile Seizures. Practice parameter: Long-term treatment of the child with simple febrile seizures. Pediatrics 1999;103:1307–1309.

Fenichel GM. Clinical Pediatric Neurology: A Signs and Symptoms Approach. 4th ed. Philadelphia: WB Saunders, 2001.

Goetz CB. Textbook of Clinical Neurology. Philadelphia: WB Saunders, 1999.

Hancock E, et al. Treatment of infantile spasms (Cochrane Review). Cochrane Library 2002;2:CD001770.

Hirtz D. Practice Parameter: Evaluating a first nonfebrile seizure in children. Neurology 2000;55:616–623.

Painter MJ, Scher MS, Stein AD, et al. Phenobarbital compared with phenytoin for the treatment of neonatal seizures. N Engl J Med 1999;341:485–489.

Provisional Committee on Quality Improvement, Subcommittee on Febrile Seizures. Practice parameter: the neurodiagnostic evaluation of the child with a first simple febrile seizure. Pediatrics 1996;97:769–775.

Sillanpaa M, Shinnar S. Status epilepticus in a population-based cohort with childhood-onset epilepsy in Finland. Ann Neurol 2002;52:303–310.

Snead OC. How does ACTH work against infantile spasms? Bedside to bench. Ann Neurol 2001;49:288–289.

Swaiman KF, Ashwal S, eds. Pediatric Neurology, Principles and Practice. 3rd ed. St. Louis: Mosby, 1999.

Brenda Waber, RD, CSP, CNSD, LDN, Colleen Yanni, MS, RD, LDN,
Maria R. Mascarenhas, MBBS, and the CHOP Committee of Dietitians

ASSESSMENT OF NUTRITIONAL STATUS

Information gathering, growth assessment, estimation of needs, determination of risk factors, identification of goals, recommendation, and education

Assessment
- Diet history:
  - Usual intake including types and portion sizes of foods consumed
  - For breast-feeders, minutes on each breast and frequency
  - Food aversions, allergies, or religious/ethnic restrictions
  - Oral supplements or tube feedings
  - Herbal, vitamin, or mineral supplements
  - Access to food or special circumstances and current history
  - Note specific conditions that may affect absorption, metabolism, digestion
  - Deficiencies from inadequate intake or comorbidities
  - Note any diagnoses that may increase the caloric needs of the patient (fever, respiratory difficulty, etc.)
- Gastrointestinal history including stooling patterns, nausea, vomiting
- Medications and potential food/drug interactions:
  - Note side effects of drugs that may cause electrolyte wasting, change in stool patterns or malabsorption.
  - Note whether the drug's efficacy is reduced by food or food interferes with absorption or mechanism of action.
- Laboratory values:
  - Most notable for electrolytes, albumin and prealbumin, iron studies, and liver and lipid panels if pertinent
- Growth parameters:
  - Length/height, weight, head circumference (if younger than 3 years)
  - Optional: triceps skinfold, arm muscle area, mid arm circumference, lower leg length or knee height (when unable to obtain accurate length/height)
  - Plot on Center for Disease Control National Center for Health Statistics growth chart or Specialty Chart (prematurity, low birth weight, disease specific, etc) until 20 years of age.
  - Typical growth velocity presented in Table 20.1.

Stunting and Wasting
- Wasting is an indicator of acute malnutrition.
- Stunting is an indicator of chronic malnutrition.

Waterlow Criteria for Grading Malnutrition
- Wasting (as percentage of median weight for height): 90% to 110%, normal; 80% to 89%, mild; 70% to 79%, moderate; less than 70%, severe
- Stunting (as percentage of median height for age): 95% or greater, normal; 90% to 94%, mild; 85% to 89%, moderate; less than 85%, severe

Body Mass Index
- Body mass index (BMI) = Weight/(Height)^2 × 10,000
  - Use weight in kg
  - Use height in cm
- Used for children older than 2 years of age for assessment of obesity

Table 20.1: Growth Velocity

Age	Weight (g/d)	Length (cm/mo)
<3 mo	25–35	2.6–3.5
3–6 mo	15–21	1.6–2.5
6–12 mo	10–13	1.2–1.7
13 yr	4–10	0.7–1.1
4–6 yr	5–8	0.5–0.8
7–10 yr	5–12	0.4–0.6

- BMI 85% to 95% = at risk for becoming overweight
- BMI > 95% = overweight

Estimating Nutrition Needs

There are a variety of methods to estimate energy (calorie) needs.

- The recommended daily allowances (RDA) guideline is recommended for infants and may be used as an estimate for healthy children for both calories (Table 20.2) and protein (Table 20.3).
- The World Health Organization (WHO) equation (Table 20.4) provides a more detailed calculation of energy requirements for children and adolescents to provide the resting energy expenditure (REE). The REE is then modified by activity levels and stress factors, which are important considerations in hospitalized children.
- Once the REE is calculated, an activity or stress factor must be incorporated to take into consideration additional calorie needs under special circumstances. (REE × [Activity or Stress Factor] = estimated caloric needs)
  - REE × 1.3: well-nourished child at bed rest with mild-to-moderate stress
  - REE × 1.5: normally active child with mild to moderated stress; inactive child with severe stress (trauma, sepsis, cancer) or child with minimal activity and malnutrition requiring catch-up growth
  - REE × 1.7: active child requiring catch-up growth or active child with severe stress

Table 20.2: RDA Guidelines for Daily Calories

Age	Kcal/kg
0–6 mo	108
6–12 mo	98
1–3 yr	102
4–6 yr	90
7–10 yr	70
Males:	
11–14 yr	55
15–18 yr	45
Females:	
11–14 yr	47
15–18 yr	40

Table 20.3: Daily Recommended Intake for Protein

Age	AI (g/kg/day)	EAR (g/kg/day)	RDA (g/kg/day)
0–6 mo	1.52	—	2.2
7–12 mo	—	1.1	1.5
1–3 yr	—	0.88	1.10
4–8 yr	—	0.76	0.95
9–13 yr	—	0.76	0.95
Boys: 14–18 yr	—	0.73	0.85
Girls: 14–18 yr	—	0.71	0.85

AI, adequate intake (protein intake sufficient if above this level); EAR, estimated average requirement (half of the healthy individuals in this group would meet their protein requirements at this level); RDA, recommended daily allowance (risk of inadequate intake is very small at this level).

Obese Population
- When calculating calorie needs for an obese patient, use an adjusted body weight (BW) instead of the actual BW in the WHO equation.
- Adjusted BW = Ideal BW + 0.25 × (Actual BW – Ideal BW)

Catch-Up Growth
- Calorie requirements for catch-up growth can be calculated using the RDA Guideline table (see Table 20.2) and the following equation:

> Daily calorie requirement for catch-up growth = RDA × calories for weight age × Ideal weight for actual height / actual weight

Table 20.4: WHO Equation for Resting Energy Expenditure

Age	Kcal/Day
Males:	
0–3 yr	(60.9 × Wt) – 54
>3–10 yr	(22.7 × Wt) + 495
>10–18 yr	(17.5 × Wt) + 651
>18–30 yr	(15.3 × Wt) + 679
Females:	
0–3 yr	(61.0 × Wt) – 51
>3–10 yr	(22.5 × Wt) + 499
>10–18 yr	(12.2 × Wt) + 746
>18–30 yr	(14.7 × Wt) + 495

Wt = weight in kilograms.

- Protein requirements for catch-up growth can be calculated using the DRI for Protein table (see Table 20.3) and the following equation:

$$\text{Protein requirements for catch-up growth} = \frac{(\text{Protein for Weight Age} \times \text{Ideal Weight for height})}{\text{Actual Weight}}$$

  - Use weight in kilograms.
  - Weight-age = kcal/kg/day = age at which present weight would be at the 50th percentile on the growth chart.
  - To determine ideal weight for actual height, use the patient's height to find the 50th-per-centile point on the height curve, and then drop down vertically to the weight curve to the corresponding 50th-percentile point on the weight curve. Follow that point horizontally to determine the corresponding weight.

ENTERAL NUTRITION

Tube Feeding

Tube feeding should be considered if the patient has a functional gastrointestinal (GI) tract but is unable/unwilling to consume sufficient calories/protein intake for weight maintenance/growth. Feedings may be intermittent or continuous.

- Due to risk of bacterial contamination, hang time of formula should not exceed 4 hours for hospitalized patients (especially neonates).

Continuous Feeds

- Advantages of continuous feeds:
  - Enhanced tolerance and absorption (short bowel patients)
  - Used for nocturnal supplemental feedings (with daytime oral intake)
  - Decreased abdominal distention
  - Physiologic for small bowel feeds
- Disadvantages of continuous feeds:
  - Decreased mobility (tied to pump)
  - Risk of bacterial contamination if feeds at room temperature for long period
  - May be difficult to monitor tolerance if feeding is post pyloric as residuals are not checked from the small bowel.
- Suggested initial regimen and advancement for continuous feeding:
  - For age 1 month to 7 years: *initial regimen*, 0.5–2 mL/kg/hr; *advance by* 0.5–1 mg/kg/hr every 4 to 24 hours as tolerated
  - For age greater than 7 years: *initial regimen*, 10–20 mL/hr; *advance by* 10–20 mL/hr every 4 to 8 hours as tolerated
  - Individual tolerance must be closely monitored.

Intermittent (bolus) feeds

- Advantages of bolus feeds:
  - Easier to monitor tolerance/residual gastric volumes
  - Physiologic for gastric feeds: similar pattern to mealtimes
  - Enhances mobility: not tied to pump
- Disadvantages of bolus feeds:
  - Aspiration risk due to volume of feeding in stomach
  - May worsen gastroesophageal reflux
  - May impinge on respiratory effort with large bolus feeds
- Suggested initial regimen and advancement refer to Table 20.5; individual tolerance must be closely monitored.

Monitoring

- BUN/creatinine: if high check for increased protein content of formula, decreased renal func-tion, or inadequate fluid intake.
- GI tolerance:
  - *Constipation:* possible impaction, inadequate fluid intake, inactivity, inadequate fiber intake.

Table 20.5: Guidelines for Intermittent Enteral Feeding Regimens

Age	Initial	Advance by
1 mo–7 yr	2–5 mL/kg/feed every 3–4 hr *Usually full strength*	Advance volume by 5–10 mL/feed every 3–12 hr as tolerated OR if hypertonic formula is used increase caloric density q 8–24 hours as tolerated. Do not advance both volume and caloric density at the same time.
>7 yr	90–120 mL/feed every 3–4 hr *Usually full strength*	Advance volume by 30–60 mL q 4–8 hours as tolerated OR if hypertonic formula is used increase caloric density every 8–24 hr as tolerated. Do not advance both volume and caloric density at the same time.

- *Diarrhea:* hyperosmolar medication or formula, infusion too rapid, intolerance to particular component of formula, tube migration (i.e., from stomach to duodenum with bolus feeds), inadequate fiber intake, low albumin, impaction leading to overflow diarrhea, possible bacterial contamination of formula.
- *Vomiting:* possible delayed gastric emptying; GER; tube in distal esophagus; gastritis; intolerance to particular component of formula (i.e., allergy); infusion too rapid; behavioral component
- Hydration status: urine specific gravity, input and output, check if meeting free water requirements
- Glucose homeostasis: if high blood glucose, consider possible infection, check carbohydrate intake, and check if on steroid therapy
- Anthropometrics: weight, height, and head circumference (as appropriate for age); adjust calorie/protein intake accordingly

Mechanical problems
Clogged Tube
- Usually avoided by scheduled water flushes, especially after interruption of feeds or following instillation of medications
- Attempt to flush with water using progressively larger syringes (e.g., 1-mL, 3-mL, 5-mL, 10-mL, and 20-mL)
- Enzyme preparation for dissolving clog: Viokase8 (1 tab) + sodium bicarbonate (325 mg) + water (5 mL). Crush tabs together and add water, using 2.5 mL push/pull to instill solution (may take 10 minutes to instill). Leave in place for 20 to 30 minutes; if no results after 30 minutes, may repeat ONE time.
- If attempts to clear clog fail, consider replacement of tube.

Leaking around Gastrostomy Site
- Prevent by minimizing tube movement
- Do not upsize tube
- Protective skin care is important.
- Consider calling service that placed device to decide if further action needed.
- Check water in balloon (refer to original volume).

Granulomas at Gastrostomy Tube Site
- Consider silver nitrate or stoma adhesive application, especially if bleeding.
- Migration of mucosa through stoma is a problematic complication that may require temporary removal of tube or surgical revision of site. Surgical consultation is recommended.

PARENTERAL NUTRITION

Peripheral parenteral nutrition (PPN): used in peripheral veins and therefore is limited to maximum dextrose concentration of 10% (in some circumstances, 12.5%) and osmolality less than 1000 mOsm/L. It is intended for nutritional support of less than 10 days' duration.

Central parenteral nutrition: used in central veins which allows for higher dextrose concentrations and greater than 1000 mOsm/L. It is used when the anticipated need is greater than 7 to 10 days.

Laboratory Studies
- *Initial laboratory studies* (within 48 hours of PN initiation): CBC, electrolytes, calcium, phosphorus, magnesium, triglycerides, alanine transaminase (ALT), gamma-glutamyl transferase (GGT), total and conjugated bilirubin, albumin, prealbumin. Severe abnormalities in electrolytes should be corrected before initiating PN.
- *Daily or every-other-day laboratory studies:* electrolytes, phosphorus, magnesium, calcium, and triglycerides until stable and at full kcal and protein goal
- *Weekly laboratory studies* (once stable): electrolytes, calcium, phosphorus, magnesium, triglycerides, cholesterol, ALT, GGT, albumin, prealbumin, total and conjugated bilirubin
- Long-term PN and minimal enteral nutrition: check vitamin status, trace elements, cholesterol, iron panel, CBC, and reticulocyte count

Parenteral Nutrition Components
- *Carbohydrates:* given as dextrose (glucose)
  - Calorie density: 3.4 kcal/g
  - Glucose infusion rate (GIR) (mg/kg/min): start with GIR of 5 mg/kg/min (infants) or 2 mg/kg/min (child):

$$GIR = (TPNF^* \times Dextrose\ Conc \times 1000\ mg/g)/(Wt\ (kg) \times 1440\ min/day)$$

*TPNF = total amount of parenteral nutrition fluids to be administered daily
(TPNF = total daily fluid requirement minus other enteral or nonnutritional parenteral fluids administered). Dextrose conc = 0.10 for 10% solution, 0.15 for 15% solution, etc.
  - Increase by 2.5% to 5.0% dextrose each day (max GIR: 12 mg/kg/min)
  - Monitor urine for glucose when PN is started and after changing GIR
  - Check serum glucose if positive glucosuria and reduce GIR as appropriate
- *Protein:* given as amino acids
  - Calorie density: 4 kcal/g
  - Initiate protein as per Table 20.6, then advance daily by 1.0 g/kg/day to goal.
- *Fat:* given as lipid (also known as intralipid or IL)
  - Calorie density: 2 kcal/mL of 20% solution (20 g/100 mL)
  - Minimum 3% to 5% total calories to prevent essential fatty acid deficiency
  - Initial rate of lipid administration: refer to Table 20.7 (unless contraindicated), then advance daily by 1.0 g/kg/day to goal.
  - Volume of lipid solution needed is calculated as follows:

$$Weight\ (kg) \times desired\ grams\ IL/kg\ per\ day \times 100\ mL/20\ g\ IL = mL\ of\ 20\%\ IL$$

  - Lipid should generally not exceed 3.0 g/kg/day or 50% of total daily calories (infants max: 60%).
  - Consider reducing lipid if triglyceride level is greater than 400–500 mg/dL in children and adolescents and greater than 200–250 mg/dL in infants. Carnitene may be added to improve lipid tolerance.
- *Minerals and electrolytes:* refer to Tables 20.8 and 20.9

Table 20.6: Protein Requirements for Parenteral Nutrition

Weight	Initiate Protein (g/kg/day)	Goal Protein (g/kg/day)
0–5 kg	2.0	3.0–3.5
5–20 kg	1.0–1.5	2.0–2.5
20–40 kg	1.0	2.0
>40 kg	0.8–1.0	2.0*

*A maximum of 150 g of protein/day is recommended.
(Reprinted with permission from the Children's Hospital of Philadelphia Formulary)

Table 20.7: Lipid Administration

Weight	Initiate Lipid (g/kg/day)	Goal Lipid (g/kg/day)
0–5 kg	1.0–2.0	3.0
5–20 kg	1.0–1.5	1.5–2.0
20–40 kg	1.0–1.5	1.5–2.0
>40 kg	0.5–1.0	0.5–1.0

(Reprinted with permission from the Children's Hospital of Philadelphia Formulary)

Table 20.8: Parenteral Nutrition Mineral Requirements

Element	Dose < 5 kg	Dose 5–40 kg	Dose > 40 kg	Maximum
Chromium	0.2 µg/kg	0.2 µg/kg	8 µg	15 µg
Copper	20 µg/kg	20 µg/kg	800 µg	1500 µg
Manganese	1 µg/kg	1 µg/kg	40 µg	150 µg
Selenium	2 µg/kg	2 µg/kg	80 µg	120 µg
Zinc	400 µg/kg	125 µg/kg	5000 µg	16,000 µg

(Reprinted with permission from the Children's Hospital of Philadelphia Formulary)

Parenteral Energy Intake
- 10% to 20% lower than estimated enteral needs due to reduced energy cost for digestion/absorption (see estimating nutritional needs earlier in chapter)
- Guidelines: carbohydrates, 45% to 60%; protein, 8% to 15%; fat, 25% to 50%

Special Circumstances: Parenteral Nutrition Cycle Regimen
- The infusion rate of PN solutions with greater than 10% dextrose should be decreased by 50% during the last hour of the infusion to prevent rebound hypoglycemia.
- Cycling is used in long-term PN patients. In infants weighing more than 3 kg, PN may be cycled if the patient is receiving continuous feeds to avoid hypoglycemia.
- Decreasing the administration time from 24 hours to 8 to 18 hours allows more normal daily activity and may help lower the risk of PN-associated steatosis.

Table 20.9: Parenteral Nutrition Electrolyte Requirements

	Full–term Infants 0–5 kg mEq/kg/day	Children 5–20 kg mEq/kg/day	20–40 kg mEq/kg/day	Adolescents/Adults > 40 kg mEq/day
Acetate	PRN*	PRN*	PRN*	PRN*
Ca²⁺	1.0–4.0	0.5–1.0	10–25†	10–20
Cl⁻	2.0–5.0	2.0–5.0	2.0–3.0	80–150
Mg	0.3–0.5	0.3–0.5	0.3–0.5	10–30
Phos	2.0–4.0	1.0–2.0	1.0–1.5	30–60
K⁺	2.0–4.0	2.0–3.0	1.5–2.5	40–60
Na⁺	2.0–5.0	2.0–6.0	2.0–3.0	80–150

*As needed for acidosis.
†mEq/d for Ca^{2+} in this age group.
(Reprinted with permission from the Children's Hospital of Philadelphia Formulary)

CHOP Committee of Dieticians

Brenda Waber, RD, CSP, CNSD, LDN, Colleen Yanni, MS, RD, Kristin Andolaro, RD, LDN, Jessica Arvay, RD, LDN, Susan Boyden, MS, RD, LDN, Darla Bradshaw, RD, LDN, CNSD, Cagla Bulgun, RD, LDN, Lori Enriquez, RD, CSP, CNSD, Christy Franz, RD, Rachelle Lessen, MS, RD, IBCLC, Nancy Moore, RD, LDN, Monica Nagle, RD, CNSD, LDN, Jennifer Ranalli, RD, Rebecca Thomas, RD, Michelle Verona Williams, MS, RD, CNSD, Samantha Zucker, RD, LDN, CNSD, CDE

Resources

Baker RD, Baker SS, Davis AM. Pediatric Parenteral Nutrition. New York: Chapman & Hall, 1997.

Conkin C, Gilger M, Jennings H, et al., eds. The Baylor Pediatric Nutrition Handbook for Residents. 2nd ed. Houston: Baylor College of Medicine, 2001.

Davis A. Pediatrics. In: Contemporary Nutrition Support Practice. 2nd ed. Philadelphia: W.B. Saunders, 2003:347–364.

Dietary Reference Intakes for Energy, Carbohydrate, Fiber, Fat, Fatty Acids, Cholesterol, Protein, and Amino Acids (macronutrients). Washington DC: National Academy Press, 2002:358.

Fomon SJ, Haschke F, Ziegler EE, Nelson SE. Body composition of reference children ages birth to 10 years. Am J Clin Nutr 1982;35:1169–1175.

Gottschlich MM, Fuhrman MP, Hammond KA, et al. The Science and Practice of Nutrition Support—A Case-Based Core Curriculum. Dubuque, IA: Kendall/Hunt, 2001.

Hendricks KM, Duggan C, Walker WA. Manual of Pediatric Nutrition. 3rd ed. Hamilton, Ontario: BC Decker, 2000.

Institute of Medicine of the National Academies. Dietary Reference Intakes for RDA. 10th ed. National Academy of Sciences. Washington DC: National Academy Press, 1989:33–36.

Jew RK, Mascarenhas M, Thorpe J, Manning ML. Pharmacy Handbook and Formulary—The Children's Hospital of Philadelphia. Hudson, Ohio: Lexi-Comp, 2001.

Registered Dietitians, Department of Clinical Nutrition, Children's Hospital, Columbus, Ohio. Infant Formulas and Selected Nutritional Supplements. Columbus: Children's Hospital, 1999.

Samour, PQ, Helm KK, Lang CE. Handbook of Pediatric Nutrition, 2nd ed. Gaithersburg, MD: Aspen Publishers, 1999.

World Health Organization. Energy and Protein Requirements. WHO Technical Report Series. No. 724. Geneva Switzerland: World Health Organization, 1985.

Malignancies

ABDOMINAL MASSES
A. WILMS' TUMOR

Wilms' tumor or nephroblastoma, the most common pediatric primary renal tumor, is a malignant tumor of renal precursor cells.

Epidemiology
- There are 460 cases/year in the United States (~5% of childhood cancer)
- Mean age is 42 months for unilateral tumors and 30 months for bilateral tumors with 80% diagnosed by age 5 years
- Associated anomalies can include aniridia, hemihypertrophy, cryptorchidism, and hypospadias.
- Associated syndromes can include Beckwith-Wiedemann (macroglossia, omphalocele, genitourinary [GU] anomalies, hemihypertrophy and exophthalmos; see Genetics chapter), Denys-Drash syndrome (degenerative kidney disease and pseudohermaphroditism), WAGR syndrome (sporadic Wilms', aniridia, GU anomalies, and retardation), and Perlman syndrome (unusual facies, islet cell hypertrophy, macrosomia, and hamartomas).

Etiology
- Hypothesized to result from functional loss of tumor suppressor genes
- Two-hit hypothesis proposed in 1970s:
  - First genetic mutational event can be pre-zygotic: if so, the tumor could be hereditary and those individuals are at risk for the development of more than one tumor because all cells have had this event. Only one more event is required for tumor development.
  - For sporadic or non-inherited tumors: results from two independent, somatic mutations in one cell. If so, these patients are *unlikely* to develop more than 1 tumor.
- Genetic regions involved in Wilms' tumor development have been identified on chromosome 11p13 (WT1 and WT2).

Clinical Manifestations
- Most common: asymptomatic flank mass often noticed by family member bathing the child
- Also can present with pain, gross hematuria, and fever
- Microscopic hematuria in one third of patients
- Hypertension in 25% of patients
- Tumor hemorrhage and resultant anemia in 10%
- Varicoceles can be seen in males with spermatic vein compression
- von Willebrand disease in 8%
- Metastases at presentation in 10% to 15%
- Note any signs of syndromes associated with Wilms' tumor including aniridia, facial abnormalities of Beckwith-Wiedemann syndrome, hemihypertrophy, or GU anomalies (see Genetics chapter)
- Most common patterns of spread: penetration through the renal capsule, extension into adjacent vasculature including the inferior vena cava, regional nodes, lungs and liver; clear cell variant to bones and brain

Diagnostics
- Laboratory evaluation: CBC, renal and liver function testing, and urinalysis

- Abdominal ultrasound: evaluates tumor texture, origin, size and excludes vascular tumor invasion by vena caval blood flow
- Abdominal CT scan to assess tumor invasion of adjacent structures
- Chest x-ray: exclude pulmonary metastases (controversial whether abnormalities seen on chest CT but not on chest x-ray are truly metastatic disease)
- If clear cell sarcoma or rhabdoid tumor of the kidney (not a true Wilms' tumor), obtain bone scan, skeletal survey, and MRI of head postoperatively
- Favorable prognosis: small tumor size, patient age less than 2 years, favorable histology, no lymph node metastases or capsular/vascular invasion

Management

If tumor histology demonstrates anaplasia, clear cell sarcoma of the kidney, or rhabdoid tumor, the treatment may differ significantly.

Surgical
- Removal of the primary tumor without rupture through an anterior approach
- If unable to remove the whole tumor safely (massive size or intravascular invasion), biopsy only
- Thorough abdominal exploration and accurate assessment of tumor spread for staging, including the contralateral kidney

Chemotherapy for Favorable Histology Tumors
- Stage I (tumor limited to kidney and completely excised): Dactinomycin/vincristine for 6 months
- Stage II (regional tumor extension, but completely resected): Dactinomycin/vincristine for 6 months
- Stage III (residual tumor present, but confined to the abdomen): Dactinomycin/vincristine/ doxorubicin for 6 months and radiation therapy as outlined subsequently.
- Stage IV (metastatic disease): as stage III
- Stage V (bilateral disease): special considerations depending on extent of disease in each kidney

Radiation
- Stage III: Radiation to tumor bed, extending across vertebral column to avoid scoliosis
- Stage III as a result of peritoneal spill: whole abdominal XRT
- Stage IV: Radiation to primary disease site (only if stage III and to lung, liver, or other metastases)

ABDOMINAL MASSES
B. NEUROBLASTOMA

A malignant tumor derived from neural crest cells that can be found anywhere along the sympathetic chain, including the adrenal medulla. Variations in location and histologic differentiation result in a wide range of biologic and clinical characteristics. The International Neuroblastoma Staging System (INSS) classification system is used for staging:

Stage 1: Localized disease with complete resection
Stage 2A: Localized disease with gross residual disease
Stage 2B: Localized disease with ipsilateral nodes
Stage 3: Invasion across the midline (directly or via nodal extension)
Stage 4: Disseminated disease
Stage 4S: Distinct stage with favorable outcome: localized tumor (1, 2A, 2B) with dissemination to skin, liver, or bone marrow in patients younger than 1 year of age

Epidemiology
- Neuroblastoma (NBL) is the most common extracranial solid tumor in children and the most common malignancy of infancy (8% to 10% of all childhood cancer).
- There are 600 new cases/year in the United States.
- At diagnosis, 90% of patients are younger than 5 years old; median age is 17 months.

Etiology
- Genetic: associated with Hirschsprung disease, central hypoventilation, and neurofibromatosis-1 (NF-1) in sporadic and familial cases suggestive of a global neural crest disorder (neuro-cristopathy); familial in 1% to 2% (autosomal dominant)

Clinical Manifestations
- Can occur at any site along the sympathetic chain:
  - Abdominal (65%); adrenal (40%); paraspinal (25%)
  - Adrenal more common in children
  - Thoracic and cervical more common in infants
  - Metastases: regional nodes, bone marrow, bone, liver, skin and, rarely, lung and brain
- High thoracic and cervical tumors may present with Horner syndrome (ptosis, myosis, anhidrosis).
- Any paraspinal mass can present with nerve/spinal cord compression.
- Classic signs and symptoms include fever, weight loss, limp, periorbital ecchymosis/proptosis, bone pain or irritability in infants, pancytopenia.
- Can present with hypertension more often secondary to renal vascular compression rather than catecholamine release.
- Infants can present with skin involvement (stage 4S) with bluish, non-tender subcutaneous nodules.
- Uncommon, but unique paraneoplastic manifestations include:
  - Opsomyoclonous (myoclonic jerking and random eye movement) or cerebellar ataxia presumed to be secondary to anti-neural antibodies
  - Intractable, secretory diarrhea associated with vasoactive intestinal peptide (VIP) secretion

Diagnostics
- CBC with differential, electrolyte panel, LFTs, ferritin, and lactate dehydrogenase (LDH)
- Minimal criteria for establishing a diagnosis of neuroblastoma include:
  - Bone marrow involved with tumor AND increased urine VMA/HVA
        OR
  - Tumor tissue biopsy with NBL +/− increased urine catecholamines
- Urine VMA and HVA (elevated in 90% to 95%)
- Bone marrow aspirate and biopsy (bilateral)
- Tissue biopsy for histology, DNA ploidy, and MYCN analysis
- CT scan of chest/abdomen/pelvis, bone scan, MIBG scan

Management
Surgical
- At diagnosis: to determine resectability and avoid sacrifice of vital structures. If not resectable, biopsy only. Sample regional nodes and areas of gross or radiologic evidence of metastases (i.e., liver)
- For local control: used for tumor resection after chemotherapy if not resectable at time of diagnosis.

Radiation
- Used in neonates with stage 4S disease and respiratory distress secondary to hepatospleno-megaly when chemotherapy is unsuccessful
- Used at varying times for patients with locoregional disease for local control
- Used in conjunction with stem cell transplant or palliation of bone disease

Chemotherapy
Main therapeutic modality for intermediate and high-risk patients

General Treatment (risk-related therapy)
- *Low risk*: (all stage 1 patients, all stage 2 except younger than 1 year with unfavorable patho-logic and biologic characteristics, stage 4S with favorable pathologic/biologic characteristics)
  - Surgical removal
  - If 4S: biopsy and observe unless respiratory distress

- *Intermediate risk*: (stage 3 infants with favorable biology, stage 3 patients >1 year of age with favorable pathology/biology, stage 4 infants with favorable biology)
  - Moderate intensity chemotherapy
  - Avoid radical surgery and radiation therapy for majority of patients
- *High risk*: (stage 4 patients >1 year, stage 3 with unfavorable pathology/biology, stage 2 with unfavorable pathology/biology, stage 4S with unfavorable biology)
  - Induction therapy with multiple cycles of intensive, combination chemotherapy
  - Local control with surgery with or without radiation therapy
  - Consolidation with autologous stem cell transplantation
  - Maintenance therapy for minimal residual disease (13-cis retinoic acid)

Prognostic Factors
- Age greater than 2 years and increased stage are the most important factors predictive of unfavorable disease outcome.
- Pathologic: undifferentiated tumors with high mitotic rate (unfavorable)
- Serum: elevated serum markers including neuron-specific enolase (NSE), LDH, and ganglioside GD_2 have prognostic value in some patients.
- Genetic: MYCN amplification (unfavorable), hyperdiploid (favorable), chromosomal deletion of allelic loss (unfavorable) and other biologic markers have been proposed as prognostic markers.

BONE TUMORS

Osteosarcoma (OS) is a malignant bone tumor arising from mesenchymal cells. It is unique in its production of immature bone (osteoid) by cell stroma.

Ewing sarcoma (ES) is part of a family of tumors comprising a histologic spectrum ranging from undifferentiated small round blue cells to differentiated cells resembling peripheral neuroectodermal tissue (PNETs).

Epidemiology
See Table 21.1.

Clinical Manifestations
- Pain over involved site with or without associated soft tissue mass
- Can have erythema, warmth, or swelling that mimics infection
- Can result in pathologic fracture
- Average duration of pain is 3 to 6 months.
- If paraspinal in location (ES), can present with symptoms of back pain or cord compression
- Constitutional symptoms are more common in ES (fever, weight loss).
- Metastases:
  - Osteosarcoma: 15% to 20% at diagnosis (lung, bone most common)
  - Ewing's sarcoma: 20% at diagnosis (lung, bone, marrow, which are more common in those with central location ES vs. extremity)

Diagnostics
Osteosarcoma
- History and physical exam
- Laboratory studies are often not helpful.
- Plain x-ray: characteristic findings include periosteal new bone formation with the formation of Codman's triangle, soft tissue mass, and/or soft tissue ossification.
- MRI for primary tumor site
- Evaluation for metastatic disease: chest CT and bone scan
- Note: open biopsy should be performed by an experienced orthopedic surgeon (ideally should be the surgeon who will perform later definitive surgery). Incision and technique are extremely important and can affect the subsequent surgery as well as the patient's prognosis if not performed properly.

Table 21.1: Epidemiology of Osteosarcoma and Ewing Sarcoma

Characteristic	Osteosarcoma	Ewing Sarcoma
Incidence	6th most common childhood cancer and most common bone cancer; 2500 cases/year in United States	1% of all childhood cancers; one-third of all pediatric bone cancers
Race	Slightly more common in white patients	More common in white patients
Gender	Males > females	Males > females
Age	Peak during adolescent growth spurt	Most common in the second decade of life, but does occur in young children
Primary location	Metaphysis of long bones: distal femur, proximal tibia, proximal humerus	Evenly split between extremities (midshaft diaphyseal long bones) and central axis (pelvis, ribs, vertebrae)
Genetics	Increased risk in patients with retinoblastoma both with and without prior radiation therapy, role of p53 mutation, Li-Fraumeni familial cancer syndrome	t(11;22) translocation in 88%–95% of tumors
Environmental	Ionizing radiation, alkylating agents, Paget's disease	
Viral	Unknown	
Other	Patients are taller than their peers	Not commonly associated with other congenital diseases of childhood

Ewing Sarcoma
- History and physical exam
- Laboratory studies including CBC and chemistries
- Plain x-ray: usually reveals a destructive diaphyseal bone lesion sometimes accompanied by periosteal reaction; may note associated soft tissue mass
- CT or MRI of primary site
- Evaluation for metastatic disease: chest CT, bone scan, bone marrow evaluation including bilateral aspirates and biopsies

Prognostic Factors
- Osteosarcoma: extent of disease at diagnosis (metastatic disease unfavorable), OS in association with Paget disease (unfavorable), location of disease (axial skeleton unfavorable as more difficult resection), tumor size (>15 cm unfavorable), young age (<10 years unfavorable), gender (males unfavorable), response of tumor to chemotherapy (<90% necrosis at time of surgery unfavorable)
- Ewing sarcoma: most important adverse prognostic factor is the presence of metastatic disease on imaging at diagnosis. Other factors include primary site of disease (pelvis unfavorable), larger tumor size (unfavorable), initial poor response to therapy (unfavorable) and age (older age unfavorable).

Management
Osteosarcoma
- *Presurgical chemotherapy:* allows evaluation of tumor responsiveness to chemotherapy in a uniform manner, eradication of micrometastases early instead of waiting until post-operative recovery and demonstrated improvement in outcome. It is usually given for 2 to 3 months before definitive surgery. First line agents include cisplatin, doxorubicin, and high-dose methotrexate. Chemotherapy is continued after recovery from the surgical procedure.
- *Surgery:* removal of all gross and microscopic tumor is essential to prevent local recurrence. Surgical procedures include either amputation or limb-salvage procedures (allografts, vascularized grafts, endoprostheses, rotationplasty). The type of surgical procedure depends on tumor location, size, presence of metastatic disease, age, skeletal development, lifestyle preference, and desired activities.
- *Radiation therapy:* not used because OS is unresponsive to radiation

Ewing Sarcoma
- *General:* every patient is assumed to have micrometastatic disease at diagnosis and the primary treatment involves combination chemotherapy. Goal is to decrease primary tumor volume for both eventual local control and immediate control of micrometastatic disease. First line agents include vincristine, Adriamycin, cyclophosphamide, ifosfamide, and etoposide.
- *Local control:* both surgery and radiation therapy are used for primary tumor control. The approach depends on the site (whether bone is expendable such as the fibula) and whether radiation would cause significant growth or functional difficulty. Each potential site of disease is associated with varied options for surgery and radiotherapy. Final decision balances the need for complete tumor eradication with the goal of maintaining function.

BRAIN TUMORS

Epidemiology
- Second most common group of all pediatric malignancies (~20% of total)
- Incidence peaks in first decade
- Male predominance
- Supratentorial tumors are most common in patients younger than 1 year and older than 11 years.
- Infratentorial tumors are more common in patients 1 to 11 years of age.
- Embryonal histology is more common in children (medulloblastoma, PNETs, pineoblastoma); high-grade tumors (glioblastoma multiforme) are less common
- Conditions that place children at increased risk include:
  - Genetic disorders (<10% of cases): NF-1, NF-2, tuberous sclerosis, von Hippel-Lindau, Turcot syndrome, Gorlin syndrome, Li-Fraumeni syndrome
  - Ionizing radiation: patients with history of CNS radiation for leukemia or total body irradiation with stem cell transplantation
  - Immunosuppression: higher risk of CNS lymphoma in Wiskott-Aldrich syndrome, ataxia-telangiectasia, AIDS and solid organ transplant patients
- Relative frequency of pediatric brain tumors: low grade supratentorial astrocytoma (22%); brainstem glioma (17%); medulloblastoma (PNET) (14%); other gliomas (14%); high grade supratentorial astrocytoma (14%); craniopharyngioma (8%); ependymoma (8%); rhabdoid tumor (2%)

Clinical Manifestations
- *Supratentorial* (cerebrum, basal ganglia, thalamus/hypothalamus, pituitary pineal, optic): increased intracranial pressure (ICP) (seizures, visual loss, hemiparesis, headache, emesis); new need for glasses; difficulty in school; behavioral difficulty, personality changes; failure to thrive; change in dominant hand; diencephalic syndrome (failure to thrive with increasing appetite and good mood); endocrinopathies such as diabetes insipidus, short stature; Parinaud's syndrome (paralyzed upward gaze, absent pupillary light reflex and convergence nystagmus)

- *Infratentorial (cerebellum, brainstem):* ataxia, clumsiness, worsening handwriting, dysarthria; nystagmus; head tilt; cranial nerve palsy; increased ICP from ventricular compression; morning vomiting without nausea; extreme vomiting if near area postrema
- *Nonspecific signs and symptoms:* change in activity level, change in appetite with associated weight gain or loss, delayed or precocious puberty, macrocephaly in infants, vomiting, complaints consistent with spinal cord involvement such as back pain or bowel/bladder dysfunction (see Oncologic Emergencies section)

Diagnostics
- CT scan of brain with and without contrast (especially in unstable patients)
- Brain MRI with gadolinium
- Spinal MRI to evaluate for drop metastases
- Newer modalities include magnetic resonance spectroscopy (MRS) and positron emission tomography (PET), but are not uniformly used.
- Lumbar puncture (only after scan and evaluation for increased intracranial pressure) for glucose, protein, culture, cytology, and markers such as α-fetoprotein and β-HCG

Management
- Initial care may involve management of increased intracranial pressure (see Neurology chapter), respiratory or cardiovascular stabilization, and involvement of neurosurgical and critical care services.
- Therapy for the tumor usually consists of a combination of surgery, chemotherapy and radiation (which may be delayed in children younger than 5 years). An ideal approach includes an experienced, multidisciplinary team including a pediatric neurosurgeon, oncologist, radiation oncologist, neurocognitive specialist, endocrinologist, and neuro-ophthalmologist.
- *Surgery:* balance between preservation of function and maximization of tumor removal. For some tumors (JPA), surgery alone is adequate therapy. Diffuse tumors are not amenable to resection, but biopsy and identification of the tumor are often critical and may be achieved using CT- or MRI-guided stereotactic surgical techniques.
- *Chemotherapy:* used in combination and specific to tumor type. Active agents include alkylating agents (cyclophosphamide, ifosfamide, thiotepa, BCNU, cisplatin, carboplatin, and temozolamide), antimetabolites (methotrexate, cytarabine), and plant alkaloids (vincristine, etoposide). For aggressive or recurrent tumors, high-dose (marrow ablative) chemotherapy with stem cell rescue has been used.
- *Radiation therapy:* goal is to increase radiation dose to the target while sparing surrounding cells. Techniques include conformal therapy, intensity modulation, dosing, and fractionation. Proton beam therapy is being used increasingly in children for its precise targeting and fewer side effects. Age, comorbidities, and balance of early and late toxicity must be considered.

LEUKEMIA

Predominance of immature hematopoietic precursors classified according to cell lineage as lymphocytic (ALL) or myelogenous (AML)

Epidemiology/Etiology
See Table 21.2.

Clinical Manifestations
See Table 21.3.

Diagnostics
- CBC with differential and review of peripheral smear to evaluate for blasts
- Bone marrow aspirate and biopsy (send for morphology, immunophenotype, cytogenetics)
- Complete metabolic panel, LDH, uric acid, calcium, magnesium, phosphorus
- Coagulation studies to exclude disseminated intravascular coagulation (DIC)
- Blood, urine, and viral cultures if infection is suspected
- Chest x-ray (PA and lateral) to evaluate for mediastinal mass

Table 21.2: Epidemiology of Acute Lymphocytic and Acute Myelogenous Leukemia

Characteristic	ALL	AML
Incidence	2500–3000 cases/year (75%)	350–500 cases/year (15%–20%)
Peak age	4 yr	Increased in adolescence
Race	White > African American	Equal (APML more common in Hispanic population)
Gender	Male > Female	Equal
Genetics	Trisomy 21, Bloom syndrome, Fanconi anemia, ataxia-telangiectasia, Schwachmann's syndrome, neurofibromatosis, twins, siblings at increased risk	Trisomy 21 (AML much more likely < 3 yr), Bloom syndrome, Fanconi anemia, ataxia telangiectasia, Kostmann's syndrome, NF-1, Diamond-Blackfan syndrome, Li Fraumeni
Noninherited		Aplastic anemia, MDS, PNH
Pathogenesis		
• Environment	Ionizing radiation	Ionizing radiation, benzene, epidophyllotoxins, alkylating agents (nitrogen mustard, melphalan, cyclophosphamide)
• Viral	EBV and L3 ALL	None
• Immuno-deficiency	Wiskott-Aldrich, congenital hypogammaglobulinemia, ataxia telangiectasia	

- Viral titers for varicella zoster virus
- Echocardiogram with pulmonary function testing if mediastinal mass
- Lumbar puncture to evaluate for CNS disease: be wary of this procedure in any patient with severe thrombocytopenia or coagulation abnormalities.
- No patient with a mediastinal mass should undergo sedation for a diagnostic procedure until they are evaluated by echocardiography, pulmonary function tests (if necessary), and anesthesiology.

Management (ALL)
- Alkalinization (see Management of Tumor Lysis Syndrome)
- Allopurinol and close monitoring for tumor lysis syndrome especially in T cell acute lymphocytic leukemia (ALL), patients with a mediastinal mass, high white blood cell (WBC) count, or evidence on physical exam of high tumor burden (see Oncologic Emergencies section)
- Evaluation for occult infection and coverage with broad-spectrum antibiotics if presence of fever (see Oncologic Emergencies section)
- Hyperleukocytosis occurs in 9% to 13% of patients; most common with ALL, T cell ALL with a mediastinal mass and hypodiploid ALL. It may require pheresis if WBC greater than 300,000 to 400,000/mm^3. Observe patient for mental status changes, headache, blurry vision, dizziness, seizures, stroke, cerebral hemorrhage, retinal vessel distention, dyspnea, hypoxia, priapism, or acidosis secondary to hyperviscosity in regional vessels. Packed red blood cell (RBC) transfusions lead to increased viscosity and, therefore, should be avoided when possible (goal to keep hemoglobin less than 10 g/dL). Transfuse platelets if less than 20,000/mm^3 to prevent hemorrhage.

Table 21.3: Comparison of the Clinical Presentation of Acute Lymphocytic and Acute Myelogenous Leukemia

Characteristic	ALL	AML
Marrow failure: • Anemia (g/dL)	Hb < 7 (43%) Hb 7–11 (45%) Hb > 11 (12%)	Hb < 9 (50%)
• Thrombocytopenia (per mm^3)	Plt < 20,000 (20%) Plt 21,000–99,000 (47%) Plt > 100,000 (25%)	Plt < 100,000 (75%)
• Neutropenia (per mm^3)	WBC < 10,000 (53%) WBC 10,000–49,000 (30%) WBC > 50,000 (17%)	WBC > 100,000 (20%)
Fever	60%	30%–40%
Mediastinal mass	10% (mostly in T cell)	
Central nervous system involvement	5%	2%
Chloromas		Common in M4, M5 subtype Common in periorbital area
Testicular involvement	2%–5%	Rare
Disseminated intravascular coagulation		Common especially in APML
Bone pain	20%	20%
Hepatosplenomegaly	60%–65%	50%
Other		Leukemia cutis (10%) • Neonates • Blueberry muffin spots Gingival hypertrophy (15%)

- Therapy (ALL)
  - *Induction:* goal is to induce remission; first 28 days of therapy; remission in 95%; evaluate for disease response at day 7 +/– 14 as failure to achieve early response necessitates intensification of therapy; combination therapy with vincristine (VCR), steroids, intrathecal (IT) methotrexate (MTX) and asparaginase + daunomycin for high-risk patients.
  - *Consolidation:* goal is to consolidate remission and treat the CNS; intensified treatment after induction using non-cross reactive agents and continued IT chemotherapy; intensified therapy for high-risk patients
  - *Interim maintenance:* less intense therapy after induction/consolidation using VCR, 6MP, and MTX.
  - *Delayed intensification (DI):* repetition of induction/consolidation; shown to increase survival; current study evaluating the efficacy of 2 instead of 1 DI regimen for standard risk patients.
  - *Maintenance:* remainder of therapy with monthly IV VCR and steroid pulse, daily oral 6MP, weekly oral MTX, and IT MTX every 3 months.
  - *Radiation:* part of therapy for patients with CNS or testicular disease
  - Total length of therapy: slightly over 2 years for girls and 3 years for boys

Management (AML)
- Correct coagulation abnormalities and DIC.
- Hyperleukocytosis occurs in 5% to 22% of patients. Most common symptoms for patients with acute myelogenous leukemia (AML) are pulmonary leukostasis and CNS hemorrhage. Patients may require pheresis for hyperleukocytosis at a lower WBC count than for patients with ALL because AML cells are larger and stickier. Keep hemoglobin less than 10 g/dL because this increases blood viscosity. Transfuse platelets for less than 20,000/mm³ to prevent hemorrhage.
- Therapy (AML)
  - *Induction:* anthracycline (daunomycin, doxorubicin, mitoxantrone) with Ara-C +/– 6TG. Remission is seen in 70% to 85% of patients after induction. Therapy is profoundly immunosuppressive and patients are at significant risk for infection. Current study guidelines mandate that patients remain hospitalized until blood count recovery, which is usually 4 to 6 weeks.
  - *Bone marrow transplant:* if longer than 3 months of remission can be achieved, matched sibling bone marrow transplant is recommended, although only 40% of patients have a matched related donor. If no donor is available, patients continue on a standard chemotherapy regimen
  - *Special treatment and prognostic considerations given to acute promyelcytic leukemia (APML) and Down syndrome–associated AML:*
    — APML: treatment with anthracycline/cytarabine and all-trans retinoic acid (ATRA) with ~80% overall survival.
    — AML with Down syndrome: chemotherapy is given in a less intense manner with excellent overall survival.

Prognostic Features
- ALL: factors associated with a poor prognosis include age greater than 10 years or less than 1 year, WBC count greater than 50,000/mm³ at diagnosis, and failure to respond to induction therapy. Patients with T cell ALL require more intense therapy. Other factors include hypodiploidy or t(9;22), t(8;14), t(1;19), or t(4;11) translocations.
- AML: factors associated with a poor prognosis include WBC greater than 100,000/mm³, secondary AML/myelodysplastic syndrome, and monosomy 7. Other potential adverse factors include splenomegaly, FAB M4 or M5, and patients requiring more than one course for complete remission.

LYMPHOMA

Hodgkin disease (HD) (40%): pleomorphic lymphocytic invasion of the lymphoreticular system by malignant multinucleated giant cells (Reed-Sternberg cells)

Types: nodular sclerosing (40% to 70%); mixed cellularity (30%); lymphocyte predominant (10% to 15%); lymphocyte depleted (5%)

Non-Hodgkin lymphoma (NHL) (60%): collection of malignant cells deriving from the lymphoreticular system including all lymphomas not able to be classified as Hodgkin disease.

Types: Burkitt (50%); lymphoblastic (35%); large cell (15%)

Epidemiology/Etiology
See Table 21.4.

Clinical Manifestations
Hodgkin Disease
- Painless, rubbery, cervical lymphadenopathy is present in 80% of patients
- Mediastinal mass in 60% and more common in adolescents
- Systemic symptoms in 20% to 30% ("B" symptoms): unexplained fever greater than 38°C; weight loss (unintentional and greater than 10% of body weight over preceding 6 months); drenching night sweats
  - Other symptoms: anorexia, fatigue, pruritus

Table 21.4: Comparison of the Epidemiology and Etiology of Hodgkin Disease and Non-Hodgkin Lymphoma

Characteristic	Hodgkin Disease	Non-Hodgkin Lymphoma
Age	Bimodal: 20–30 and > 50 years; Developing countries: peak in adolescence	Incidence increases with age
Gender	Male > female	Male > female
Geographic	Types vary in developed and developing countries	Increased Burkitt's lymphoma in Africa
Genetics	Suggestive: siblings, twins	
Environment	Small sibship size, low-density housing, higher maternal education	No evidence
Viral	Associated with EBV	Associated with EBV
Immune	Ataxia telangiectasia, Wiskott-Aldrich, Bloom syndrome	Ataxia telangiectasia, Wiskott-Aldrich, Bloom syndrome, SCID, CVID, X-linked lymphoproliferative disease, HIV
Other	Immune dysregulation often present at diagnosis and after treatment is completed	

CVID, common variable immunodeficiency; EBV, Epstein-Barr virus; HIV, human immunodeficiency virus; SCID, severe combined immunodeficiency.

Non-Hodgkin Lymphoma
- Lymphoblastic: T cell lymphoma is most often associated with mediastinal mass (50% to 70%). B cell lymphoma often involves bone, isolated node, and skin. Super vena cava syndrome can be associated.
- Burkitt's: often rapidly growing and can be associated with tumor lysis syndrome
  - Sporadic: abdominal tumors associated with nausea/vomiting or intussusception. Other locations include tonsils, bone marrow (20%), and CNS (uncommon)
  - Endemic: locations include jaw, orbit, maxilla
- Anaplastic large cell lymphoma: slowly progressive disease with fever and weight loss. Common involvement includes nodes, skin, and bone. Bone marrow and CNS involvement is rare.

Diagnostics
- CBC with differential, ESR, direct agglutination test if anemia (autoimmune cytopenias associated with HD)
- Comprehensive metabolic panel, magnesium, phosphorus
- Lactate dehydrogenase, uric acid, alkaline phosphatase, ferritin
- Chest x-ray to rule out mediastinal involvement before anesthesia for biopsy
- Biopsy of accessible node or mass after anesthesia clearance and evaluation of cardiac and pulmonary function
- Bone marrow aspirate and biopsy with flow cytometry, cell markers/immunophenotyping, and cytogenetics. Only perform in patients with HD if "B" symptoms or bony pain.

- CT scan of the neck, chest, abdomen, and pelvis. Gallium or PET scan if available. Bone scan only in HD if symptoms of bone pain.
- Lumbar puncture for cytology in NHL; not part of staging for HD

Management

Hodgkin Disease

- Risk-adapted therapy to decrease late effects while maintaining efficacy.
  - Favorable presentation: absence of "B" symptoms and bulky, mediastinal adenopathy
  - Unfavorable presentation: presence of "B" symptoms, bulky mediastinal or peripheral adenopathy, high stage (IIIB, IV) disease
- Radiation therapy: used in involved fields for the majority of children with HD. Decisions are based on patient age, tumor burden, and potential for late effects.
- Chemotherapy: use of non-cross reactive drugs with non-overlapping toxicities. Multiple combinations are used; intensity depends upon risk group

Non-Hodgkin Lymphoma

- Burkitt: chemotherapy is the mainstay of treatment, unless tumor is localized and complete surgical resection is possible. Therapy is intense and given over a short period of time (4 to 6 months) using drugs including cyclophosphamide, prednisone, vincristine, methotrexate, cytarabine, doxorubicin, and etoposide. Patients with CNS involvement are known to have a poorer prognosis.
- Lymphoblastic: combination chemotherapy is used and is quite similar to ALL therapy as the diseases are immunophenotypically similar, but with a different distribution of disease (nodal vs. marrow)
- Anaplastic large cell lymphoma: combination chemotherapy is used and many regimens have demonstrated success. Children are most commonly treated on B cell lymphoma protocols.

Late Effects of Treatment of Hodgkin Disease

- Secondary malignant neoplasms (SMN): breast cancer is most common; others include thyroid, gastric, colon, and AML
- Cardiac toxicity secondary to radiation therapy and anthracyclines
- Pulmonary toxicity secondary to radiation therapy and bleomycin
- Infertility in males secondary to alkylating agents
- Premature ovarian failure in females
- Thyroid dysfunction as a result of radiation therapy
- Musculoskeletal effects of radiation therapy: thoracic soft tissues and vertebral bodies

RHABDOMYOSARCOMA

Tumor derived from primitive mesenchyme that may develop into muscle, fat, fibrous tissue, bone, or cartilage. Two staging systems are used:

- Clinical group system that depends upon extent of disease and surgical result (e.g., gross total resection vs. microscopic residual disease vs. gross residual disease)
- TNM staging system, which depends on site of involvement (some favorable and others unfavorable), size and extension of tumor, nodal involvement, and presence of metastatic disease

Epidemiology

- Third most common extracranial neoplasm
- In the United States, 250 new cases/year
- Males affected more often than females
- Two thirds of cases in children younger than 6 years of age
- Sites of involvement vary by age:
  - Infants may present with the botryoid variant growing like a cluster of grapes in a hollow structure like the vagina or bladder.
  - Children younger than 8 years present with orbital, head, and neck tumors.
  - Adolescents tend to present with extremity lesions.

- Associations: Li-Fraumeni syndrome, NF-1, adrenocortical cancers, breast cancer syndromes, and Beckwith-Wiedemann syndrome
- Maternal use of marijuana or cocaine has been shown to have a three and five times increased risk, respectively, of progeny rhabdomyosarcoma (RMS)
- Types of rhabdomyosarcoma (RMS): embryonal (>50%); alveolar (21%); botryoidal (6%); undifferentiated (8%)

Pathophysiology
- Embryonal RMS: often show loss of heterozygosity at chromosome 11p15
- Alveolar RMS: 70% with characteristic translocation t(2;13). This fusion product is important in regulating transcription in early neuromuscular development

Clinical Manifestations
- Most common presentations:
  - Mass lesion without a prior history of associated trauma
  - Disturbance in normal function due to mass effect
- Metastatic disease:
  - Present in less than 25% at the time of diagnosis
  - Most common sites: lymph node, lung, bone marrow, bone, brain
- Head and neck RMS: 25% in orbit, 50% parameningeal and 25% in either scalp, face, buccal mucosa, oropharynx, neck. Presenting symptoms depend on location and may include proptosis, ophthalmoplegia, visual disturbances, or chronic sinus obstruction. If intracranial growth of a skull base tumor occurs, RMS may result in headache/vomiting.
- Genitourinary RMS most commonly involves bladder or prostate gland. Presenting symptoms include dysuria, hematuria, pain, obstruction of the urinary outflow tract, or constipation. Testicular RMS often presents with painless unilateral enlargement. Genitourinary RMS is most often embryonal.
- Extremity RMS is most commonly associated with pain, tenderness, and erythema of the affected limb, and most are alveolar.
- Less common sites: biliary tract, perineal, perianal, intrathoracic and retroperitoneal areas

Diagnostics
- History and physical exam
- Imaging of primary site: can include ultrasound, CT, or MRI (especially for head, neck, pelvic, and extremity tumors)
- Biopsy and resection without mutilation when possible
- CBC with differential, comprehensive metabolic panel including renal function and liver function testing
- Evaluation for metastases: CT chest, bone marrow aspirate and biopsy, bone scan

Management
Treatment involves surgical removal (if possible), radiation therapy for local control of the primary tumor and chemotherapy for decreasing gross disease and micrometastases:
- *Surgery:* always use unless impaired function or cosmetic result. Aggressive surgery or wide excision should not be used in the female genital tract, orbit, bladder, or biliary tract.
- *Radiation therapy:* dose, fractionation, and therapy for certain tumor locations (orbit/cranial tumors) are variable and controversial. In general, radiation therapy should be given for patients with large tumors, alveolar/undifferentiated histology and in sites other than the genitourinary tract.
- *Chemotherapy:* combination depends upon patient risk that is determined by combinations of the prognostic factors listed above. Most commonly used agents include vincristine, actinomycin D, cyclophosphamide, ifosfamide, and etoposide.
- *Favorable prognostic factors:*
  - Absence of metastatic disease
  - Site: favorable sites include orbit, eyelid, other non-parameningeal head/neck, and non-bladder/nonprostate GU locations.
  - Surgical resectability: complete excision is favorable.

- Histology (embryonal vs. alveolar): embryonal is most often favorable
- Age: age less than 10 years tends to be more favorable.
- Response to treatment: those without an early and complete response do not survive.

Oncologic Emergencies

FEVER AND NEUTROPENIA

Fever: a single temperature taken orally that is greater than 38.5°C or three temperatures greater than 38.0°C in a 24-hour period.

Neutropenia: an absolute neutrophil count (ANC) less than 500 cells/mm³ or less than 1000 cells/mm³ and falling.

Epidemiology
- Cancer and the immunocompromised host:
  - Cancer can increase infectious risk by inherent immunosuppression (leukemia) or by a mass creating obstruction of an organ (bladder, biliary tree, etc.) and subsequent development of infection.
  - Therapy disrupts normal barriers to infection including myelosuppression, disruption of the mucosal epithelium, local tissue breakdown, skin disruption, and the presence of foreign bodies such as a central venous catheter.
- Many febrile, neutropenic patients have an occult infection.
- When pathogens are documented, bacteria are the most common (85% to 90%).
- Infections with fungi are most common in patients exposed to chronic broad-spectrum antibiotics or with prolonged neutropenia.
- High risk features: inpatient at the time of diagnosis, uncontrolled cancer, comorbidities (hypotension, tachypnea, hypoxemia, mucositis), prolonged neutropenia (>5 days), higher fever, lower absolute neutrophil count.

Clinical Manifestations
- Careful history and meticulous physical exam: sites requiring close attention during the exam include the teeth and gums, pharynx, abdomen, lung, perineum, skin, and site of central venous line insertion.
- Signs and symptoms of infection including induration or erythema of the skin, oropharynx, perirectal or catheter-exit site may be absent in the neutropenic patient. Additionally, collection of body fluids (urine, CSF) may not demonstrate pleocytosis, but should be considered for culture.

Diagnostics
- At least one set of blood cultures from each lumen of the central venous catheter and ideally from a peripheral site before initiation of antibiotics
- If catheter site is inflamed or draining, send Gram stain and culture for bacteria and fungi
- If lesion is persistent or chronic, send acid-fast stain and culture
- CT scan (head/sinuses, chest, abdomen) for evaluation of fungal disease with white blood cell count recovery in patients who have prolonged febrile neutropenia or in patients on long-standing broad-spectrum IV antibiotics who develop a new fever

Management
Empiric Therapy
- Since gram-positive or gram-negative organisms can cause infection, empiric therapy must be broad spectrum and bactericidal. Antibiotic choice depends on the individual institutional resistance patterns and the combinations used are quite varied. Typical empiric combinations include:
  - Monotherapy with cefepime, ceftazidime, or imipenem/meropenem
  - Two drug therapy with a third- or fourth-generation cephalosporin or an anti-pseudomonal penicillin + an aminoglycoside
  - Consider addition of vancomycin for gram-positive coverage (see below)

- Recommendations for empiric use of vancomycin include high institutional rate of gram-positive organisms leading to severe infection; clear central line infection; receipt of intensive chemotherapy known to result in severe mucositis (SCT, AML); prior quinolone prophylaxis; recent infection sensitive to vancomycin; colonization with vancomycin-sensitive organisms; patients presenting with hypotension
- If there are signs of a specific infection on exam, add appropriate coverage (i.e., gram-positive coverage for skin infection or anaerobic coverage for perirectal or oral infection)
- If no organism can be identified, broad coverage (usually with a third- or fourth-generation cephalosporin) should continue until the patient is afebrile with evidence of bone marrow recovery seen as an increase in ANC of 200 to 500 cells/mm^3 on 2 consecutive days.
- *Empiric* antifungal coverage should be started in patients who have persistent febrile neutropenia (>3 to 5 days) or a new fever while on broad-spectrum empiric antibacterial coverage.
- *Remove central venous catheters if* there is evidence of a subcutaneous tunnel infection, periportal infection, fungemia, atypical mycobacteremia, or persistently positive bacterial blood cultures, despite IV antibiotics.
- Some centers are studying the management of low-risk patients with fever and neutropenia with oral antibiotics, but this is NOT yet the standard of care.
- Fever with a true infection may not develop in patients receiving steroids as part of their therapy or for chronic symptom management. Empiric antibiotic coverage should be considered in afebrile patients taking steroids who are neutropenic and have signs or symptoms suggestive of infection.

NAUSEA AND VOMITING

General Guidelines
- Understand the emetogenic potential of each drug in the chemotherapy regimen or the site of radiation. Emetogenic potential common agents:
  - *High:* carboplatin, cisplatin, cyclophosphamide (high dose), cytarabine (high dose), doxorubicin (high dose), ifosfamide, methotrexate (high dose), radiation (total body, brain, craniospinal)
  - *Moderate/high:* cyclophosphamide (low dose), cytarabine (moderate dose), intrathecal cytarabine, etoposide, actinomycin-D
  - *Moderate:* asparaginase, lower dose doxorubicin or cytarabine
  - *Low:* bleomycin, 6MP, hydroxyurea, busulfan, thioguanine, vincristine, low-dose (oral) methotrexate
- Consider special situations: anticipatory nausea and cisplatin-delayed nausea/vomiting, which can occur up to 5 days after drug administration
- Consider oral before IV anti-emetics
- Patients receiving 1-day chemotherapy regimens should receive oral anti-emetics before chemotherapy.
- Always administer anti-emetics "around the clock" rather than symptomatically for patients actively receiving chemotherapy.
- Bone marrow transplant patients usually receive anti-emetics until 24 hours after the last dose of chemotherapy or irradiation.

Potential Regimens Based on Current or Anticipated Degree of Nausea
- Low: no anti-emetics recommended
- Moderate: promethazine 0.5 mg/kg/dose IV (maximum = 25 mg) or prochlorperazine 0.05–0.15 mg/kg/dose IV (maximum = 10 mg) + diphenhydramine 1 mg/kg/dose every 6 hours as needed (maximum = 50 mg)
- Moderate/high: ondansetron 0.3 mg/kg/dose PO/IV every day (maximum = 16 mg) + dexamethasone PO/IV every day (see Table 21.4, maximum = 8 mg)
- High: ondansetron 0.45 mg/kg/dose PO/IV every day (maximum = 24 mg) + dexamethasone PO/IV every 12 hours (see Table 21.4, maximum = 8 mg)

Table 21.5: Dexamethasone Dosing for Nausea Management in Children with Cancer	
Weight (kg)	**Dexamethasone Dose**
<10 kg	0.15 mg/kg/dose
10–20	2 mg
21–40	4 mg
≥41 kg	8 mg

Breakthrough Nausea/Vomiting
Greater than three episodes of emesis or retching within 24 hours. May add any of the following:
- Dexamethasone 5 mg/m²/dose IV/PO every 12 hours (maximum = 8 mg) (Table 21.5)
- Droperidol 0.05–0.06 mg/kg/dose IV every 6 hours as needed (maximum = 5 mg)
- Lorazepam 0.02–0.04 mg/kg/dose PO (maximum = 2 mg) the night before or the morning of chemotherapy
- Metoclopramide 1 mg/kg/dose IV/PO every 4 to 6 hours given with diphenhydramine 1 mg/kg/dose IV/PO every 6 hours (maximum = 50 mg)
- Ondansetron 0.45 mg/kg/dose PO/IV every day (maximum = 24 mg)
- Promethazine 0.5 mg/kg/dose IV every 6 hours as needed (maximum = 25 mg) or prochlorperazine 0.05 mg/kg/dose IV every 6 hours as needed (maximum = 10 mg) + diphenhydramine 1 mg/kg/dose (maximum = 50 mg)

SPINAL CORD COMPRESSION

A mass that compromises the integrity of the spinal cord, conus medullaris, or cauda equina (also see Neurology chapter)

Etiology
- Tumor in the epidural or subarachnoid space
- Metastatic spread to the cord parenchyma or the vertebrae with secondary cord compression
- Extension of paravertebral tumor through the intervertebral foramina leading to epidural compression
- Subarachnoid spread down the spinal cord from a primary CNS tumor

Epidemiology
- Acute compression of the spinal cord develops in 3% to 5% of children with cancer.
- Back pain develops in 5% to 10% that must be differentiated from spinal cord compression.
- Sarcomas (especially Ewing) account for ~50% of cases. Other commonly involved tumors include neuroblastoma, leukemia, and lymphoma.

Pathophysiology
- Physical compression of the spinal cord, conus, or cauda equina leads to impaired blood flow, which results in venous hypertension and vasogenic cord edema, hemorrhage, ischemia, and eventually, infarction

Clinical Manifestations
- Back pain with localized tenderness is presenting sign in 80% of patients.
- Radicular pain
- Abnormalities of bowel or bladder dysfunction (i.e., incontinence, retention)
- Most have objective motor loss.

Diagnostics
- Spine radiographs: may be helpful, but are abnormal in less than 50% of cases
- Radionuclide bone scanning: more sensitive than plain films, but are not appropriate with evolving neurological dysfunction

- MRI with and without gadolinium: detects presence and extent of epidural involvement, intra-parenchymal spread of tumor, and small lesions compressing nerve roots in the cauda equina
- Cerebrospinal fluid analysis: important in the evaluation of subarachnoid disease and meningeal leukemia or carcinomatosis, but is not appropriate before the initial imaging.

Management

- History: night-waking, weakness, pain, tingling, bowel or bladder dysfunction
- Perform detailed neurologic exam
- If patient has focal spinal tenderness or neurologic deficit, determine the nature of symptoms and if they are progressive.
- If neurologic symptoms are evolving, discuss initiation of steroids (see below) with an oncologist and perform MRI with and without gadolinium.
- If evidence of spinal cord compression by imaging, consider surgery, local radiation or chemotherapy only after careful discussion with all disciplines as initial management decisions can have a profound effect on future therapy and patient function.
- Dexamethasone:
  - For progressive dysfunction with significant physical deficits, administer 1–2 mg/kg/day as loading dose followed by 1.5 mg/kg/day divided every 6 hours.
  - For mild stable deficits, administer 0.25–1 mg/kg/dose every 6 hours

SUPERIOR VENA CAVA SYNDROME AND SUPERIOR MEDIASTINAL SYNDROME

Signs and symptoms that result from compression, obstruction, or thrombosis of the superior vena cava (SVC). Superior mediastinal syndrome (SMS) includes SVC syndrome (SVCS) with associated tracheal compression.

Etiology

- Malignant (90%): most commonly seen with non-Hodgkin lymphoma, Hodgkin disease, T cell ALL, and germ cell tumors
- Non-malignant: vascular thrombosis secondary to central venous line, thrombotic complications of cardiovascular surgery for congenital heart disease, infectious masses (i.e., tuberculosis, histoplasmosis, aspergillosis), bronchogenic cyst; hamartoma; ganglioneuroma

Pathophysiology

- The SVC is a thin-walled vessel surrounded by lymph nodes and the thymus. Tumor or infection in the nodes or thymus can compress the SVC, causing venous stasis.
- The trachea and right main stem bronchus in infants and children are smaller than that in adults and minimal compression/swelling can result in obstructive symptoms. Compression, clotting, and edema decrease air flow and reduce venous return from the head, neck, and upper thorax, leading to the signs and symptoms of SVCS and SMS.

Clinical Manifestations

- 75% of children with mediastinal masses have respiratory symptoms that are aggravated when the patient is supine.
- Signs: edema and/or cyanosis of the face, neck, and upper extremities; plethoric appearance; conjunctival suffusion; cervical and thoracic venous distention; wheezing; stridor; pleural/pericardial effusion
- Symptoms: cough, dyspnea, dysphagia, orthopnea, hoarseness, wheezing, stridor, chest pain, anxiety, headache, confusion secondary to carbon dioxide retention

Diagnostics

- Chest x-ray demonstrates mass
- Laboratory evaluation:
  - CBC: pancytopenia, leukocytosis, blasts on smear (leukemia, lymphoma), left shift (infection)
  - Chemistry panel: potassium, calcium, phosphorus, creatinine, uric acid, LDH (can be elevated with leukemia, lymphoma)
  - α-fetoprotein, β-HCG: elevated in germ cell tumors

- Urine catecholamines: elevated in neuroblastoma
- ESR: can be elevated with lymphoma
• Assess risk for general anesthesia/surgery:
  - If respiratory distress at presentation: high risk for anesthesia
  - If even minimal symptoms, full evaluation is necessary before sedation: CT scan, echocardiography, pulmonary function testing including a volume flow loop to assess reserve
  - *Sedation or general anesthesia in patients with a mediastinal mass may be contraindicated because they can decrease respiratory drive and result in respiratory failure, decreased venous return, and circulatory collapse.*

Management
Clinical Decision-Making
• If CBC and other studies confirm diagnosis, begin tumor-specific treatment.
• If no diagnosis is made after initial noninvasive studies, continue evaluation and assess risk of patient for anesthesia to safely obtain tumor tissue.
• If patients is at low risk for anesthesia, perform diagnostic procedures and begin tumor-specific treatment
• If patient is at high risk for anesthesia, treat empirically with chemotherapy or radiation based on the most likely disease, although this is can complicate the eventual diagnostic procedure. Empiric therapy should only be done after consultation with an oncologist if possible.

General Management Issues
• Control the airway, give oxygen, AVOID INTUBATION IF POSSIBLE
• Extreme care in handling the patient: minimize stress, sedation, and avoid the supine position
• If tissue diagnosis is not possible, empiric therapy may be necessary.
• Empiric use of steroids, radiation therapy and chemotherapy can all affect masses and lymph nodes making subsequent tissue diagnosis more difficult, but these interventions are sometimes medically indicated.

TUMOR LYSIS SYNDROME

Metabolic abnormalities that result from dying tumor cells and the rapid release of intracellular metabolites into circulation that exceeds the excretory capacity of the kidneys. Tumor lysis syndrome often occurs at presentation or within 12 to 72 hours after the start of chemotherapy. The classic triad involves hyperuricemia, hyperkalemia, and hyperphosphatemia:

• Hyperuricemia: results from the release of nucleic acids from malignant cell breakdown. Uric acid is soluble at physiologic pH, but precipitates in the acidic environment of the kidney and can lead to acute renal failure.
• Hyperkalemia: potassium is the principal intracellular cation and serum levels can also increase with acute renal failure. High serum potassium can lead to cardiac arrest in minutes to hours.
• Hyperphosphatemia: lymphoblasts have four times the content of phosphate as normal lymphocytes; leads to hypocalcemia by decreasing production of calcitriol, decreasing absorption of calcium from the GI tract and from precipitation; if $Ca^{+2} \times PO_4^{-3}$ product reaches 60, calcium phosphate crystals form and precipitate in the microvasculature, leading to acute renal failure.

Etiology
• Most common: Burkitt lymphoma, lymphoblastic lymphoma, ALL (T cell)
• Predisposing factors: tumors with high growth fraction and sensitivity to chemotherapy, bulky tumors, high pre-therapy uric acid or LDH, poor urine output, high WBC count

Clinical Manifestations
• Usually have no signs or symptoms; most commonly occurs in the 24 hours after starting treatment
• May present with vomiting or diarrhea
• May present with evidence of hypocalcemia: muscle weakness, spasms, tetany, seizures, renal failure

Diagnostics

- CBC
- Serum chemistries: electrolyte panel (especially potassium, calcium, and phosphate), creatinine, uric acid
- Urinalysis: pH and specific gravity
- ECG: may show peaked T-waves, prolonged PR interval and/or QRS widening in hyperkalemia (K > 7 meq/L), or prolonged QT_c interval in hypocalcemia
- Chest x-ray: to evaluate for mediastinal mass
- Abdominal ultrasound: consider if abdominal mass or renal failure

Management

- *Hydration:*
  - Increase urine flow and glomerular filtration rate
  - D5 1/4NS + $NaHCO_3$ 25–40 meq/L without potassium to run at least two times maintenance rate. If patient has renal failure and cannot be hydrated appropriately, consider dialysis.
  - Maintain urine output greater than 100 to 250 $cc/m^2/hr$
  - Maintain urine pH 7.0 to 7.5 and adjust fluid rate or $NaHCO_3$ additive appropriately. Note: an excessively high urinary pH can cause precipitation of hypoxanthine or calcium phosphate stones.
  - Consider mannitol (0.5–1.0 g/kg) if oliguria is unresponsive to increased hydration and patient has reasonable renal function.
  - Close monitoring of weight/fluid status
- *Monitoring:* electrolytes, creatinine, uric acid every 4 to 6 hours; CBC count every 6 hours if significant leukocytosis; cardiac monitoring if hyperkalemia or hypocalcemia; urine pH and output
- *Hyperuricemia:*
  - Allopurinol: xanthine oxidase inhibitor that prevents uric acid synthesis (10 mg/kg/day divided three times daily)
  - Urate oxidase (Rasburicase): converts uric acid to allantoin, which is much more soluble; can rapidly decrease level of uric acid and is available in IV formulation; used more commonly in adults and the minimal experience in children is to give only one dose (100 U/kg); causes significant hemolysis in patients with G6PD deficiency
- *Hyperkalemia:*
  - Insulin: increases cellular uptake of potassium (co-administer with glucose to avoid hypoglycemia)
  - Kayexalate: a resin that exchanges sodium for potassium in the GI tract; promotes excretion of potassium in stool
  - Calcium gluconate: stabilizes the myocardium
- *Hyperphosphatemia:*
  - Amphogel promotes the excretion of phosphate in stool.
  - Insulin and glucose shift phosphorus from the extracellular space into the intracellular compartment.
- *Hypocalcemia:* do not treat unless symptomatic. Calcium administration in the face of hyperphosphatemia can precipitate metastatic calcifications.
- *Indications for dialysis:* hyperkalemia (potassium > 6 mEq/L); hyperphosphatemia (phosphate > 10 mg/dL); uremia; respiratory distress (volume overload); oliguria or anuria; severe, uncontrolled hypertension.

Resources

Baker D, Children's Oncology Group: Phase III Study of Combination Chemotherapy in Children with Intermediate-Risk Neuroblastoma. COG-A3961, Clinical Trial, Temporarily closed.

Golden CB, Fenusner JH. Malignant abdominal masses in children: quick guide to evaluation and diagnosis. Pediatr Clin North Am 2002;49:1369–1392.

Hughes WT, Armstrong D, Bodey GP, et al. 2002 guidelines for the use of antimicrobial agents in neutropenic patients with cancer. Clin Infect Dis 2002;34:730–751.

Keating RF, Goodrich JT, Packer RJ, eds. Tumors of the Pediatric Central Nervous System. New York: Thieme Medical, 2001.

Kapoor M, Chan G. Fluid and electrolyte abnormalities. Crit Care Clin 2001;17:503–529.

Lanzkowsky P. Manual of Pediatric Hematology and Oncology. 3rd ed. San Diego: Academic Press, 2000.

Matthay KK, Villablanca JG, Seeger RC, et al. Treatment of high-risk neuroblastoma with intensive chemotherapy, radiotherapy, autologous bone marrow transplantation, and 13-cis-retinoic acid. Children's Cancer Group. N Engl J Med 1999;341:1165–1173.

Miller SL, Hoffer FA. Malignant and benign bone tumors. Radiol Clin North Am 2001;39:673–699.

Naring S, et al. Anesthesia for patients with a mediastinal mass. Anesthesiol Clin North Am 2001;19:559–579.

Nathan DG, Orkin SH. Nathan and Oski's Hematology of Infancy and Childhood. 5th ed. Philadelphia: WB Saunders, 1998.

Pizzo PA, Poplack DG, eds. Principles and Practice of Pediatric Oncology. 4th ed. Philadelphia: Lippincott Williams & Wilkins, 2002.

Pui CH, Campana D, Evans WE. Childhood acute lymphoblastic leukemia: current status and future perspectives. Lancet Oncol 2001;2:597–607.

Raney RB. Rhabdomyosarcoma and undifferentiated sarcoma in the first two decades of life: a selective review of intergroup rhabdomyosarcoma study group experience and rationale for Intergroup Rhabdomyosarcoma Study V. J Pediatr Hematol Oncol 2001;23:215–220.

Schiff D. Spinal cord compression. Neurol Clin 2003;21:67–86.

Strother DR. Children's Oncology Group: Phase III Study of Primary Surgical Therapy in Children With Low-Risk Neuroblastoma, COG-P9641, Clinical trial, Active.

Ulrich NJ, Pomeroy SL. Pediatric brain tumors. Neurol Clin 2003;2:897–909.

Velez MC. Lymphomas. Pediatr Rev 2003;24:380–386.

Wittig JC, Bickels J. Osteosarcoma: A multidisciplinary approach to diagnosis and treatment. Am Fam Phys 2002;65:1123–1132.

Ophthalmology 22

Judit Saenz-Badillos, MD, Stefanie L. Davidson, MD

GLAUCOMA

Irreversible optic nerve damage, usually due to increased intraocular pressure

Epidemiology and Etiology
Primary Glaucoma
- *Primary infantile glaucoma* (congenital glaucoma): 1:10,000 to 1:15,000; 90% sporadic
- Caused by developmental defect in the structure of the anterior chamber
- Can be associated with systemic syndromes such as Sturge-Weber, neurofibromatosis type 1, Marfan, Stickler
- Also associated with ocular syndromes such as aniridia, Peters' syndrome

Secondary Glaucoma
- Secondary glaucomas of childhood are more common.
- *Traumatic:* trauma may damage the angle of the eye and can cause glaucoma related to a hyphema acutely (see Hyphema) or years after trauma secondary to angle recession.
- *Inflammatory:* caused by clogging of the trabecular meshwork from inflammatory debris; e.g., uveitis associated with juvenile rheumatoid arthritis
- *Steroid-induced:* can be caused by topical, systemic, or inhaled forms of glucocorticoids by decreasing aqueous outflow
- *Aphakic:* absence of the natural lens usually secondary to cataract extraction; 8% to 41% chance of developing glaucoma
- *Intraocular neoplasms* such as juvenile xanthogranuloma, retinoblastoma

Pathophysiology
- Intraocular pressure (IOP) is maintained by the balance of aqueous humor production by the ciliary body and drainage by the trabecular meshwork.
- When this drainage system is impaired, IOP increases.
- Elevated IOP causes loss of the nerve fiber layer of the retina and eventual blindness if left untreated.

Clinical Manifestations
- Children younger than 3 years present with photophobia, epiphora (tearing), blepharospasm (repetitive closure of the lids), and buphthalmos (enlarged eye, "cow's eye").
- Children older than 3 years may have asymptomatic glaucoma until advanced, irreversible visual loss occurs.
- Check ocular size, corneal size, and visual acuity.
- *Haab's striae:* breaks in the Descemet's membrane (basement membrane of the cornea) that occur as the cornea enlarges. They are seen as horizontal lines on the cornea and develop in children younger than 3 years.
- *Cupping of the optic nerve:* cup to disc ratio greater than 0.3 is suggestive of glaucoma.
- Look for evidence of associated syndromes

Diagnostics
- *Tonometry:* pressure greater than 20 mm Hg in a calm infant is diagnostic
- *Gonioscopy:* assesses the angle anatomy
- Measure corneal diameter and axial length to follow response to treatment: normal corneal diameter is 9.5 to 10.5 mm in newborns and 11 to 12 mm in adults

Management
Medical
- *Topical Therapy:* beta-blockers (e.g., Timolol maleate), carbonic anhydrase inhibitors (e.g., dorzolamide, brin-olamide) and prostaglandins (latanoprost)
- *Oral therapy:* acetazolamide

Surgical
- Primary congenital glaucoma is a surgical disease.
- 80% of children can be cured with:
  1. *Goniotomy:* an incision is made in the trabecular meshwork with a needle inserted into the anterior chamber. This improves trabecular outflow and reduces IOP. This procedure can only be performed if the cornea is clear.
  2. *Trabeculotomy ab externo:* external dissection of Schlemm's canal to increase exit of aqueous fluid. This is the procedure of choice in the presence of a cloudy cornea (corneal edema).

When primary infantile glaucoma fails above surgeries and other types of glaucomas fail medical management then:

  3. *Trabeculectomy:* filtration procedure creating a communication between the anterior chamber and subconjunctival space to redirect aqueous away from trabecular meshwork
  4. *Glaucoma drainage device:* similar purpose to trabeculectomy but uses an implant
  5. *Photocyclocoagulation and cyclocryotherapy:* destroys the ciliary body, thereby reducing production of aqueous fluid; usually a last resort

HYPHEMA

Blood in the anterior chamber of the eye

Epidemiology
- Serious trauma to the eyes causes hyphema one third of the time.
- Annual incidence of 17 to 20 per 100,000; mostly younger than 20 years old

Pathophysiology
- Trauma breaks vessels in the eye, causing blood to leak into the anterior chamber and leads to increased intraocular pressure.
- Bleeding stops when a clot forms.
- Re-bleeding risk is highest on days 3 to 5 when the clot weakens.

Clinical Manifestations
- Patients present with a history of eye trauma, eye pain, and vision loss.
- Children may be somnolent.
- Some patients have history of bleeding disorders, sickle cell disease, or anticoagulation therapy.
- Blood in the anterior chamber appears as a dark meniscus in the aqueous humor on top of the iris. The cornea may also be stained with blood.

Diagnostics
- Small hyphemas may only be seen with a slit lamp.
- Assess visual acuity and intraocular pressure
- Consider a sickle cell preparation in African Americans who are at greater risk for acute glaucoma with hyphema

Management
- Ophthalmology should be consulted on all patients with hyphema.
- Bed rest with head elevation for blood resorption
- Admission and sedation for young, active children
- Topical mydriatics (e.g., homatropine) and steroids

- Glaucoma medications for elevated intraocular pressure
- Protect the eye with a metal shield but do not apply a patch. This allows the patient to report changes in vision.
- *Consider surgical management if:* elevated intraocular pressure unresponsive to medications, patients with sickle cell disease, corneal blood staining
- *Surgical procedures:* anterior chamber washout and clot removal

LEUKOKORIA

From Greek meaning "white pupil"

Epidemiology
- Congenital cataracts are most common cause: 11/2500 live births
- Retinoblastoma in 1/15,000 people; extremely rare before 6 years of age

Differential Diagnosis
- *Cataracts* (lens opacity) are most common cause of leukokoria.
- *Retinoblastoma* is the most concerning diagnosis.
- *Retinal dysplasia* is a developmental anomaly, present at birth.
- *Coats disease* is an idiopathic condition of retinal vascular changes and exudation.
- *Cicatricial retinopathy of prematurity*
- *Leukemic ophthalmopathy*

Pathophysiology
- The vascular choroid is a retinal structure that reflects white light, thereby forming the normal "red reflex."
- White light passes through the cornea, aqueous humor, pupil, lens, and vitreous to get to the retina. Any abnormal light intake by any of these structures may lead to a white reflex.

Clinical Manifestations
- *Red reflex exam:* a direct ophthalmoscope at an arm's length from the infant's eyes should be used in a dark room. A normal exam has no white spots or opacities, and has bilateral and equal color, intensity, and clarity.

Diagnostics
- A patient with leukokoria needs prompt and complete evaluation.
- Ultrasound and CT of the eye to rule out retinoblastoma
- MRI may demonstrate sellar and parasellar involvement, but is less useful for intraocular tumors.

Management
- Depends on etiology of leukokoria
- Retinoblastoma requires prompt treatment because untreated children will die in 2 to 4 years from expansion into the brain.
- Children with congenital cataracts should be tested for congenital infections (TORCH) and for metabolic diseases.
- Laser photocoagulation for leaking vessels in Coats disease

ORBITAL FRACTURE

Fracture of one or more of the orbital bones due to trauma, including aggression, falls, motor vehicle accidents, and sports

Differential Diagnosis
- Bruised extraocular muscles, cranial nerve palsy, and orbital edema all present with double vision.
- Eye trauma may result in hyphema, retinal detachment, vitreous hemorrhage, dislocated lens, and/or choroidal rupture.

Pathophysiology
- The orbit is composed of seven bones: maxilla, zygoma, lacrimal, ethmoid, palatine, sphenoid, and frontal
- The walls of the orbit are thin; the rims are thick.
- Most fractures occur in the posteromedial floor, near the infraorbital groove.
- The infraorbital groove crosses the floor of the orbit and contains the infraorbital nerve V2, which provides sensation to the cheek and upper alveolus/teeth.

Clinical Manifestations
- Patients may be asymptomatic or present with periorbital ecchymosis, pain on vertical gaze, double vision, eyelid swelling after nose blowing, and decreased sensation in the V2 cranial nerve distribution.

Diagnostics
- Plain x-rays are often used but are falsely negative in 50% of cases.
- Thin cut coronal CT is the study of choice; MRI depicts bones poorly, and therefore should not be used.
- Ultrasound has a sensitivity of 85%.

Management
Non-surgical
- Ice treatments for 48 hours; elevation of head in bed
- Nasal decongestants, oral steroids, antibiotic coverage for sinus flora (e.g., Augmentin)
- Avoid aspirin, minimize coughing, no nose blowing

Surgical
- Surgery is recommended within 1 to 3 weeks if patient has diplopia, enophthalmos (2 to 3 mm or more), soft tissue herniation into maxillary sinuses, or if greater than 50% of orbital floor is fractured.
- Some physicians consider hypoesthesia in the V2 cranial nerve distribution and intraorbital emphysema as reasons for surgery.
- Most common surgical approach is transconjunctival. A graft may be used if necessary.

Resources

American Adademy of Pediatrics. Section on Ophthalmology, Red Reflex Subcommittee. Red reflex examination in infants. Pediatrics 2002;109:980–981.

Behrman R, Klegman R, Jenson H. Nelson Textbook of Pediatrics. 16th ed. Philadelphia: WB Saunders, 2000.

Beck A. Diagnosis and management of pediatric glaucoma. Ophthal Clin North Am 2001;14:501–512.

Brady S, McMann MA, Mazzoli RA, et al. The diagnosis and management of orbital blowout fractures: update 2001. Am J Emerg Med 2001;19:147–154.

Catalano JD. Leukokoria—the differential diagnosis of a white pupil. Pediatr Ann 1983;12:498–505.

Hamid R, Newfield P. Pediatric eye emergencies. Anesthesiol Clin North Am 2001;19:257–264.

Kuhn F, Mester V. Anterior chamber abnormalities and cataracts. Ophthamol Clin North Am 2002;15:195.

Ravinet E, Mermoud A, Brignoli R. Four years later: a clinical update on Latanoprost. Eur J Ophthalmol 2003;13:162–175.

Yanoff M. Ophthalmology. St. Louis: Mosby, 1999.

Walton DS. Pediatric Ophthalmology. New York: Thieme Medical, 2000.

Denise M. Bell, MD, Jennifer Minarcik Hwang, MD,
Stephen Ludwig, MD, John M. Flynn, MD

Fractures

CLAVICLE FRACTURES

Most frequently fractured bone in the pediatric population

Mechanism of injury: birth trauma, fall on outstretched arm, fall onto shoulder

Most fractures are midshaft, with incomplete fractures being more common in younger children.

Clinical Manifestations
- Birth trauma: pseudoparalysis in immediate postnatal period or bony callus in asymptomatic infant around day 10 of life
- Child will support affected side with opposite hand and tilt head toward affected side
- Point tenderness +/– bony deformity
- Shoulder range of motion frequently limited by pain

Diagnostics
- Plain radiographs: anteroposterior (AP) view of clavicle usually sufficient; 30-degree cephalic view if high index of suspicion and negative anteroposterior view

Management
- Infants: avoid laying on affected side; safety pin shirt sleeve to shirt for comfort
- Figure-of-eight splint: helps bring clavicle to length (theoretical), relieves muscle spasm, minimizes motion; sling +/– swath is an alternative; duration of splint is 3 weeks in younger children and 4 weeks in adolescents and adults; risk of brachial plexus injury with long-term use of splint
- Ice and analgesia are also important
- Orthopedic follow-up necessary if bone fractured
- Advise families that palpable callus frequently develops

FEMUR FRACTURES

Femoral shaft (diaphyseal) fractures: often occur with falls in young children, but occur with high-energy trauma in adolescents; 80% due to abuse in children younger than walking age; more than 90% caused by motor vehicle accidents in adolescents

Distal femoral (physeal) fractures: usually seen with knee injuries; mechanism involves indirect stress on knee from vehicular accident or sports, fall onto a flexed knee, direct trauma or birth trauma (breech)

Femoral neck fractures: uncommon in children

Clinical Manifestations
Femoral Shaft
- Inability to ambulate; extreme pain
- Variable swelling and gross deformity
- Compartment syndrome is rare; occurs with severe hemorrhage
- Hypotension rarely caused by isolated femur fracture

Distal Femur
- Usually unable to bear weight
- Knee flexion due to hamstring spasm
- May see gross deformity with angular deformity
- Point tenderness over physis
- Often presents with history of "pop" and knee effusion or soft tissue swelling in adolescents

Diagnostics
- Radiographs for femoral shaft fracture: anteroposterior and lateral views; obtain knee and hip films to rule out associated injuries
- Radiographs for distal femur fractures: AP, lateral, and oblique views; used to diagnose nondisplaced fractures; CT may be useful for assessing articular involvement

Management
Femoral Shaft
- Age birth to 2 years: early spica cast; Pavlik harness in infants; usually good healing by 4 weeks in infants
- Age 2 to 6: less than 2 cm overriding, early spica cast; greater than 2 cm overriding, traction followed by spica cast; flexible intramedullary nail is for children 6 to skeletal maturity
- Skeletally mature: distal femoral traction followed by intramedullary nail. Risk of avascular necrosis if intramedullary nail used in children with open physes.
- Consider external fixation for open fractures or multiple injuries.
- Criteria for reduction: overriding less than 2 cm for age less than 10 years or less than 1 cm for age greater than 10 years; angulation less than 10° in sagittal plane or greater than 10° in frontal plane; rotation greater than 10°
- Operative management: multiple trauma or head injury; open fracture; pathologic fracture; vascular injury

Physeal Fractures
- Type I or nondisplaced: simple immobilization: long leg or spica cast with 15° to 20° knee flexion; aspiration for symptomatic relief of knee effusion
- Type II: closed reduction if possible; require percutaneous pin/wire fixation if unstable
- Types III, IV, and irreducible type II: open reduction with internal fixation; postoperatively immobilize in long leg cast with 10° knee flexion; may ambulate with crutches in 1 to 2 days

HAND FRACTURES

Tuft fracture: crushing force to distal phalanx; considered open fracture if accompanied by nailbed laceration

Phalanx fracture: usually at base of phalanx; epiphyseal injury at base of proximal or middle phalanx may be accompanied by considerable rotation at line of separation

Boxer's fracture: fracture of distal metaphysis of fifth metacarpal, usually caused by punching

Clinical Manifestations
- Assess for rotational deformity by assessing the digital cascade with fingers flexed; all fingers should point to scaphoid
- Point tenderness may indicate Salter-Harris type I fracture

Diagnostics
- Plain x-rays: AP, lateral, and oblique views

Management
Immobilization
- Children with finger fractures should be referred to orthopedics
- Aluminum-foam splints work poorly in children

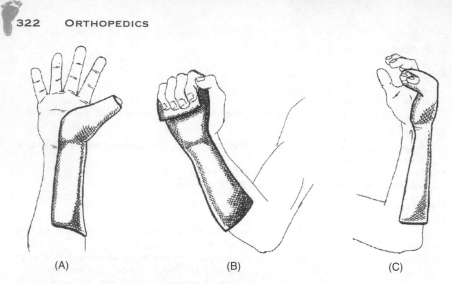

(A)   (B)   (C)

Figure 23.1 A: Thumb spica splint. B: Volar splint. C: Ulnar gutter splint.

- Position of safety: wrist in 30° extension, metacarpophalangeal joints in 70° flexion, and inter-phalangeal joints fully extended
- Must include joint on either side of fracture
- Splints for phalanx fractures (ALWAYS include adjacent finger)
  - Thumb fracture: thumb spica splint (Figure 23.1A)
  - Second or third digit fractures: volar (Figure 23.1B), dorsal, or volar/dorsal splint
  - Fourth or fifth digit fractures: ulnar gutter splint (Figure 23.1C)
- Elevate hand at or slightly above level of heart
- Avoid slings because elbow flexion restricts circulation

Boxer's Fractures
- Need reduction only if displaced, rotated, or greater than 30° to 40° angulated
- Ulnar gutter splint with orthopedic follow-up within 1 to 2 days

Referral and Follow-up of Phalanx Fractures
- Open or unstable fractures and those with joint involvement or rotational deformity should be referred to hand service in emergency department
- Other fractures can be seen in 2 to 5 days

LATERAL HUMERAL CONDYLE FRACTURES

Mechanism of injury: varus force applied to elbow in extension, usually from a fall on out-stretched hand or less commonly from a direct lateral blow to a flexed elbow with shear-ing of condyle

Fracture line starts laterally in metaphysis and proceeds through epiphysis toward elbow joint; may or may not extend into joint

Milch classification: based on where fracture line exits at articular surface; type I frac-tures occur at capitotrochlear groove and correspond to Salter-Harris type IV; type II fractures extend into the apex of the trochlea

Most commonly seen in children ages 6 to 10 years

Clinical Manifestations
- Significant swelling, lateral point tenderness, crepitus
- Assess for neurovascular compromise, especially ulnar nerve

Diagnostics
- Plain x-rays: AP, lateral, and oblique; oblique view more accurate for determining displacement
- Arthrogram: used preoperatively to assess stability

Management (all require orthopedic consult)
- Minimally displaced (0 to 2 mm): long arm cast; elbow flexed, hand supinated, wrist extended during immobilization; must see orthopedics within 5 days of injury
- Displaced fractures (2 to 4 mm): closed reduction and percutaneous pinning if articular surface intact; most need open reduction because articular surface unstable
- Displaced and rotated fractures (>4 mm): open reduction and internal fixation; cast immobilization at least 6 weeks after surgery; restoration of articular congruity most important
- Complications include nonunion, late ulnar nerve palsy, malunion, avascular necrosis, physeal arrest

MEDIAL HUMERAL EPICONDYLE FRACTURES

Mechanism of injury involves valgus force on elbow associated with contraction of flexor muscles

Little leaguer's elbow: avulsion of medial epicondyle from repeated valgus stress

Accompanies elbow dislocation in 50% of cases

Acute injury associated with athletic activities, e.g., arm wrestling

Most common in children 7 to 15 years of age

Clinical Manifestations
- Elbow held in flexion; movement resisted
- Elbow swollen, ecchymotic, tender medially
- Neurovascular assessment for possible ulnar nerve entrapment
- Positive valgus stress test at 30° flexion (rarely done on children due to pain)

Diagnostics
- Plain x-rays: fracture of epicondyle visible if ossified (age 5 in girls, age 7 in boys); widened joint space if fragment entrapped within joint; epicondyle is displaced if it is visible on lateral x-ray or if distal humerus appears smooth on AP view

Management
- Immediate orthopedic consult
- General guidelines (controversial):
  - Minimal displacement (0 to 2 mm): cast alone
  - Displaced 2 to 4 mm: cast or percutaneous pinning if unstable
  - Displaced greater than 4 mm, neurovascular injury or entrapped fragment: open reduction with internal fixation (ORIF)
  - ORIF of dominant elbow recommended for those wishing to return to throwing sports in the future
- Complications: symptomatic instability uncommon, ulnar nerve irritation, nonunion, loss of terminal elbow extension

PHYSIS (GROWTH PLATE) FRACTURES

Salter-Harris classification system: system for classifying fractures involving the proliferating cartilage cells between metaphysis and epiphysis in skeletally immature bone (Table 23.1 and Figure 23.2)

Some specific fractures involving physis do not use this classification (e.g., distal tibial physis fractures)

Clinical Manifestations
- Point tenderness over physis

Table 23.1: Salter-Harris Classification System		
Type	Fracture Description	Comment
I	Separations of growth plate without bony fracture	Most frequent in infants and toddlers; usually involve shearing, torsion, or avulsion movement
II	Fracture line extends through physis into metaphyseal bone (away from joint)	Account for 75% of physeal fractures; metaphyseal bone fragment called Thurston-Holland fragment
III	Fracture line extends through physis into epiphysis and joint	Approx. 10% of physis fractures
IV	Fracture line extends through metaphysis, physis, and epiphysis	Approx. 10% of physis fractures
V	Crush injuries to growth plate	< 1%; most frequent in knee or ankle with severe abduction or adduction injuries

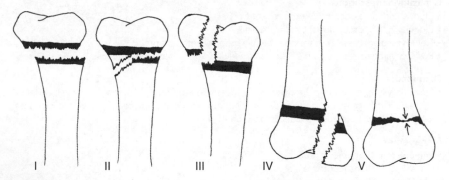

Figure 23.2   Salter-Harris classification of growth plate fractures.

Diagnostics
- May be inapparent on plain films
- Contralateral films help minimize diagnostic errors
- Ultrasound and bone scintigraphy do not alter initial management

Management
Type I and Type II without Angulation or Displacement
- Point tenderness over physis with negative x-ray should be treated as type I fracture
- Splint immobilization, intermittent icing, elevation
- Outpatient orthopedics referral
- Counsel family about potential for future growth disturbance

Displaced Types I, II and Types III, IV, V
- Orthopedics consultation in emergency department
- Gentle reduction to minimize further stress on physis; avoid repeated attempts without adequate muscle relaxation

PROXIMAL HUMERUS FRACTURES

Fractures of proximal humeral physis

Birth injuries: transphyseal (Salter-Harris I)

Consider abuse in young children

Adolescents: majority are Salter-Harris type II resulting from fall backward onto out-stretched arm

Neer Classification based on displacement: grade I: less than 5 mm; grade II: up to one third shaft diameter; grade III: up to two thirds shaft diameter; grade IV: greater than two thirds shaft diameter

Proximal fragment: abducted, flexed, internally rotated (rotator cuff and subscapularis)

Distal fragment: adducted (pectoralis major)

Clinical Manifestations
- Poorly localized tenderness of proximal humerus
- Assess for clavicle fracture
- Assess for neurovascular compromise (axillary nerve)

Diagnostics
- Plain x-rays: epiphysis ossifies at age 6 months; only see malalignment of shaft to glenoid in younger infants; x-ray entire shoulder girdle
- Ultrasound may be helpful in infants

Management
Infants
- Uniformly good results secondary to generous remodeling
- Consider reduction with traction, abduction, and flexion

Older Children and Adolescents
- Controversial; majority of series favor nonsurgical management
- Immobilization with cast or sling and swathe is standard
- Consider attempting a closed reduction in older adolescents
- Percutaneous pinning considered with greater than 30° to 40° angulation (>70° in preadolescent) or greater than 50% displacement (grades III and IV)
- Open reduction may be necessary in open fractures or neurovascular compromise; little data in literature
- Should be seen by orthopedic surgeon in 24 to 48 hours

SUPRACONDYLAR FRACTURE OF HUMERUS

Fracture of humerus proximal to transverse epicondylar line

Mechanism of injury: hyperextension of elbow during fall on outstretched arm or fall directly on flexed elbow

Extension type (95%): failure of anterior cortex +/– posterior displacement of distal fragment

Gartland classification: type I: nondisplaced; type II: displaced fracture with intact posterior cortex; type III: displaced fracture with no cortical contact

Flexion type (5%): failure of cortex posteriorly with anterior displacement of distal fragment

Typically seen in children ages 3 to 9 years of age

Risk of neurovascular injury: brachial artery or median nerve injury with posterolateral displacement; radial nerve injury with posteromedial displacement

Clinical Manifestations
- Wide range of symptoms from mild swelling and elbow pain to grossly displaced humerus
- Flexion type: arm held in flexion with empty space in area of olecranon

- Extension type: arm held in extension with S-shaped configuration of elbow and prominence at olecranon
- Avoid manipulation, which may cause further neurologic damage; good neurovascular assessment is imperative.
- Monitor for development of compartment syndrome of forearm
- Anterior interosseous nerve most sensitive to injury

Diagnostics
- Plain x-rays: AP view of extended elbow and lateral view of flexed elbow; consider oblique view if these are negative and clinical suspicion high
- Findings in extension injuries:
  - Type I: hard to detect; posterior fat pad associated with 70% chance of fracture
  - Type II: posterior tilt of distal fragment seen on lateral x-ray; anterior humeral line intersects anterior one third of capitellum or is anterior to capitellum
  - Type III: obvious displacement

Management
- Splint elbow in 30° flexion (maximum) while awaiting x-rays and definitive treatment
- Type I: cast with elbow in 90° flexion; may splint with orthopedic follow-up the next day
- Orthopedic consult in emergency department for all type II and type III
- Percutaneous pinning: used for type II and all type III (not requiring open reduction); reduction in operating room
- Indications for open reduction: irreducible fracture, vascular compromise, open fracture

Common Orthopedic Issues

COMPARTMENT SYNDROME

Increased interstitial pressure in an osseofascial compartment. Impaired blood flow to muscles and nerves in the compartment causes tissue damage. Delay in diagnosis or treatment results in ischemic necrosis and permanent myoneuronal deficits.

Epidemiology
- Most frequently seen in lower leg and forearm

Etiology
- Increased volume in compartment secondary to edema or hematoma: fractures are associated with 75% of cases of compartment syndrome. Tibial fractures are most common. Other causes of increased volume include soft tissue trauma, intraosseous infusion, sickle cell trait, coagulopathies, venomous bites, and extravasation of IV fluid
- External compression of compartment: cast or restrictive dressing; burn eschar, especially circumferential burn; limb compression during altered consciousness

Pathophysiology
- Reduced perfusion due to decreased arteriovenous pressure gradient
- Increased tissue pressure leads to increased venous pressure, decreased arteriovenous pressure gradient, decreased blood flow, and tissue ischemia.
- Arterial injury or systemic hypotension also decreases arteriovenous pressure gradient and increases risk.
- Dysfunction reversible if detected early

Clinical Manifestations
- Clinical signs traditionally described as 5 "Ps": Pain (out of proportion to injury; pain with passive movement); Paresthesias; Paresis; Pallor (late finding); Pulselessness/diminished pulses (late finding)

- Onset varies from 2 hours to 6 days after injury
- Can occur after fracture has been successfully reduced

Diagnostics
- Compartment pressure monitoring: diagnostic gold standard; indicated when compartment syndrome suspected and clinical findings are equivocal or difficult to interpret
  - Absolute pressure measurements: 0 to 10 mm Hg are normal. Greater than 20 mm Hg, capillary flow may be compromised. Greater than 30 to 40 mm Hg, muscle and nerve fibers at risk for ischemic necrosis.

Management
Medical
- Remove all restrictive dressings immediately
- Affected limb should be placed at level of heart. Elevation of limb is contraindicated because it decreases arterial flow.
- Treat hypotension to maximize perfusion
- Ice contraindicated because it may compromise microcirculation
- If pulses absent, single attempt at reduction may restore blood flow. Prolonged attempts are contraindicated.

Surgical
- Assess for and treat vascular injury
- Immediate surgical or orthopedic consultation is mandatory.
- Definitive treatment: fasciotomy relieves compartment pressure
- Absolute indications for fasciotomy: clinical signs of acute compartment syndrome that do not resolve within 30 to 60 minutes of appropriate treatment; tissue pressure within 30 mm Hg of mean arterial pressure or tissue pressure greater than 30 mm Hg with clinical picture of compartment syndrome; interrupted arterial circulation to an extremity for longer than 4 hours

DEVELOPMENTAL DYSPLASIA OF THE HIP

Instability or abnormal relationship between the femoral head and acetabulum results in hip that can be subluxated (reduced to partial contact between acetabulum and femoral head), dislocated (elimination of contact between the acetabulum and femoral head) or reduced from either of these positions by clinical maneuvers.

Epidemiology
- One in 100 infants have some hip instability on exam
- On exam, 1.5/1000 have hip dislocation
- Left hip is three times more likely to be affected than the right hip
- Risk factors: family history, female, first-born, white or Native American, breech presentation, oligohydramnios, other positional deformities, musculoskeletal abnormalities

Pathophysiology
- A normal hip requires balanced growth of the femoral head and the cartilage that comprises the acetabulum. Acetabular dysplasia results from absent or asymmetric modeling forces of the femoral head.
- Without the femoral head applied to the acetabulum, the acetabulum is abnormally shallow. The femoral neck becomes valgus (away from midline) and anteverted (tilted forward). The adductor and iliopsoas muscles shorten and fibrofatty tissue grows into the acetabulum.

Clinical Manifestations
- Early diagnosis (birth to 6 months) based on two maneuvers:
  - Ortolani maneuver: abduction of the hip while applying traction to the greater trochanter in an attempt to relocate a femoral head displaced from the acetabulum results in a "click of entry"
  - Barlow maneuver: flexion and adduction of the hip while palpating the femoral head in an attempt to sublux/dislocate the femoral head from the acetabulum results in a "click of exit"

- Late diagnosis based on secondary soft tissue, muscular, and bony changes: limited abduction of hip; asymmetry of the gluteus, thigh, or labia; limb length inequalities; if bilateral dislocations, waddling gait and hyperlordosis of lumbar spine

Diagnostics
- Largely a clinical diagnosis based on physical manifestations
- Ultrasonography can be used to assess initial hip morphology, track progress during treatment, guide reduction attempts, and assess hip motion (dynamic assessment)
- X-ray is used after 6 months of age

Management
- Greater than 50% of hips unstable at birth spontaneously stabilize by ~2 weeks of age
- Early treatment is optimal
- Splinting: all devices place hip in abduction; the most common device is the Pavlik harness; duration of treatment is 6 to 12 weeks
- Children older than 6 months unlikely to be helped by Pavlik harness
- Treatment of late identified DDH: traction, closed reduction under anesthesia with serial spica casts, open reduction with surgical manipulation
- Complications: avascular necrosis of the femoral head, growth impairment in proximal femur, degenerative joint disease

LEGG-CALVÉ-PERTHES DISEASE

Idiopathic avascular necrosis of the femoral head in a skeletally immature child

Epidemiology
- Typically affects children ages 4 to 8 years
- Boys:girls = 4:1
- Bilateral involvement in 20% of cases
- Limited data suggest that passive smoke exposure, thrombophilia, or hypofibrinolysis may increase risk

Pathophysiology
- Fragile blood supply to anterior portion of proximal femoral epiphysis
- Hypothesized that vascular insufficiency results from multiple insults rather than a single event

Clinical Manifestations
- Painless limp
- If painful, often mild and intermittent localizing in the anterior or proximal thigh, groin, or knee
- Flexion contracture of the involved leg with lower extremity held in slightly externally rotated position
- Limited abduction of the hip (typically 20° to 30° at diagnosis; normal is 45°); limited internal rotation of the hip
- Adductor muscle spasm (early) and contracture (late)
- Proximal thigh atrophy, delayed bone growth, mild short stature

Diagnostics
- X-ray: AP and frog-leg lateral views of the pelvis
- Continuum of disease based on radiographic finding: 1) fracture of subchondral region; 2) fragmentation/resorption; 3) reossification; 4) healed or residual stage
- Multiple systems exist to further classify radiographic findings.
- Bone scan may reveal an inadequate blood supply: consider if early x-rays are normal

Management
Principles
- Self-limited process of 1 to 2 years in which the femoral head always revascularizes, so treatment focuses on preserving hip motion and a spherical femoral head to minimize degenerative joint disease

- Primary principle is "containment": using the acetabulum as a spherical mold to re-shape the femoral head
- Intervention if loss of "containment" within the acetabulum, bone age greater than 6 years at diagnosis (consider intervention in girls greater than 5 years), necrosis of greater than 50% of femoral head, or collapse of lateral pillar

Interventions
- NSAIDs, limiting activity, crutches, range of motion exercises
- Occasionally, temporary traction to relieve pain
- Bracing offers no advantage
- Pelvic or femoral osteotomy may be needed to achieve "containment," especially in children closer to skeletal maturity.

TRANSIENT SYNOVITIS (Toxic Synovitis)

Sudden onset of unilateral hip pain and physical findings in a non-toxic child

Epidemiology
- Most common cause of hip pain in childhood
- Typically affects children 3 to 8 years of age; males affected more often than females (2:1)
- Risk factors: obesity, intercurrent or recent illness

Etiology
- Etiology unclear, frequently follows upper respiratory tract infection

Clinical Manifestations
- Unilateral hip pain: may manifest as groin, hip, anterior thigh, or knee pain; limp; occasional refusal to bear weight
- Afebrile or low grade temperature (<38°C)
- "Position of comfort:" mildly flexed and externally rotated
- Restricted abduction and internal rotation on exam
- Minimal pain on "log roll" test (gentle rotation of leg with hip and knee in extension)

Diagnostics
- Diagnosis of exclusion: AP and frog-leg lateral films are normal; WBC, ESR, and CRP may be mildly elevated
- Hip ultrasound reveals fluid in asymptomatic contralateral hip in 25% of cases.
- Joint aspiration in child with fever, hip pain, and elevated ESR or CRP to exclude septic arthritis; usually less than 10,000 WBC/mm^3 with toxic synovitis (see septic arthritis in Infectious Diseases)

Management
- Most cases resolve completely in 1 to 2 weeks. Recurrence in 10% to 20%.
- Avoid weight-bearing; encourage bedrest
- NSAIDs
- No need for antibiotics or steroids
- Joint aspiration provides dramatic pain relief but joint effusion rapidly reaccumulates; therefore, reserve for diagnostic purposes.

Resources

Fractures
Della-Giustina K, Della-Giustina DA. Emergency department evaluation of pediatric orthopedic injuries. Emerg Med Clin North Am 1999;17:895–922.

Marx JA, ed. Rosen's Emergency Medicine: Concepts and Clinical Practice. 5th ed. St. Louis: Mosby, 2002.

Overly F, et al. Common pediatric fractures and dislocations. Clin Pediatr Emerg Med 2002;3:106–117.

Casas J, et al. Femoral fractures in children from 4 to 10 years: conservative treatment. J Pediatr Orthop 2001;10:52–62.

Koval KJ, Zuckerman JD. Handbook of Fractures. 2nd ed. Philadelphia: Lippincott, Williams and Wilkins, 2002.

Morris S, Cassidy N, Stephens M, et al. Birth-associated femoral fractures. J Pediatr Orthop 2002;22:27–30.

Stans AA, Morrissy RT, Renwick SE. Femoral shaft fractures in patients age 6 to 16 Years. J Pediatr Orthop 1999;19:222–228.

Mahabir RC, Kazemi AR, Cannon WG, Courtemanche DJ. Pediatric hand fractures. Pediatr Emerg Care 2001;17:153–156.

Do T, Herrera-Soto J. Elbow injuries in children. Curr Opin Pediatr 2003;15:68–73.

Lins RE, Simovitch RW, Waters PM. Pediatric elbow trauma. Orthop Clin North Am 1999;30:119–132.

Villarin LA Jr, Belk KE, Freid R. Emergency department evaluation and treatment of elbow and forearm injuries. Emerg Med Clin North Am 1999;17:843–858.

Canale ST, ed. Campbell's Operative Orthopedics. 9th ed. St Louis: Mosby, 1998.

Perron AD, Hersh RE, Brady WJ, Keats TE. Orthopedic pitfalls in the ED: Galeazzi and Monteggia fracture-dislocation. Am J Emerg Med 2001;19:225–228.

Perron AD, Miller MD, Brady WJ. Orthopedic pitfalls in the ED: pediatric growth plate injuries. Am J Emerg Med 2002;20:50–54.

Della-Giustina K, Della-Giustina DA. Emergency department evaluation of pediatric orthopedic injuries. Emerg Med Clin North Am 1999;17:895–922.

Beringer DC, Weiner DS, Noble JS, Bell RH. Severely displaced proximal humeral epiphyseal fractures: a follow-up study. J Pediatr Orthop 1998;18:31–37.

Common Orthopedic Issues

American Academy of Pediatrics. Early detection of developmental dysplasia of the hip. Pediatrics 2000;105:896–905.

Canale ST, ed. Campbell's Operative Orthopedics. 9th ed. St Louis: Mosby, 1998.

Morrissy RT, et al. Lovell & Winter's Pediatric Orthopaedics. 5th ed. Philadelphia: Lippincott, Williams and Wilkins, 2001.

POSNA. The Core Curriculum. Developmental dysplasia of the hip (older infant). Available at: http://www.posna.org/index?service=page/coreCurriculum&article=DDHOlderInfant.html. Accessed on December 1, 2003.

POSNA. The Core Curriculum. Developmental dysplasia of the hip (walking age). Available at: http://www.posna.org/index?service=page/coreCurriculum&article=DDHWalking.html. Accessed on December 1, 2003.

Wall EJ. Legg-Calvé-Perthes' disease. Curr Opin Pediatr 1999;11:76–79.

Del Beccaro MA, Champoux AM, Bockers T, Mendelman PM. Septic arthritis versus transient synovitis of the hip: value of screening laboratory tests. Ann Emerg Med 1992;21:1418–1422.

Ehrendorfer S, LeQuesne G, Penta M, et al. Bilateral synovitis in symptomatic unilateral transient synovitis of the hip: an ultrasonographic study in 56 children. Acta Orthop Scand 1996;67:139–142.

Marc Eisen, MD, PhD, Steven D. Handler, MD, MBE

ADENOTONSILLAR HYPERTROPHY

Enlargement of palatine tonsils and adenoid lymphoid tissue that contributes to obstruction of the upper airway (UA)

- Results in continuum of snoring, sleep disordered breathing, UA resistance syndrome, and obstructive sleep apnea (OSA)

Epidemiology
- Volume of lymphoid tissue increases from 6 months of age to puberty; peak of OSA in preschool years, when tissue makes up greatest proportion of UA
- Associated with craniofacial and neuromuscular disorders

Pathophysiology
- Upper airway obstruction is multifactorial; includes hypertrophied lymphoid tissue, compliance and elasticity of pharyngeal soft tissue, facial morphology, and changes to the pharyngeal musculature during sleep.
- Cyclic airway obstruction during sleep causes hypoxia and hypercapnia, leading to arousals and restoration of respiration.
- Repeated arousals interrupt rapid eye movement sleep, which can lead to daytime and nighttime problems.

Clinical Manifestations
- Mouth breathing, dry lip mucosa, hyponasal speech
- Nighttime: snoring, apnea, restless sleep, enuresis, nightmares
- Daytime: somnolence, behavioral changes, learning difficulties, mouth breathing, growth disturbances
- Possible craniofacial abnormalities: dental malocclusion, pharyngeal soft tissue anatomy, shape and size of tongue and uvula
- Degree of tonsillar enlargement: tonsil within fossa = 0; less than 25% obstruction = 1+; less than 50% obstruction = 2+; less than 75% obstruction = 3+; greater than 75% obstruction = 4+

Diagnostics
- Lateral neck radiograph to assess adenoid size and airway caliber; however, volume of tonsils and adenoids do not correlate well with severity of OSA
- ECG in cor pulmonale reveals right heart strain or right ventricular hypertrophy
- Polysomnography is definitive test for OSA
- Home video or audio sleep recording may be helpful

Management
Medical
- Systemic or topical steroids may shrink lymphoid tissue, but long-term effectiveness is questioned.
- Noninvasive positive pressure ventilation (e.g., nasal continuous positive airway pressure)
- Weight loss for patients with morbid obesity

Surgical
- Indications for adenoidectomy and tonsillectomy: alveolar hypoventilation (obstructive sleep apnea), cor pulmonale, nasal obstruction causing discomfort in breathing and severe distortion of speech (adenoidectomy only), or dysphagia (tonsillectomy only). Removal for recurrent peritonsillar abscess or chronic tonsillitis is controversial.

- Complications of surgery include postoperative hemorrhage, dehydration, and post-obstructive pulmonary edema
- Tracheostomy may be needed (temporary or permanent), especially for children with complex medical/surgical issues.

BRANCHIAL CLEFT ANOMALIES

Persistence of branchial cleft resulting in cysts, sinuses, or fistulae of the lateral neck

- *Cyst:* persistent lateral neck mass; usually painless unless it is infected
- *Sinus:* external opening to neck along the anterior border of the sternocleidomastoid muscle (SCM), extending along the tract. May trap/drain external fluid.
- *Fistula:* opening externally in neck and internally in tonsilar fossa

Epidemiology

- Branchial cleft anomalies are present from birth, but are often not recognized until acute infection of the structure in the first decade of life
- 90% arise from the second branchial cleft

Etiology

- Anomalies develop from ectodermal remnants in the tract of the second branchial cleft, which arises from the anterior-superior border of the SCM, passes between the internal and external carotids and over the 10th and 12th cranial nerves to end at the tonsillar fossa.
- These anomalous structures may become infected.

Differential Diagnosis

- Differential diagnosis affected by location (Figure 24.1)
- Congenital: hemangioma, cystic hygroma, thyroglossal duct cyst, SCM pseudotumor of infancy (fibromatosis coli), remnant of branchial arch cartilage, enlarged or ectopic thyroid, epidermoid cyst (usually lateral), neurofibroma (usually lateral), lipoma

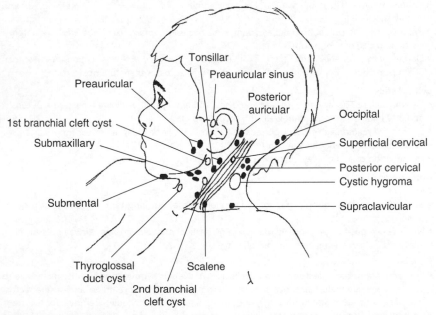

Figure 24.1 Typical locations of cystic and solid neck masses. Key: o = Cysts/sinuses; • = lymph nodes.

- Following trauma: hematoma, subcutaneous emphysema
- Infectious: reactive adenopathy, adenitis (see Infectious Diseases chapter), Kawasaki, infectious mononucleosis syndrome, toxoplasmosis, sarcoid
- Malignant: leukemia, lymphoma, neuroblastoma, Langerhans cell histiocytosis, others

Clinical Manifestations
- Cystic neck mass or opening anterior to mid-portion of SCM
- Usually nontender, firm, mobile, and located just beneath the skin
- May have tenderness, redness, or swelling if infected
- Internal opening of fistula may be visible near tonsillar fossa
- Key point: Midline mass that moves upward with tongue protrusion or swallowing suggests thyroglossal duct cyst

Diagnostics
- CT (preferred) or MRI usually delineates the structure
- Ultrasound can establish cystic versus solid masses (Figure 24.1)
- Rarely, instillation of radiopaque material is needed to demonstrate the extent of the fistula or sinus.

Management
- Complete surgical excision is the definitive treatment of choice, preferably performed when structure is not acutely inflamed.
- Acute infection/abscess is treated with systemic antibiotics (e.g., ampicillin-sulbactam, amoxicillin-clavulanate, or clindamycin) and, if needed, incision and drainage.

CLEFT LIP/PALATE

Cleft Lip
Complete = extends into floor of the nose

Incomplete = extends part way through the lip

Microform = notch in vermillion border

Cleft Palate
Always involves uvula

Unilateral or bilateral

Severity depends on degree of soft and hard palate involvement

Epidemiology
- One in 1000 white births; 1:400 Japanese births; 1:3000 African births
- Cleft lip: 80% unilateral, 20% bilateral. 75% have associated cleft palate
- Facial clefting associated with approximately 300 syndromes
- Both genetic and environmental factors appear to be responsible for clefting.

Pathophysiology
- Embryology: palatogenesis occurs between 5th and 12th week of gestation
- Clefting results from incomplete closure of upper lip, the two halves of the hard palate, and the overlying soft palate.
- Feeding difficulties are due to inability to create adequate negative oral pressure with sucking.
- Airway difficulties may require nasal airway and positioning to maximize airway patency; tracheostomy for severe cases.
- Conductive hearing loss and middle ear disease are due to eustachian tube dysfunction. Most require pressure equalization tubes.
- Speech problems found in most cleft palate patients.
- Other congenital abnormalities common

Management
Multidisciplinary approach: surgeon, dentist, speech pathologist, audiologist, geneticist, social worker, nurse, nutritionist, psychologist

Feeding
- Specially designed nipples such as Habermann feeder or Mead-Johnson cleft bottle.
- Frequent burping required due to increased air swallowing.
- Nasogastric feeding may be required, but minimize to avoid oral aversion.
- Gastrostomy tube is last resort.

Surgical
- Cleft lip repair usually performed between 6 and 12 weeks of age.
- Lip adhesion may be performed as initial procedure.
- Cleft palate repair: goal includes separation of nasal from oral cavity and a competent velopharyngeal valve, elongation of the palate, and restoration of palate musculature. All are aimed at yielding adequate speech results.
- Cleft palate repair typically completed by 12 to 18 months of age.

EPISTAXIS

Nose bleed

Pathophysiology
- Anterior septum (Little's area) is most common site due to vascularity (Kiesselbach's plexus) and exposure (dry air, trauma)
- Epistaxis from trauma (digital or impact), inflammation, dryness, or less often, tumor, vascular abnormality, or coagulopathy

Clinical Manifestations
- Active bleeding or dry blood +/– identifiable source
- Mucosa: dry, cracked, pale, boggy, prominent vessels
- Localize active bleeding: anterior, posterior, unilateral or bilateral
- Check for masses, polyps, foreign bodies
- Signs of underlying bleeding disorder: petechiae, ecchymosis
- Hypertension: unusual cause in children
- History: bruising, bleeding, or family history of same; use of anticoagulants or platelet inhibitors

Diagnostics
- None routinely required but clinical situation may warrant the following:
- Hematologic and coagulation studies
- Sinus CT or MRI if malignancy suspected
- Arteriography or MR angiography if vascular anomaly suspected or embolization is considered

Management
Medical
- Hold pressure on nostrils
- Phenylephrine (0.25%) or oxymetazoline (0.05%; Afrin) spray to affected nostril for local vasoconstriction
- Anterior nasal packing with ointment-coated sponges
- Posterior packing (gauze, nasal tampons/balloons) rarely needed except for severe trauma or tumor bleeding
- Antibiotics (e.g., cephalexin, clindamycin, amoxicillin-clavulanate) while packing in place due to risk of toxic shock syndrome and sinusitis
- Treat underlying process (e.g., allergic rhinitis, bleeding diathesis)
- ENT consult for severe epistaxis, suspicion of occult nasal lesion, or underlying hemorrhagic diathesis
- For chronic epistaxis: moisten/lubricate with saline spray, petrolatum, antibiotic ointment

Surgical
- Chemical cautery (e.g., silver nitrate) of bleeding site
- Electrocautery of bleeding site (do *not* cauterize both sides of nasal septum due to risk of septal ischemia and perforation)

- Limited septoplasty
- Embolization, laser excision, or arterial ligation in severe cases (e.g., tumor, vascular malformation)

FOREIGN BODY ASPIRATION/INGESTION

Epidemiology
- Highest incidence in children 1 to 3 years of age
- Twice as common in boys as in girls
- Most common foreign body (FB): vegetative matter (aspiration), coin (ingestion)

Etiology
- Toddlers have less control of swallowing and immaturity in laryngeal elevation and glottic closure
- Mental retardation and seizure disorder are predisposing factors

Clinical Manifestations
- History of FB in mouth or close to child or unobserved period before appearance of symptoms
- May be asymptomatic for weeks or months before presentation
- Airway FB: wheezing, unexplained coughing spells, significant respiratory distress, pneumonia, decreased breath sounds in obstructed lobe/lung
- Upper airway symptoms: hoarseness, aphonia, stridor, inspiratory wheeze
- Lower airway symptoms: expiratory wheeze, asymmetric aeration of lung fields
- Ingested FB: drooling, throat pain, dysphagia, odynophagia, localizable anterior neck pain, respiratory distress due to compression of the airway from esophageal FB

Diagnostics
- Posteroanterior and lateral chest and neck films together are used to localize radiopaque objects in airway.
- Chest CT if erosion or extraluminal extension suspected
- *Aspiration:* acutely, failure of affected lobe to deflate may be seen on inspiratory/expiratory (hyperinflation on expiratory film) or lateral decubitus (air trapping in dependent lung) chest x-ray. Subacutely or chronically, the chest x-ray may show resorptive post-obstructive atelectasis, compensatory emphysema of nonobstructed lobes, pneumonia, pneumothorax, shift of mediastinum during expiration, or abscess.
- *Ingestion:* esophageal air may delineate tissue density FB on plain film. Barium swallow may identify radiolucent esophageal FB
- *Repeated episodes:* consider evaluation of swallowing function (presence of gag reflex, observed feedings, modified barium swallow with speech therapy), or esophageal anatomy (upper endoscopy, barium swallow)

Management
Complete airway obstruction is an absolute emergency. Perform the Heimlich maneuver on children older than 1 year of age, and back blows/chest thrusts on children younger than 1 year of age.
- Endoscopy can be both diagnostic and therapeutic. General anesthesia is required.
- Rigid bronchoscope: allows visualization of the trachea and bronchi, with removal of the FB through the scope. Ventilation occurs through the scope.
- Rigid esophagoscopy: allows visualization of the entire esophagus with removal of the FB through the scope.
- FBs that cannot be removed endoscopically may require thoracotomy for direct removal.

LARYNGOMALACIA

Congenital flaccid larynx

Epidemiology
- Most common laryngeal anomaly in neonates
- Accounts for 65% to 75% of neonatal stridor

Etiology
- Exact etiology unknown
- Theories include hypotonia or incoordination of laryngeal or supralaryngeal structures
- Gastroesophageal reflux may be contributing factor

Pathophysiology
- Supraglottic collapse can be caused by prolapse of arytenoid mucosa, foreshortened aryepiglottic folds, or posterior displacement of epiglottis.
- With normal growth, the symptoms initially worsen, then gradually resolve between 6 and 18 months.

Clinical Manifestations
- Onset of "noisy breathing" or inspiratory stridor within the first few weeks of life, which worsens with agitation and/or supine positioning
- Inspiratory stridor that is typically positional, louder when child is supine or during sleep; also with agitation or exertion (e.g., feeding, crying, laughing)
- Normal cry is typical (expiratory process)
- Evidence of increased work of breathing: nasal flaring, retractions, pectus excavatum

Diagnostics
- Flexible nasopharyngolaryngoscopy: confirms diagnosis; reveals omega-shaped epiglottis and posterior collapse of supraglottis with prolapse of cuneiform cartilage into glottis during inspiration.
- Airway fluoroscopy may reveal supraglottic collapse, but less useful test than direct visualization.
- For severe cases, rigid laryngoscopy and bronchoscopy under general anesthesia may be warranted.
- Evaluation for concurrent congenital anomalies is important.

Management
Medical
- Depends on severity of symptoms
  - Mild: no feeding problems; symptoms not progressive
  - Moderate: feeding difficulties but thriving; progressive stridor
  - Severe: apnea, cyanosis, failure to thrive
- Treatment of gastroesophageal reflux may help airway symptoms
- *Mild/Moderate:* conservative management with reassurance to family that condition is self-limited, yet complete resolution may take up to 18 months. CPR education for caretakers. Home pulse-oximetry monitoring may be indicated.
- *Severe:* surgery may be necessary.

Surgical
- Supraglottoplasty: excision of the obstructive aryepiglottic folds or redundant supraglottic tissues.
- Tracheotomy: occasionally indicated in most severe cases

TRACHEOSTOMY

Trache**os**tomy: the actual hole in the trachea following tracheotomy

Trache**ot**omy: the surgical incision in the trachea used to gain access to the airway

Indications for Tracheostomy
- Ventilator dependency (40%)
- Extrathoracic obstruction (30%)
- Neurologic dysfunction (20%)
- Intrathoracic obstruction (10%)

Tracheostomy versus Prolonged Endotracheal Intubation
- Risks of prolonged intubation include injury to glottis, subglottis, and trachea due to pressure of tube.
- Endotracheal tubes can easily become blocked due to small lumen of pediatric tubes.
- Endotracheal tube irritation can be minimized by deflating cuff and restricting patient movement.
- Typical recommendation is for tracheostomy after 2 weeks of intubation in child, longer in neonates
- Advantages of tracheostomy: hospital discharge on ventilator support, avoid damage to larynx and subglottis, easier replacement if decannulated
- Disadvantages of tracheostomy: need for frequent cleaning, suctioning, and humidification; surgical risks; risk of general anesthesia

Complications of Tracheostomy
- Intraoperative complications: hemorrhage, subcutaneous emphysema, pneumomediastinum, pneumothorax
- Early postoperative complications: tracheostomy tube plugging, decannulation, tracheitis
- Late postoperative complications: erosion of the anterior tracheal wall, which may lead to tracheo-innominate fistula, tracheoesophageal fistula, tracheal granulomas, suprastomal collapse

Tracheostomy Care
- Cuffless tubes preferred in young children to prevent pressure on tracheal wall
- Softer, pliable tubes are less likely to cause pressure damage
- Tracheostomy tube size corresponds to the inner diameter in mm. Outer diameter is variable and depends on manufacturer and/or material.
- Humidified air is supplied to prevent drying of tracheal mucosa
- Trained caregiver, suctioning equipment, and replacement tube should always be available to maintain airway patency.

Changing Tracheostomy Tubes
- Surgeons typically make first change and survey stoma for patency
- Further changes can be made by other caregivers
- All tracheostomy changes best made with neck extended, with good lighting and suction available

VOCAL CORD PARALYSIS

Unilateral or bilateral paralysis of the vocal folds

Epidemiology
- 10% of all congenital laryngeal lesions
- Rarely an isolated lesion in children
- Unilateral vocal cord paralysis (VCP) is more common on left

Etiology
- 50% congenital, 50% acquired
- Usually one manifestation of multisystem abnormality, most frequently involving CNS (usually at brainstem level)
- Central nervous system causes (e.g., Arnold-Chiari malformation, closed head injury)
- Progressive peripheral nerve disorders (e.g., myasthenia gravis)
- Iatrogenic: thoracic or neck surgery (injury to the recurrent laryngeal nerve), endotracheal intubation
- Neoplasia or inflammation are very unusual causes in children
- Idiopathic in 35% to 47% of cases

Pathophysiology
- Abductors and adductors of vocal cords are controlled by the recurrent laryngeal nerve, a branch of the vagus nerve, which can be damaged anywhere along the path from the brainstem to the larynx.
- Unilateral VCP is more commonly due to peripheral nerve injury.
- Bilateral VCP is more likely due to CNS cause.
- Direct injury to glottic tissues can occur during endolaryngeal instrumentation.

Clinical Manifestations
- Unilateral vocal cord paralysis: weak cry, breathy voice, aspiration, and/or feeding difficulties, ineffective cough, recurrent pneumonia, hoarseness
- Bilateral vocal cord paralysis: stridor, respiratory distress, aspiration, and/or feeding difficulties; may have normal cry
- Evaluate severity of respiratory impairment: work of breathing, respiratory rate, oxygen saturation
- Search for associated congenital anomalies or predisposing trauma

Diagnostics
- Flexible laryngoscopy: cornerstone of diagnosis; can usually be done at bedside without sedation
- MRI and/or CT to evaluate CNS and course of vagus nerve
- Barium swallow to assess swallowing function, risk of aspiration, or associated abnormal mediastinal anatomy

Management
Three Goals of Management
1. *Safe airway*
   - Tracheostomy: necessary for 20% to 50% of bilateral VCP; rarely necessary for unilateral VCP
   - Spontaneous resolution is common, so period of observation is essential
   - Lateralization of VC may be needed for unresolved bilateral VCP
2. Intelligible speech
3. Prevention of aspiration
   - May require G-tube temporarily.

Resources

Agarwala S, Bhatnagar U, Mitra DK. Coins can be safely removed from the esophagus by Foley's catheter without fluoroscopic control. Indian Pediatr 1996;33:109.

Bailey BJ, Calhoun K, eds. Head and Neck Surgery: Otolaryngology. 3rd ed. Philadelphia: Lippincott, Williams & Wilkins, 2001.

Freiman MA, McMurray JS. Unique presentation of a bronchial foreign body in an asymptomatic child. Ann Otol Rhinol Laryngol 2001;110:495–497.

Kenealy JF, Torsiglieri AJ, Tom LW. Branchial cleft anomalies: a five-year retrospective review. Trans Penn Acad Ophthalmol Otolaryngol 1990;42:1022–1025.

Laurikainen E, Erkinjuntti M, Alihanka J, et al. Radiological parameters of the bony nasopharynx and the adenotonsillar size compared with sleep apnea episodes in children. Int J Pediatr Otorhinolaryngol 1987;12:303–310.

Manning SC, Stool SE. Foreign bodies of the pharynx and esophagus. In: Bluestone CD, Stool SE, et al., eds. Pediatric Otolaryngology. 4th ed. Philadelphia: WB Saunders, 2003:1324–1337.

Murray AD, Mahoney EM, Holinger LD. Foreign bodies of the airway and esophagus. In: Richardson MA, ed. Otolaryngology Head & Neck Surgery. 3rd ed. St. Louis: Mosby, 1998:377–387.

Olney DR, Greinwald JHJ, Smith RJH, Bauman NM. Laryngomalacia and its treatment. Laryngoscope 1999;109:1770–1775.

Rosin DF, Handler SD, Potsic WP. Vocal cord paralysis in children. Laryngoscope 1990;100:1174–1179.

Seibert RW, Wiet GJ, Bumsted RM. Cleft lip and palate. In: Richardson MA, ed. Otolaryngology Head & Neck Surgery. 3rd ed. St. Louis: Mosby, 1998:133–173.

Torsiglieri AJ, Tom LW, Ross AJ, et al. Pediatric neck masses: guidelines for evaluation. Int J Pediatr Otorhinolaryngol 1988;16:199–210.

Wetmore RF, Muntz HR, McGill TJ, eds. Pediatric Otolaryngology: Principles and Pathways. New York: Thieme, 2000.

Nicholas Tsarouhas, MD (with contributions from Linda L. Brown, MD,
Lauren Daly, MD, Reza Daugherty, MD, Marla J. Friedman, DO,
Karen J. O'Connell, MD, Vivian Hwang, MD)

ENDOTRACHEAL INTUBATION

Indications
- Airway protection; cardiac, respiratory or neurologic failure; severe burns; multiple trauma; head injury
- See inside back cover for rapid sequence intubation medications.

Equipment
Mnemonic: "MSOAP"
- *M-Meds:* Intubation adjuncts, sedatives, paralytics, resuscitation meds, anti-convulsants
- *M-Monitors:* cardiorespiratory (CR) monitor, pulse-oximeter, blood pressure (BP), CO_2 detector
- *S-Suction:* Yankauer (rigid catheter), "spaghetti" (soft catheter)
- *O-Oxygen:* Tank or "wall" supply, delivery tubing
- *A-Airway Equipment:* Endotracheal tubes, stylets, laryngoscope blades, bag/valve/mask apparatus, masks, nasopharyngeal airway, oropharyngeal airway, tape, benzoin
- *P-Personnel*

Choosing an Endotracheal Tube
- Diameter of endotracheal tube (ETT) same as infant's external nares or fifth finger
- Formula for ETT diameter:

[Age (years) + 16]/4 or [Age (years)/4] + 4

- Use uncuffed ETT if younger than 8 years of age and cuffed ETT if older than 8 years of age

Choosing a Laryngoscope Blade
- Preemie: "0" straight
- Zero to 3 months: "1" straight
- Three months to 3 years: "1.5" straight
- Three to 12 years: "2" straight/curved
- Older than 12 years: "3" straight/curved

Technique
- Check all equipment and monitors. Preoxygenate with 100% O_2. Administer selected pharmacologic agents (see inside cover).
- If stable cervical (C)-spine, place patient's head in sniffing position. If unstable C-spine, use in-line stabilization with gentle jaw thrust.
- If using stylet, tip should not extend beyond end of ETT.
- Have assistant apply cricoid pressure (Sellick maneuver).
- Open mouth using scissor-finger technique with right hand (thumb on mandibular dental ridge, index or middle finger on maxillary dental ridge).
- Holding laryngoscope in left hand, insert blade on the right side of the patient's mouth, and sweep tongue toward the midline. Gently but firmly pull up along the axis of the handle of the laryngoscope. Do not rotate (lever) the instrument by rotating the wrist.
- Visualize glottic opening (characteristic inverted V of vocal cords)
- Introduce ETT with right hand from the right side of mouth (not through sight line) and pass tip of tube through the vocal cords.
- Depth of insertion: internal diameter of the ETT × 3 (length to corner of mouth), or double lines on tube just past vocal cords

- *Confirmation of proper placement*: Listen for equal breath sounds; observe chest wall for equal rise; look for "misting" in ETT; use CO_2 detector
- Temporarily secure ETT to patient with benzoin and tape. Obtain chest x-ray to confirm placement (tip just above carina). Definitively secure ETT by splitting tape lengthwise; secure one arm to upper lip and wrap second arm around ETT. Repeat with second piece of tape.

FEMORAL VENOUS CATHETERIZATION

Indications
- Administration of fluids or drugs to treat circulatory failure, administration of drugs that are unsafe through peripheral access, measurement of central venous pressure or mixed venous blood gases, long-term access

Equipment
- *Sterile field:* Antiseptic solution (povidone-iodine), gauze, towels, gloves, gown, mask
- *Monitoring equipment:* CR monitor, pulse oximeter, blood pressure monitor, central venous pressure (CVP) transducer
- *Sedation/Analgesia:* Consider 1% lidocaine subcutaneous AND fentanyl, morphine, midazolam, ketamine, or etomidate (see anesthesia section)
- *Catheter kit:* Should include central venous catheter, dilator, guidewire, heparinized saline, 5-cc sterile syringe with needle.
- *Misc. equipment:* Suture material (3.0 or 4.0 silk), needle driver, number 11 blade scalpel, transparent polyurethane dressing

Catheter Size: Flow rate is proportional to the fourth power of radius and inversely proportional to length, so largest diameter/shortest length catheter should be used.

- *General guide to catheter sizing (French):* 0 to 6 months: 3F; 6 months to 2 years: 3–4F; 3 to 6 years: 4F; 7 to 12 years: 4–5F

Technique
1. *Initial Preparation:* monitor and sedate as necessary. Position patient with hip elevated, abducted, and externally rotated.
2. *Locate the femoral vein:* from lateral to medial: femoral Nerve, Artery, Vein, Empty space, Lymphatics (mnemonic: NAVEL)
   - *Child with a pulse:* vein lies 1 to 2 cm medial to femoral arterial pulse and 1 to 2 cm below inguinal ligament.
   - *Pulse weak or absent:* vein lies approximately halfway between pubic symphysis and anterior superior iliac spine, and 1 to 2 cm below inguinal ligament.
3. *Final preparation:* locally infiltrate lidocaine at intended site of puncture. Don sterile gloves, mask, and gown. Prepare area with sterile technique and sterile drapes. Flush all ports of catheter with heparinized saline.
4. *Advancing needle:* attach needle to 5-cc syringe. Enter skin at 45 degrees over anticipated location of femoral vein. Slowly advance needle towards the umbilicus while applying slight negative pressure. Re-angle or slightly alter direction if no blood return. (Do NOT pass level of inguinal ligament.) Enter and withdraw the needle slowly to prevent multiple vascular lacerations. If unsuccessful after several attempts, flush the needle and syringe with saline to eject any possible skin plugs.
5. *Insertion of guidewire:* Once freely flowing venous blood return is noted, stabilize the needle and carefully remove the syringe. Occlude the needle lumen with your thumb to prevent air embolism or significant blood loss. Insert guidewire with the "J curve" first, ensuring that the back end of the wire is always visible and held tightly. Withdraw the needle over the wire. Carefully grasp the wire at the skin insertion site as soon as the needle exits from the skin.
6. *Advance and secure the catheter:* use a no. 11 blade scalpel to make small skin incision along path of wire with sharp edge of blade pointing away from the wire. Pass the dilator over the wire. Remove the dilator and pass the catheter over the wire until the hub is flush with the skin. Rotate

the catheter during insertion to facilitate passage through the skin and subcutaneous tissues. Remove the wire, leaving the catheter in place. Suture the catheter to the patient's skin using the flanges on the catheter. Apply a transparent polyurethane dressing.

7. *Confirm venous placement:* a) Venous blood flow is not pulsatile. b) Blood gas analysis yields venous PaO_2. c) Pressure transducer can distinguish venous from arterial pressures. d) An abdominal x-ray can confirm tip position if CVP monitoring is desired; the tip should be below the level of the right atrium.

INTRAOSSEOUS LINE PLACEMENT

Indications
- Immediate vascular access for cardiopulmonary arrest or shock; intravenous access difficult or not possible
- Typically used in children younger than 6 years of age
- May administer fluids, blood products, medications
- Aspirated blood can be sent for electrolytes, type and cross, and blood culture, but is not reliable for blood count.

Equipment
Sterile gloves, drapes, gauze; antiseptic solution (povidone-iodine); 1% lidocaine; syringes (3, 5, 10 cc); 22- or 25-gauge needles; saline flush in 10-cc syringe; IV fluid/blood "pressure bag" (optional); intraosseous (IO) or bone marrow aspiration needle with trocar

- A 20-gauge spinal needle can be used if IO needle not available

Placement Sites
1. *Proximal tibia:* tibial plateau (anterior, medial flat surface of tibia), 1 to 2 cm below the tibial tuberosity. Preferred site
2. *Distal femur:* midline on femoral plateau (lower third of femur), approximately 3 cm above the lateral condyle or 1 to 2 cm above the superior border of the patella
3. *Distal tibia:* 1 to 2 cm above the medial malleolus. Easier to use in children older than 3 years of age.

Technique
- In awake patients, inject 1% lidocaine into skin and periosteum.
- Prepare skin with antiseptic solution (povidone-iodine).
- Stabilize extremity with non-dominant hand. (Keep hand away from opposite side of insertion site to avoid self-stabbing!)
- Hold IO needle with hub resting in the palm; Stabilize needle with thumb and index finger placed 1 to 2 cm from the tip.
- Insert needle perpendicular to the bony cortex or slightly angled (10 to 15 degrees) away from the growth plate. Use steady back and forth rotational motion while gradually increasing pressure until a sudden decrease in resistance is felt. Immediately release pressure to prevent piercing opposite end of bone.
- Advance the needle 1 cm and then remove the trocar. If the needle is secure in the bone, it should stand without support.
- Confirm intramedullary placement with aspiration of blood or bone marrow and easy infusion of fluids without extravasation.
- Secure needle with tape bridge. Avoid bulky dressings.

LACERATION REPAIR

Indication
- Restore integrity and function of injured tissues while minimizing scar formation and infection.

Equipment

1. *Basics:* bed, light, mask, sterile gloves, povidone-iodine solution
2. *Irrigation:* 20- to 60-mL syringes, sterile saline, splash guard
3. *Suture tray:* needle holder, nontraumatic tissue forceps, tissue scissors, hemostats, sterile gauze
4. *Suture material:*
   • Nonabsorbable: monofilament nylon, polypropylene
   • Absorbable: Vicryl, fast-absorbing gut
   • Size: Face: 6-0 or 5-0; Scalp, trunk, extremities: 4-0; Sole of foot, over large joints: 4-0 or 3-0

General Technique

1. *Local Anesthesia:*
   • *"LET" gel:* contains lidocaine, epinephrine, and tetracaine. Apply for 15 to 20 minutes up to three times or until skin blanches. Avoid areas where vasoconstriction is contraindicated.
   • *1% Lidocaine (10 mg/mL):* Infiltrative anesthetic; maximum dose: 5 mg/kg; onset: 2 to 5 minutes; duration: 50 to 120 minutes.
   • *1% Lidocaine with Epinephrine (1:200,000):* Infiltrative anesthetic; maximum dose: 7 mg/kg; onset: 2 to 5 minutes; duration: 60 to 180 minutes; contraindicated in digits, penis, pinna, tip of nose
   • *Sodium Bicarbonate:* Buffers local anesthetic to improve potency and reduce pain. Mix 1 part NaHCO$_3$ to 10 parts lidocaine.
2. *Wound Preparation:*
   • Exploration: provide hemostasis; explore for foreign body.
   • Débridement: Remove devitalized or heavily contaminated tissue
   • Hair: may clip. Alternatively, use petroleum jelly to keep unwanted scalp hair away from wound. Do not shave eyebrows.
   • Irrigation: Irrigate with normal saline using 20- 60-mL syringe and splash-guard. Use 100–200 mL for average 2-cm laceration. Clean wound periphery using povidone-iodine solution.
3. *Apply Suture Using Needle Holder:*
   • For better control, hold loaded needle holder near the tip. Do NOT keep fingers in rings of the needle holder while sewing.
   • Enter skin with needle perpendicular to surface. Retrieve needle after each pass with needle holder or forceps.
4. *Instrument Tie:* tighten knot so than skin edges just come together, making sure that wound edges are everted to minimize scar formation (Figure 25.1). Repeat single loop tie, in an over and under manner, for a total of four throws. Cut both ends of suture allowing adequate length (at least 1 cm) to retrieve suture at time of removal.
5. *Suture Removal:* Neck: 3 to 4 days; face, scalp: 5 days; upper extremities, trunk: 7 to 10 days; lower extremities: 8 to 10 days; joint surface: 10 to 14 days

Suture Techniques

1. *Simple Interrupted Sutures:* Enter skin with needle directed downward or angled slightly away from wound edge (see Figure 25.1).

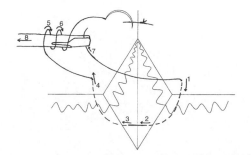

Figure 25.1   Simple interrupted suture.

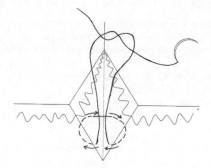

Figure 25.2 Inverted subcutaneous suture.

2. *Inverted ("Buried") Subcutaneous Sutures:* Used to counteract tension on wound. Insert needle from within wound at fat-dermal junction (Figure 25.2).
3. *Vertical Mattress Sutures:* Combines a deep and superficial stitch into one suture (Figure 25.3). Used in wounds of high tension or where difficult to tie an inverted subcutaneous suture.
4. *Horizontal Mattress Sutures:* Reinforces subcutaneous tissue and relieves tension from wound edges. Useful as deep layer in relatively shallow lacerations and in areas with minimal subcutaneous tissue (Figure 25.4).
5. *Half-buried or Corner Suture:* Useful in flap closure. Enter skin below and just lateral to the point of V-shaped flap (Figure 25.5).
6. *Simple (Continuous) Running Suture:* Limited to linear, clean, low tension wounds. Saves time but breakage unravels entire stitch (Figure 25.6).

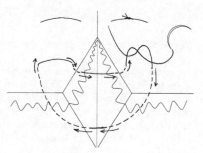

Figure 25.3 Vertical mattress suture.

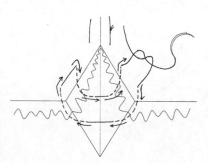

Figure 25.4 Horizontal mattress suture.

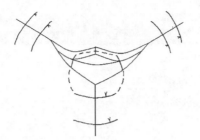

Figure 25.5 Half-buried (corner) suture.

Alternatives to Sutures
Tape ("Steri-Strips")
- *Indications:* linear lacerations under minimal tension; useful for reinforcing or refining other repairs; not useful for wounds requiring meticulous approximation or for moist or hairy areas
- *Technique:* clean and dry skin surrounding laceration. Apply adhesive (benzoin) to surrounding skin, and wait 90 seconds for it to become "tacky." Place tape strips perpendicularly across wound leaving some space for oozing. Place extra tape strips across ends of previous strips and parallel to wound.

Staples
- Best for scalp wounds. Requires special staple remover.
- *Technique:* Prepare wound in same manner as for sutures. Have assistant evert wound edges with tissue forceps or finger pressure. Place staples by applying steady firm pressure to stapling device.

Tissue adhesives ("Dermabond")
- Best for linear wounds with minimal tension
- Allows rapid, painless closure of wounds. No removal needed.
- *Technique:* Once wound is clean and dry, assistant holds wound edges together with forceps. Apply adhesive along surface of wound with light brushing stroke at least three times, waiting 2 seconds between each stroke. (Avoid applying adhesive to inside of wound.) Hold wound for 45 to 60 seconds to obtain adequate bonding.

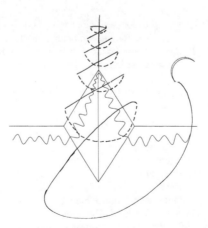

Figure 25.6 Simple (continuous) running suture.

Table 25.1: Tetanus Prophylaxis

Prior Tetanus Toxoid Doses	Clean, Minor Wound	Dirty Wounds
Uncertain or < 3 doses	DTaP or Td	DTaP or Td & TIG
3 or more (last > 10 yrs ago)	Td	Td
3 or more (last 5–10 years ago)	None	Td
3 or more (last < 5 years ago)	None	None

DTaP, diphtheria, tetanus, acellular pertussis; Td, tetanus, diphtheria; TIG, human tetanus immune globulin.

- Do not use in hairy areas, in the mouth, or near the eyes of young children. Do not apply ointment over adhesive.
- Wears off in 5 to 10 days

Post-Laceration Repair Management
- Apply topical antibiotic ointment. Cover with dry sterile gauze.
- *Antibiotics* may be indicated for "high risk wounds." Consider first-generation cephalosporin (e.g., cephalexin). Consider erythromycin if penicillin/cephalosporin allergic. Consider amoxicillin-clavulanic acid for mammalian bites.
- *High Risk Wounds:* contaminated wound, wound with foreign body, human and cat bite, crush injury, stellate laceration, very long wound, intraoral laceration, wound of hands, feet, or perineum, open fracture, exposed joints and tendons, immunocompromised patient, exposed cartilage, contamination from adjacent nasal passages, delayed repair, tetanus-prone wounds (Table 25.1)

LUMBAR PUNCTURE

Indications
- Suspicion of CNS infection, suspicion of subarachnoid hemorrhage, measurement of opening pressure, treatment of pseudotumor cerebri, diagnosis of CNS metastases

Equipment
- Sterile gloves, antiseptic solution (povidone iodine), lumbar puncture (LP) tray, CR monitor and pulse-oximeter, cardiorespiratory resuscitative equipment, "EMLA" topical anesthetic cream
- *Lumbar puncture tray:* generally includes drapes, sponges, lidocaine 1%, 3-cc syringe for lidocaine injection, adhesive bandage strip, collecting tubes, manometer; may include spinal needle.
- *Needle size:* generally 22 gauge; younger than 1 year: 1.5 inch; 1 year to adolescent: 2.5 inch; adolescent/obese patient: 3.5 inch

Technique
1. *Preparing and positioning the patient:*
   - Apply EMLA cream to puncture site for 30 minutes
   - Begin monitoring, consider sedation
   - Two positions commonly used:
     - *Lateral recumbent:* Assistant cradles young infant into fetal position. In older child, assistant holds patient in knee-chest position. The upper back can be flexed gently: avoid flexing the neck, which may lead to fatal respiratory compromise.
     - *Sitting position:* Patient sits with feet over side of bed with neck/upper body flexed forward over pillow on lap or on bedside tray (usually reserved for older children).

- Locate the puncture site by palpating the upper aspects of the posterior superior iliac crests. A line between the two crests will intersect approximately at top of L4 at midline. The L3-L4 and L4-L5 interspaces are both suitable LP sites.
- Prepare the area with antiseptic solution starting at the intended puncture site and swabbing in enlarging circles. Apply sterile drapes. Anesthetize the interspace with lidocaine 1%.
2. *Inserting the needle:* Ensuring the shoulders are perpendicular to the bed, slowly insert the bevel-up, styletted needle, aiming slightly cephalad, toward the umbilicus. As the needle moves beyond the ligamentum flavum/dura into the cerebrospinal fluid (CSF) space, a loss of resistance may be appreciated ("pop"). If the "pop" is not appreciated, the physician must remove the stylet every few millimeters (after the first 1 to 2 cm) to observe for CSF flow.
3. *Use of manometer:* The opening pressure is the highest recorded level the CSF reaches in the column. Normal opening pressure is 5 to 20 cm H_2O. The reading is falsely high in a struggling patient.
4. *Finishing procedure:*
   - Collect 1 cc fluid in each tube and send tubes to lab as follows: Tube 1, Gram stain/culture; tube 2, protein/glucose; tube 3, cell counts; tube 4, any additional studies
   - Replace stylet and remove needle. Clean site and apply strip bandage or sterile dressing.

PNEUMOTHORAX: NEEDLE DECOMPRESSION

Indication
- Tension pneumothorax, which may present with deviated trachea, diminished or asymmetric breath sounds, diminished chest wall expansion, or sudden cardiopulmonary decompensation

Equipment
- 16- or 18-gauge angiocatheter; 5- to 10-mL syringe; three-way stopcock; antiseptic solution; lidocaine (1%)

Technique
- Do not delay if tension pneumothorax suspected
- Place patient in supine position and elevate head of bed to 30 degrees.
- Swab area with antiseptic solution.
- Apply local anesthesia with 1% lidocaine if time permits.
- Insert a 16- or 18-gauge angiocatheter attached to a syringe perpendicular to the midclavicular line on the upper edge of the third rib. Gently aspirate on the syringe as the needle is advanced into the lower portion of the second intercostal space. A loss of resistance in the syringe indicates evacuation of air.
- Advance the catheter over the needle into the pleural space, and remove the needle. Attach a one-way drainage device to the catheter or intermittently draw back on a syringe connected to the catheter with a three-way stopcock.
- Consider immediate chest radiograph and tube thoracostomy

SUPRAPUBIC BLADDER ASPIRATION

Indications
- Sterile collection of urine in children younger than 2 years of age; urinary tract anomaly; contamination of urethra by stool

Equipment
- Sterile gloves, povidone-iodine antiseptic, sterile gauze; 3- or 5-mL syringe, 25-gauge 1-inch needle (preterm infants), 22-gauge 1.5-inch needle (term infants), specimen cup, bandage

Technique
- Wait at least 1 hour after last void. Place the infant supine and restrain in frog-leg position. Occlude urethral opening.
- Identify insertion site: midline, 1 to 2 cm above pubic symphysis.
- Clean skin with povidone-iodine three times.

- Attach syringe to needle. Insert needle in a cephalad direction angled 20 degrees from the vertical. Maintain gentle negative pressure on syringe until urine is obtained.
- If unsuccessful, consider hydration or ultrasound to identify full bladder before re-attempt.
- Transfer urine sample to sterile cup. Clean povidone-iodine from skin, and cover site with bandage.

TUBE THORACOSTOMY

Indications
- Pneumothorax, hemothorax, previous needle decompression of tension pneumothorax, recurrent or large pleural effusions, empyema, chylothorax

Equipment
- Antiseptic solution, sterile gloves, drapes, gauze, Vaseline impregnated gauze, tape, 1% lidocaine, no. 11 and no. 15 scalpels, curved Kelly clamps, suture material, sterile scissors, needle driver, drainage apparatus (e.g., Pleurovac), chest tube
- *Age-appropriate chest tube size:* premature: 10 to 14F; neonate: 12 to 18F; 6 months: 14 to 20F; 1 to 2 year: 14 to 24F; 4 to 7 year: 20 to 32F; older than 10 year: 28 to 38F

Technique
- Consider analgesia and sedation (see Analgesia and Sedation chapter).
- Place patient in the supine or lateral decubitus position with affected side elevated. Gown and glove in a sterile manner. Prepare with antiseptic solution and drape with sterile towels.
- Inject 1% lidocaine into the skin and deeper subcutaneous tissues starting one interspace below the planned insertion site. Therefore, inject directly over the seventh rib below the sixth intercostal space if the fifth intercostal space will be used for entry into the pleural space. Draw back on the syringe before injection of the lidocaine to confirm that the needle is not in the pleural or vascular space. When the needle contacts the superior aspect of the rib, the periosteum should also be infiltrated.
- Use the scalpel to make a 0.5 to 2 cm horizontal incision on top of the rib where the initial wheal of lidocaine was injected. Insert a closed Kelly clamp (curved clamp) into the incision. Perform blunt dissection with the clamp by opening and closing it while advancing toward the top of the adjacent cephalad rib; one rib above where the initial incision was made.
- When the superior aspect of the selected rib is contacted with the clamp, advance steadily over the top until a loss of resistance is felt as the pleural space (at the fifth intercostal space) is entered. Open the clamp widely to create a larger opening for the tube. Remove the clamp with the tips open. Insert a finger into the incision to confirm successful placement into the pleura.
- Insert the chest tube by grasping it with the curved clamp and guiding it through the incision. Alternatively, insert the curved clamp, open the tips, and direct the tube through the opening. Advance tube until all side holes are within the pleural space.
- Connect the chest tube to the drainage system. Suture the tube in place. Apply sterile petroleum gauze around the skin site, apply a layer of sterile gauze, and tape securely.
- Confirm placement with chest x-ray.

UMBILICAL VESSEL CATHETERIZATION

Indications
- Frequent arterial or venous blood gases, continuous monitoring of arterial or central venous blood pressures, emergency vascular access, administration of fluids and medications, exchange transfusion

Equipment
- Umbilical artery catheter (UAC), umbilical vein catheter (UVC), three-way stopcock, radiant warmer, cardiac monitor, pulse oximetry, supplemental oxygen source, antiseptic solution (povidone-iodine), soft restraints, sterile towels, sterile gauze, scalpel: no. 11 or 15, forceps:

curved, non-toothed (Iris forceps or vessel dilator), forceps: straight, Crile, hemostats: at least four pairs, scissors, suture: 3.0 or 4.0 silk on curved or straight needle, umbilical tape (approximately 15 inches), syringe: 10cc with sterile saline (with or without heparin 0.5 to 1 U/mL), gown, gloves, mask
- *UAC Sizing:* Infants less than 2 kg: 3.5 to 4F, infants greater than 2 kg: 5F
- *UVC Sizing:* Smaller lumens: 5F, larger lumens: 8F

Technique
- Restrain infant in supine, frog-legged position. Keep infant warm with overhead warmers, and place on cardiac monitor/pulse oximetry with supplemental oxygen available.
- Don gown, gloves, and mask. Using sterile technique, wash cord and skin with antiseptic solution. Drape with sterile towels.
- Loosely tie umbilical tape at base of cord to prevent bleeding. Cut cord with scalpel to length of 1 to 2 cm.
- Stabilize cord with forceps or hemostats: grasp one edge of cord with curved hemostat or grasp opposite sides with 2 hemostats and evert edges.
- Identify the vessels: one central, cephalad, larger lumen, thin-walled vein; two smaller lumen, thick-walled arteries
- Dilate lumen for 1 cm using curved, non-toothed, Iris forceps.
- Flush catheter with sterile saline or heparinized sterile saline.
- Hold catheter 1 cm from tip with toothless forceps and insert into vessel lumen with gentle pressure. Blood return signifies proper insertion. Turn stopcock handle toward infant to stop flow. Advance to desired length (see below). Mark appropriate length with tape. Temporarily secure line placement with "purse-string suture" through cord and around catheter.
- Maintaining the sterile field, confirm proper placement with radiograph of chest and abdomen. Once the sterile field is broken, do not advance the catheter. It may be withdrawn.
- Finish securing catheter with purse-string suture and tape bridge.
- *To remove catheter:* Place umbilical tape loosely around stump to control bleeding. Remove catheter gradually over 3 to 4 minutes, allowing vessels to segmentally constrict and/or clot to form.

Positioning and Insertion Length
"High" Umbilical Artery Catheter
- Used in non-emergent situations and in small infants (<750 g)
- Catheter tip placed just above diaphragm at spinal level T6-T9
- Measure shoulder-to-umbilical length, if less than 13 cm, insert catheter that distance plus 1 cm, if greater than 13 cm, insert catheter that distance plus 2 cm.
- Alternatively, UAC length (cm) = [3 × birth weight (kg)] + 9

"Low" Umbilical Artery Catheter
- Used in emergent situations
- Catheter tip positioned below diaphragm, just above aortic bifurcation at spinal level L3-L5.
- Insert catheter until blood return obtained, then advance an additional 1 cm.
- Alternatively, UAC length (cm) = birth weight (kg) + 7

Umbilical Vein Catheter
- Normally, catheter tip is placed above diaphragm at the junction of the inferior vena cava and right atrium
- In emergent situations, catheter is passed cephalad for 4 to 5 cm until blood return obtained.
- To estimate normal UVC length: Length (cm) = shoulder-to-umbilicus length (cm) × 0.6

Resources
Bell LM. Suprapubic bladder aspiration. In: Dieckmann RA, Fiser DH, Selbst SM, eds. Pediatric Emergency & Critical Care Procedures. St. Louis: Mosby, 1997:417–419.

Brownstein DR, Rivara FP. Emergency medical services for children. In: Nelson WE, ed. Nelson Textbook of Pediatrics. Philadelphia: WB Saunders, 1996:232–239.

Edlich R, Rodenheaver G, Thacker J. Emergency wound management. In: Tintinalli J, Ruiz E, Krome R, eds. Emergency Medicine, A Comprehensive Study Guide. 4th ed. New York: McGraw-Hill, 1996:267–301.

Fleisher G, Ludwig S. Textbook of Pediatric Emergency Medicine. 4th ed. Philadelphia: Lippincott Williams & Wilkins, 2000.

Gray JE, Ringer SA. Common neonatal procedures. In: Cloherty JP, Stark AR, eds: Manual of Neonatal Care. 4th ed. Philadelphia: Lippincott-Raven, 1998.

Henretig F, King C. Textbook of Pediatric Emergency Procedures. Baltimore: Williams & Wilkins, 1997.

Lynch R, Lungo J, Loftis L, et al. A procedure for placing pediatric femoral venous catheter tips near the right atrium. Pediatr Emerg Care 2002;18:130–132.

Amy Kim, MD, Anthony L. Rostain, MD, MA

AGITATION/AGGRESSION

Etiology
Multiple conditions can cause a patient to act in an agitated or aggressive manner: alcohol and substance abuse, primary psychiatric disorders, psychosis, personality disorders, severe conduct disorder, autism, pervasive developmental delay (PDD), mental retardation, delirium, temporal lobe seizure, other "organic" causes (steroid-induced, herpes simplex virus [HSV] encephalitis)

Clinical Manifestations
- *Mental Status Exam:* level of alertness and concentration; psychotic symptoms; presence of suicidal or homicidal ideation
- *Signs of intoxication:*
  - Alcohol: alcohol on breath, dysarthria, incoordination, ataxia
  - Amphetamine: dilated pupils, altered pulse or blood pressure
  - Cocaine: dilated pupils, hypertension, tachycardia
  - Hallucinogens: dilated pupils, tachycardia, sweating, palpitations, tremors, incoordination
  - Phencyclidine (PCP): nystagmus, hypertension, tachycardia, ataxia, dysarthria, muscle rigidity, seizures

Diagnostics
- Urine or serum drug screen
- Consider other studies as clinically indicated

Management
Information Gathering
- Interview patient, parents, outpatient psychiatrist/therapist
- Mental status exam and physical exam
- Diagnostic tests if indicated
- Identify and treat the underlying cause of the agitated behavior

Prevention/De-escalation Strategies
- Provide a safe and nonthreatening environment
- Time-out
- Decrease sensory stimulation (dim lights, speak softly)
- Attempt to redirect patient (talking, offering alternate strategy)
- Consider 1:1 supervision, chemical or physical restraints

Chemical Restraints
Refers to the use of medication to achieve behavioral control or sedation. Always attempt to offer oral (PO) medications first.
- *Antipsychotic Medications:* haloperidol PO/IM/IV, risperidone PO. May cause side effects (refer to Psychosis: Adverse Effects of Antipsychotics)
- *Benzodiazepines:* lorazepam PO/IM/IV. In some patients, may cause disinhibition with increased behavioral dyscontrol
- *Antihistamines:* diphenhydramine PO/IM/IV. May give with haloperidol as prophylaxis for neuroleptic-induced dystonia. In some patients, may cause disinhibition with increased behavioral dyscontrol

Physical/Mechanical Restraints
- Should only be used when a patient's behavior becomes so violent or aggressive that it endangers his/her own safety or that of others.
- Examples include four-point restraints, papoose board, wrist-to-waist, physical holds by staff or security.
- While restrained, patient should be continually monitored (every 15-minute checks of vital signs, extremity range of motion, and circulation) and attention given to nutrition, hydration, and elimination needs.
- Parents or guardians should be informed as soon as possible.
- Restraints should be discontinued as soon as patient's behavior is controlled and is no longer a threat to self or others.
- Debrief the patient regarding why restraints were used, future alternative strategies, and provide opportunity for patient to apologize or make amends.
- All accredited facilities should have a formal policy regarding the use of restraints that adhere to HCFA guidelines. Become familiar with it.

PSYCHOSIS

Psychotic symptoms include:

Formal thought disorder: disorganized or incoherent speech, illogical thought, loose associations

Positive symptoms: auditory or visual hallucinations, delusions

Negative symptoms: flattened affect, alogia, avolition

Differential Diagnosis
- Mood disorders (depression, bipolar affective disorder)
- Substance-Induced (alcohol, amphetamine, D-lysergic acid diethylamide [LSD], PCP)
- Schizophrenia, autism, PDD, mental retardation
- "Organic" causes (delirium, steroid-induced, thyroid disease, systemic lupus erythematosus, temporal lobe epilepsy, HSV encephalitis)

Pathophysiology
- Abnormal monoaminergic activity in the central nervous system (CNS)

Clinical Manifestations
- Younger children's delusions tend to be less complex, less fixed
- They may believe they have superpowers
- Adolescent's delusions may be paranoid, grandiose, bizarre
- May present agitated or disruptive
- *Mental Status Exam:* psychotic symptoms, mood and affect (depression, anxiety, irritability, and lability), presence of suicidal or homicidal ideation, level of judgment
- Signs of intoxication

Diagnostics
- Urine or serum drug screen
- Thyroid-stimulating hormone
- Consider EEG, lumbar puncture, head CT or MRI

Management
Information Gathering
- See "Agitation/Aggression"

Evaluate for safety
- Impaired judgment risks injury of self/others
- Disruptive behavior/agitation risks injury to self/others
- Admit patient if there are safety concerns

If Patient Requires Admission
- Admit to appropriate level of care until medically stable
- Consider 1:1 supervision of patient for monitoring of safety
- Consult child psychiatrist
- Consider antipsychotic medication
- Evaluate for inpatient psychiatric care

Antipsychotic Medications
- Atypical drugs, associated with lower incidence of extrapyramidal symptoms (EPS): risperidone, olanzapine, quetiapine
- Typical drugs: haloperidol
- Common side effects: sedation, weight gain, orthostatic hypotension
- Extrapyramidal symptoms: acute dystonic reaction (treat with diphenhydramine, benztropine), neuroleptic-induced parkinsonism, akathisia (treat with beta-blocker, benzodiazepine)
- Neuroleptic malignant syndrome: life-threatening condition characterized by hyperthermia, muscle rigidity, altered mental status, choreoathetosis, tremors, and autonomic dysfunction (arrhythmias, hypertension, sweating)
- Anticholinergic effects (confusion, agitation, constipation, blurred vision, urinary retention)

SUICIDALITY

Thoughts, threats, events, or actions characterized by the desire to cause death or harm to oneself. Suicidal ideation (SI) may be ambiguous or strong.

Epidemiology
- An estimated 10% of US adolescents and 1% of preadolescents attempt suicide at least once
- Third leading cause of death among adolescents
- Females attempt suicide more often than males; males complete suicide more often than females (due to more lethal methods)
- Firearms in the home are associated with a higher risk of completed suicide

Etiology/Risk Factors
- Alcohol and substance abuse and/or intoxication
- Primary psychiatric disorders, most commonly depression, bipolar affective disorder, conduct disorder
- Developmental and preclinical personality disorders associated with impulsivity or aggression
- Biologic factors: often there is a family history of psychiatric illness, suicidal behavior, substance abuse
- Stressful life events: particularly exposure to violence, physical and sexual abuse
- Sexual orientation: lesbian, gay, bisexual, transgender, and questioning (LGBTQ) youth have higher rates of suicide attempt and completion because of social isolation

Differential Diagnosis
- Accidental versus intentional injury
- High versus low risk of injury

Pathophysiology
- Associated findings include: lower cerebrospinal fluid serotonin levels, alterations in hypothalamic-pituitary function, disturbed sleep

Clinical Manifestations
- Methods may include drug ingestions, shooting, hanging, suffocation, stabbing, drowning, burning, running into traffic, intentional motor vehicle accidents
- *Mental Status Exam:* current suicidal ideation/intent/plan, psychotic symptoms, mood and affect (depression, anxiety, irritability, and lability), level of insight and judgment
- Signs of intoxication

Management
Information Gathering
- Interview patient, parents, outpatient psychiatrist/therapist
- History of suicide attempts?
- Accessibility of methods (pills/medications locked? Firearms at home?)
- Risk factors: substance abuse, new or acute stressors, LGBTQ youth

Evaluate Suicide Threat/Attempt
- Prior attempts
- Amount of planning
- Method used
- Potential for lethality
- Desire for death as an outcome
- Awareness of death as a likely outcome
- Likelihood of discovery

If Patient Requires Admission
- Admit to appropriate level of care until medically stable
- Consider 1:1 supervision of patient for monitoring of safety
- Repeated interview and assessment until SI is diminished
- Consult child psychiatrist
- Consider psychiatric medication
- Evaluate for inpatient psychiatric care

If Stable for Discharge
- Have patient contract for safety
- Parents must agree to make guns, firearms, medications, alcohol, and drugs unavailable to patient
- If patient has outpatient psychiatrist, therapist, or pediatrician; contact them before discharge
- Otherwise, provide references for appropriate outpatient psychiatric resources
- Instruct family to contact physician/psychiatrist, or return to emergency department if concerned that patient may be at risk for harming self

Resources

American Academy of Pediatrics, Committee on Adolescence. Suicide and suicide attempts in adolescents. Pediatrics 2000;105:871–874.

Centers for Disease Control and Prevention. Suicide among children, adolescents and young adults: United States, 1980–1992. MMWR 1995;44:289–291.

Findling R, Schulz SC, Reed MD, Blumer JL. The antipsychotics: a pediatric perspective. Pediatr Clin North Am 1998;45:1205–1232.

Horowitz LM, Wang PS, Koocher GP, et al. Detecting suicide risk in a pediatric emergency department: development of a brief screening tool. Pediatrics 2001;107:1133–1137.

Lewis M, ed. Child and Adolescent Psychiatry A Comprehensive Textbook. 3rd ed. Philadelphia: Lippincott, Williams & Wilkins, 2002.

Masters K, Bellonci C, Bernet W, et al. Practice parameter for the prevention and management of aggressive behavior in child and adolescent psychiatric institutions, with special reference to seclusion and restraint. J Am Acad Child Adolesc Psychiatry 2002;41(suppl):4S–25S.

Meehan P. Attempted suicide among young adults: progress toward a meaningful estimate of prevalence. Am J Psychiatry 1992;149:41–44.

Sater N, Constantino J. Pediatric emergencies in children with psychiatric conditions. Pediatr Emerg Care 1998;14:42–50.

David Hehir, MD, Michael F. Maraventano, MD,
Suzanne Dawid, MD, PhD, Howard B. Panitch, MD

Pulmonary Diseases and Syndromes

ACUTE RESPIRATORY DISTRESS SYNDROME

An acute, severe lung injury ($PaO_2/F_iO_2 < 200$ mm Hg) of non-cardiac origin (pulmonary wedge pressure < 18 mm Hg) associated with evidence of bilateral parenchymal densities on chest radiograph.

- Acute lung injury: less severe form of lung injury defined by PaO_2/F_iO_2 less than 300 mm Hg

Epidemiology
- Mortality depends on etiology and pre-morbid conditions: trauma 2% to 45%; sepsis 45% to 65%; immunosuppression 70%; post-cardiopulmonary resuscitation 90%

Etiology
- Most common etiologies: shock, sepsis, drowning, pneumonia, aspiration, smoke inhalation, lung contusion, multiple fractures/trauma, head injury
- Occurs more commonly in immunocompromised hosts

Pathophysiology
Acute respiratory distress syndrome (ARDS) follows a predictable progression of histologic and clinical stages:

1. **Exudative stage:** epithelial and endothelial injury, noncardiogenic pulmonary edema, and neutrophil migration lead to impaired gas exchange, surfactant deficiency, and decreased lung compliance
2. **Proliferative stage:** pulmonary vascular remodeling leads to progressive pulmonary fibrosis.
3. **Fibrotic stage:** decreased lung compliance, pulmonary hypertension, and poor alveolar gas exchange

Clinical Manifestations
- The initial presentation varies with specific insult and may include cyanosis, tachypnea, dyspnea, and rales on auscultation.

Diagnostics
- Arterial blood gas: profound hypoxemia, usually refractory to supplemental oxygen; hypercarbia; acidosis
- Indicators of end-organ damage and multiorgan failure: liver function tests, coagulation studies, cardiac enzymes
- Chest x-ray: diffuse bilateral parenchymal densities; may be normal early in course.
- Chest CT: may reveal densities in dependent areas of lung
- Lung function: decreased total lung volume, decreased functional residual capacity (FRC), large intrapulmonary shunt fraction (Q_s/Q_T), decreased pulmonary compliance

Management
Management involves supportive ventilation and correction of underlying causes while treating co-morbidities and limiting complications.

- *Ventilation:* goal is to achieve adequate alveolar gas exchange while limiting complications by using low tidal volume to avoid alveolar overdistention, low FiO_2 to reduce oxidant injury, and

high positive end-expiratory pressure (PEEP) to limit barotrauma and maximize lung recruitment:
- Minimize tidal volume: goal 4 to 6 mL/kg
- Permissive hypercapnia: goal $PaCO_2$ 45 to 65 mm Hg, but levels of 80 mm Hg and above may be tolerated if needed
- PEEP: 5 to 15 cm H_2O
- Limit peak inflating pressure (PIP) to less than 30 to 35 cm H_2O
- Goal SaO_2 88% to 92%; attempt to use "non-toxic" F_iO_2 of less than 60% to keep PaO_2 greater than 60 mm Hg
- Goal pH 7.25 to 7.40

- *Consider alternate modes, adjuncts:* inverse inspiratory-to-expiratory ratio ventilation; pressure-regulated volume control (PRVC); airway pressure release ventilation (APRV); high frequency oscillation; prone positioning; nitric oxide; surfactant; extracorporeal life support
- *Supportive treatment:*
  - Limited fluid resuscitation ensures adequate tissue perfusion while limiting alveolar edema. Measures to decrease oxygen demand are helpful.
  - Inotropic support; support hematocrit; diuretics; sedation and paralysis; antipyretics
- *Experimental therapies:* steroids, nitric oxide, liquid ventilation
- *Manage comorbidities:* renal failure, cardiac failure, hepatic failure, CNS failure, disordered coagulation
- *Manage complications:* Ventilator-associated pneumonia, barotrauma, bacterial tracheitis, sepsis, respiratory deconditioning, central line infections, central line thrombosis, decubitus ulcer formation

CYSTIC FIBROSIS

An autosomal recessive defect in the cystic fibrosis transmembrane conductance regulator (CFTR) gene, located on the long arm of chromosome 7. Abnormal cell membrane chloride/water transport results in viscid mucus secretions and elevated sweat chloride levels. Progressive chronic pulmonary disease and exocrine pancreatic insufficiency are the primary clinical manifestations.

Epidemiology
- Carrier frequency in certain white populations as high as 1 in 25
- More than 1000 mutations of the CFTR gene have been identified
- ΔF508 is most common mutation in Northern European-white population and accounts for approximately 70% of CFTR mutations in the United States

Pathophysiology
- Failure of epithelial cells to conduct chloride and the associated water transport abnormalities result in viscid secretions in the respiratory tract, pancreas, gastrointestinal tract, liver/gallbladder, and genitourinary tracts.
- Decreased clearance of viscid secretions causes obstruction of progressively larger airways starting with bronchioles.
- Bacterial colonization causes chronic airway inflammation and destruction progressing from bronchiolitis and bronchitis to bronchiolitis obliterans, bronchiolectasis, bronchiectasis, bronchiectatic cysts, and emphysematous bullae. Loss of normal airway architecture causes obstructive changes with air trapping and hyperinflation.

Clinical Manifestations
Respiratory Tract
- Cough is the most consistent symptom.
- Infants and young children: tachypnea, chronic or recurrent episodes of wheezing, respiratory distress with crackles and wheeze, and/or nonproductive cough; recurrent lower respiratory tract infections; respiratory cultures grow *Staphylococcus aureus*, *Escherichia coli*, or *Klebsiella* spp.

- Older children and adolescents: progressive respiratory symptoms including mucopurulent cough worse in morning and with activity, exercise intolerance, and hemoptysis (occasionally massive). Physical exam findings include increased anteroposterior chest diameter, hyperresonance, persistent crackles, cyanosis, and digital clubbing. Respiratory cultures usually grow *Pseudomonas aeruginosa*
- Progressive lung pathology includes bronchiectasis, atelectasis, fibrosis, and occasionally pneumothorax. Right heart failure is usually a late consequence of chronic hypoxemia but can present secondary to acute respiratory failure.
- Pansinusitis is common and chronic, but acute sinusitis is less common.
- Nasal polyps can be a presenting finding.
- Allergic bronchopulmonary aspergillosis can occur.
- Colonization with *Burkholderia cepacia* occasionally correlates with more rapid disease progression.

Gastrointestinal Tract
- Obstructive symptoms due to paucity of intestinal water and large malabsorptive stools: newborns may present with no stool in first 24 to 48 hours of life, abdominal distention, bilious emesis, and meconium ileus. Infants may present with rectal prolapse in association with straining. Children and adolescents may present with constipation, emesis, abdominal distention, and distal intestinal obstructive syndrome (DIOS).
- Pancreatic insufficiency: malabsorption, fat soluble vitamin (A, D, E, K) deficiencies, recurrent pancreatitis, diabetes mellitus
- Biliary tract: persistent neonatal direct hyperbilirubinemia, obstructive biliary cirrhosis
- Failure to thrive (infants)/maintain growth parameters (children)
- Physical exam: rectal prolapse, protuberant abdomen, decreased muscle mass, delayed Tanner staging, hepatosplenomegaly

Genitourinary
- Average delay in sexual maturity of approximately 2 years
- Males: atretic epididymis, vas deferens and seminal vesicles secondary to failure of Wolffian development and inspissation of secretions; obstructive azoospermia and infertility; normal sexual function; higher incidence of anatomic defects including hernia and undescended testes
- Females: increased rate of secondary amenorrhea with pulmonary exacerbations; tenacious cervical mucus leads to increased risk of cervicitis; pregnancy tolerance is correlated with lung function.

Metabolic Abnormalities
- Higher risk for acute salt and volume depletion with gastroenteritis or dehydration (hyponatremic dehydration) and chronic hypochloremic metabolic alkalosis due to increased losses of sodium and chloride in sweat
- History of "tasting salty" or salt crystallization on forehead

Diagnostics
Both history/physical findings AND laboratory confirmation are required to make the diagnosis of cystic fibrosis (CF) (Table 27.1).

Table 27.1: Cystic Fibrosis Diagnostic Criteria	
Patient History	**Evidence of CFTR Gene Dysfunction**
1. One or more characteristic phenotypic features	1. Elevated sweat chloride
2. Sibling with cystic fibrosis	2. Identification of mutations in each CFTR gene known to cause cystic fibrosis
3. Positive newborn screen	3. Characteristic abnormalities in ion transport across the nasal epithelium

- Tests for abnormal CFTR are used to confirm a diagnosis in a patient with one or more clinical features consistent with the CF phenotype, a history of CF in a sibling and/or a positive newborn screen.
  - Sweat test (by pilocarpine iontophoresis): sweat chloride concentration of more than 60 mmol/L on two separate occasions with adequate amounts (>100 mg) of sweat collected; values of 40 to 60 mmol/L are considered borderline and the test must be repeated.
  - Identification of two CF mutations: finding two CFTR mutations in association with clinical symptoms is diagnostic, but negative results on genotype analyses do not exclude the diagnosis.
  - Nasal potential difference measurements
- Tests suggesting CFTR dysfunction (these supporting findings need confirmation with a diagnostic test)
  - Newborn screen: blood test for immunoreactive trypsinogen
  - Exocrine pancreatic insufficiency
  - Seventy-two–hour stool fat collection
  - Invasive pancreatic enzyme measurements (impractical)
  - Vitamin A and E levels and prothrombin time as evidence of fat malabsorption
  - Semen analysis: obstructive azoospermia is suggestive of CF
  - Bronchoalveolar lavage fluid positive for *Pseudomonas aeruginosa*
  - Sputum microbiology positive for *S. aureus* or *P. aeruginosa*, especially the mucoid form
- Clinical data used to follow clinical course
  - Chest x-ray: hyperinflation, atelectasis, and peribronchial thickening are initial findings. Advanced findings include bowed sternum, cyst or nodule formation, extensive bronchiectasis, dilated pulmonary artery, pneumothorax, and scarring.
  - Chest CT: may be used for evaluation of acute processes
  - Sinus films: pan-opacification + failure of frontal sinus development
  - Pulmonary function testing: initially can be normal. Early changes indicate an obstructive pattern whereas advanced disease displays a combined obstructive and restrictive pattern due to fibrosis. A decrease of 10% from baseline FEV1 may prompt hospital admission.
- Laboratory evaluation during an acute exacerbation:
  - Fluid balance, renal function, liver function, glucose, magnesium (especially in patients with a history of frequent IV aminoglycoside use)
  - Complete blood cell count with differential
  - PT/international normalized ratio to rule out coagulation disorder secondary to vitamin K deficiency
  - Aminoglycoside and theophylline levels if appropriate
  - Serum total IgE level if history of or concern for allergic bronchopulmonary aspergillosis
  - Consider vitamin and mineral levels (A, E, zinc, D-25-OH)
  - HgbA1c if signs or history of diabetes mellitus
  - Obtain sputum culture, cough swab, or deep throat culture before starting antibiotics and second sample after chest physiotherapy. Repeat sputum cultures on day 7 of admission.
  - Urinalysis to look for glucosuria

Miscellaneous Diagnostics
- 72-hour fecal fat collection and assay with food diary
- DEXA (bone density scan)
- Audiology exam

Management
Respiratory Management of Pulmonary Exacerbation
- Antibiotics: empiric parenteral administration of two antipseudomonal antibiotics for 14 to 21 days (e.g., aminoglycoside and beta-lactam antibiotic such as gentamicin + imipenem, ticarcillin-clavulanate, or piperacillin-tazobactam). Specific therapy should be based on the identification and susceptibility testing of bacteria isolated from sputum. Administration of aerosolized antibiotics (e.g., tobramycin) delivers high concentrations of medication directly to the site of infection.

- Nonpharmacologic secretion clearance:
  - Chest physiotherapy with postural drainage
  - High-frequency chest wall oscillation with an inflatable vest or airway oscillator
- Pharmacologic secretion clearance:
  - Bronchodilator therapy (beta-2-agonist) if increase of 10% or more in FEV1 in response to inhaled bronchodilator is noted
  - Anti-inflammatory therapy (e.g., cromolyn, inhaled corticosteroids) is often added.
  - Theophylline only if inadequate responses to other forms of bronchodilator therapy
  - Inhaled human recombinant DNAse can reduce the viscoelasticity of sputum.
  - N-acetylcysteine is a mucolytic but can be toxic to endothelium.

Nutritional Management
- Diet: most have increased caloric needs. Children and adolescents require a high calorie, high protein, and extra salt diet.
- Pancreatic exocrine enzyme replacement
- Vitamins A, D, E, and K in doses used for malabsorption

HEMOPTYSIS

The expectoration of blood or blood-tinged sputum. The immediate danger is from suffocation, not from exsanguination.

- *Massive* or *Major:* >240 cc in 24 hours or >100 cc per day for several days
- *Minor:* smaller volumes
- Life-threatening hemoptysis is typically defined as greater than 8 cc/kg/day.

Etiology
- Minor hemoptysis: direct mucosal injury (shearing forces dislodging mucus from airway wall, direct trauma from suction catheters, etc.)
- Massive hemoptysis: usually from bronchial artery (high pressure system) to pulmonary artery anastomosis
- Infection is the most common etiology of hemoptysis in children.
- Bleeding from tracheostomy
- Foreign body aspiration, especially long standing
- Congenital heart disease with pulmonary vascular obstruction or enlarged collateral bronchial circulation
- Cystic fibrosis
- Tuberculosis
- Immune-mediated: Henoch-Schönlein purpura, Wegener's granulomatosis, polyarteritis nodosa, Goodpasture syndrome, systemic lupus erythematosus
- Less frequent: pulmonary sequestration, pulmonary embolism, neoplasm

Diagnostics
- Assess adequacy of ventilation
- Orthostatic pulse and blood pressure to estimate blood loss
- CBC, PT, PTT
- Purified protein derivative (PPD) test
- If indicated: rheumatologic markers including anti-nuclear antibody, doubel-stranded DNA, ESR, CRP, complement levels, anti-neutrophil cytoplasmic antibodies, IgG levels
- Sputum Gram stain and culture
- Chest x-ray
- Chest CT: limited utility in defining structural abnormalities or masses. Spiral CT may be useful if pulmonary embolus is suspected.
- Angiography in cases of severe refractory hemoptysis
- Fiberoptic bronchoscopy is best performed after bleeding has subsided.

- Rigid bronchoscopy allows for suctioning and better visualization of the airway and is best performed after bleeding has subsided, unless airway compromise demands immediate instrumentation.
- Bronchoalveolar lavage or biopsy may show organisms in infection and hemosiderin-laden macrophages in pulmonary hemosiderosis.

Management
- Management is typically supportive except in the case of massive hemoptysis, and is otherwise directed at treating the underlying cause of bleeding.
- Secure the airway and assure adequacy of ventilation
- Support circulating volume with crystalloid until red cell transfusion
- Treat the underlying etiology
- In the case of massive hemoptysis, emergency bronchoscopy may be required. Sites of bleeding can be slowed by either balloon catheter tamponade or with the use of topical oxymetazoline, epinephrine, or cold saline.
- If bleeding cannot be controlled, emergency arteriography may help to localize the area of bleeding and can allow selective embolization.

OBSTRUCTIVE SLEEP APNEA

A syndrome of disordered breathing during sleep. Children with obstructive sleep apnea (OSA) exhibit patterns of sleep interrupted by breath holding, grunting, and/or snoring, which may result in daytime behavior problems, cognitive impairment, failure to thrive, hypertension, and right heart failure.

Epidemiology
- Occurs at all ages, although may be more common in preschoolers
- Prevalence in school age children from 2% to 12%

Etiology
- Risk factors: adenotonsillar hypertrophy, obesity, craniofacial anomalies, neuromuscular disorders, trisomy 21, chronic lung disease, sickle cell disease

Clinical Manifestations
- Most common symptom of clinically significant OSA is simple snoring.
- Other common manifestations: labored breathing, restless sleep, apnea while asleep, daytime sleepiness, daytime behavior problems, cognitive deficits
- Severe presentations: cor pulmonale, failure to thrive, mental retardation
- Possible exam findings: adenotonsillar hypertrophy, craniofacial abnormalities, hypertension, loud pulmonary component of S2

Diagnostics
- *Full polysomnography* requires overnight admission to a sleep laboratory and can reveal abnormalities in gas exchange that occur during rapid eye movement sleep. It is the only method that quantifies ventilatory and sleep abnormalities.
- *Partial polysomnography* has a poor negative predictive value; if negative, full polysomnography is necessary.
- *Other useful adjunctive tests*: pulse oximetry, audio or videotaping, and abbreviated polysomnography or nap sleep study. The positive predictive value of these adjunctive studies are high; however, if results are negative, full nocturnal polysomnography should be performed.
- *Adjunctive tests*: ECG to evaluate for right ventricular hypertrophy; elevated serum bicarbonate reflects chronic hypoventilation.

Management
Acute
- Positioning: upright, sniffing position. In the case of hypotonia or tracheomalacia, prone positioning may relieve obstruction.
- Nasal airway: use pre-formed nasal trumpet or trimmed down endotracheal tube (ETT). Oxygen and positive pressure may be delivered through a nasopharyngeal ETT.

- Antibiotics: if acute infection
- Anti-inflammatories: may help reduce swelling. Consider dexamethasone, oxymetazoline nasal spray, nebulized racemic epinephrine or fluticasone nasal spray
- Epinephrine: use in cases of severe refractory obstruction
- Tracheal intubation: reserved for refractory cases

Chronic
- *Continuous positive airway pressure*: used in patients with specific surgical contraindications, minimal adenotonsillar tissue, persistent OSA after adenotonsillectomy or for those who prefer nonsurgical alternatives
- *Adenotonsillectomy*: most common treatment for pediatric OSA

Mechanical Ventilation and Pulmonary Assessment

BLOOD GAS INTERPRETATION

Step 1: Acidemia or Alkalemia?
- Alkalemia: pH greater than 7.40
- Acidemia: pH less than 7.40

Step 2: Metabolic or Respiratory?
- Primary respiratory alkalemia: pH greater than 7.40 and $PaCO_2$ less than 40
- Primary metabolic alkalemia: pH greater than 7.40 and $PaCO_2$ greater than 40
- Primary respiratory acidosis: pH less than 7.40 and $PaCO_2$ greater than 40
- Primary metabolic acidosis: pH less than 7.40 and $PaCO_2$ less than 40

Step 3: Is the problem acute or chronic and is there a secondary problem? In other words, are changes in pH greater than expected from the primary disorder alone?
- For respiratory acidemia/alkalemia, a 10-mm Hg change in $PaCO_2$ causes 0.08 change in pH in acute setting or 0.03 in chronic setting.
- For metabolic acidemia/alkalemia, a 10-mEq/L change in HCO_3 causes 0.15 change in pH.

Step 4: Is the compensation adequate?
- For metabolic acidosis, expect a decrease in $PaCO_2$ of 1 to 1.5 mm Hg for every decrease in HCO_3 of 1 mEq/L
- For metabolic alkalosis, expect an increase in $PaCO_2$ of 0.5 to 1 mm Hg for every increase in HCO_3 of 1 mEq/L
- For acute respiratory acidosis, expect an increase in HCO_3 of 1 mEq/L for every increase in $PaCO_2$ of 10 mm Hg
- For acute respiratory alkalosis, expect a decrease in HCO_3 of 1 to 3 mEq/L for every decrease in $PaCO_2$ of 10 mm Hg
- For chronic respiratory acidosis, expect an increase in HCO_3 of 4 mEq/L for every increase in $PaCO_2$ of 10 mm Hg
- For chronic respiratory alkalosis, expect a decrease in HCO_3 of 2 to 5 mEq/L for every decrease in $PaCO_2$ of 10 mm Hg

Step 5: In metabolic acidosis, calculate the anion gap.

$$\text{Anion Gap} = Na - (Cl + HCO_3)$$

- Normal anion gap less than 12 mEq/L
- In normal gap metabolic acidosis, hyperchloremic acidosis results from the loss of HCO_3 in the gut or kidneys.
- Anion gap acidosis results from addition of nontitratable acid to the system. Etiologies include lactic acidosis (e.g., caused by hypotension, prolonged seizures), diabetic ketoacidosis, starvation ketoacidosis, uremia, ingestions such as iron, isoniazid, methanol, ethanol, salicylates, NSAIDs, cyanide, and ethylene glycol.

Step 6: If there is an anion-gap metabolic acidosis, is there a second metabolic problem? Calculate the delta gap . . .
- To determine if there is a second metabolic derangement (metabolic alkalosis or non-gap acidosis) use the following equation:

$$\text{corrected } HCO_3 = \text{measured } HCO_3 + (\text{anion gap} - 12)$$

- Where corrected $HCO_3 = 24$. If the result is higher than 24, a concurrent metabolic alkalemia exists, whereas a result lower than 24 indicates a concurrent non-gap acidemia.

MECHANICAL VENTILATION

Definitions
- *Amplitude* (ΔP): in high frequency ventilation (HFV), ΔP represents the change in pressure above and below the MAP.
- *Compliance* (C): the elasticity of the lungs and chest wall. Compliance can be expressed in terms of pressure and volume so that $C = \Delta V / \Delta P$.
- *Expiratory Time* (T_E): time of the respiratory cycle spent in expiration.
- *Fractional Inspiratory Oxygen Concentration* (F_iO_2): concentration of oxygen delivered.
- *Functional Residual Capacity* (FRC): resting lung volume.
- *Hertz* (Hz): in HFV, represents the frequency of ventilation where 1 Hz = 60 breaths per minute.
- *Inspiratory Time* (T_I): time of the respiratory cycle spent in inspiration
- *Mean Airway Pressure* (MAP): average pressure transmitted to the airway during a respiratory cycle
- *Minute Ventilation* (MV): "cardiac output" of the lungs, where MV is the product of tidal volume and respiratory rate: $MV = V_T \times RR$.
- *Peak Inspiratory Pressure* (PIP): highest pressure measured during the respiratory cycle.
- *Positive End-Expiratory Pressure* (PEEP): airway pressure maintained above atmospheric at end-expiration during mechanical ventilation; prevents alveolar collapse between ventilator breaths. High PEEP may impair cardiac output by reducing venous return, or improve cardiac output by reducing left ventricular afterload.
- *Rate* (RR): number of breaths delivered per minute.
- *Tidal Volume* (V_T): volume of gas delivered during a respiratory cycle.

Indications for Mechanical Ventilation
- General indications: improve alveolar ventilation, improve arterial oxygenation, decrease metabolic cost of breathing, provide respiratory support for neuromuscular insufficiency, lower intracranial pressure, control ventilation and oxygenation in circulatory failure
- Specific Indications: apnea; acute respiratory failure with $PaCO_2$ greater than 55 mm Hg; vital capacity less than 15 mL/kg; cyanosis or PaO_2 less than 70 mm Hg despite F_iO_2 greater than 0.6; $AaDO_2$ greater than 300 mm Hg with $F_iO_2 = 1$; loss of airway protective reflexes

Modes of Mechanical Ventilation
Supported Ventilation
- *Continuous Positive Airway Pressure (CPAP):* supplies a constant airway pressure above atmospheric pressure during both inspiratory and expiratory phases of spontaneous ventilation. This increases FRC.
- *Bi-level Positive Airway Pressure (BIPAP):* supplies two levels of continuous positive pressure; can be set to deliver patient-triggered positive pressure breaths; delivered via endotracheal or tracheostomy tube, face mask, or nose mask.
- *Pressure Support:* a patient-initiated breath is supported to a pre-set pressure by the ventilator and terminated based on characteristics of the patient's respiratory system. This mode enhances the patient's native respiratory drive, reducing respiratory work while allowing the

patient to determine respiratory rate as well as the length and depth of breaths. Pressure support is often used in conjunction with assisted ventilation as a tool for weaning.

Mandatory Ventilation

- *Pressure control*: the ventilator delivers flow in a decelerating flow pattern at a set respiratory rate and peak pressure. The tidal volume and minute ventilation vary from breath to breath depending on lung compliance. This mode is useful in children with depressed respiratory drives and where a uniform pressure is desirable or where a large leak around a tracheostomy tube exists. Advantages include limiting barotrauma due to a set PIP, and less turbulent flow due to a decelerating flow pattern.
- *Volume control*: flow is delivered with a square wave pattern to a set V_T and rate, allowing the pressure needed to generate the set V_T to vary as the compliance and resistance of the system changes. Advantages include lower MAP due to square wave pattern, limited volutrauma due to set tidal volume, and limited alveolar collapse with set tidal volume.
- *Pressure-regulated volume control (PRVC)*: flow is delivered with a decelerating wave form to a set tidal volume while limiting the PIP. This allows the ventilator to respond to changes in compliance and resistance in the system, thereby limiting volu and barotrauma.
- *High-frequency ventilation* (high-frequency oscillatory ventilation [HFOV] or high-frequency jet ventilation [HJV]): delivers low tidal volume breaths (1 to 3 mL/kg) at very high rates (3 to 15 Hx = 180 to 900 breaths per minute). HFOV settings are mean airway pressure, Hertz, and amplitude or power. Indications include severe neonatal respiratory distress syndrome (RDS), ARDS, and severe air leak syndromes.

Assisted Ventilation

- *Synchronized intermittent mandatory ventilation (SIMV)*: the most frequently used mode of ventilation in most pediatric institutions. SIMV allows spontaneous breathing between ventilator breaths that are delivered in either pressure control or volume control mode. Mechanical breaths can be programmed to trigger with patient-initiated breaths or independent of the patient's respiratory effort.
- *Airway pressure release ventilation (APRV)*: allows spontaneous ventilation while maintaining MAP with a high level of CPAP for a preset time (T high) and a "release" that intermittently drops the MAP to a lower CPAP level for a shorter period of time (T low). This is designed to open and maintain collapsed alveoli and enhance ventilation of lungs with poor compliance without excessive PIP.

Initial Ventilator Settings

Initial settings depend on the age and indication. Premature infants with surfactant deficiency require short inspiratory times with higher than average pressures. Children with cyanotic heart disease have compliant lungs and require less pressure. *The following should be used as a general guide: evaluation of the patient's response and care by physicians experienced with managing the mechanically ventilated child are critical to ensure the settings provide an appropriate level of support.*

Conventional Ventilation

- *Mode*: decide if the patient should be fully supported with no ability to breathe spontaneously (control), or with some ability to breathe over the set rate (assist/control); if the patient should be partially supported with each breath (SIMV with pressure support); or if the patient should be allowed to breathe spontaneously without support between mandatory breaths (IMV or SIMV)
- *Rate (per minute)*: Typical starting ventilator rates assuming minimal spontaneous respiration: 30 to 40 neonates, 20 to 30 infants, 15 to 20 children. If allowing for the patient to take some spontaneous breaths, begin supporting at one half to two thirds of the normal respiratory rate for age. In general, children with lung disease require respiratory rates at the higher end of the range, and children who are intubated for other indications such as head trauma and circulatory collapse require lower rates. One notable exception is children with asthma, who require lower rates with long expiratory times to fully exhale.
- F_iO_2: set at 1.0 (or last known effective F_iO_2) and wean to desired SaO_2

- *Positive end-expiratory pressure:* Three to 5 cm H_2O, depending on clinical scenario. Neonates with severe lung disease may require PEEP as high as 8 cm H_2O or more. Older children with ARDS may require PEEP as high as 12 to 15 cm H_2O.
- *V_T:* set to 10–15 mL/kg; if low tidal volume strategy is desired wean to goal of 4 to 6 mL/kg as tolerated
- *T_i (inspiratory time):* neonates 0.3 to 0.4 seconds; infants 0.4 to 0.7 seconds; children 0.5 to 1.0 seconds. Shorter inspiratory times are favored in heterogeneous disease (e.g., ARDS, asthma).
- *I/E ratio:* 1:2, with longer E times in obstructive disease
- *Positive inspiratory pressure:* In pressure control mode, set pressure control (PC) to achieve adequate chest wall movement.

High Frequency Ventilation
- *Hertz:* Set at 10 to 15 Hz in neonates; may need 5 to 7 in severe ARDS
- *Mean airway pressure (MAP):* Set 1 to 4 cm H_2O higher than that needed on conventional ventilation. Wean slowly once recruitment established.
- *Amplitude:* Set to level with best chest wall movement

Adjusting Ventilator Settings
Ventilator settings are manipulated in order to provide ideal oxygenation and CO_2 clearance while limiting complications (Table 27.2).

- Conventional ventilation: to increase CO_2 exchange, increase either RR or V_T. To increase oxygenation, increase MAP or F_iO_2. MAP increase can be achieved by increasing PEEP, PIP, or inspiratory time.
- High-frequency ventilation: to increase CO_2 exchange, increase amplitude or decrease hertz. Increase oxygenation by increasing F_iO_2 or MAP.

Weaning Ventilation
The most common weaning modes are SIMV, PSV, and T-piece trials.
- *Weaning with SIMV:* gradually wean rate of ventilator breaths by 2 to 5 breaths per minute to a minimal level (5 breaths per minute). If tolerated, switch to CPAP mode. Decrease CPAP/PEEP to 2 to 3 cm H_2O (infants) or 5 cm H_2O (children). If tolerated, wean off support. This method may increase the metabolic cost of breathing for the patient during the weaning process.

Table 27.2: Some Possible Effects of Ventilator Changes

Change	$PaCO_2$	PaO_2
↑ RR	↓	No change or ↑
↑ PIP	↓	↑
↑ PEEP	↑, No change, or ↓	↑, No change, or ↓
↑ I time	↓	↑, No change, or ↓
↑ F_iO_2	No change	↑
↑ Amp	↓	No change
↑ Hz	↑	No change
↑ MAP	↓	↑

- *Weaning with PSV (two options):*
  - Place patient on SIMV mode with PS. Initiate short trials of only PS, gradually lengthening the time off SIMV until the patient is maintained only on minimal PS.
  - Place patient on full PSV mode to produce a fully supported tidal volume. Gradually wean down the PS until the patient is minimally supported. If tolerated, wean off support.

Indicators of Readiness to Wean

- *Negative Inspiratory Force (NIF):* measures maximum negative deflection during inspiration of 1 breath after occlusion of airway. Used to assess adequacy of spontaneous breaths. A NIF less than −15 in an adult has 97% sensitivity for weaning failure. There is poor positive predictive value for this test in children.
- *Measured vital capacity:* adequate vital capacity is 10 to 15 mL/kg.
- *Spontaneous tidal volume:* at least 4 mL/kg
- *Minute ventilation:* at least 15 L/min
- *Respiratory rate:* physiologic (lack of rapid shallow breathing); in adults, a respiratory frequency/tidal volume ratio <105 during a spontaneous breathing trial is associated with weaning success (rapid shallow breathing index)
- Able to maintain PaO_2 greater than 60 mm Hg on F_iO_2 less than 0.35
- *Rapid shallow breathing index (RSBI) (see formula listed below):* RSBI of 8 or less has both a sensitivity and specificity of 74% in predicting successful extubation (Thiagarajan et al.). In children, RSBI occasionally used in clinical practice.

$$RSBI = RR \text{ (in breaths/min.)}/V_T \text{ (in mL/kg)}$$

PULMONARY FUNCTION TESTS

Definitions
PFTs are used to diagnose, assess severity, and assess response to therapy in pulmonary disease. To assess reversible airway obstruction or bronchodilator responsiveness, the patient is given an inhaled bronchodilator and the test is repeated. Histamine, methacholine, exercise, isocapneic cold dry air, and hypertonic or hypotonic aerosol challenges may also help assess airway reactivity. Key definitions (Figures 27.1 and 27.2):

- *Body plethysmograph:* apparatus for measurement of FRC, RV, TLC, and airway resistance
- *Capacity:* addition of two or more volumes
- *Expiratory reserve volume (ERV):* volume that can be exhaled from V_T to RV
- *FEV1:* volume that is forcefully exhaled in one second
- *FEV 25–75:* average forced expiratory flow over the mid portion of the FVC
- *FEV1/FVC:* ratio of FEV1 to FVC, expressed as a percentage
- *Forced Vital Capacity (FVC):* volume that can be maximally forcefully exhaled
- *Functional Residual Capacity (FRC):* volume in the lungs at the end of a relaxed normal breath (RV + ERV)
- *Inspiratory Capacity (IC):* volume taken into the lungs on a full inspiration (IRV + V_T)
- *Inspiratory Reserve Volume (IRV):* volume that can be inhaled above the V_T
- *Peak Expiratory Flow (PEF):* peak flow rate during expiration
- *Residual Volume (RV):* volume remaining in the lungs after maximal expiration (FRC-ERV; TLC-VC)
- *Spirometer:* apparatus for measuring lung volumes (except RV) and flow rates. Spirometry is used to plot a volume–time curve and a flow–volume loop.
- *Total lung capacity (TLC):* total volume of gas in the lungs at full inspiration (VC + RV; IC + FRC; IRV + V_T + ERV + RV)
- *Tidal volume (V_T):* volume of a normal breath
- *Vital capacity (VC):* maximal volume that can be expired from a full inspiration (IRV + TV + ERV; TLC-RV)

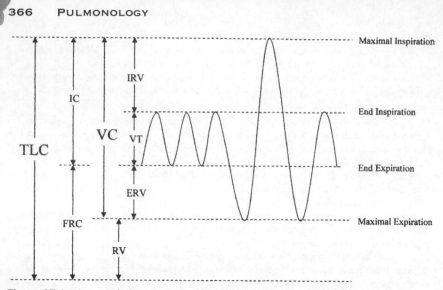

Figure 27.1 Lung volumes. TLC, total lung capacity; FRC, functional residual capacity; IC, inspiratory capacity; VC, vital capacity; RV, residual volume; IRV, inspiratory residual volume; VT, tidal volume; ERV, expiratory reserve volume.

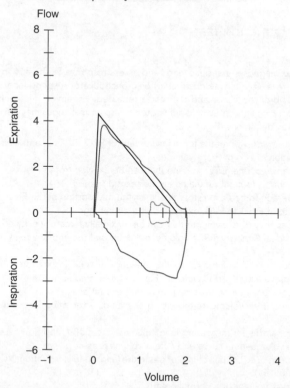

Figure 27.2 Normal flow-volume loop. During expiration, the normal loop can be straight or slightly convex to the volume (x-) axis. The small loop represents the flow-volume curve during tidal breathing. Curvy loop (light grey), patient measurement; triangular loop (black), computer-generated predicted loop.

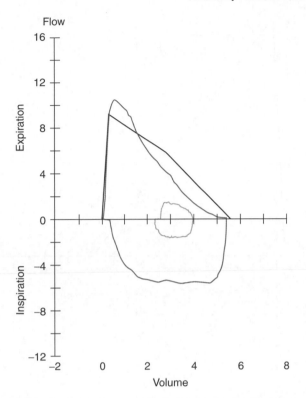

Figure 27.3   Obstructive flow volume curve. During expiration, the obstructive curve is concave to the volume axis. A normal peak flow (as in this case) does not preclude an obstructive process. Curvy loop (light grey), patient measurement; triangular loop (black), computer-generated predicted loop.

Obstructive Lung Disease
Obstruction to airflow during expiration leads to gas trapping, increased RV, decreased, increased, or normal VC, and increased to normal TLC (Figure 27.3). Common causes include asthma, bronchiolitis, chronic bronchitis, cystic fibrosis, and bronchiectasis. Spirometry reveals a low FEV1 (<80% predicted), low FVC (<80% predicted), low FEV1/FVC (<75% predicted), decreased FEV 25–75, and an expiratory flow–volume curve that is concave to the volume axis.
- Small airway obstruction is represented by low FEV 25–75.
- Response to bronchodilators with a greater than 12% increase in the FEV1 and/or FVC considered significant.
- Methacholine challenge that results in a decrease in FEV1 20% or greater from baseline at a dose less than 25 mg/dL, or exercise or cold dry air challenge that results in 15% or greater decrease in FEV1 from baseline are used to diagnose airway hyperreactivity.

Restrictive Lung Disease
Restrictive lung diseases cause reductions in lung volumes due to decreased lung compliance, decreased chest wall compliance, or muscle weakness. Etiologies include interstitial lung disease, neuromuscular diseases, and chest wall abnormalities. TLC is decreased whereas flow rates are proportionally normal or slightly increased. Spirometry reveals a low FEV1 (< 80% predicted), low FVC (<80% predicted), normal FEV1/FVC ratio, and "miniaturized" appearance to flow–volume curve (Figure 27.4).

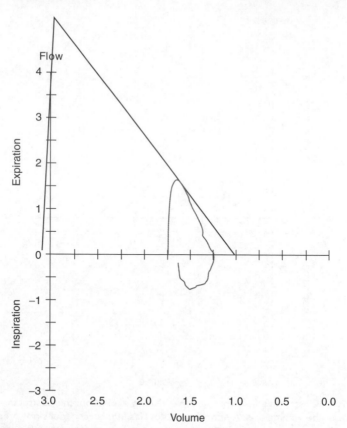

Figure 27.4 Restrictive flow volume curve. The diagonal line represents the reference line. In a restrictive process, the flows are normal when corrected for low lung volumes. Curvy loop (light grey), patient measurement; triangular loop (black), computer-generated predicted loop.

Resources

Pulmonary Diseases and Syndromes

Atabai K, Matthay MA. Acute lung injury and the acute respiratory distress syndrome: definitions and epidemiology. Thorax 2002;57:452–458.

American Academy of Pediatrics, Section on Pediatric Pulmonology, Subcommittee on Obstructive Sleep Apnea Syndrome. Clinical practice guideline: diagnosis and management of childhood obstructive sleep apnea syndrome. Pediatrics 2002;109:704–712.

Bates DV, ed. Respiratory Function in Disease. 3rd ed. Philadelphia: WB Saunders, 1989.

Batra PS, Holinger LD. Etiology and management of pediatric hemoptysis. Arch Otolaryngol Head Neck Surg 2001;127:377–382.

Belligan GJ. The pathogenesis of ALI/ARDS. Thorax 2002;57:540–546.

Flemons WW. Obstructive sleep apnea. N Engl J Med 2002;347:498–504.

Koch C, Hoiby N. Pathogenesis of cystic fibrosis. Lancet 1993;341:1065–1069.

Ramsey BW. Management of pulmonary disease in patients with cystic fibrosis. N Engl J Med 1996;335:179–188.

Redding GJ. Current concepts in adult respiratory distress syndrome in children. Curr Opinion Pediatr 2001;13(3):261–266.

Rosenstein BJ, Cutting GR. The diagnosis of cystic fibrosis: A consensus statement. J Pediatr 1998;132:589–595.

Schechter MS, and the American Academy of Pediatrics, Section on Pediatric Pulmonology, Subcommittee on Obstructive Sleep Apnea Syndrome. Technical report: diagnosis and management of childhood obstructive sleep apnea syndrome. Pediatrics 2002;109:e69.

Sheikh S, Sisson B, Senler SO, Eid N. Moderate hemoptysis of unknown etiology. Pediatr Pulmonol 1999;27:351–355.

Mechanical Ventilation and Pulmonary Assessment

Chernick V, Boat TF, ed. Disorders of the Respiratory Tract in Children. 6th ed. Philadelphia: WB Saunders, 1998.

Clausen JL, ed. Pulmonary Function Testing Guidelines and Controversies. New York: Harcourt Brace Jovanovich, 1982.

Cordingley JJ, Keogh BF. Ventilatory management of ALI/ARDS. Thorax 2002;57:729–734.

Goldstone J. Difficult weaning. Thorax 2002;57:986–991.

Hillman BC, ed. Pediatric Respiratory Disease: Diagnosis and Treatment. Philadelphia: WB Saunders, 1993.

Rogers M, Helfaer M, ed. Handbook of Pediatric Intensive Care. 3rd ed. New York: Lippincott, Williams and Wilkins, 1999.

Rogers M, Nichols D. Textbook of Pediatric Intensive Care. 3rd ed. New York: Lippincott, Williams and Wilkins, 1996.

Thiagarajan RR, Bratton SL, Martin LD, et al. Predictors of successful extubation in children. Am J Resp Crit Care Med 1999;160:1562–1566.

Pamela G. Fitch, MD, Elise R. DeVore, MD,
Jeffrey C. Klick, MD, Jon M. Burnham, MD

DERMATOMYOSITIS (Juvenile Dermatomyositis)

Most common pediatric inflammatory myopathy. Diagnostic criteria as follows (Bohan and Peter):

Definitive juvenile dermatomyositis (JDM): rash plus at least three criteria; probable JDM: rash plus two criteria

- Heliotrope rash (eyelids)
- Gottron's papules (extensor surfaces)
- Progressive symmetric proximal muscle weakness
- Elevated skeletal muscle enzymes (creatine kinase [CK], aspartate transaminase [AST], aldolase, lactate dehydrogenase [LDH])
- Electromyography consistent with myopathy
- Biopsy evidence of myositis or muscle abnormalities on MRI

Epidemiology
- Incidence: ~2 to 3 cases/million children
- Peaks at 6 years and 11 to 12 years of age; female:male = 2:1
- White predominance in the United States (71%)

Etiology
- Potential infectious triggers: group A beta-hemolytic *Streptococcus*, coxsackievirus B, parvovirus, others
- Human leukocytic antigen and tumor necrosis factor–alpha (TNF-α) alleles may predispose a child to JDM
- Molecular mimicry is suspected
- Sun exposure may trigger onset of rash

Pathophysiology
- Perivascular inflammation, mostly mononuclear cells
- Swelling and blockage of capillaries, tissue infarction, perifascicular atrophy
- Chronic inflammation ensues with fibrosis and microscopic calcification

Clinical Manifestations
- *Proximal muscle weakness* (neck flexors, shoulders, abdomen, thighs): Gower sign, difficulty climbing stairs or combing hair
- *Skin:* heliotrope rash (violaceous rash of eyelids), facial erythema, possibly in malar distribution, papulosquamous eruption on extensor surfaces, particularly over interphalangeal joints (Gottron's papules), shawl sign (erythematous rash in a shawl distribution), cutaneous calcinosis and ulceration
- *Nail folds:* capillary drop-out, vessel dilation, cuticular hypertrophy
- *Arthritis:* effusions, limited range of motion, pain, deformity
- *Mucocutaneous:* oral ulcers, gingival inflammation
- *Pulmonary:* shortness of breath, cough, crackles can be consistent with interstitial lung disease or aspiration pneumonia
- *Gastrointestinal:* dysphagia, ulceration, perforation, bleeding, constipation, diarrhea, abdominal pain

- *Other manifestations:* lipodystrophy, polyneuropathies, retinal exudates and cotton wool patches
- *Other complications:* calcinotic lesions may spontaneously drain, causing local inflammatory response and superinfection; can form exoskeleton; diabetes mellitus secondary to steroid use; rare arrhythmias and cardiomyopathy; growth failure; osteoporosis

Diagnostics
- CBC: lymphopenia, anemia
- ESR and CRP: normal or high
- Elevated muscle enzymes: creatine kinase, aldolase, AST, LDH
- Anti-nuclear antibodies: positive in 60% to 70%; rheumatoid factor: negative
- Neopterin and von Willebrand factor antigen: elevations correlate with disease activity
- Anti-RNP (may indicate systemic lupus erythematosus [SLE] overlap), anti-PM-Scl (associated with SLE or scleroderma), anti-Jo-1 (associated with interstitial lung disease)
- Urinalysis to rule out renal involvement
- MRI with T2-weighted images: localizes active disease sites
- Chest x-ray: evaluate for infiltrates
- High-resolution chest CT: evaluate for interstitial lung disease
- Modified barium swallow: detect palato-esophageal dysfunction
- Plain films: detect calcinosis
- ECG: may see arrhythmias, cardiomyopathy
- Muscle biopsy: myositis, perifascicular necrosis with degenerating and regenerating fibers
- Electromyography: fibrillations, insertional irritability
- Pulmonary function tests: often decreased secondary to respiratory muscle weakness, restrictive lung disease

Management
- Mild disease: corticosteroids (2 mg/kg/day then taper), methotrexate, +/– hydroxychloroquine
- Moderate-severe disease: add pulse corticosteroids (30 mg/kg/day, up to 1000 mg) x 3, IVIG (2 g/kg IV every 3 to 4 weeks)
- Refractory disease: cyclosporine A, cyclophosphamide, TNF-α inhibitors (etanercept, infliximab)
- Interstitial lung disease: cyclophosphamide, pulse corticosteroids
- Sunscreen: minimum sun protection factor of 15 with ultraviolet A and ultraviolet B protection
- Nutritional supplements: vitamin D and calcium
- Physical and occupational therapy
- Immunizations: no live vaccines for individuals on high dose steroids or antimetabolites. Inactivated influenza and pneumococcal vaccination are indicated. Delay MMR 11 months after last IVIG treatment if it is not contraindicated.

HENOCH-SCHÖNLEIN PURPURA

Immune complex-mediated small vessel systemic necrotizing vasculitis of undetermined etiology mainly affecting the skin, joints, gastrointestinal (GI) tract, and kidneys: 1990 American College of Rheumatology classification criteria (need two of four for disease): age younger than 20, palpable purpura, bowel angina, biopsy evidence.

Epidemiology
- Most common childhood vasculitis in the United States
- Age range commonly 2 to 12 years; peak: 4 to 7 years
- Incidence: 3 to 17/100,000
- Seasonal variation with peak incidence in winter and spring

Pathophysiology
- Small vessel vasculitis affecting capillaries and pre- and post-capillary vessels
- Mediated by immune complexes (IgA, IgG, and activated complement C3) that are deposited in end organs causing inflammation
- May be associated with antecedent respiratory infection (GABHS, mycoplasma, parvovirus, other viral pathogens)

Clinical Manifestations
- Classic triad: nonthrombocytopenic purpuric rash, arthritis, urinary sediment
- Typical symptoms:
  - *Rash:* most common presenting symptom; non-blanching, purpuric lesions developing in gravity or pressure dependent areas, usually distal to the elbows and waist. Early lesions may appear erythematous, petechial, or urticarial, evolving into hemorrhagic or ecchymotic lesions; may ulcerate; can see Koebner phenomenon
  - *Musculoskeletal:* arthralgia/arthritis are second most common manifestation; periarticular or articular pain with impaired mobility and minimal joint warmth and effusion, typically affecting the ankles, knees, elbows, wrists, digits; subcutaneous edema
  - *Gastrointestinal:* hemorrhage, intussusception, bowel perforation possible; presents with pain, vomiting, loose stool, melena, hematemesis; hepatosplenomegaly may be present
  - *Renal:* affects 20% to 60% of patients with Henoch-Schönlein purpura (HSP); increased risk in presence of bloody stool; may lead to end-stage renal disease. Manifestations include microscopic or macroscopic hematuria with or without proteinuria, hypertension, glomerulonephritis, ureteritis, urethritis, and cystitis
  - *Rare manifestations:* genitourinary: scrotal swelling/hemorrhage mimicking testicular torsion, testicular torsion (rare); CNS: headache, seizures, hemorrhage, cerebrovascular thrombosis, focal deficits, and peripheral neuropathies; pulmonary: interstitial disease, alveolar hemorrhage, and respiratory failure; cardiovascular: carditis, myocardial infarction
- Vital signs: possible low-grade fevers; hypertension due to renal disease; tachycardia due to anemia or pain
- Duration of symptoms: average 4 weeks if untreated; range: 3 days to 2 years
- Recurrence: up to 33%

Diagnostics
- White blood cells (normal to slightly elevated); hemoglobin (normal to slightly low); platelet count (normal to elevated); PT/PTT (normal)
- ESR: normal to elevated
- BUN and creatinine: elevated with renal disease
- Albumin: decreased with proteinuria and GI losses, malnutrition, and inflammation
- Urinalysis: proteinuria and/or hematuria; RBC casts
- Stool: may be Hemoccult positive
- Immunologic: elevated IgA (type 1) levels in 50%; ANCA (IgA type) may be positive; c-ANCA and p-ANCA negative
- Plain abdominal radiograph, barium studies, and ultrasound may be useful for assessment of abdominal obstruction and intussusception.
- Skin biopsy: can be diagnostic as light microscopy will show leukocytoclastic vasculitis and IgA deposition on immunofluorescence
- Renal biopsy: useful if proteinuria/hematuria is significant or does not resolve; normal to severe crescentic glomerulonephritis with immune complex deposits
- Arthrocentesis: useful to exclude infectious arthritis

Management
- Acetaminophen for analgesia; avoid NSAIDs if GI or renal involvement
- Steroids: indicated for renal involvement, abdominal and musculoskeletal pain. For severe disease, consider pulse solumedrol up to 30 mg/kg/day up to 3 days then daily treatment for 1 to 2 weeks with 2-week taper. For mild or moderate disease, consider prednisone or solumedrol 2 mg/kg/day up to 60 mg/day for 1 to 2 weeks with 2-week taper.

- Cytotoxic therapy: should be considered in patients with severe nephritis and pulmonary or CNS manifestations
- Antibiotics: may be useful in preventing relapses given that GABHS may be a common infectious trigger.
- Supportive care: severe pain may require narcotics. Severe GI involvement may require nothing-by-mouth status, nasogastric suction, and total parenteral nutrition, although response to steroids is often dramatic with prompt initiation of therapy.

JUVENILE RHEUMATOID ARTHRITIS

Chronic synovial inflammation of unknown etiology with onset before 16 years of age and leading to arthritis in one or more joints for at least 6 weeks. Type defined by symptoms in first 6 months:

- Oligoarticular: involvement of four or fewer joints (40% to 50%)
- Polyarticular: involvement of five or more joints (30% to 40%)
- Systemic: characterized by fever, rash, and arthritis (10% to 15%)

Epidemiology
- Most common chronic childhood rheumatologic disease
- Girls affected with oligo- and polyarthritis twice as often as boys
- Incidence: 10 to 15/100,000 in children less than 16 years old

Etiology
- Genetic and environmental factors suspected
- HLA associations exist
- Associated with immunodeficiencies: IgA deficiency, 22q11 del
- Possible viral trigger: for example, rubella, parvovirus B19

Differential Diagnosis of Chronic Arthritis
- *Oligoarthritis:* Lyme disease, mycobacterial infection, leukemia, bone or synovial tumor, sarcoid, spondyloarthropathies, Legg-Calvé-Perthes disease, slipped capital femoral epiphysis, pigmented villonodular synovitis, cystic fibrosis, congenital arthropathies, metabolic disorders, foreign body
- *Polyarticular arthritis:* Lyme disease, systemic lupus erythematosus and related disorders, dermatomyositis, sarcoidosis, vasculitis, spondyloarthropathies
- *Systemic onset arthritis:* septic arthritis, Lyme disease, EBV, parvovirus B19, acute rheumatic fever, leukemia, lymphoma, Langerhans cell histiocytosis, SLE, sarcoidosis, Kawasaki disease, neonatal onset multisystem inflammatory disease, periodic fever syndromes

Pathophysiology
- Synovitis with villous hypertrophy and hyperplasia
- T cell activation and recruitment into joint synovium leads to release of pro-inflammatory cytokines by multiple cell types
- Pannus formation in late disease, causing progressive erosion of cartilage and bone

Clinical Manifestations
- General: fatigue, low-grade fevers, anorexia, weight loss, failure to thrive, limp, joint swelling (may be asymptomatic), hepatosplenomegaly, pain with inactivity, evanescent urticarial rash, lymphadenopathy, morning stiffness
- Oligoarticular: usually involves knees, ankles, fingers, wrists, or elbows; systemic symptoms unusual
- Polyarticular: may involve large and small joints, spares distal interphalangeal joints
- Systemic onset: high fevers one to two times/day for at least 2 weeks, temperature often returns to normal or subnormal and is accompanied by erythematous macular rash on trunk and proximal limbs; serositis (pericarditis and/or pleuritis); pericardial tamponade may ensue.

- Musculoskeletal: swelling/effusion; limited range of motion; warm; contracture/deformity; +/− limb length discrepancies and wasting of surrounding muscles (gastrocnemius or quadriceps); cervical spine extension and rotation may be limited.
- Arthritis of temporomandibular joint may cause failure to thrive secondary to pain. Micrognathia and/or hemifacial atrophy may ensue.
- Ophthalmologic: pupil irregularities, synechiae, band keratopathy; uveitis: oligoarticular more often than polyarticular, rare in systemic onset; may lead to visual loss, cataract, glaucoma
- Macrophage activation syndrome is a potentially life threatening complication seen with systemic onset juvenile rheumatoid arthritis (JRA). Symptoms may include fever, hepatosplenomegaly, lymphadenopathy, bruising, mucosal bleeding, respiratory distress, encephalopathy, liver failure, coagulopathy, and renal involvement.
- Other complications: growth disturbances, osteoporosis, pseudoporphyria with NSAID use

Diagnostics
- ESR and CRP: normal or high in oligoarticular or polyarticular disease; high with systemic onset disease
- CBC: leukocyte count normal or high; platelets may be elevated
- Anti-nuclear antibodies: positive in 40% to 85% of oligoarticular and polyarticular disease; rarely positive in systemic onset disease; positive ANA associated with increased risk for developing uveitis
- Rheumatoid factor: positive in a minority of patients with polyarticular JRA, useful for prognostic purposes only
- Urinalysis: abnormal results may suggest alternative diagnosis
- Joint fluid aspirate: usually 2000 to 50,000 WBC/uL (but may be higher); neutrophils may predominate; glucose normal to slightly low; elevated protein
- Radiologic studies are helpful to rule out other disease processes, such as tumors, and to establish baseline for evaluation of joint erosions.
- If cervical spine range of motion limited, order cervical lateral flexion and extension spinal films to assess for atlantoaxial instability and subaxial ankylosis prior to surgery, intubation, sports participation

Management
- Oligoarticular JRA: treatment of choice is intra-articular corticosteroids for persistent joint inflammation; NSAIDs (e.g., naproxen 15–20mg/kg/day, divided twice daily); if no response then use methotrexate
- Polyarticular JRA: methotrexate, TNF-α inhibitors (e.g. etanercept, infliximab), NSAIDs, intra-articular corticosteroids
- Systemic onset JRA: corticosteroids, methotrexate, TNF-α inhibitors, cyclosporine, NSAIDs, intra-articular corticosteroids; cyclophosphamide for refractory disease
- Regular ophthalmology examinations: slit-lamp examination to diagnose silent uveitis
- Dietary evaluation: ensure adequate calcium, vitamin D
- Physical therapy: to maintain joint function
- Occupational therapy: if hands and wrists involved
- Immunizations: no live vaccines for individuals on high dose steroids or antimetabolites. Inactivated influenza and pneumococcal vaccination are indicated.

KAWASAKI DISEASE

An acute, febrile vasculitis of childhood defined by 5 days of fever and four of the following: conjunctivitis, mucous membrane changes, peripheral extremity changes, polymorphous rash, cervical adenopathy. Atypical Kawasaki disease may present with fewer than four criteria.

Epidemiology
- Incidence: United States: ~12 per 100,000; Japan: ~112 per 100,000
- ~80% of cases before 5 years of age

Differential Diagnosis
- *Viral:* measles, EBV, adenovirus, enterovirus, parvovirus B19
- *Bacterial:* scarlet fever, staphylococcal scalded skin syndrome, toxic shock syndrome, *Yersinia pseudotuberculosis*, typhoid fever
- *Allergic:* drug reaction, serum sickness, Stevens-Johnson syndrome
- *Rheumatologic:* systemic JRA, polyarteritis nodosa, Reiter syndrome
- *Toxic:* mercury poisoning

Pathophysiology
- Etiology unknown
- Vasculitis of medium-sized arteries including coronary arteries, and arterioles, capillaries, and venules.
- Edema of endothelial and smooth muscle cells; inflammatory infiltration of vascular wall.

Clinical Manifestations
- Three phases: acute febrile phase (7 to 14 days), subacute phase (10 to 24 days), and convalescent phase (>24 days)
- Fever: high and spiking
- Conjunctival injection: bilateral, bulbar, generally nonpurulent
- Peripheral extremity changes: edema, erythema, desquamation
- Mucous membrane changes: injected pharynx, dry fissured lips, strawberry tongue
- Polymorphous rash: may be maculopapular, scarlatiniform, erythema multiforme, prominence in groin area
- Cervical adenopathy: 1.5 cm or greater, generally unilateral
- Coronary artery aneurysms: develop in ~15% to 25% of patients not treated within 10 days of onset, but in less than 5% of treated patients
- Other manifestations: extreme irritability, aseptic meningitis, cranial nerve palsy, pancarditis, gallbladder hydrops, hepatitis, hepatosplenomegaly, arthralgias, arthritis, urethritis, uveitis

Diagnostics
- Elevated ESR and CRP
- Complete blood cell count: WBC normal or leukocytosis (WBC >15,000/mm^3 in ~50%); normocytic anemia; thrombocytosis after first week
- Mildly elevated ALT, AST, GGT, bilirubin, alkaline phosphatase
- Urinalysis: sterile pyuria in 70%, catheter sample may miss urethritis so consider clean-catch specimen to detect associated pyuria
- Cerebrospinal fluid: pleocytosis with lymphocyte predominance in 25% to 50% of patients who undergo lumbar puncture
- Chest x-ray: may show pneumonitis, cardiomegaly
- ECG: may show arrhythmia, ischemia, low voltage
- Echocardiogram: may show coronary artery ectasia or aneurysms, pericardial effusion, valvular abnormalities, diminished ventricular function
- Slit lamp examination: anterior uveitis in majority (85%) of patients

Management
- *Intravenous immunoglobulin (IVIG):* 2 g/kg over 10 to 12 hours; if still febrile after 24 hours, may consider a repeat dose of 1–2 g/kg
- *Aspirin:* 80–100 mg/kg/day divided into four doses; when afebrile for 24 hours, decrease dose to 3–5 mg/kg every day. Discontinue aspirin if follow-up echocardiogram and ESR are normal.
- *Steroids:* some authors suggest prednisone or methylprednisolone for persistent symptoms after two doses of IVIG. Studies are ongoing.
- *Disposition:* close follow-up with pediatric cardiologist; follow-up echocardiogram at 6 to 8 weeks to monitor for coronary artery aneurysms

RHEUMATIC FEVER

Post-infectious sequela of group A streptococcal (GAS) pharyngitis. Diagnosis is based on the "Jones" criteria (two major or one major and two minor PLUS evidence of prior GAS infection).

- *Major criteria:* carditis, migratory polyarthritis, chorea, erythema marginatum, subcutaneous nodules
- *Minor criteria:* fever, arthralgias, prolonged PR interval, elevated acute phase reactants (ESR and CRP)
- *Evidence of prior GAS infection:* positive throat culture result, positive rapid strep test result, or increasing antistreptolysin-O or anti-DNaseB titers
- *Exceptions to Jones criteria* (diagnoses are presumptive until all other diagnoses are excluded): chorea as sole manifestation, indolent carditis, recurrence of rheumatic fever
- Should be distinguished from post-streptococcal reactive arthritis, a GAS-associated reactive arthritis that does not fulfill Jones criteria, and is less likely to cause cardiac disease

Epidemiology
- Most common in 5 to 15 year olds
- Annual incidence less than 1/100,000 until the mid to late 1980s when new outbreaks occurred
- Carditis more common in young children; arthritis more common in adults

Etiology
- Usually develops 2 to 3 weeks following an untreated group A streptococcal pharyngitis
- Not caused by streptococcal skin infections

Pathophysiology
- Immune complexes may cause nondestructive synovitis and reversible reactions in basal ganglia that cause chorea.
- Extracellular GAS toxin may target organs such as the heart and brain.
- Autoimmunity and cell-mediated cytotoxicity may cause valvular inflammation.

Clinical Manifestations
- Arthritis: migratory, typically affects knees, ankles, elbows; joints may be swollen, warm, tender, limited range of motion; joint involvement more severe and common in teenagers; does not cause chronic disease
- Subcutaneous nodules: firm and painless; over extensor surfaces of joints, occipital region, thoracic or lumbar spinous processes
- Erythema marginatum: pink/red blanching rash with raised borders, central clearing, not pruritic or indurated, facial sparing
- Heart disease in 40% to 80% of patients: affects mitral valve and aortic valve most commonly. Valves scar with typical "fish mouth" abnormality or calcified tissue.
- Chorea: involuntary, purposeless movements, often unilateral; associated with muscle weakness and emotional lability usually disappears over weeks to months; rarely recurs. "Milkmaid sign": patient's grip strengthens and weakens

Diagnostics
- Evidence of prior infection: increased antistreptolysin-O, anti-DNAaseB, positive throat culture result, recent history of scarlet fever
- ESR and CRP usually elevated
- CBC: normocyctic, normochromic anemias
- Joint fluid: sterile, WBC count may be in septic range
- X-rays of affected joints: normal or effusion present
- Chest x-ray: may see cardiomegaly
- ECG: may see heart block (usually 1st degree), cardiomegaly
- Echocardiography: may see mitral and/or aortic valve regurgitation

Management
- GAS infection: penicillin (10 days oral therapy or single IM injection of benzathine penicillin G)
- Arthritis: salicylates (90–120 mg/kg/day)
- Carditis: salicylates; corticosteroids are indicated if congestive heart failure present (2.5 mg/kg/day for 2 to 3 weeks with taper)
- Chorea: haloperidol or diazepam
- Secondary prophylaxis: benzathine penicillin G (1.2 million units IM every 3 to 4 weeks); oral penicillin (250 mg twice daily) not as effective given non-adherence. In penicillin-allergic patients: sulfadiazine (0.5 g every day if <60 lb; 1g every day if >60 lb) or erythromycin (250 mg twice daily).

SYSTEMIC LUPUS ERYTHEMATOSUS

A multisystem autoimmune disease caused by pathologic production of autoantibodies and tissue deposition of immune complexes, and characterized by global immune dysregulation.

Epidemiology
- 15% to 25% present in first two decades of life, often in puberty
- Female:male = 5–10:1, with a more equal ratio before puberty
- African American:White = 3:1
- Incidence: 2 to 8 per 100,000; Prevalence: 15 to 50 per 100,000

Etiology
- Genetic predisposition (HLA haplotype associations)
- Immune system dysregulation
- Environmental stimuli (ultraviolet light, drugs, herpesvirus infections)
- Hormonal factors

Pathophysiology
- Autoantibodies are directed against nuclear and cytoplasmic antigens. Organ-specific antibodies to cell surface antigens are also present.
- Disease can be secondary to pathogenic autoantibodies (renal disease, thrombocytopenia, antiphospholipid antibody syndrome, neonatal lupus and fetal loss, CNS disease), pathogenic immune complexes (secondary to quantity and size, tissue tropism, and decreased clearance), and T lymphocyte dysregulation (skin disease).

Clinical Manifestations
Many children have nonspecific symptoms for months before diagnosis, often presenting with fatigue, malaise, easy bruising, arthritis, rash, Raynaud's phenomenon, and weight loss before other characteristic findings occur.

- *Mucocutaneous:* malar rash, discoid rash, alopecia, photosensitivity, Raynaud's phenomenon, periungual erythema
- *Musculoskeletal:* arthralgia and arthritis are frequent at presentation. Arthritis is often polyarticular, and often affects the proximal interphalangeal and metacarpophalangeal joints
- *Pleuropulmonary:* pleuritis and pleural effusions. Pneumonitis presents similarly to bacterial pneumonia. Consider infection as a cause of pulmonary infiltrates in patients with SLE, particularly when immunocompromised.
- *Cardiovascular:* pericarditis, pericardial effusions, myocarditis, verrucous endocarditis, atherosclerosis, and dyslipoproteinemia
- *Gastrointestinal:* nausea, diarrhea, and abdominal discomfort. Acute crampy pain may signal mesenteric vasculitis. Peritonitis, acute pancreatitis, pseudo-obstruction, and intestinal perforation are less common.
- *Renal:* affects up to 50% of patients at initial diagnosis and up to 90% of patients eventually. It is the primary cause of morbidity and mortality

- *Neurologic (20% to 35%):* mild cognitive dysfunction, seizures, and psychosis are common. Also seen are severe headache, ataxia, intracerebral hemorrhage, cranial nerve palsy, and cerebral vascular accident. Neuropsychiatric testing may confirm cognitive impairment, depression, emotional lability, and difficulty concentrating.
- *Hematologic:* anemia (of chronic disease or hemolysis), thrombocytopenia, and leukopenia (usually lymphopenia). Antiphospholipid syndrome (APS) may be present, leading to recurrent fetal loss, vascular thrombosis, bleeding, and valvular heart disease.
- *Ocular:* retinal vasculitis (blindness can develop over several days) and less commonly conjunctivitis, episcleritis, optic neuritis, and the sicca syndrome secondary to secondary Sjögren syndrome.
- *Neonatal lupus:* congenital heart block, hepatitis, cytopenias, and erythema annulare
- *Miscellaneous endocrinopathies:* autoimmune thyroid disease, diabetes mellitus, menstrual irregularities, and dysregulation of calcium metabolism
- *Acute life-threatening complications:* vasculitic crisis, infection, catastrophic vascular occlusion, renal failure, pulmonary hemorrhage

Diagnostics
1997 American College of Rheumatology Criteria for the Diagnosis of Systemic Lupus Erythematosis (need 4 of 11)

- Skin: 1. Malar rash; 2. Discoid lupus rash; 3. Photosensitivity; 4. Oral or mucocutaneous ulcerations
- Organ: 5. Nonerosive arthritis; 6. Nephritis (proteinuria, cellular casts); 7. Seizures/psychosis; 8. Pleuritis or pericarditis
- Blood: 9. Cytopenia; 10. *Positive immunoserology; 11. Positive ANA

  *Antibodies to dsDNA, antibodies to Sm nuclear antigen, antiphospholipid antibodies (anti-cardiolipin antibodies, lupus anticoagulant, or confirmed false-positive serologic test for syphilis)

Initial Laboratory Evaluation
- Complete blood cell count: thrombocytopenia, autoimmune hemolytic anemia, leuko/lymphopenia
- Metabolic panel: elevated creatinine, hypoalbuminemia suggests renal disease with proteinuria; may see hepatitis
- Urinalysis: proteinuria, cellular casts suggests nephritis
- Amylase/lipase if significant abdominal pain present
- Complement: low CH50, C3, C4
- Anti-nuclear antibody profile: ANA rarely negative in a SLE patient. Anti–double-stranded DNA is specific for SLE and suggests renal disease. Anti-Smith is SLE-specific. Anti-ribonuclear protein (RNP) is seen in SLE and mixed connective tissue disease (high titer). Anti-SCL 70 is seen in scleroderma and overlap syndromes. Anti-SSA and -SSB are seen in Sjögren syndrome. Anti-Jo1 raises suspicion for interstitial lung disease in a variety of autoimmune disorders.
- Antiphospholipid syndrome evaluation: PTT and dilute Russell viper venom time elevated with a functional lupus anticoagulant. Anti-cardiolipin antibodies are also part of laboratory criteria for antiphospholipid syndrome (also need clinical event to fulfill criteria). Anti-ß2-glycoprotein 1 antibodies are not part of the laboratory criteria but are also seen.
- Renal biopsy if significant proteinuria (greater than 1 g/24 hours), hematuria, cellular casts, hypertension, or renal function impairment
- Biopsy of skin rash if diagnostic precision required
- Arthrocentesis and culture if concerned about septic arthritis
- Blood culture if febrile. Patient may be functionally immunosuppressed secondary to hypocomplementemia and/or immunosuppressive medications.
- Chest x-ray and pulmonary function tests, ECG, and echocardiogram for baseline evaluation or if indicated clinically
- Brain imaging if focal CNS examination, severe headaches, psychiatric symptoms; EEG if concerned about seizures

Management

Pharmacologic Management
- Symptom-specific management is key
- Must balance benefits of therapy with adverse effects
- *Corticosteroids:* for ongoing disease activity. Initial dose is up to 2 mg/kg/day or 60 to 80 mg/day with a taper over 3 to 6 months, usually to maintenance dose or off as tolerated.
- *High dose (pulse) methylprednisolone:* for life- or organ-threatening disease; dose is 30 mg/kg/day up to 1 g IV usually for 3 days
- *Cyclophosphamide:* for severe organ-specific complications such as neuropsychiatric disease and glomerulonephritis
- *Azathioprine or mycophenolate mofetil:* for maintenance of renal remission or steroid sparing
- *Methotrexate:* for arthritis, refractory cutaneous disease, thrombocytopenia
- *IVIG:* for severe thrombocytopenia
- *NSAIDs:* for arthralgia, arthritis, myalgia, serositis, headache (use with care in individuals with renal dysfunction)
- *Antimalarial (hydroxychloroquine):* for dermatitis, constitutional symptoms, arthralgia, arthritis (check glucose-6-phosphate level before initiating therapy in persons at risk for deficiency)
- *Topical or intralesional steroids:* for skin lesions
- *Angiotensin-converting enzyme inhibitor:* for hypertension and/or proteinuria
- *Low dose aspirin:* for lupus anticoagulant or presence of antiphospholipid antibodies
- *Anticoagulation:* for thrombotic event (deep venous thrombosis, pulmonary embolism, arterial thrombus, recurrent fetal loss)

Health Maintenance
- Monitor serum cholesterol, low-density lipoprotein, high-density lipoprotein, and triglycerides
- Encourage regular exercise, weight loss, smoking cessation, and low-fat diet
- Calcium and vitamin D are recommended for patients on chronic steroids. Regular DEXA scans to monitor bone density.
- Obstetric/gynecologic: Avoid estrogen-containing oral contraceptive pills if possible, or use low estrogen formulations. Awareness of neonatal SLE risk is important, particularly in patients positive for anti-Ro/SSA and anti-La/SSB.
- Sun avoidance and protection (minimum sun protection factor of 30 with UVA/B protection)
- Avoid live vaccines if immunocompromised
- Influenza and pneumococcal vaccination are recommended
- Specialized nursing, social work, physical and occupational therapy, psychology, and nutritional counseling

Resources

Behrman RE, et al., eds. Nelson Textbook of Pediatrics. 16th ed. Philadelphia: WB Saunders, 2000.

Boon SJ, McCurdy D. Childhood systemic lupus erythematosus. Pediatr Ann 2002;31:407–416.

Burnham JM, Meyers KEC. Systemic lupus erythematosus. In: Kaplan BS, Meyers KEC, eds. Pediatric Nephrology and Urology: the Requisites. Philadelphia: Mosby, 2004:191–202.

Burns JC, Kushner HI, Bastian JF, et al. Kawasaki disease: a brief history. Pediatrics 2000;106:E27.

Cassidy JT, Petty RE. Textbook of Pediatric Rheumatology. 4th ed. Philadelphia: WB Saunders, 2000.

Dajani AS, Taubert KA, Gerber MA, et al. Diagnosis and therapy of Kawasaki disease in children. Circulation 1993;87:1776–1780.

Fauci A, et al., eds. Harrison's Principals of Internal Medicine. 14th ed. New York: McGraw-Hill, 1998.

Gaasch WH. Guidelines for the diagnosis of rheumatic fever: Jones criteria. Clin Cardiol 1992;268:2069–2073.

Gibofsky A, Zabriskie JB. Clinical manifestations and diagnosis of acute rheumatic fever. UpToDate, 2000.

Holman RC, Curns AT, Belay ED, et al. Kawasaki syndrome hospitalizations in the United States, 1997 and 2000. Pediatrics 2003;112:495–501.

Ilowite NT. Current treatment of juvenile rheumatoid arthritis. Pediatrics 2002;109:109–115.

Keenan GF. Henoch-Schonlein purpura. In: Liacouras C, Altschuler S, eds. Clinical Pediatric Gastroenterology. Philadelphia: Churchill-Livingstone, 1998:197–204.

Melish ME. Kawasaki syndrome. Pediatr Rev 1996;17:153–162.

Morrissy R, Weinstein S, eds. Lovell and Winter's Pediatric Orthopedics. 4th ed. Philadelphia: Lippincott-Raven Publishers, 1996.

Pachman LM. Juvenile dermatomyositis: immunogenetics, pathophysiology, and disease expression. Rheumatol Dis Clin North Am 2002;28:579–602.

Ramanan AV, Feldman BM. Clinical features and outcomes of juvenile dermatomyositis and other childhood onset myositis syndromes. Rheumatol Dis Clin North Am 2002;28:833–857.

Robson WLM, Leung AKC. Henoch-Schonlein purpura. Adv Pediatr 1994;41:163–194.

Ruddy S, et al., eds. Kelly's Textbook of Rheumatology, 6th ed. Philadelphia: WB Saunders, 2001.

Schneider R, Passo MH. Juvenile rheumatoid arthritis. Rheumatol Dis Clin North Am 2002;28:503–530.

Stollerman G. Rheumatic fever in the 21st century. Clin Infect Dis 2001:806–814.

Terai M, Shulman ST. Prevalence of coronary artery abnormalities in Kawasaki disease is highly dependent on gamma globulin dose but independent of salicylate dose. J Pediatr 1997;131:888–893.

Tizard EJ. Henoch-Schonlein purpura. Arch Dis Child 1999;80:380–383.

Amy L. Winkelstein, MD, Mercedes Blackstone, MD,
Suzanne Dawid, MD, PhD, Michael Nance, MD (with contributions
from James P. Franciosi, MD, MS, Leonard J. Levine, MD,
Gary Frank, MD, MS)

Neonatal Surgery

CONGENITAL DIAPHRAGMATIC HERNIA

Disorder characterized by pulmonary hypoplasia due to intrauterine compression of the developing lungs by herniated viscera.

Epidemiology
- Incidence is 1:2500 of live births; female:male 2:1
- 7% to 10% gestations end in fetal demise
- Defects more common on left side (70% to 85%) than bilateral (5%)
- Associated with anomalies (20% to 30%) including: central nervous system (CNS) lesions, esophageal atresia, omphalocele, cardiovascular (CV) lesions, and syndromes (trisomy 13, 18, 21, Brachmann-de Lange, Pallister-Killian)

Etiology
- Unknown currently
- Embryologic theory: postulates the lack of closure of the posterolateral pleuroperitoneal canals in the 8th week of gestation which separates the thoracic and abdominal cavities
- Portions of the diaphragm and pulmonary parenchyma arise from thoracic mesenchyme and if disrupted may lead to absence of part of hemidiaphragm and pulmonary hypoplasia.
- Majority of cases sporadic although there is other evidence to suggest a possible familial link.

Differential Diagnosis
- Cystic adenomatoid malformation, cystic teratoma, pulmonary sequestration, bronchogenic cyst, neurogenic tumors, primary lung sarcoma

Pathophysiology
- Herniation of abdominal contents into thoracic cavity through posterolateral foramen of Bochdalek
- Diaphragmatic defect may be small or may include entire hemidiaphragm.
- Pulmonary vasculature has increased muscularization of pulmonary arterioles and decreased branching of vessels.

Clinical Manifestations
- Respiratory distress within first hours of life secondary to severe pulmonary hypoplasia and associated pulmonary hypertension
- Pneumothorax
- On exam: absence of breath sounds; bowel sounds in chest; scaphoid abdomen; increased anterior-posterior diameter of chest; shifted heart sounds
- At least 10% are diagnosed beyond neonatal period with acute gastrointestinal (GI) symptoms.

Diagnostics
- Prenatal ultrasound able to detect defect as early as 25th week
- Echocardiography and amniocentesis to detect other anomalies
- Chest x-ray
- Inject contrast into stomach to reveal intestines above diaphragm.

Management
Initial Medical Management
- Initial resuscitation includes correction of hypoxia, hypercarbia, acidosis, hypothermia as they increase pulmonary vascular resistance and worsen pulmonary hypertension
- Nasogastric tube to decompress the stomach and decrease bowel distension that can compromise cardiopulmonary function
- Echocardiography to determine cardiac anomalies and determine severity of pulmonary hypertension and shunting
- Permissive hypercapnia and gentle ventilation may improve survival and decrease need for extracorporeal membrane oxygenation (ECMO).
- Surfactant has not been clearly shown to improve outcomes
- Response to nitric oxide is inconsistent
- Persistent right-to-left shunting may require ECMO

Surgical Management
- Repair typically performed at age 3 to 15 days since major acute problem is pulmonary hypoplasia with associated pulmonary hypertension (not herniation of abdominal viscera into chest).
- Abdominal surgical approach (favored) allows for repair of associated malrotation.
- In utero reduction of herniated viscera has been successfully performed and may be more common in the future.

Prognosis
- Poor prognosis seen with associated major anomaly, symptoms prior to 24 hours, distress requiring ECMO, delivery in nontertiary center.
- Survival 72% to 97% with initial stabilization, then surgical repair
- Long-term sequelae may include neurodevelopmental problems, gastroesophageal reflux, nutritional deficiencies, skeletal anomalies, and bronchopulmonary dysplasia.

ESOPHAGEAL ATRESIA AND TRACHEOESOPHAGEAL FISTULA

Anatomic lesions, which may be congenital or acquired and involve a blind pouch of the esophagus, are often associated with a fistula to the trachea.

Epidemiology
- Esophageal atresia seen in 1:3000 to 4500 live births.
- 90% of infants with esophageal atresia have an associated tracheo-esophageal fistula (TEF).
- Associated with trisomy 18 or 21.
- 30% of affected infants are born prematurely.
- Associated anomalies in greater than 50%: musculoskeletal (rib and vertebral anomalies), CV, GI (duodenal atresia, intestinal malrotation), GU (choanal atresia): *VATER* association (Vertebral and Vascular, Anal, Tracheal, Esophageal, Radial and Renal) or *VACTERL* association (Vertebral, Anal, Cardiac, Tracheal, Esophageal, Renal, Limb), CHARGE association (Coloboma, Heart disease, choanal Atresia, Retarded growth and development, Genital hypoplasia, and Ear anomalies)

Pathophysiology
- *Esophageal atresia with distal TEF*: most common type (>85% cases). Proximal esophagus is dilated and thickened, and ends around level of third thoracic vertebra. Fistula at distal esophageal segment enters back wall of lower trachea.
- *Isolated esophageal atresia without TEF*: 3% to 5% of cases. Proximal esophageal pouch ends around third thoracic vertebrae and distal pouch is usually short
- *Isolated TEF without atresia*: 3% to 6% of cases. "H" type fistula; level of thoracic inlet. Majority of fistulas are single.
- *Esophageal atresia with proximal fistula*: 2% of cases; narrow and short fistula
- *Esophageal atresia with fistulas to upper and lower tracheal segment*: 3% to 5% of cases. Similar to most common type with additional short, narrow fistula from proximal pouch to trachea.

Clinical Manifestations
- May present shortly after birth with excessive secretions and need for frequent suctioning because infant is unable to swallow secretions
- May have aspiration events
- Feeding leads to immediate regurgitation with choking, coughing, and sometimes cyanosis
- Association with polyhydramnios

Diagnostics
- Continuity of esophagus is demonstrated by passage of a 10F or 12F orogastric tube with an abrupt stop at 9 to 13 cm from upper gum line.
- X-ray will show coiled catheter in upper esophageal pouch
- Air in abdomen on x-ray confirms a distal TEF; gasless abdomen is evidence of esophageal atresia.
- Contrast studies of upper esophagus are not routinely necessary.
- Echocardiogram and renal ultrasound to evaluate for associated abnormalities
- "H"-type is more difficult to diagnose and often presents with history of recurrent pneumonia.
- Rigid bronchoscopy provides definitive diagnosis.

Management
- Surgical repair is either primary or staged.
- Signs prognostic for primary repair: clear lungs on auscultation and x-ray, no undefined cardiac abnormality, arterial PaO_2 greater than 60 mm Hg in room air.
- Staged repair: usually involves initial ligation of fistula and placement of gastrostomy tube for feeding followed by future esophageal anastomosis.
- Contrast swallow should be done day 3 to 10 after anastomosis to evaluate for continuity. Oral feedings are then initiated.
- *Complications*: gastroesophageal reflux, dysphagia, anastomotic stricture, tracheomalacia, airway obstruction, vascular compression, reflex apnea
- Morbidity and mortality in neonates are related to pulmonary complications

GASTROSCHISIS

Derived from Greek word meaning "belly cleft," a defect in the abdominal wall lateral to the intact umbilical cord

Epidemiology
- Incidence 1:10,000 to 15,000; more common in term infants
- Associated with young maternal age, low socioeconomic status, social instability, maternal smoking, alcohol use, medications (aspirin, ibuprofen, acetaminophen, pseudoephedrine)
- Occasionally associated with intestinal atresia or cryptorchidism
- Long-term survival over 85%

Etiology
- Postulated to be result of vascular accident during embryogenesis
- Recent studies suggest a possible inherited tendency

Pathophysiology
- In utero, abdominal viscera herniate through lateral abdominal defect (usually to the right) and float in the amnion
- Normal bowel rotation and fixation do not occur

Clinical Manifestations
- Herniation of viscera through lateral abdominal wall defect
- Intact umbilical cord
- Absence of peritoneal sac covering bowel

Management
- Delivery may be vaginal or cesarean section.
- Protect exposed viscera with saline-moistened sterile wraps or plastic bag immediately
- May need fluids 2.5 to 3.0 times above maintenance rate because of increased losses
- 75% are candidates for primary surgical closure.
- Remaining 25% have prosthetic, extra-abdominal compartment or "silo," which allows for gradual manual reduction.
- Most patients are weaned off ventilator within 24 hours of repair.
- Postoperative complications include prolonged ileus, parenteral nutrition–related cholestatic liver disease, sepsis, necrotizing enterocolitis.

OMPHALOCELE

A central defect of the umbilical ring through which bowel and abdominal viscera herniate. The abdominal contents are covered with a membrane composed of the inner layer of peritoneum fused to outer layer of amnion.

Epidemiology
- Occurs in 1:4000 to 7000 live births
- Up to 50% of affected infants have associated karyotypic anomaly (for example: trisomy 13 or 18)
- Associated with Beckwith-Wiedemann and pentalogy of Cantrell (combination of severe defects of the sternum, heart, diaphragm, and abdominal wall)
- Greater than 50% have other malformations: CV anomalies most common; also renal, skeletal, neural tube, sternum, diaphragm, bladder
- 10% have "giant" omphalocele where liver and intestine herniate through an 8- to 10-cm defect

Pathophysiology
- Failure of migration and fusion of embryonic folds
- Failure of the gut to migrate from the yolk sac to the abdomen
- Extruded abdominal contents are covered by a two-layered membrane; umbilical cord inserts into membrane.

Diagnostics
- Detected in second trimester ultrasound
- Amniocentesis: to evaluate for associated chromosomal abnormalities

Management
- May be delivered vaginally or via cesarean section
- Cover exposed membranous sac with sterile saline soaked dressings to prevent heat and fluid losses
- Correct fluid and electrolytes preoperatively
- Extra-uterine echocardiogram before surgical repair to evaluate for cardiac defect
- Surgical primary repair when possible. Placement of a "silo" for sequential reduction when primary repair not possible.

General Surgery

APPENDICITIS

Inflammation of the appendix caused by obstruction of the appendiceal lumen. Classically difficult to diagnose in children, because typical signs and symptoms may be absent in more than half of the patients presenting to the emergency department.

Epidemiology
- Approximately 1 in 15 people will have appendicitis in their lifetime

- Peak incidence in adolescence, uncommon in children younger than 5 years of age
- Slight male predominance

Differential Diagnosis
- Mesenteric adenitis, bacterial enterocolitis (especially with *Yersinia enterocolitica* and *Campylobacter jejuni*), intussusception, Meckel's diverticulitis, urinary tract infection, right lower lobe pneumonia, testicular torsion, and gynecologic etiologies such as ectopic pregnancy, ovarian torsion, and pelvic inflammatory disease

Pathophysiology
- The appendix is a blind pouch that can be obstructed by fecaliths, hypertrophied lymphoid follicles, parasites, or foreign bodies.
- Can also have bacterial invasion without previous obstruction
- This closed-loop obstruction causes edema, inflammation, and vasocongestion, which lead to necrosis and perforation.
- Once this process starts, children are more prone to earlier perforation and development of peritonitis than adults.

Clinical Manifestations
- Classically, pain which begins in periumbilical region and moves to right lower quadrant, nausea, vomiting, anorexia, and fever
- Can have dysuria
- In children, particularly younger than 2 years, clinical signs can be more vague and misleading and can include irritability, upper respiratory infection symptoms, lethargy, abdominal rigidity, or refusal to walk
- Perforation usually occurs 36 to 48 hours after symptom onset and should be considered in context of patient with persistent symptoms, high fevers, and peritoneal signs.
- Abdominal tenderness: typically periumbilical pain that migrates to the right lower quadrant (RLQ); can also be diffuse
- Bowel sounds usually normal or hyperactive, occasionally hypoactive
- Coughing, driving over a bump, or standing on the toes and dropping the heels may worsen the pain
- Presence of one or more of the following may suggest appendicitis (few pediatric studies):
  - Rovsing's sign: palpation of left lower quadrant (LLQ) causes pain in RLQ
  - Psoas sign: patient flexes right hip against resistance. Increased abdominal pain indicates positive sign.
  - Obturator sign: raise patient's right leg with the knee flexed. Rotate the leg internally at the hip. Increased abdominal pain indicates a positive sign.
- Rectal exam can show rectal masses, abdominal abscesses, or right-sided rectal tenderness
- Guarding and rebound more likely with perforation

Diagnostics
- Difficult to diagnose, particularly in young children
- 10% to 30% negative appendectomy rate
- Can be diagnosed on basis of history and physical exam alone, but adjunctive radiologic studies often helpful
  - Abdominal flat plate films have limited utility. Findings include fecalith, localized ileus, soft tissue mass, splinting, loss of peritoneal fat stripe, or free air
  - Ultrasound can be diagnostic; sensitivity and specificity vary among studies. Findings include increased appendiceal diameter or thickened wall, target sign, echogenicity surrounding the appendix, appendicolith, pericecal or perivesical free fluid
  - CT has sensitivity of 87% to 100% (increased with oral and rectal contrast) and specificity of 83% to 97%. Findings include fat streaking, increased appendiceal diameter, cecal apical thickening. Prospective study by Garcia Pena and colleagues suggests protocol of CT with rectal contrast in children with equivocal clinical findings and normal ultrasounds. This protocol has ~90% positive predictive value.

- No laboratory study sensitive and specific for appendicitis
- Should obtain urine pregnancy test in females of reproductive age
- CBC, urinalysis, CRP frequently ordered
- Often see leukocytosis and high percentage of neutrophils on CBC with differential; one of these is elevated in 90% to 96% of cases, but specificity of these studies is unclear

Management
- Patient should have nothing by mouth
- Fluid resuscitation as needed for dehydration or sepsis
- Broad-spectrum IV antibiotics that cover enteric aerobes and anaerobes in cases of perforation or sepsis (e.g., ampicillin-sulbactam ± aminoglycoside, ticarcillin-clavulanate, ampicillin + gentamicin + metronidazole, or ciprofloxacin + metronidazole)
- Standard of care is urgent appendectomy in uncomplicated appendicitis; cases with known perforation may require prolonged period of antibiotics.
- Administration of prophylactic antibiotics in uncomplicated cases of acute appendicitis is controversial, often left to surgeon's discretion.
- In uncomplicated appendicitis, laparoscopic appendectomy appears to be more cost effective than open surgery and reduces length of hospital stay. Unclear whether same benefits apply to small children.

HIRSCHSPRUNG'S DISEASE

Congenital aganglionic megacolon; abnormal innervation of the bowel beginning in the internal anal sphincter and extending proximally

Epidemiology
- Incidence 1:5000 live births; males:females 4:1
- Most common cause of lower intestinal obstruction in neonates
- Associated with Down syndrome, Laurence-Moon-Bardet-Biedl syndrome, Waardenburg syndrome, and CV abnormalities
- Uncommon among full-term infants

Etiology
- Multifactorial genesis and complex pattern of inheritance

Pathophysiology
- Absence of ganglion cells in the bowel wall, which extends proximally from the anus for variable distance
- Arrest of neuroblast migration from proximal to distal bowel
- Limited to the rectosigmoid colon in 75% of patients and involves the entire colon in 10% of patients
- Histologically, absence of Meissner and Auerbach plexus and hypertrophied nerve bundles
  - Increased nerve endings in aganglionic bowel results in increased acetylcholinesterase

Clinical Manifestations
- Often presents with delayed passage of meconium; 99% of normal full-term infants pass meconium within 48 hours of birth.
- Constipation is presenting symptom later in life.
- Bowel dilatation leading to increased intraluminal pressure, resultant decreased blood flow and deterioration of the mucosal barrier may lead to stasis and proliferation of bacteria with subsequent enterocolitis.
- Failure to pass stool leads to dilatation of proximal bowel and abdominal distention.
- On exam: palpable fecal mass in left lower abdomen but absence of stool in rectum
- Rectal exam reveals normal anal tone but is often followed by massive release of gas and feces.

Diagnostics

Anorectal Manometry
- Measures the pressure of the internal anal sphincter while a balloon is distended in the rectum
- In individuals without disease, rectal distention initiates a reflex drop in internal sphincter pressure. In individuals with the disease, pressure does not drop and may actually increase.
- Accuracy is greater than 90% but is difficult to use in young infants. This test is less commonly used compared to the barium enema (see subsequent section).
- A normal response excludes diagnosis but an equivocal or paradoxical response requires rectal biopsy.

Roentgenographic (Barium Contrast Enema)
- First-line study for suspected Hirschsprung disease at many centers
- Transitional zone seen after 1 to 2 weeks of age as a funnel-shaped area of intestine by barium contrast enema

Rectal Biopsy
- Obtained no closer than 2 cm to dentate line because there is a normal area of hypoganglionosis at anal verge
- Need submucosa to accurately evaluate
- Specimen is stained for acetylcholinesterase.
- Aganglionosis shows hypertrophied nerve bundles.

Management
- Initially, decompression with nasogastric tube; repeated emptying of rectum using rectal tubes and irrigations
- Definitive treatment is surgical resection: Swenson's technique, Duhamel-Grob technique, Rehbein-anterior resection, Soave-endorectal pull-through.
- Postoperative complications: recurrent enterocolitis, stricture, prolapse, perianal abscesses, fecal soiling

INGUINAL HERNIA

A protrusion into the groin of contents of the abdominal cavity, most commonly small bowel, into a persistently patent processus vaginalis. There are three types: indirect, direct, and femoral. Indirect hernias enter the inguinal canal through the internal inguinal ring and are by far the most common in children (>95%). Femoral hernias are rare in children.

Epidemiology
- Incidence of approximately 1% to 5% in children; male:female 6:1
- More common in premature infants; typically present in infancy.
- Approximately 10% of inguinal hernias are complicated by incarceration
- Likelihood of incarceration decreases sharply with time; the risk is greatest during the first 6 months of life.
- More often right-sided but bilateral in approximately 10%
- Patients with abdominal wall defects, connective tissue disorders, chronic respiratory disease, or undescended testes are at higher risk. Processes causing increased intra-abdominal pressure such as ascites, ventriculo-peritoneal shunting, or peritoneal dialysis can lead to high incidence of previously unrecognized inguinal hernias.

Differential Diagnosis
- Lymphadenopathy, lymphoma, undescended or retractile testes, hydrocele, testicular torsion
- May be difficult to differentiate hydrocele from inguinal hernia. Hydroceles typically transilluminate, but hernias may as well. Unlike hydroceles, neck of hernia can often be felt at the inguinal ring. Also, hydroceles may get larger over the course of the day, but cannot be fully reduced and do not fluctuate in size.

Pathophysiology
- Embryologically, the processus vaginalis is a diverticular portion of the peritoneum, which herniates through the abdominal wall and into the inguinal canal. The testes descend into the scrotum by the 29th week of gestation external to the processus vaginalis. The processus vaginalis usually fuses and is obliterated by the time a pregnancy reaches term or shortly thereafter. Partial or complete failure to obliterate results in a range of inguinal anomalies from hydroceles to hernias.
- With increased intra-abdominal pressure, bowel (or ovary in females) can slip into this communication with risk for possible incarceration (being unable to reduce the hernia), strangulation (compromised blood supply), and subsequent necrosis.

Clinical Manifestations
- Most children are asymptomatic until incarceration occurs.
- Characterized by intermittent groin, scrotal, or labial swelling that spontaneously reduces; more prominent with Valsalva
- Incarcerated hernia presents with signs of obstruction (emesis, poor feeds, abdominal distention, lack of bowel movements).
- Examine testes first because retractile testes can be mistaken for hernias.
- Classically, an inguinal bulge is noted at the inguinal ring or a scrotal/labial swelling that is reducible or changes in size.
- Causing infant to cry or having older child stand can increase intra-abdominal pressure to make diagnosis easier.
- With time, area surrounding an incarcerated hernia will become indurated, tender, and erythematous.

Management
- Once an asymptomatic inguinal hernia is diagnosed, the patient should be scheduled for an elective operative repair.
- An incarcerated hernia must be immediately reduced to avoid strangulation, necrosis, and perforation. Manual reduction is done by placing a calm child in Trendelenburg position and applying gentle upward pressure while trying to milk herniated tissues back into peritoneal cavity.
- Consider analgesia and sedation for difficult or painful reductions. Unsuccessful reductions require immediate surgical repair.
- In cases of successful manual reduction, prompt surgical repair can be electively scheduled as outpatient with strict instructions to return to emergency department in case of reincarceration.
- In cases where intestinal obstruction is present, patient needs nasogastric tube, laboratory studies, fluid resuscitation, and immediate surgical consultation.
- Controversy exists about routine contralateral inguinal exploration at time of repair of affected side.

INTUSSUSCEPTION

An invagination of a proximal portion of the bowel and its mesentery (the intussusceptum) into an adjacent distal bowel segment (the intussuscipiens)

Epidemiology
- Majority of cases occur between three months and two years with peak incidence between 3 and 9 months of age
- 2:1 male to female ratio
- Occasionally associated with cystic fibrosis (CF) and Henoch-Schönlein purpura (HSP)
- Seasonal incidence with peaks in winter and summer
- Occurs in neonates, older children, and adults but usually secondary to a pathologic lead point

Etiology
- Cause is unknown in approximately 90% of cases
- Incidence follows peak seasons of viral gastroenteritis. Postulated theory is that Peyer's patches become inflamed secondary to viral infection and serve as a lead point.
- Pathologic lead points in cases where cause is identified include Meckel diverticulum, intestinal polyps, B cell lymphoma, submucosal hemangioma, carcinoid tumor, and *Ascaris lumbricoides* infestation.
- Certain conditions such as CF, HSP, Peutz-Jeghers syndrome, and hemolytic-uremic syndrome predispose to lead points.
- Can also occur as a postoperative complication following a laparotomy
- Tetravalent rotavirus vaccine (Rotashield) associated with an increased rate of intussusception, prompting withdrawal from the market in 1999

Differential Diagnosis
- Gastroenteritis, incarcerated hernia, Meckel diverticulum, malrotation with midgut volvulus
- For patients who present with lethargy, consider vast differential for change in mental status

Pathophysiology
- Proximal portion of bowel and its mesentery telescopes into distal portion—usually ileocolic, but can be ileoileal or colocolic as well.
- Constriction of the mesentery causes engorgement of the intussusceptum and venous congestion with eventual bowel necrosis.

Clinical Manifestations
- Classic triad is intermittent colicky abdominal pain, vomiting, and "currant jelly" stools (due to mucosal sloughing).
- However, this triad is present in less than half of cases and grossly bloody stool is often a late finding.
- Pain typically occurs in screaming spells every 20 to 30 minutes during which the child draws up his/her legs. Children often look healthy and even playful between these episodes.
- Emesis becomes bilious as obstruction progresses.
- Up to 10% of patients present with only lethargy or hypotonia.
- Can be febrile and have other abnormal vital signs
- Even in infants without grossly bloody stools, stools will be guaiac-positive in approximately 75% of cases.
- Sausage-shaped mass in the right upper quadrant
- *Dance sign*: Absence of bowel sounds in the RLQ (present in approximately 85% of cases but can be difficult to discern)
- Abdomen often distended; bowel sounds high-pitched or normal

Diagnostics
- Plain abdominal x-ray: can see paucity of intestinal gas, minimal stool in the colon, small bowel obstruction, and right upper quadrant soft tissue mass; however, plain films may be normal
- Upright or decubitus film: rule out intraperitoneal air
- Barium or water-soluble contrast enemas: gold standard study for diagnosis and treatment of intussusception, which classically has a "coiled spring" appearance. Air contrast enemas have been shown to be as effective as barium enemas in diagnosis and treatment and can decrease the risks associated with a potential perforation.
  - Obtain surgical consultation before attempted reduction because 1) risk of intestinal perforation during reduction and 2) failed reduction attempt requires surgical correction.
  - Barium contraindicated if clinical peritonitis or free air on abdominal x-ray
- Ultrasound: possible role in unstable patients in emergency department; may see pseudokidney sign, target sign, or complex hyperechoic mass
- May see nonspecific lymphocytosis and electrolyte abnormalities consistent with dehydration

Management

- Patient should not eat (NPO). Begin antibiotics (e.g., ampicillin-sulbactam, cefazolin) and fluid resuscitation in preparation for barium or air enema.
- Surgery and anesthesiology staff should be standing by in case radiologic reduction is unsuccessful. In this event, laparotomy is performed with manual reduction and appendectomy.
- Enemas are successful in 60% to 90% of patients, but are less successful in patients that have had symptoms for more than 48 hours or when bowel obstruction is obvious on plain films.
- Recurrence of intussusception after barium or air reduction can occur in up to 10% of cases, and usually within the first 24 hours.
- If the intussusception recurs, repeated radiologic reduction may be attempted once before surgical reduction. Recurrence is rare following surgical resection (~2%).

MALROTATION AND MIDGUT VOLVULUS

Malrotation, an abnormal midgut development, results in anomalous positioning of the small intestine, cecum, and ascending colon. The intestines are not correctly attached to the mesentery and abnormal bands of tissue are present (Ladd bands). A midgut volvulus occurs when the malrotated intestine twists on the axis of the superior mesenteric artery (SMA) compromising intestinal blood flow.

Epidemiology

- Detected in 0.2% of live births, but in 1% to 2% of autopsy studies
- Approximately 30% of cases detected by 1 week of age, 60% by 1 month, and 90% by 1 year. Remaining 10% may present at any age.
- Up to 70% of patients have associated anomalies that include abdominal heterotaxia, omphalocele, gastroschisis, congenital diaphragmatic hernia, intestinal atresia, Hirschsprung disease, anorectal anomalies, situs inversus, atrial septal detect, ventricular septal detect, transposition of the great vessels, dextrocardia, anomalous systemic or pulmonary venous return, asplenia, and polysplenia.

Differential Diagnosis

Bilious (green or yellow) emesis in a neonate is a midgut volvulus until proven otherwise!

- Malrotation is in the differential diagnosis for failure to thrive, cyclic vomiting, chronic abdominal pain, intermittent apnea, testicular torsion, and incarcerated hernia.

Pathophysiology

- Normally, in the fifth to sixth week of development, intestinal size exceeds the space of the abdominal cavity causing them to protrude into the umbilical cord. As the embryo grows, the midgut structures (duodenum, jejunum, ileum, ascending colon, and half of the transverse colon) reposition in the abdominal cavity, rotating 270 degrees around the SMA.
- Malrotation occurs when the normal counterclockwise rotation of the midgut is incomplete.

Clinical Manifestations

- Varies from acute intestinal obstruction to chronic, intermittent abdominal pain.
- Delayed presentation of a midgut volvulus and significant intestinal necrosis includes shock (septic or hypovolemic) with hematochezia or melena and abdominal distention.
- With a midgut intestinal obstruction, the abdomen should be flat or scaphoid. Abdominal distention suggests a more distal small bowel or colonic obstruction.
- Abdominal wall distention, edema, erythema, and crepitus suggest gangrenous or necrotic bowel. *Bowel viability is time-dependent.*

Diagnostics

- Abdominal radiograph: Gastric and duodenal dilation with a paucity of distal gas suggests a midgut obstruction.

- *An upper GI series is the best test to diagnose intestinal malrotation*:
  - The stomach lies left of the midline and the duodenum makes the shape of the letter C (C-loop) crossing the abdomen from left to right to left again, joining the jejunum at the ligament of Treitz.
  - In malrotation, the C-loop and ligament of Treitz lie on the right and do not cross the midline.
- Ultrasound and CT scan may be used. A midgut volvulus on ultrasound has a "barber pole" or "whirlwind" appearance of the small intestine wrapping clockwise around the axis of the SMA.

Management
- Given the potential for volvulus and obstruction, any patient with a diagnosis of malrotation requires operative intervention.
- Ladd procedure: counterclockwise volvulus reduction, lysis of adhesive bands, conservative (necrotic) bowel resection, *appendix removal*, and repositioning of small intestine to RLQ and cecum to left lower quadrant.
- May need repeat operations to assess bowel viability (24 to 48 hours)
- Postoperative course may be complicated by wound infection, shock, sepsis, intra-abdominal abscess, small bowel obstruction, recurrent volvulus, bowel necrosis, intussusception, short gut syndrome, strictures, and dysmotility.

PERIRECTAL ABSCESS

Infection of the perirectal area via spread from the anal crypts to the anal ducts and glands

Epidemiology
- 68% to 90% of affected children are male.
- 90% of children are younger than 2 years of age.
- Occurs most frequently in children who have had previous rectal surgery, immunodeficiency from chemotherapy, HIV, diabetes mellitus, or Crohn's disease

Etiology
- Small tears in the anal mucosa may lead to infection, or infection may arise from the anal glands and extend into the anal crypts.
- When cultured, abscesses usually are polymicrobial. Most frequent organisms isolated are *Escherichia coli*, *Klebsiella pneumoniae*, *Staphylococcus aureus*, and anaerobes (e.g., *Bacteroides* species)

Clinical Manifestations
- 42% of children younger than 2 years of age have history of diarrhea.
- Fever (81%), rectal pain (69%), rectal mass (40%), pain on sitting (27%), pain with defecation (21%), abnormal gait (19%)
- On exam, there is erythematous, painful swelling in the perirectal area with or without fluctuance or drainage.

Management
- Most patients require surgical drainage or needle aspiration followed by antibiotic therapy (e.g., cephalexin, amoxicillin-clavulanate) and sitz baths.
- Current recommendation for immunosuppressed children with rectal abscesses is to treat with broad spectrum antibiotics initially (e.g., ticarcillin-clavulanate) and to consider surgical drainage if there is fluctuance, progression of soft tissue infection, or evidence of sepsis.
- IV antibiotic therapy (e.g., cefazolin, ampicillin-sulbactam) may be required for non-immuno-suppressed patients with extensive abscesses or evidence of systemic disease.

PNEUMOTHORAX

Collection of extrapulmonary air within the chest

Epidemiology/Etiology
- Often due to penetrating or blunt thoracic trauma
- Can result from disruption of pulmonary parenchyma, injury to tracheobronchial tree, or esophageal rupture
- Occurs in 5% of children hospitalized for asthma.
- Occurs in 10% to 25% of patients older than 10 years old with CF
- Iatrogenic: tracheotomy, subclavian line placement, thoracentesis, transbronchial biopsy
- Bilateral pneumothoraces are rare beyond neonatal period.
- Tension pneumothorax will develop in up to 20% of patients with simple pneumothorax.
- Other: lymphoma or other malignancies, staphylococcal pneumonia

Differential Diagnosis
- Localized/generalized emphysema, extensive emphysematous bleb, large pulmonary cavity, cystic formation, diaphragmatic hernia, gaseous distention of stomach

Pathophysiology
- Tension pneumothorax: a one-way valve created by initial trauma allows air to enter the pleural space but not to leave. This collection of air causes collapse of the ipsilateral lung and compression of the contralateral lung. Mediastinal structures may shift, and there may be a decrease in venous return to the heart and cardiovascular compromise.
- Primary spontaneous pneumothorax: occurs in patients without trauma or underlying lung disease (e.g., Ehlers-Danlos disease, Marfan syndrome)
- Secondary spontaneous pneumothorax: arises secondary to underlying lung disorder but without trauma. Examples include pneumonia with empyema, pulmonary abscess, gangrene, infarct, rupture of cyst, rupture of emphysematous bleb, foreign body

Clinical Manifestations
- Onset may be abrupt; may be asymptomatic; severity of symptoms depends on extent of lung collapse
- Pain, dyspnea with respiratory distress, cyanosis, splinting on involved side, agitation, increased pulse rate
- Respiratory distress: retractions, tachypnea, cyanosis
- Crepitus
- Decreased breath sounds on auscultation of affected lung
- Percussion of area involved is tympanitic
- Larynx, trachea, and/or heart may be shifted to unaffected side

Diagnostics
- Chest x-ray: expiratory views emphasize the contrast between lung markings and area of pneumothorax. Tension pneumothorax limits expansion of contralateral lung.

Management
Medical
- Small (less than 15%) or moderate sized pneumothorax in healthy child may spontaneously resolve within 1 week without intervention
- Because a small pneumothorax can quickly progress to a tension pneumothorax, even asymptomatic trauma patients with pneumothorax should be admitted for observation
- Administration of 100% oxygen may increase nitrogen pressure gradient between pleural air and blood
- Analgesia: consider respiratory depressant effects of codeine, morphine

Surgical
- Tube thoracostomy: indicated for symptomatic patients and those receiving positive pressure ventilation. Tube is placed at the midaxillary line at level of the fifth intercostal space (approximately nipple level) over the top of the rib.
- Needle decompression for tension pneumothorax: needle is placed in midclavicular, second intercostal space of the ipsilateral side; an immediate release of air is noted, and tube thoracostomy must be performed (see Pneumothorax Needle Decompression in Chapter 25)
- Recurrent pneumothorax: may use sclerosing agent that induces an adhesion between the lung and chest wall (tetracycline, talc, silver nitrate)
- Open thoracotomy: allows for plication of blebs, closure of fistula, stripping of pleura, basilar pleural abrasion

PYLORIC STENOSIS

Enlarged pylorus with increased muscular thickness, which generally leads to gastric outlet obstruction and bilious emesis

Epidemiology
- Occurs in approximately 3 to 6 per 1000 infants
- Male:female 4:1; more common in white infants
- 10% to 20% of infants of mother with history of pyloric stenosis

Etiology
- Hereditary and environmental factors thought to be involved.
- Other factors: abnormal muscle innervation, erythromycin therapy during first 2 weeks of life, maternal stress in third trimester, and B and O blood groups
- Underlying defect is redundant pyloric mucosa which produces edema, obstruction, and secondary muscular hypertrophy.

Clinical Manifestations
- 2 to 5 weeks of age most common
- Nonbilious vomiting is initial symptom.
- Weight loss and dehydration
- Patients are often hungry and eager to feed.
- 2-cm olive-shaped mass may be palpated in the midepigastrium beneath the liver edge
- Gastric peristaltic wave may be visible.
- Jaundice occasionally present

Diagnostics
- Clinical diagnosis possible in 60% to 80% of patients.
- Electrolyte panel: hypochloremic metabolic alkalosis due to loss of gastric HCl (may be acidotic if severe dehydration)
- Abdominal x-ray: dilated stomach bubble
- Abdominal ultrasound: radiologic study of choice (sensitivity around 90%)
- Upper GI series: sensitive and specific, but risk for aspiration. Barium studies may show elongated pyloric channel, bulge of pylorus into antrum, and parallel streaks of barium in the channel.

Management
Medical
- Initial IV fluids: 5% dextrose with normal saline
- Risk of hyponatremia if hypotonic saline is used.
- Potassium chloride can be added to IV fluids when urine output is established.
- Correction of alkalosis to bicarbonate less than 30 essential to prevent postoperative apnea.

Surgical
- Delay surgery until adequate rehydration and electrolyte correction established (approximately 24 hours).
- Ramstedt pyloromyotomy is procedure of choice. This involves splitting the pylorus without cutting through the mucosa.
- Approach is laparoscopic or through small incision

Urologic Surgery

OVARIAN TORSION

Twisting of the ovary or adnexa resulting in venous and lymphatic congestion and eventual loss of arterial perfusion with resulting ovarian necrosis

Epidemiology
- Rare in children, occurs predominantly in neonates and early adolescence

Etiology
- Torsion typically occurs in the setting of enlarged ovaries containing either follicular cysts or tumors; however, normal ovaries can also torse.
- Torsion is the most common complication of ovarian tumors in children occurring in 3% to 16% of patients. Ovarian tumors that undergo torsion are more commonly benign.

Differential Diagnosis
- Appendicitis, gastroenteritis, ruptured ovarian cyst, ectopic pregnancy, pelvic inflammatory disease, tubo-ovarian abscess, nephrolithiasis

Pathophysiology
- Ovarian mass (follicle, cyst, tumor) acts as a lead point for twisting of the ovary on its vascular supply.
- Right ovarian torsion is more common than left (3:2).
- Initially, venous and lymphatic drainage are compromised, leading to an enlarged ovary. If prolonged (greater than 8 hours), arterial supply is affected and necrosis, gangrene, and peritonitis can result.
- Neonatal ovarian torsion typically occurs in ovaries with large (>5 cm) follicular cysts that are believed to develop in response to exposure to maternal hormones. Torsion can occur either in utero or postnatally.

Clinical Manifestations
- Presentation is highly variable: abdominal pain (100%); vomiting (73%); fever (22%); palpable abdominal mass (20%); dysuria (14%)
- Patients note pain on abdominal (RLQ, LLQ) and pelvic exam.

Diagnostics
- Pelvic ultrasound with Doppler: the preferred imaging modality. Can show echogenic pelvic mass and absence of blood flow. Normal US and Doppler flow does not exclude ovarian torsion. If clinical suspicion is high, prompt surgical evaluation.
- Pelvic CT scan: helpful if ultrasound unavailable and can help to rule out other abdominal processes.
- β-HCG: quantitative to rule out ectopic pregnancy and germ cell tumors
- α-fetoprotein: order if tumor diagnosed; abnormal with teratoma or endodermal sinus tumors

Management
- Prompt exploratory laparotomy (preferably by 8 hours from start of symptoms) with detorsion or salpingo-oophorectomy.
- Management of a normal torsed ovary that is edematous and hemorrhagic is controversial. Recent trends suggest detorsion and careful observation may preserve fertility in the ovary.

- Ovariopexies should be considered in patients with a normal ovary that has torsed because these patients are at an increased risk of retorsion and contralateral ovarian torsion. Effect on future fertility is unknown.

TESTICULAR TORSION

Surgical emergency of males in which testis and spermatic cord twist, leading to acute ischemia of testis

Epidemiology
- One in 4000 males under 25 years old; not common in newborns
- Peaks at 1 year of age and onset of puberty (weight of testes)

Etiology
- Most common in individuals with "bell-clapper deformity" in which the tunica vaginalis extends up to the spermatic cord, suspending the testes freely within the tunica cavity.
- Deformity is frequently bilateral and can be detected by examining testes for a horizontal lie.
- Undecended testes are ten times more likely to torse.
- Intravaginal torsion (associated with bell-clapper deformity) is typically seen in adolescents.
- Extravaginal torsion (torsion of the cord and coverings) tends to occur in neonates secondary to highly mobile testes.
- Can result from contraction of cremasteric muscle after sex, trauma, cold, or exercise; can occur at rest

Differential Diagnosis
- Torsion of appendix testis, epididymitis, orchitis, scrotal trauma, incarcerated inguinal hernia, HSP, idiopathic scrotal edema, varicocele

Pathophysiology
- Spermatic cord twists within the tunica vaginalis.
- Arterial blood flow interrupted: leads to ischemia
- Prolonged torsion: leads to infarction and necrosis
- Recurrent episodes if spontaneously untwists before significant damage done (one-third of patients have had past transient episodes)
- Can result in abnormal spermatogenesis and infertility

Clinical Manifestations
- Acute onset testicular pain (89%); vomiting (39%), dysuria or frequency (5%), history of similar pain or swelling (36%)
- Scrotal pain can radiate to the abdomen, thigh, flank.
- Usually afebrile, no dysuria or penile discharge
- On exam: swollen and tender testis, scrotal edema and erythema, high-riding testicle (twisted cord) with horizontal lie, thickened tender spermatic cord, absent cremasteric reflex, palpable secondary hydrocele
- Fever and erythema are late signs.

Diagnostics
- Doppler ultrasonography is study of choice, but very operator-dependent. Blood flow on Doppler does not rule out torsion.
- 99m-Technetium radioisotope scan (rarely available)

Management
- Surgical emergency: obtain immediate consultation
- Detorsion: cord is untwisted and the testis wrapped in warm saline–soaked gauze while reperfusion is assessed. Necrotic testes are removed, orchiopexy (attach testes to tunica vaginalis) viable testicle. Orchidopexy of the contralateral testis
- Testis removed if not viable because of the risk of infertility secondary to the development of anti-sperm antibodies.

Resources

Neonatal Surgery

Adzick NS, Nance ML. Pediatric surgery (first of two parts). N Engl J Med 2000;342:1651–1657.

Ashcraft KW, et al., eds. Pediatric Surgery. 3rd ed. Philadelphia: WB Saunders, 2000.

Liu LMP, Pang LM. Pediatric emergencies. Anesth Clin North Am 2001;19:265–286.

Weber TR, Au-Fliegner M, Downward CD, Fishman SJ. Abdominal wall defects. Curr Opin Pediatr 2002;14:491–497.

General Surgery

Abramson JS, Baker CJ, Fisher MC, et al. Possible association of intussusception with rotavirus vaccination. American Academy of Pediatrics. Committee on Infectious Diseases. Pediatrics 1999;104:575.

Adzick NS, Nance ML. Medical progress: pediatric surgery (first of two parts). N Engl J Med 2000;342:1651–1657.

Arditi M, Yogev R. Perirectal abscess in infants and children: report of 52 cases and review of the literature. Pediatr Infect Dis J 1990;9:411–415.

Ashcraft KW, et al., eds. Pediatric Surgery. 3rd ed. Philadelphia: WB Saunders, 2000.

Behrman R, Kliegman H, Jenson H, eds. Nelson's Textbook of Pediatrics. 16th ed. Philadelphia: WB Saunders, 2000.

Birkhahn R, Fiorini M, Gaeta TJ. Painless intussusception and altered mental status. Am J Emerg Med 1999;17:345–347.

Bliss D, Silen M. Pediatric thoracic trauma. Crit Care Med 2002;30:409–415.

D'Agostino J. Common abdominal emergencies in children. Emerg Med Clin North Am 2002;20:139–153.

Davenport, M. Surgically correctable causes of vomiting in infancy. BMJ 1996;312:236–239.

Dennehy PH, Bresee JS. Rotavirus vaccine and intussusception: where do we go from here? Infect Dis Clin North Am 2001;15:189–207.

Fleisher G, Ludwig S, ed. Textbook of Pediatric Emergency Medicine. 4th ed. Philadelphia: Lippincott, Williams & Wilkins; 2000.

Garcia Peña BM, Mandl KE, Kraus SJ, et al. Ultrasonongraphy and limited computed tomography in the diagnosis and management of appendicitis in children. JAMA 1999;282:1041–1046.

Garcia Peña BM, Cook EF, Mandl KE. Selective imaging strategies for the diagnosis of appendicitis in children. Pediatrics 2004;113:24–28.

Marcus RH, Stine RJ, Cohen MA. Perirectal abscess. Ann Emerg Med 1995;25:597–603.

Rothrock SG, Pagane J. Acute appendicitis in children: emergency department diagnosis and management. Ann Emerg Med 2000;36.

Samuel M. Pediatric appendicitis score. J Pediatr Surg 2002;37:877–881.

Schwartz et al., eds. Principles of Surgery. 7th ed. New York: McGraw-Hill, 1999.

Shimanuki Y, Aihara T, Oguma E, et al. Clockwise whirlpool sign at color Doppler US: an objective and definite sign of midgut volvulus. Radiology 1996;199:261–264.

Townsend. Sabiston Textbook of Surgery. 16th ed. Philadelphia: WB Saunders, 2001.

Urologic Surgery

Anderson MM, Neinstein LS. Scrotal Disorders in Adolescent Health Care: A Practical Guide. 4th ed. Philadelphia: Lippincott, Williams & Wilkins, 2002.

Bellinger MF. Urologic diseases. In: Zitelli BJ, Davis HW, eds. Atlas of Pediatric Physical Diagnosis. 3rd ed. St. Louis: Mosby-YearBook, 1997.

Cuckow PM, Frank JD. Torsion of the testis. BJU Int 2000;86:349–353.

Graif M, Itzchak Y. Sonographic evaluation of ovarian torsion in childhood and adolescence. AJR Am J Roentgenol 1988;150:647–649.

Hamrick HJ, Fordham LA. Ovarian cyst and torsion in a young infant [Letter]. Arch Pediatr Adolesc Med 1998;152:1245–1246.

Kass EJ, Lundak B. The acute scrotum. Pediatr Clin North Am 1997;44:1251–1266.

Klein BL, Ochsenschlager DW. Scrotal masses in children and adolescents: A review for the emergency physician. Pediatr Emerg Care 1993;9:351–361.

Kokoska ER, Keller MS, Weber TR. Acute ovarian torsion in children. Am J Surg 2000;180:462–465.

Lee EJ, Kwon HC, Joo HJ, et al. Diagnosis of ovarian torsion with color Doppler sonography: depiction of twisted vascular pedicle. J Ultrasound Med 1998;17:83–89.

Marx JA, et al. Rosen's Emergency Medicine: Concepts and Clinical Practice. 5th ed. St. Louis: Mosby, 2002.

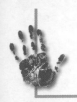

Rebecca Collier, MD, Diane P. Calello, MD, Fred M. Henretig, MD

Decontamination and Enhanced Elimination

ACTIVATED CHARCOAL

- Used in most pediatric ingestions to decrease drug absorption
- Should be used within a few hours of ingestion
- Technique: activated charcoal given orally or by nasogastric (NG) tube at dose of 1 g/kg (maximum, 50 g); repeat dose 0.5–1 g/kg every 4 to 6 hours, if necessary (see multiple-dose activated charcoal subsequently)
- Ideally should achieve ratio of at least 10 g charcoal per gram of drug ingested
- Multiple-dose activated charcoal (MDAC): some recommend repeat doses after large ingestion (listed in management section for specific drugs)
  - May improve results by decreasing enterohepatic recirculation
  - Use caution with sorbitol: may result in electrolyte abnormalities
- Does not bind metals (iron, lithium, lead)
- Contraindicated in caustic or hydrocarbon ingestion and in patients without protected airway (altered mental status or unconscious)

CATHARTICS (SORBITOL, MAGNESIUM CITRATE)

- Use is controversial
- Sometimes given with charcoal to hasten elimination
- Can be used for drugs that do not bind to charcoal
- Contraindicated in patients with ileus, intestinal obstruction, or renal insufficiency
- DO NOT use mineral oil or castor oil because these may increase toxin absorption

GASTRIC LAVAGE

- Gastric lavage commonly used in emergency departments
- Efficacy not proven, but most effective if done within 1 hour of ingestion
- Technique: place patient on left side with head lower than body. Use large bore orogastric tube. Lavage with normal saline until return of fluid is clear. Fifty to 100 cc per cycle should be used, and up to 200 cc in adolescents.
- May delay administration of charcoal
- Contraindicated in patients with altered mental status (inability to protect airway), hydrocarbon or caustic ingestion, or possibility of foreign body ingestion

HEMODIALYSIS

- Usually reserved for life-threatening poisoning or when renal failure results from overdose; consult pediatric nephrologist
- Blood is pumped through dialysis machine.
- Toxins diffuse passively from blood into dialysate solution.
- Patient must be anticoagulated.

HEMOPERFUSION

- Blood is pumped through column containing a material that directly absorbs the toxin/drug.
- Usually achieves better clearance than hemodialysis
- Anticoagulation is required.

SYRUP OF IPECAC

NO LONGER RECOMMENDED

WHOLE BOWEL IRRIGATION

- Uses: iron ingestions, massive ingestions, ingestion of sustained-release or enteric coated preparations, and when charcoal cannot be used, such as in lithium ingestion
- Technique: give preparation via NG tube until stool is clear
- Use polyethylene glycol solution, such as GoLYTELY at 500 cc/hour in children and 2 L/hour in adolescents
- Contraindicated in patients with ileus or intestinal obstruction, caustic ingestions, as well as in patients who are unable to protect airway (may require intubation)
- Charcoal may be less effective when used together with whole bowel irrigation (WBI)

Specific Poisonings

ACETAMINOPHEN

Over-the-counter analgesics (e.g., Tylenol), over-the-counter (OTC) cold remedies, prescription combination medications (e.g., Percocet)

Toxicology/Pharmacology
- Most commonly ingested drug in overdose
- Metabolized by cytochrome P450 system in liver
- Toxicity is via metabolite, N-acetyl-p-benzoquinone-imine (NAPQI), which is normally conjugated with glutathione; in overdose, glutathione is depleted and metabolite causes direct hepatic cell injury and death.
- Toxic dose is 150 mg/kg in children or 6–7 g in adults.
- Fulminant liver failure develops in 3% to 4% of children with hepatotoxicity.

Clinical Manifestations
- Early (first 24 hours): asymptomatic or nausea, vomiting, malaise
- One to 3 days after ingestion: right upper quadrant abdominal pain, increase in liver enzymes; may develop jaundice; initial symptoms usually resolve
- Three to 5 days after ingestion: resolution of signs and symptoms or signs of fulminant hepatic failure with encephalopathy or coma; coagulopathy; renal failure; death from liver failure possible

Diagnostics
- Draw acetaminophen (APAP) level 4 hours after ingestion (also at 8 hours and 12 hours if extended release form or if co-ingestion with medications that delay gastric emptying) (Figure 30.1).
- Labs: aspartate aminotransferase (AST), alanine aminotransferase (ALT), glucose, PT, bilirubin, electrolytes, creatinine, arterial blood gas, urinalysis

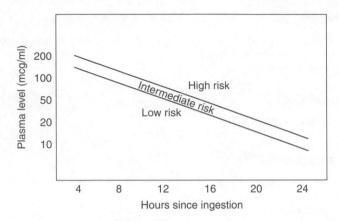

Figure 30.1 Nomogram for estimating severity of acute acetaminophen poisoning. (Modified with permission from Rumack BH, Matthew H. Acetaminophen poisoning and toxicity. Pediatrics 1975;55:871–876.)

Management
- Gastric lavage is controversial; give charcoal if within 4 hours.
- For acute ingestions, base need for subsequent treatment on nomogram (see Figure 30.1).
- N-acetylcysteine (NAC, Mucomyst) has greatest benefit in preventing liver toxicity if given within 8 hours of ingestion, but can be given as late as 24 hours after ingestion. Give dose if patient is presenting more than 8 hours after ingestion or if 4-hour level is above line on nomogram.
- N-acetylcysteine dose: loading dose is 140 mg/kg orally (PO); maintenance dose is 70 mg/kg PO every 4 hours for 17 doses.
- Cannot use nomogram to determine need for treatment in chronic ingestions; decision to treat in these cases is based on amount ingested (150–200/kg in 24-hour period) or evidence of hepatotoxicity.
- *Criteria for admission:* admit all patients with 4 hour APAP level above line on nomogram (see Figure 30.1).

AMPHETAMINES

Prescribed for narcolepsy, attention deficit hyperactivity disorder, and weight loss; found in OTC diet pills and some nasal decongestants; used illicitly as a stimulant

Toxicology/Pharmacology
- Toxic effects are via central nervous system (CNS) stimulation and catecholamine release
- Toxicity through various routes: ingestion, inhalation, or injection
- Methamphetamine is the most commonly abused amphetamine.
- Tolerance develops with chronic use; low therapeutic index

Clinical Manifestations
- Gastrointestinal: nausea, vomiting, anorexia, diarrhea
- Central nervous system: euphoria, agitation, pressured speech, seizures; stroke can occur from either hypertension or vasculitis
- Cardiac: palpitations, chest pain, hypertensive crises, arrhythmias, myocardial infarction, and circulatory collapse
- Psychiatric: psychotic state with hallucinations and paranoia
- Other: hyperthermia, sweating, tremor, difficulty urinating, dilated pupils, rhabdomyolysis

- With chronic use may see: cardiomyopathy, cerebral vasculitis, weight loss; psychiatric disturbances may be permanent

Diagnostics
- Based on history of ingestion and clinical presentation
- Urine toxicologic screen
- Laboratory studies: electrolytes, glucose, BUN, creatinine, creatine phosphokinase (CPK), urinalysis
- ECG, CT of head if concern for cerebrovascular accident (CVA)

Management
- *Decontamination:* activated charcoal; do not induce emesis
- *Symptomatic care:* hydration; treat seizures or agitation with benzodiazepines; can use haloperidol for severe agitation; treat hypertension with peripheral vasodilator (nitroprusside, phentolamine); treat hyperthermia
- Treat arrhythmias and rhabdomyolysis if they occur
- *Criteria for hospitalization:* monitor for at least 6 hours; if symptomatic, admit for observation.

ANTIHISTAMINES

Over-the-counter and prescription allergy medicines; cold and cough medicines; sleep aids; motion sickness medications

Toxicology/Pharmacology
- Antihistamines block H1 receptors
- Can cause CNS stimulation or depression
- In overdose can result in anticholinergic symptoms
- Elimination half-lives are variable, ranging from hours to days, depending on the specific drug
- Toxic dose is around three to five times the therapeutic dose

Clinical Manifestations
- Lower doses: CNS depression-sedative effect
- Higher doses: CNS stimulation-agitation, confusion, hallucinations, excitement, tremors
- Neurologic: seizures
- Cardiac: QRS widening with diphenhydramine (Benadryl), QT prolongation or torsades with terfenadine or astemizole
- Anticholinergic toxidrome: delirium, flushed skin, dry mouth, fever, tachycardia, hypertension, dilated pupils

Diagnostics
- Diagnosis based on history and presence of anticholinergic syndrome
- Can be detected on comprehensive urine toxicologic screen
- Laboratory studies: electrolytes, glucose, blood gas; ECG

Management
- Charcoal and/or gastric emptying
- Manage agitation or seizures with benzodiazepines.
- If symptoms are severe and life-threatening, can use physostigmine to treat anticholinergic effects—not routinely recommended because of toxicity.
  - Physostigmine dose: 0.02 mg/kg given over 1 to 2 minutes every 5 minutes to a maximum dose of 2 mg; can repeat if needed in 20 minutes
  - PERFORM ECG before physostigmine to rule out conduction delays.
  - DO NOT use in tricyclic overdose.
  - GIVE SLOWLY: can precipitate seizures or asystole
  - Have atropine ready if needed for cholinergic cardiac effects (bradycardia and hypotension)
  - Atropine dose is half of the amount of physostigmine given.

BETA-BLOCKERS

Most common use is for cardiac disorders, such as hypertension, angina, and arrhythmia; non-cardiac uses include migraines, essential tremor, thyrotoxicosis, glaucoma, and anxiety.

Toxicology/Pharmacology
- In treatment doses, drugs are beta-receptor–specific; in overdose, this specificity is lost.
- Sustained release preparations exist.
- Can be fatal in doses of only two to three times the therapeutic dose

Clinical Manifestations
- Cardiac: bradycardia, hypotension, atrioventricular block; asystole can occur but is rare
- Central nervous system: seizures, coma
- Bronchospasm: mostly seen in patients who have asthma
- Labs may show hypoglycemia or hyperkalemia.
- ECG may show prolonged PR interval or wide QRS if severe; sotalol ingestion can result in torsades de pointes.

Diagnostics
- Diagnosis based on history and vital signs
- Laboratory studies: electrolytes, glucose, BUN, creatinine, blood gas
- ECG

Management
- *Decontamination:* gastric lavage if large ingestion or immediate presentation; activated charcoal; can consider WBI for sustained release preparations
- *Hypotension:* treat with fluids; dopamine or epinephrine may be needed.
- *Bradycardia:* atropine; isoproterenol can be used if no response to atropine.
- Glucagon can also be used to treat hypotension and bradycardia that do not respond to previous measures.
- Magnesium for torsades de pointes
- Bronchodilators for bronchospasm
- Cardiac pacing or extracorporeal membrane oxygenation (ECMO) is reserved for patients not responding to medical management.
- Treat seizures with lorazepam (Ativan); phenobarbital can be used if patient is in status epilepticus.
- *Criteria for hospitalization:* must perform ECG monitoring for 6 hours after ingestion; all pediatric ingestions and ingestions with sustained release preparation should be admitted.

CALCIUM CHANNEL BLOCKERS

Medication for treatment of hypertension, atrial fibrillation, angina, migraines

Toxicology/Pharmacology
- Toxicity due to vasodilatory effects on both coronary and peripheral vessels, decreased contractility, slowing of the conduction system both at sinus node and through AV node
- Toxicity can occur from therapeutic use or in overdose.
- Can be fatal in small overdoses
- Most severe toxicity seen with verapamil or diltiazem
- Elimination half-life ranges from 2 to 50 hours.
- Sustained release preparations available

Clinical Manifestations
- May be asymptomatic for hours after ingestion
- Cardiac: hypotension, bradycardia (verapamil, diltiazem), reflex tachycardia (amlodipine, nifedipine)
- Other symptoms: nausea, vomiting, altered mental status

Diagnostics
- Based on history and clinical presentation
- Laboratory studies: electrolytes, glucose, BUN, creatinine, blood gas (may see hyperglycemia, metabolic acidosis, normal serum calcium)
- ECG shows prolonged PR interval with normal QRS

Management
Decontamination
- Gastric lavage: only if within 1 hour and will not delay charcoal administration
- Activated charcoal: consider multiple-dose (MDAC) in large sustained-release ingestions
- Whole bowel irrigation for sustained release preparations

Treating Hypotension
- Fluids
- Calcium chloride (20 mg/kg IV) or calcium gluconate (50–75 mg/kg IV)
- Dopamine, epinephrine, or norepinephrine for refractory hypotension
- Insulin and glucose infusions may be effective.

Other Therapies
- Atropine for bradycardia
- Cardiac pacing for failed medical management
- In life-threatening overdoses, consider ECMO

Criteria for Hospitalization
- Observe for 24 hours
- Monitor for at least 24 hours if large ingestion or any sized sustained release

CARBAMAZEPINE

Medication used for seizures (Tegretol, Carbatrol), neuropathic pain, some psychiatric disorders

Toxicology/Pharmacology
- Blocks sodium channels in the brain, preventing high-frequency firing; at high doses, also blocks cardiac sodium channels.
- Some mild anticholinergic activity
- Absorption can be erratic partially due to anticholinergic-induced delayed gastric emptying.
- Peak level reached from 4 to 24 hours
- Metabolized via P450 to active compound, so drug level may not reflect magnitude of clinical toxicity

Clinical Manifestations
- Central nervous system: ataxia, mydriasis, nystagmus, altered mental status, nausea, vomiting, dystonic posturing, coma, seizures
- Cardiac: sinus tachycardia, atrioventricular block, bradycardia, QRS or QT prolongation, hypotension
- Chronic toxicity: syndrome of inappropriate antidiuretic hormone secretion, leukopenia, thrombocytopenia
- Can have delay in onset of symptoms due to delayed absorption

Diagnostics
- Based on history and clinical signs
- Obtain immediate carbamazepine level; repeat levels every 4 to 6 hours; levels above 40 mg/L associated with severe toxicity in adults; toxic level is even lower in children
- Laboratory studies: CBC, electrolytes, glucose, ABG
- ECG

Management

- Treatment based on clinical status, not drug levels
- Supportive care
- Activated charcoal
- Massive ingestion: can consider MDAC or whole bowel irrigation
- Life-threatening toxicity: charcoal hemoperfusion
- Treat seizures with benzodiazepines and phenobarbital, NOT phenytoin (has same intracellular mechanism as carbamazepine)
- *Criteria for hospitalization:* observe asymptomatic patients for 6 hours; admit symptomatic patients to monitored bed if levels or clinical picture are concerning.

CARBON MONOXIDE

Fire (indoor charcoal or house fire), automobile exhaust, gasoline engines operating in enclosed spaces (car in garage), faulty furnaces or gas stoves, woodburning stoves, inhaled spray paint; also, the main ingredient in paint remover is metabolized to carbon monoxide

Toxicology/Pharmacology

- Children are at higher risk from CO because of their higher metabolic and respiratory rates.
- Toxicity results from the fact that CO binds hemoglobin with higher affinity than oxygen, which results in decreased saturation and decreased delivery to tissues.
- CO also can bind myoglobin, resulting in cardiac toxicity by decreasing contractility.
- Mild symptoms of toxicity can be seen at carboxyhemoglobin levels of 5% and death at levels of 50%.

Clinical Manifestations

- Most mild exposures present with flu-like symptoms, headache, dizziness, nausea, and/or weakness
- More severe exposure can present with syncope, seizures, coma, cardiac ischemia or infarction, dysrhythmias, pulmonary edema, or death.
- Physical exam findings can include tachycardia, hypotension or hypertension, tachypnea, and pallor.
- Classic description of cherry red skin is actually a late finding.

Diagnostics

- Carbon monoxide hemoglobin (COHgb) levels: remember, pulse-oximetry may be normal
- CBC, BUN, creatinine, cardiac enzymes, glucose, pregnancy test
- Chest x-ray
- ECG to look for ischemia or dysrhythmias
- Obtain history of risk factors for CO poisoning (heaters, etc.)

Management

- Give 100% oxygen to reduce half-life of carboxyhemoglobin.
- Can consider hyperbaric oxygen in several situations: COHgb greater than 25%, pregnancy, significant cardiac or neurologic symptoms
- Continue therapy until COHgb less than 5% to 10%
- Delayed neurologic symptoms (DNS) may develop days to weeks after exposure; symptoms may include headache, disorientation, dementia, apraxia, peripheral neuropathy, ataxia, chorea, or Parkinson-like signs. 25% of these patients may have permanent neurologic findings. Hyperbaric oxygen may decrease the significance of DNS.
- *Criteria for hospitalization:* adults with COHgb greater than 25%; children with COHgb greater than 15%; all patients with metabolic acidosis, ECG changes, neuropsychiatric symptoms, abnormal thermoregulation, PaO_2 less than 60 mm Hg

CAUSTICS

Acids or alkali; oven or drain cleaner; powdered laundry and dishwasher detergents; hair relaxers; button batteries; industrial products

Toxicology/Pharmacology
- Can cause burns when inhaled or ingested, but also with skin and eye contact
- Acids result in coagulation necrosis and more superficial damage
- Alkali causes liquefactive necrosis, which is deeper and usually more severe. These deep burns are more likely to result in perforation or predispose to later stricture formation.

Clinical Manifestations
- Stridor, hoarseness, dyspnea, aphonia, vomiting or drooling
- May be asymptomatic initially
- Symptoms do not reliably predict presence or absence of esophageal injury.
- Usually present with burning of exposed areas
- Airway edema and obstruction can be delayed up to 48 hours in alkali exposures.
- Acids and alkali both can cause esophageal injury; however, acid ingestions usually also cause damage to stomach with risk for gastric perforation and peritonitis. Alkali ingestions are more likely to damage esophagus with possibility of perforation and resulting mediastinitis.
- Can present with acute GI bleed or acute gastric perforation
- Third-degree esophageal burns at risk for developing strictures

Diagnostics
- Based on history of exposure and symptoms
- Important to determine if substance was only irritant or if actually a corrosive (call poison control center, check pH)
- Laboratory studies: CBC, type and screen, electrolytes, glucose, blood gas
- Chest x-ray and abdominal x-rays to look for free air

Management
- Stabilize airway: may need intubation under direct visualization (fiberoptic); blind intubation can worsen damage or cause perforation
- IV access; keep patient NPO
- NO GI decontamination, NO Ipecac, NO lavage
- Perform endoscopy as soon as possible to determine extent of burn.
- Surgery consult in all patients with significant burns
- Corticosteroids may be beneficial in some esophageal burns to prevent strictures (controversial).
- Pain control
- Antibiotics: if evidence of perforation or if steroids are used
- Histamine-2 blocker to reduce gastric acid formation
- *Criteria for hospitalization:* All patients with caustic ingestions

CLONIDINE

Medication to treat hypertension and attention deficit hyperactivity disorder; has been used to treat withdrawal symptoms from opioids and nicotine

Toxicology/Pharmacology
- Binds to and stimulates central alpha-2 receptors resulting in decreased sympathetic outflow
- Can also bind to peripheral alpha-1 receptors resulting in vasoconstriction
- Can be fatal in small doses
- Rapidly absorbed and distributed, so symptoms appear soon after ingestion

Clinical Manifestations
- Neurologic: can have altered mental status with irritability, lethargy, or coma; can also see seizures
- Respiratory depression, occasionally necessitating endotracheal intubation, apnea
- Cardiac: most commonly see hypotension and bradycardia, but can also see tachycardia, transient hypertension, or dysrhythmias, such as AV block or Wenckebach
- Other: miosis, pallor, hypothermia

Diagnostics
- Based on history and physical finding
- Drug levels not available
- Laboratory studies: electrolytes, glucose, blood gas
- ECG

Management
- Activated charcoal
- Treatment primarily supportive
- Hypotension: give fluids; if refractory can also use dopamine or epinephrine
- Bradycardia: treat with atropine
- The hypertension that uncommonly occurs rarely needs to be treated
- Naloxone is sometimes effective in reversing respiratory, cardiac, and neurologic effects
- *Criteria for hospitalization:* observe asymptomatic patients for 6 hours; admit all symptomatic patients

COCAINE

Used medically as local anesthetic; one of the most popular street drugs

Toxicology/Pharmacology
- Toxic effects are via CNS stimulation and inhibited catecholamine uptake
- Can get toxicity through various routes: ingestion, inhalation, or injection
- Toxic dose is highly variable
- "Body packers" swallow cocaine-filled packets or condoms in attempt to hide or smuggle drugs. Toxicity results when packets break open, releasing drugs into GI tract.

Clinical Manifestations
- Central nervous system: euphoria, agitation, psychosis, seizures, stroke
- Cardiac: hypertension, tachycardia, arrhythmias including ventricular fibrillation, myocardial infarction
- Respiratory: bronchospasm, pneumothorax, pneumomediastinum
- Other: dilated pupils, hyperthermia, rhabdomyolysis, renal failure, nasal septum perforation

Diagnostics
- Based on history of use and clinical presentation
- Urine toxicologic screen
- Laboratory studies: electrolytes, glucose, BUN, creatinine, CPK, urinalysis
- ECG
- Chest x-ray if respiratory symptoms present
- Head CT if suspect stroke
- Abdominal x-rays if suspect "body packer"

Management
- *Decontamination:* give activated charcoal if cocaine taken orally; if suspect "body packer" give MDAC and consider WBI
- *Supportive care:* benzodiazepines are used to decrease agitation, tachycardia, hypertension, and for seizures. If severe hypertension, DO NOT use beta-blocker alone, which can cause paradoxical increase in blood pressure and increased coronary vasospasm; use vasodilator alone, or combination of beta-blocker and peripheral vasodilator; treat hyperthermia.

- Treat arrhythmias and rhabdomyolysis if they occur.
- *Criteria for hospitalization:* admit patient with ECG changes, seizures, or neurologic deficits; "body packers"

DIGOXIN

Medication used to treat congestive heart failure; also found in plants (oleander, rhododendron, foxglove)

Toxicology/Pharmacology
- Inhibits sodium-potassium ATP pump, increases vagal tone, and slows AV conduction
- Toxicity can occur from chronic use or with overdose
- Doses as small as 1 mg can be toxic in children
- Absorption and redistribution occur rapidly; therefore, digoxin levels can decrease rapidly after ingestion
- Elimination half life is 30 to 50 hours

Clinical Manifestations
- Symptoms include nausea, vomiting, lethargy, visual changes (halos or changes in color vision)

Diagnostics
- Stat digoxin level; therapeutic level is 0.9–1.2 ng/mL
- May not correlate with severity of intoxication
- Laboratory findings include hyperkalemia or with chronic toxicity may see hypokalemia if concurrent diuretic use
- Other laboratory studies: electrolytes, calcium, magnesium, BUN, creatinine
- ECG findings: premature ventricular contractions (PVCs); sinus bradycardia; first-, second-, or third-degree heart block; atrial fibrillation; ventricular arrhythmias; accelerated junctional tachycardia; paroxysmal atrial tachycardia with block

Management
- Decontamination; activated charcoal with cathartic
- Correct electrolyte abnormalities
- DO NOT give calcium to correct hyperkalemia, because this may worsen ventricular arrhythmias; can use bicarbonate or insulin and glucose
- Treat bradycardia with atropine
- Treat ventricular tachycardia with lidocaine
- Digoxin specific Fab (Digibind): given in cases of life-threatening arrhythmias, severe hyperkalemia (>5 mEq/L or 5.5 mEq/L, depending on source), worsening clinical status
  - If amount of digoxin ingested is known, the dose is 38 mg Digibind to bind 0.5 mg digoxin
  - Otherwise, number of Digibind vials to administer = [(serum digoxin level in ng/mL) × (body weight in kg)]/100
- Potential side effects include hypersensitivity reactions, decreased potassium, worsening of heart failure
- *Criteria for hospitalization:* admit patients with hypokalemia, hyperkalemia, arrhythmia; patients with normal digoxin levels, no electrolyte abnormalities, and a normal ECG can be discharged after 6 hours of observation.

ETHANOL

Beer, wine, liquors; used as solvent, topical antiseptic; ingredient in perfume, cologne, mouthwash; used as antidote in treatment of methanol and ethylene glycol overdoses

Toxicology/Pharmacology
- Acts as a direct CNS depressant by binding to GABA receptors
- Ethanol can also have effects on cardiac muscle, thyroid, and liver.
- Ethanol is metabolized by the liver.

- Hypoglycemia in children results from ethanol inhibiting gluconeogenesis
- Levels at which symptoms appear are highly variable

Clinical Manifestations
- Mild acute toxicity: nausea, vomiting, euphoria, incoordination, ataxia, nystagmus, impaired judgment; hypoglycemia and seizures seen in younger age group
- More severe acute toxicity: coma, respiratory depression, metabolic acidosis; can have death from apnea
- Presentation may be different in infants and children and consists only of coma, hypothermia, hypoglycemia, and metabolic acidosis. These may be seen at levels of 50 to 100 mg/dL.
- Chronic toxicity: Liver—hepatitis, cirrhosis, portal hypertension, ascites; GI—GI bleeding from varices, gastritis, esophagitis; Cardiac—can get cardiomyopathy, dysrhythmias from electrolyte abnormalities; Neurologic—hepatic encephalopathy, cerebral atrophy, Wernicke encephalopathy, Korsakoff psychosis

Diagnostics
- Blood glucose STAT
- Laboratory studies: electrolytes, BUN, creatinine, liver enzymes, PT, blood gas
- Ethanol level
- Chest x-ray if suspicious for aspiration

Management
- *Supportive care:* assess airway and establish access; treat hypoglycemia, seizures, hypothermia
- *Decontamination:* gastric lavage if presenting within 2 hours of ingestion; activated charcoal should be given only if concern for co-ingestion.
- Hemodialysis effective, but rarely needed
- *Criteria for hospitalization:* in acute ingestions, observe until mental status is at baseline. Admit those with ethanol level greater than 100 mg/dL (toddlers), or greater than 200 mg/dL (adolescents), hypoglycemia. With chronic ethanol use, observe patient for signs of withdrawal, which can be severe and include seizures.

ETHYLENE GLYCOL

Main ingredient in antifreeze; occasionally used by alcoholics in place of liquor

Toxicology/Pharmacology
- Metabolized by alcohol dehydrogenase to toxic glycoaldehyde, glycolic, glyoxylic, and oxalic acids, causing metabolic acidosis
- Oxalic acid chelates serum calcium, causing hypocalcemia and calcium oxalate precipitation.
- Toxicity appears rapidly after ingestion.

Clinical Manifestations
- Early: patient may appear intoxicated; GI toxicity
- Later:
  - Cardiac: long QT, arrhythmias (from hypocalcemia), hypertension, tachycardia
  - Neurologic: seizures, coma, cerebral edema
  - Renal failure from calcium oxalate–induced acute tubular necrosis, metabolic acidosis

Diagnostics
- Anion gap metabolic acidosis, elevated osmolar gap
- Hypocalcemia
- Ethylene glycol levels are available, but may be falsely low if already converted to toxic metabolite
- Other laboratory studies: electrolytes, glucose, BUN, creatinine, liver enzymes, urinalysis, blood gas

- ECG
- Urine: antifreeze contains fluorescein, so urine may fluoresce under Wood's lamp; can see calcium oxalate crystals

Management
- *Supportive:* cardiac monitoring; correct hypocalcemia with calcium gluconate; correct acidosis with sodium bicarbonate
- *Decontamination:* NO emesis; NO charcoal; DO gastric lavage if presents within 1 hour
- *Antidote:* ethanol for ethylene glycol level greater than 20 mg/dL; ADH has higher affinity for EtOH and prevents formation of toxic metabolite. Fomepizole can also be used in adults but safety is not well established in children.
- *Other:* pyridoxine, folate, and thiamine prevent toxic metabolite formation. Hemodialysis can be used to enhance elimination; indicated in renal failure or in cases of severe electrolyte abnormalities
- *Criteria for hospitalization:* any known ingestion of ethylene glycol; clinical or laboratory abnormalities suggestive of ethylene glycol toxicity

HYDROCARBONS

Solvents, degreasers, fuels, pesticides, gasoline, kerosene, lighter fluid

Toxicology/Pharmacology
- Categories of hydrocarbons: aliphatic (petroleum distillates, furniture polish), aromatic (benzene, toluene, xylene), halogenated, and hydrocarbons that serve as a vehicle for other substances
- Toxicity can be due to inhalation, skin absorption, or ingestion with systemic toxicity (in aromatic, halogenated hydrocarbons or those with toxic additives)
- As little as 1 cc of fluid aspirated can lead to severe pneumonitis

Clinical Manifestations
- Respiratory symptoms usually result from aspiration: tachypnea, dyspnea, cyanosis, grunting, cough; can progress to severe pneumonitis and acute respiratory distress syndrome
- Pneumonitis can appear up to 24 hours after exposure.
- Neurologic symptoms usually result from systemic toxicity: seizures, lethargy, coma
- Gastrointestinal symptoms usually result from ingestion: nausea, vomiting, liver failure
- Cardiac: dysrhythmias
- Can also get fever, leukocytosis, or hemolysis
- Skin or eye contact can result in burns or corneal injury.

Diagnostics
- Based on history of exposure
- If respiratory symptoms, check ABG and chest x-ray.
- If concern over significant ingestion, check electrolytes, glucose, BUN, creatinine, liver enzymes, and an ECG.

Management
- In general, NO charcoal, NO lavage, NO induction of emesis
- Exceptions to this rule: if hydrocarbon contains a toxic substance (heavy metal, insecticide, camphor) or if massive amount is ingested then consider lavage after intubating to protect airway
- May need to use charcoal if there is a co-ingestion
- Supportive respiratory care: supplemental oxygen, continuous positive airway pressure, intubation as needed
- Extracorporeal membrane oxygenation has been used successfully in some patients.
- Antibiotics and steroids are not routinely indicated.

- Epinephrine is contraindicated (increased risk of ventricular fibrillation).
- *Criteria for hospitalization:* all symptomatic patients and those with abnormal chest x-rays. If asymptomatic, monitor for 6 hours. Symptoms can begin up to 24 hours after exposure

IRON

Ingredient in both pediatric and adult multivitamins; adult preparations have greater toxicity due to more elemental iron per tablet

Toxicology/Pharmacology
- In overdose, transferrin becomes saturated and unbound iron causes injury to cells.
- Toxicity can be due to direct corrosive injury or to impaired cellular metabolism.
- Toxic dose is 20 to 30 mg/kg of elemental iron.

Clinical Manifestations
Four Stages
1. Direct injury to GI mucosa results in vomiting and diarrhea, both of which can be bloody. Massive blood loss resulting in shock and death may result.
2. Gastrointestinal symptoms are seen to resolve over the next 12 to 24 hours. In mild ingestions, this may indicate recovery.
3. Up to 48 hours after ingestion, systemic symptoms may begin with GI bleeding, metabolic acidosis, coagulopathy, liver failure, seizures, shock, and possibly death.
4. Pyloric stenosis may occur from scarring 4 to 6 weeks after ingestion.

Diagnostics
- Based on history of exposure and symptoms
- Laboratory studies: STAT iron level if possible, should be done 4 to 6 hours after ingestion and then repeated 8 to 12 hours after ingestion to evaluate possibility of delayed absorption; level greater than 350 µg/dL likely to have toxicity; level greater than 500 µg/dL suggests more severe toxicity.
- CBC, electrolytes, glucose, BUN, creatinine, liver function tests, PT/PTT, type and cross-match; elevated WBC (>15,000 mm^3) and glucose (>150 mg/dL) are suggestive of ingestion.
- Abdominal radiograph at presentation and again after whole bowel irrigation

Management
- *Decontamination:* if less than 30 minutes since ingestion, can give ipecac if no concern for aspiration; can also consider gastric lavage; WBI if iron tablets seen on abdominal films (DO NOT use phosphate-containing solutions); activated charcoal is NOT EFFECTIVE
- *Supportive care:* treat hypotension with fluids; may need to give blood products to treat GI blood loss
- Chelation with continuous IV deferoxamine for severe toxicity; dose is 10–15 mg/kg/hour with maximum dose of 6 g/day; chelation treatment results in pink/orange appearance of urine; discontinue when asymptomatic with normal laboratory studies and normal appearance of urine; be aware of possible hypotension as side effect
- *Criteria for hospitalization:* symptomatic patients; patients with iron level greater than 500 or if iron tablets seen on abdominal radiographs; asymptomatic patients should have iron levels repeated at 8 to 12 hours—if levels normal and still asymptomatic, can be discharged

ISOPROPYL ALCOHOL

Solvent, antiseptic, disinfectant; main ingredient in rubbing alcohol; often ingested by alcoholics as a substitute for liquor

Toxicology/Pharmacology
- Less toxic than other alcohols
- Toxicity can result from ingestion, inhalation, or via absorption through skin.

- Causes CNS depression; large doses can also cause direct vasodilation resulting in hypotension.
- Metabolized via alcohol dehydrogenase to acetone, which is also a CNS depressant

Clinical Manifestations
- Gastrointestinal: abdominal pain, vomiting, hemorrhagic gastritis
- Central nervous system: slurred speech, ataxia, stupor, coma, respiratory arrest
- Cardiac: myocardial depression
- Respiratory: tracheobronchitis

Diagnostics
- Based on history of ingestion, presence of osmolar gap without metabolic acidosis (unlike other toxic alcohols)
- Odor of acetone may be detected
- Ketones (acetone) present in blood and urine

Management
- Supportive care
- Activated charcoal: poor adsorption, but may be helpful
- For large, recent ingestions, may consider gastric lavage
- Hemodialysis indicated for hemodynamic instability (very rare)
- *Criteria for hospitalization:* any patient with symptomatic isopropanol ingestion; symptoms do not rely as heavily on toxic metabolites as other alcohols so symptoms emerge soon after ingestion.

LEAD

Most common in paints used in houses built in and before the 1950s; also found in pipes, electric cable, gasoline as additive, bullets, batteries, glaze used for ceramics

Toxicology/Pharmacology
- Majority of toxicity results from chronic exposure
- Toxicity from enzyme inhibition, resulting in blocked heme synthesis
- Can also effect neurotransmitter functioning

Clinical Manifestations
- Most children are actually asymptomatic
- Gastrointestinal: can be nonspecific; abdominal pain, vomiting, constipation, anorexia
- Neurologic: seen at higher lead levels (>70 μg/dL); irritability, lethargy, ataxia, seizures, encephalopathy or death; may have increased intracranial pressure
- Renal: clinical picture similar to Fanconi; aminoaciduria and glycosuria

Diagnostics
- Venous whole blood lead level
- CBC will show microcytic anemia with basophilic stippling
- Elevated free erythrocyte protoporphyrin
- Long bone radiograph: may see lead lines
- Abdominal radiographs: may see opacities
- Avoid lumbar puncture if possible due to potential of increased ICP

Management
- *Prevention:* screening should start at 9 to 12 months of age at well-child visit.
- *Decontamination:* for acute ingestion, consider inducing vomiting or doing gastric lavage. Activated charcoal does not bind lead. Perform WBI if there are findings (paint chips) on abdominal radiographs.
- *Supportive care:* control seizures; manage increased ICP
- With chronic exposure, it is important to identify the source and remove child

- Need for subsequent treatment based on blood lead levels: should be less than 10 μg/dL; for level greater than 20 μg/dL, consider chelation; for level greater than 45 μg/dL, start oral chelation; for level greater than 70 μg/dL, hospitalize for two-drug chelation therapy and observation
- *Chelation:* lead level 45 to 69 μg/dL can be treated with oral chelation with Succimer or with IV CaEDTA; lead level greater than 69 μg/dL or signs of encephalopathy should be treated with BAL and CaEDTA (give BAL first and then both together 4 hours later)
- *Succimer (DMSA):* dose is 1050 mg/m^2/day (or 30 mg/kg/day) divided every 8 hours for 5 days, then 700 mg/m^2/day (or 20 mg/kg/day) divided every 12 hours for 14 days
- *Calcium EDTA:* 1000 mg/m^2/day IV divided every 12 hours for 3 to 5 days; for lead level greater than 69 μg/dL or signs of encephalopathy, use 1500 mg/m^2/day as a continuous infusion for first 48 hours; maintain adequate hydration
- *Dimercaprol or British anti-Lewisite (BAL):* used if lead level greater than 69 μg/dL or signs of encephalopathy; dose is 75 mg/m^2 per dose IM every 4 hours for 3 to 5 days; give first dose alone, then give BAL with CaEDTA; at 48 hours get lead level to decide whether to continue chelation; DO NOT use BAL in patients with hepatic insufficiency, peanut allergy, or glucose-6-phosphate dehydrogenase deficiency. Use cautiously in patients with hypertension or renal insufficiency.
- *Criteria for hospitalization:* lead level greater than 69 μg/dL or signs of encephalopathy; if only option for removing child from source of lead exposure

METHANOL

Windshield washer fluid; Sterno fuel; solvents, paint remover, antifreeze; used by alcoholics as substitute for liquor

Toxicology/Pharmacology
- Metabolized by alcohol dehydrogenase to formaldehyde and formic acid, which are responsible for the toxicity
- Metabolism is slow and symptoms may be delayed for hours.
- In children, small ingestions (5 mL of 100% methanol) can result in death.

Clinical Manifestations
- Ophthalmologic: "snowfield vision," retinal toxicity, papilledema, ophthalmoplegia, loss of pupillary light reflex, blindness
- Central nervous system: inebriation, CNS depression, seizures, coma, death
- Cardiovascular: hypotension, reflex tachycardia
- These findings may not appear for up to 24 to 30 hours.

Diagnostics
- Based on history and symptoms
- Funduscopic exams may show optic disc hyperemia, venous engorgement, or papilledema
- Anion gap metabolic acidosis may be preceded by an elevated osmolar gap
- Other laboratory studies: electrolytes, glucose, BUN, creatinine, blood gas, ethanol level, lactate level

Management
- *Decontamination:* do not induce emesis; activated charcoal is NOT effective; may perform gastric lavage; treat metabolic acidosis with IV sodium bicarbonate
- *Antidote:* ethanol (alcohol dehydrogenase has higher affinity for EtOH and so prevents formation of formaldehyde and formic acid); Fomepizole competitively inhibits ADH, and has fewer side effects than EtOH.
- Folic acid helps conversion of formic acid to carbon dioxide and water.
- Hemodialysis is indicated in cases of severe metabolic acidosis or blood methanol concentrations greater than 25 mg/dL.
- *Criteria for hospitalization:* any known methanol ingestion or clinical and lab findings suggestive of methanol ingestion

OPIOIDS

Can be natural or synthetic; most commonly used to treat severe pain, can also be used as antitussive; opioid abuse can result from use of prescription medication or illegal street drugs.

Toxicology/Pharmacology
- Opioid effects result from binding directly to receptors in CNS.
- The toxic dose is highly variable.
- Tolerance develops with chronic use, except for miosis, constipation.

Clinical Manifestations
- Classic triad of pinpoint pupils, coma, and respiratory depression
- Gatrointestinal: decreased motility and increased sphincter tone can result in constipation
- Cardiac: hypotension; propoxyphene may cause arrhythmias
- Central nervous system: lethargy, respiratory depression, coma, seizures (uncommonly)
- Pulmonary: pulmonary edema
- Diphenoxylate results in delayed onset of symptoms secondary to formulation that includes atropine

Diagnostics
- Can be based on clinical findings
- Can perform urine or blood toxicologic screen
- Laboratory studies: electrolytes, glucose, BUN, creatinine, blood gas
- Chest x-ray

Management
- Decontamination: activated charcoal for oral ingestion; consider MDAC or WBI for "body stuffers"
- Supportive care: may need to intubate to maintain airway; treat hypotension, seizures, pulmonary edema if they occur
- Naloxone is an opioid antagonist; dose is 0.4–2 mg IV; may repeat if no response after 2 to 3 minutes; if effective, may need to use repeat doses or an infusion to maintain response; in addicted patient may precipitate withdrawal
- Detoxification of an addicted patient is usually done with methadone
- *Criteria for hospitalization:* in general, patients should be admitted for observation; length of observation is based on half-life of specific drug

ORGANOPHOSPHATES

Insecticides; ingredient in chemical warfare agents

Toxicology/Pharmacology
- Toxicity is a result of irreversible binding of agent to enzyme acetylcholinesterase; clinical findings are result of accumulation of neurotransmitters at muscarinic, nicotinic, and CNS receptors.
- Can be from inhalation, ingestion, or absorption from skin
- Rapid onset of symptoms after exposure
- Children and pregnant women are at increased risk of toxicity due to lower baseline cholinesterase levels.

Clinical Manifestations
- Central nervous system: headache, agitation, seizures, coma
- Nicotinic: weakness, fasciculations, increased heart rate and blood pressure; can result in death from respiratory muscle paralysis
- Muscarinic: abdominal pain, vomiting, diarrhea, urinary and fecal incontinence, bronchospasm, decreased heart rate and blood pressure (opposite from nicotinic effects), salivation, diaphoresis, miosis
- Can occasionally see a delayed, permanent, peripheral neuropathy

Diagnostics
- Diagnosis based on history of exposure and classic clinical presentation
- Not detected on urine toxicologic screens
- Can measure plasma pseudocholinesterase levels or red blood cell cholinesterase activity, but this is not very helpful unless baseline levels have been obtained
- Laboratory studies: electrolytes, glucose, BUN, creatinine, liver function tests, blood gas
- ECG

Management
- DO NOT CONTACT contaminated clothing, skin, or gastric aspirates
- *Decontamination:* contaminated clothing must be removed and discarded as toxic waste, skin should be cleaned with soap and water, NO ipecac, gastric lavage for recent ingestions, activated charcoal
- *Antidote:* atropine in doses of 0.05–0.1 mg/kg should be repeated until asymptomatic and can be given IV or IM. Pralidoxime (used in conjunction with atropine) is used specifically to treat muscle weakness—dose is 20–40 mg/kg either IV or IM; doses can be repeated every hour as needed until muscle weakness resolves
- *Criteria for hospitalization:* any patient requiring treatment

PHENOTHIAZINES

Medication used to treat nausea and vomiting, depression, and psychosis; found in many tranquilizers

Toxicology/Pharmacology
- Toxicity is due to effects on CNS, anticholinergic effects, alpha-adrenergic blocking effects
- Toxicity can be seen with therapeutic doses.

Clinical Manifestations
- *Mild toxicity:* CNS: sedation, ataxia, slurred speech; anticholinergic symptoms include constipation, urinary retention, dry mouth (except clozapine causes hypersalivation); orthostatic hypotension, tachycardia
- *Severe toxicity:* CNS: hypothermia or hyperthermia, coma, seizures, respiratory arrest; cardiac: QRS or QT prolongation, dysrhythmias, hypotension; extrapyramidal effects: torticollis, rigidity, tremor, cogwheel rigidity
- *Dystonic reactions:* can be seen regardless of amount ingested
- *Neuroleptic malignant syndrome:* rigidity, hyperthermia, rhabdomyolysis, lactic acidosis

Diagnostics
- Based on history of ingestion and symptoms
- Drug levels not available
- Laboratory studies: electrolytes, BUN, creatinine, glucose, CPK, blood gas
- Abdominal x-ray: pills can be radio-opaque
- ECG to look for conduction delays

Management
- *Decontamination:* DO NOT induce vomiting; activated charcoal
- *Supportive care:* treat dystonic reactions with either diphenhydramine (0.5–1.0 mg/kg IV or IM) or benztropine (0.02 mg/kg IV or IM for children over 3 years); treat arrhythmias; treat seizures
- May need to use pressors to treat hypotension
- *Neuroleptic malignant syndrome:* reduce hyperthermia with cooling blankets, benzodiazepines for muscular rigidity, dantrolene or bromocriptine for severe cases
- *Criteria for hospitalization:* admit patients with signs of toxicity; observe all ingestions for 6 hours

PHENYTOIN

Treatment of seizures; occasionally used as antiarrhythmic agent

Toxicology/Pharmacology
- Phenytoin increases brain concentrations of GABA, reduces high frequency neuronal firing, and affects cardiac conduction.
- Toxicity can be seen at doses of 20 mg/kg.
- Absorption can be erratic with oral doses.
- Drug is highly protein bound and toxicity can develop from decreased protein binding or displacement of drug by other drugs.
- With IV preparations, toxicity may be due to diluent, propylene glycol.

Clinical Manifestations
- Cardiac: can see tachycardia or bradycardia; hypotension (ventricular fibrillation and asystole can be seen with IV overdose)
- Neurologic: ataxia, encephalopathy, tremor, agitation, nystagmus, confusion, hallucinations; seizures are rare (must rule out co-ingestion)
- Gastrointestinal: nausea, vomiting, hepatitis
- Can also see hypersensitivity reactions
- Rapid intravenous administration can result in hypotension and arrhythmias.

Diagnostics
- Diagnosis based on history of ingestion
- STAT Dilantin level (10–20 mg/L considered therapeutic); need to recheck due to possibility of delayed absorption
- Laboratory studies: electrolytes, BUN, creatinine, glucose, albumin
- ECG if drug was given IV

Management
- Decontamination: can give ipecac if within minutes of ingestion, activated charcoal, may consider multiple dose activated charcoal
- Supportive care: treat hypotension
- *Criteria for hospitalization:* cardiac or neurologic symptoms; unable to tolerate fluids due to severity of nausea and vomiting

SALICYLATES (ASPIRIN)

Over-the-counter analgesics and cold medications; prescription combination analgesics (Vicodin); PeptoBismol (bismuth subsalicylate); liniments, oil of wintergreen (methylsalicylate)

Toxicology/Pharmacology
- Direct stimulation of respiratory center resulting in respiratory alkalosis
- Uncouples oxidative phosphorylation and inhibits Krebs cycle, causing elevated anion gap metabolic acidosis
- Directly inhibits platelet functioning
- Start to see toxicity at doses of 150 mg/kg
- Elimination half-life can be as high as 36 hours in cases of overdose because of loss of first-order kinetics as drug concentrations increase.

Clinical Manifestations
- *Acute toxicity:* mild symptoms include vomiting, tinnitus, lethargy, tachypnea; moderate symptoms include agitation, diaphoresis, fever; severe symptoms include seizures, coma, pulmonary edema
- *Chronic toxicity:* symptoms can appear at much lower serum concentrations

- Can be nonspecific with only confusion or dehydration
- Can see metabolic acidosis and pulmonary and cerebral edema
- Laboratory abnormalities: combined respiratory alkalosis and metabolic acidosis (with anion gap), early hyperglycemia followed by hypoglycemia, hypokalemia, coagulopathy
- Can be fatal

Diagnostics
- Salicylate level: therapeutic level is 15–30 mg/dL; mild toxicity (tinnitus) at levels of 30–40 mg/dL; CNS depression at levels greater than 80 mg/dL; severe toxicity at levels greater than 100 mg/dL
- Chronic toxicity may manifest at lower levels
- Obtain serial salicylate levels (every 2 to 4 hours) and blood gases until level falling into non-toxic range
- Other: electrolytes, arterial blood gas, liver function tests, CBC, PT and PTT, urinalysis (for pH and specific gravity), ECG

Management
- Activated charcoal: give within 6 hours
- Vitamin K for coagulopathy
- Patients are dehydrated! Treat fluid deficits and electrolyte abnormalities
- Alkalinize to enhance salicylate excretion and maintain serum pH greater than 7.4: give 100–150 meq sodium bicarbonate/L of D5W at two times maintenance; goal urine pH is 7.5 to 8.0.
- Maintain serum potassium greater than 4.0 mEq/L
- Hemodialysis considered for severe metabolic acidosis or electrolyte abnormalities, renal failure, persistent CNS dysfunction, pulmonary edema, salicylate levels greater than 100 mg/dL, or if deterioration despite therapy
- *Criteria for hospitalization:* admit all symptomatic patients; observe asymptomatic patients for at least 6 hours

SELECTIVE SEROTONIN UPTAKE INHIBITORS

Used to treat depression and obsessive compulsive disorder; examples include fluoxetine, paroxetine, and sertraline

Toxicology/Pharmacology
- Caused by CNS depression
- Safer than tricyclic or monoamine oxidase inhibitor (MAOI) antidepressants; death from overdose is uncommon

Clinical Manifestations
- *Neurologic:* confusion, sedation, coma
- *Respiratory depression* can occur, more likely after co-ingestion with alcohol.
- *Cardiac:* usually mild, can get tachycardia and hypotension or hypertension
- *Serotonin syndrome:* usually results from co-ingestion of SSRI with MAOI; can also be seen after starting drug, switching drugs, or recently increasing dose; presents with restlessness, hallucinations; exam significant for mental status changes, myoclonus, rigidity, hyperreflexia, ataxia, hyperthermia, hypotension or hypertension; may resemble neuroleptic malignant syndrome

Diagnostics
- Drug levels are not useful.
- Laboratory studies: electrolytes, glucose, CPK, blood gas; ECG

Management
- Decontamination
- Supportive care: hydration; alkalinize urine if signs of rhabdomyolysis; manage seizures with benzodiazepine.
- In some case reports in the literature, serotonin syndrome has been successfully treated with cryoheptadine, a serotonin receptor antagonist.

TRICYCLIC ANTIDEPRESSANTS

Used to treat depression, enuresis, neurogenic pain

Toxicology/Pharmacology
• Due to anticholinergic effects, peripheral alpha blocking effects, sodium channel blockade causing ventricular conduction delay and myocardial depression, and inhibition of norepinephrine and serotonin re-uptake
• Large volume of distribution and long elimination half-life

Clinical Manifestations
• Anticholinergic syndrome: urinary retention, delayed gastric emptying, flushed and dry skin, delirium, dilated pupils, hyperthermia
• Can get rhabdomyolysis as result of hyperthermia
• Cardiac: hypotension from peripheral vasodilation; sinus tachycardia; conduction abnormalities (prolongation of PR, QRS, or QT intervals); QRS interval greater than 0.1 seconds is predictive of significant morbidity; various arrhythmias including PVCs, ventricular tachycardia, ventricular fibrillation
• Neurologic: can range from lethargy to seizures to coma

Diagnostics
• Drug levels are usually not helpful.
• Most can be detected on urine screening
• Laboratory studies: electrolytes, BUN, creatinine, glucose, blood gas, CPK, urinalysis
• ECG

Management
• *Decontamination:* lavage, activated charcoal
• *Supportive care:* treat seizures with benzodiazepines. Norepinephrine can be used for persistent hypotension. Lidocaine can be used for persistent arrhythmias. Prevent hyperthermia. If cardiac toxicity is present, alkalinize the blood with sodium bicarbonate to maintain a pH 7.45 to 7.55.
• *Physostigmine SHOULD NOT be given.*
• *Criteria for hospitalization:* observe all ingestions at least 6 hours. If any signs of toxicity, admit for 24 hours of observation.

Resources

Abbruzzi G. Pediatric toxicologic concerns. Emerg Med Clin North Am 2002;20:223–247.

Adrogué HJ, Madias NE. Management of life-threatening acid-base disorders-second of two parts. N Engl J Med 1998;338:107–111.

Badawy M. Toxicity, Selective Serotonin Reuptake Inhibitor. Available at: http://www.emedicine.com/ped/topic2786.htm. Accessed October 31, 2002.

Belson MG, et al. Calcium channel blocker ingestions in children. Am J Emerg Med 2000;18:581–586.

Bond GR. Home syrup of ipecac use does not reduce emergency department use or improve outcome. Pediatrics 2003;112:1061–1064.

Bozeman WP, Myers RA, Barish RA. Confirmation of the pulse oximetry gap in carbon monoxide poisoning. Ann Emerg Med 1997;30:608–611

Doty C. Toxicity, Ethanol. Available at: http://www.emedicine.com/ped/topic2715.htm. Accessed on November 19, 2003.

England A. Toxicity, Alcohols. Available at: http://www.emedicine.com/emerg/topic19.htm. Accessed on January 15, 2003.

Fleisher G, Ludwig S, eds. Textbook of Pediatric Emergency Medicine. 4th ed. Philadelphia: Lippincott, Williams & Wilkins, 2000.

Handly N. Toxicity, Amphetamines. Available at: http://author.emedicine.com/emerg/ topic23.htm. Accessed January 10, 2003.

Jacobsen D, McMartin K. Antidotes for methanol and ethylene glycol poisoning. J Toxicol Clin Toxicol 1997;35:127–143.

Lemke T, Wang R. Emergency department observation for toxicologic exposures. Emerg Med Clin North Am. 2001;19:155–167.

Liebelt EL. Targeted management strategies for cardiovascular toxicity from tricyclic antidepressant overdose: the pivotal role for alkalinization and sodium loading. Pediatr Emerg Care 1998;14:293–298.

Lowenstein DH, Alldredge BK. Status epilepticus. N Engl J Med 1998;338:970–976.

Markowitz M. Lead poisoning. Pediatr Rev 2000;21:327–335.

Marx JA, ed. Rosen's Emergency Medicine: Concepts and Clinical Practice. 5th ed. St. Louis: Mosby, 2002.

McGuigan MA. Guideline for the out-of-hospital management of human exposures to minimally toxic substances. J Toxicol Clin Toxicol 2003;41:907–917.

Mechem C. Toxicity, Isoniazid. Available at: http://www.emedicine.com/emerg/topic287.htm. Accessed November 19, 2003.

Miller C. Toxicity, Phenytoin. Available at: http://www.emedicine.com/emerg/topic421.htm. Accessed November 20, 2003.

Olsen KR. Poisoning and Drug Overdose. 3rd ed. Stamford: Appleton and Lange, 1999.

Rivera-Penera T, Gugig R, Davis J, et al. Outcome of acetaminophen overdose in pediatric patients and factors contributing to hepatotoxicity. J Pediatr 1997;130:300–304.

Romero JA, Kuczler FJ. Isoniazid overdose: recognition and management. Am Fam Physician 1998;57:749–752.

Santucci K, Shah BR, Linakis JG. Acute isoniazid exposures and antidote availability. Pediatr Emerg Care 1999;15:99–101.

Schexnayder S, James LP, Kearns GL, Farrar HC. The pharmacokinetics of continuous infusion pralidoxime in children with organophosphate poisoning. J Toxicol Clin Toxicol 1998;36:549–555.

Shannon M. The demise of ipecac. Pediatrics 2003;112:1180–1181.

Smilkstein MJ, Knapp GL, Kulig KW, Rumack BH. Efficacy of oral N-acetylcysteine in the treatment of acetaminophen overdose. Analysis of the national multicenter study (1976 to 1985). N Engl J Med 1988;319:1557–1562.

Stremski ES, Brady WB, Prasad K, Hennes HA. Pediatric carbamazepine intoxication. Ann Emerg Med 1995;25:624–630.

Traum A. Carbon monoxide (CO) poisoning. Pediatr Rev 2000;20:23–24.

Treatment of Lead-Exposed Children (TLC) Trial Group. Safety and efficacy of succimer in toddlers with blood lead levels of 20–44 µg/dL. Pediatr Res 2000;48:593–599.

Watemberg NM, Roth KS, Alehan FK, Epstein CE. Central anticholinergic syndrome on therapeutic doses of cyproheptadine. Pediatrics 1999;103:158–160.

Weaver LK, Hopkins RO, Chan KC, et al. Hyperbaric oxygen for acute carbon monoxide poisoning. N Engl J Med 2002;347:1057–1067.

Woo OF. Shorter duration of oral N-acetylcysteine therapy for acute acetaminophen overdose. Ann Emerg Med 2000;35:363–368.

Appendix A:
Normal Pediatric
Vital Signs

Table 1a: Range of Normal Values for Respiratory Rate and Heart Rate in Childhood		
Age	Respiratory Rate (per min)	Heart Rate (per min)
Neonate	35–66	93–154
1 mo	34–64	121–182
3 mo	32–61	106–186
6 mo	30–56	109–169
12 mo	27–49	89–151
5 yr	16–31	65–133
10–18 yr	12–20	60–120

(Data derived in part from 1) American Academy of Pediatrics. The fourth report on the diagnosis, evaluation, and treatment of high blood pressure in children and adolescents. Pediatrics 2004;114:555–576; 2) Zubrow AB, Hulman S, Kushner H, Falkner B. Determinants of blood pressure in infants admitted to neonatal intensive care units: a prospective, multicenter study. J Perinatol 1995;15:470–479; and 3) Rusconi F, Castagneto M, Gagliardi L, et al. Reference values for respiratory rate in the first 3 years of life. Pediatrics 1994;94:350–355.)

Table 1b: Range of Blood Pressure Values for Children of Average Height*

Age		BP Percentile	Value or Range[†]
Neonate (term)	Systolic	5th	63
		50th	78
		95th	92
	Diastolic	5th	30
		50th	45
		95th	60
1–5 yr	Systolic	50th	85–95
		95th	103–112
	Diastolic	50th	37–53
		95th	56–72
6–10 yr	Systolic	50th	96–102
		95th	114–119
	Diastolic	50th	55–61
		95th	74–80
11–18 yr	Systolic	50th	104–118
		95th	121–136
	Diastolic	50th	61–67
		95th	80–87

BP, blood pressure.

*Please consult alternate sources for more precise classification of normal blood pressure since the values vary slightly by gender, age, and height.

[†]By convention, the inflatable bladder width of an appropriate size cuff covers at least 40% of the arm circumference at a point midway between the olecranon and the acromion (for more information consult the American Heart Association or search their website at http://www.americanheart.org).

(Data derived in part from 1) American Academy of Pediatrics. The fourth report on the diagnosis, evaluation, and treatment of high blood pressure in children and adolescents. Pediatrics 2004;114:555–576; 2) Zubrow AB, Hulman S, Kushner H, Falkner B. Determinants of blood pressure in infants admitted to neonatal intensive care units: a prospective, multicenter study. J Perinatol 1995;15:470–479; and 3) Rusconi F, Castagneto M, Gagliardi L, et al. Reference values for respiratory rate in the first 3 years of life. Pediatrics 1994;94:350–355.)

APPENDIX B:
NEONATAL CODE

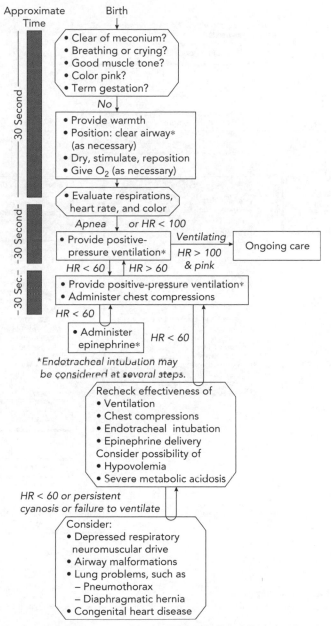

Approximate Time

Birth

- Clear of meconium?
- Breathing or crying?
- Good muscle tone?
- Color pink?
- Term gestation?

No

- Provide warmth
- Position: clear airway*
  (as necessary)
- Dry, stimulate, reposition
- Give O₂ (as necessary)

30 Second

- Evaluate respirations, heart rate, and color

Apnea   or HR < 100

- Provide positive-pressure ventilation*

Ventilating
HR > 100
& pink

Ongoing care

HR < 60   HR > 60

-30 Second- -30 Second-

- Provide positive-pressure ventilation*
- Administer chest compressions

HR < 60

- Administer epinephrine*

HR < 60

-30 Sec.-

*Endotracheal intubation may
be considered at several steps.

Recheck effectiveness of
- Ventilation
- Chest compressions
- Endotracheal intubation
- Epinephrine delivery
Consider possibility of
- Hypovolemia
- Severe metabolic acidosis

HR < 60 or persistent
cyanosis or failure to ventilate

Consider:
- Depressed respiratory
  neuromuscular drive
- Airway malformations
- Lung problems, such as
  – Pneumothorax
  – Diaphragmatic hernia
- Congenital heart disease

Appendix C:
PALS Algorithms

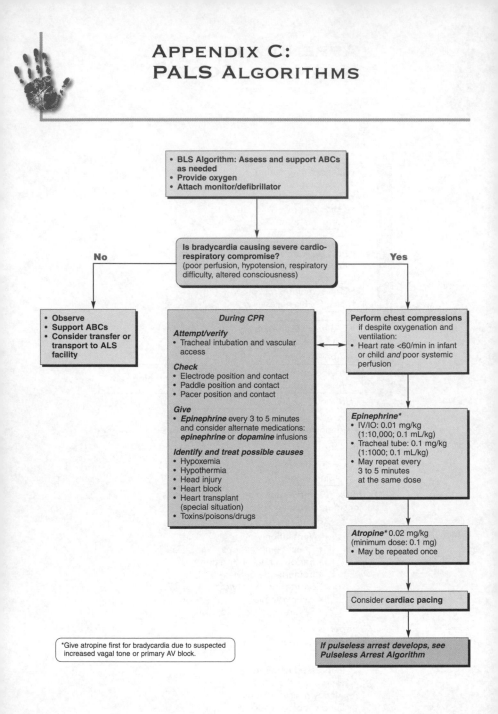

- BLS Algorithm: Assess and support ABCs as needed
- Provide oxygen
- Attach monitor/defibrillator

Is bradycardia causing severe cardio-respiratory compromise?
(poor perfusion, hypotension, respiratory difficulty, altered consciousness)

No

Yes

- Observe
- Support ABCs
- Consider transfer or transport to ALS facility

During CPR

Attempt/verify
- Tracheal intubation and vascular access

Check
- Electrode position and contact
- Paddle position and contact
- Pacer position and contact

Give
- *Epinephrine* every 3 to 5 minutes and consider alternate medications: *epinephrine* or *dopamine* infusions

Identify and treat possible causes
- Hypoxemia
- Hypothermia
- Head injury
- Heart block
- Heart transplant (special situation)
- Toxins/poisons/drugs

Perform chest compressions
if despite oxygenation and ventilation:
- Heart rate <60/min in infant or child *and* poor systemic perfusion

Epinephrine*
- IV/IO: 0.01 mg/kg (1:10,000; 0.1 mL/kg)
- Tracheal tube: 0.1 mg/kg (1:1000; 0.1 mL/kg)
- May repeat every 3 to 5 minutes at the same dose

Atropine* 0.02 mg/kg
(minimum dose: 0.1 mg)
- May be repeated once

Consider **cardiac pacing**

*Give atropine first for bradycardia due to suspected increased vagal tone or primary AV block.

If pulseless arrest develops, see Pulseless Arrest Algorithm

Pediatric Bradycardia Algorithm
(Reproduced with permission from the PALS Provider Manual. © American Heart Association, 2002)

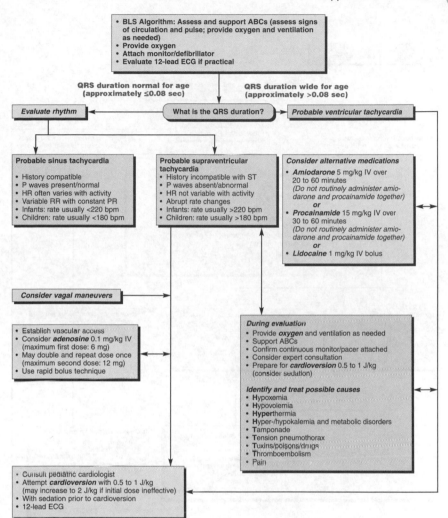

Pediatric Tachycardia Algorithm for Infants and Children with Rapid Rhythm and Adequate Perfusion

(Reproduced with permission from the PALS Provider Manual. © American Heart Association, 2002)

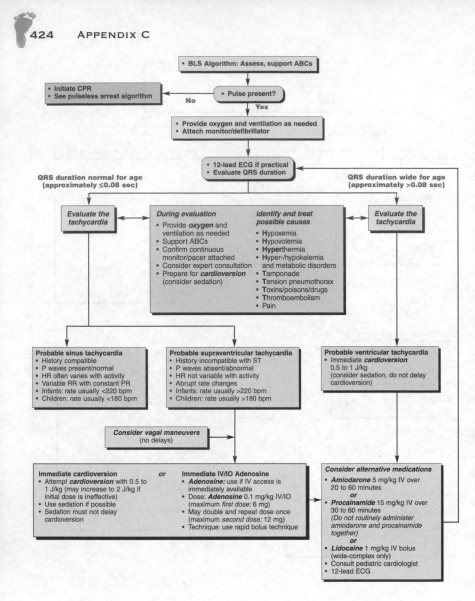

Pediatric Tachycardia Algorithm for Infants and Children with Rapid Rhythm and Poor Perfusion

(Reproduced with permission from the PALS Provider Manual. © American Heart Association, 2002)

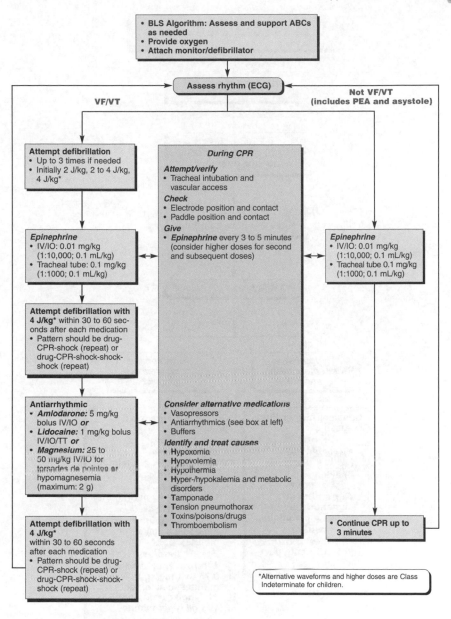

Pediatric Pulseless Arrest Algorithm

(Reproduced with permission from the PALS Provider Manual. © American Heart Association, 2002)

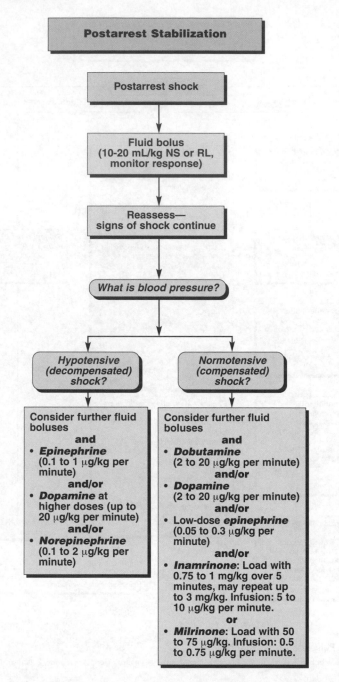

Algorithm for Stabilization of Infants and Children After Arrest
(Reproduced with permission from the PALS Provider Manual. © American Heart Association, 2002)

Index

Index note: page references with an *f* and/or *t* indicate a figure or table on the designated page.

Notes

Notes

Notes

Notes

Notes

Notes

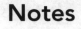

Notes

Further Praise for *The Philadelphia Guide: Inpatient Pediatrics*

"Overall, *The Philadelphia Guide: Inpatient Pediatrics* is a good book that I would recommend. The chapters cover a remarkable amount of material in a very concise manner that is easy to read and follow."

—*Pediatrics Resident, Texas Children's Hospital, Ben Taub General Hospital, Houston, Texas*

"*The Philadelphia Guide: Inpatient Pediatrics* allows a good short review of important topics. It is obvious that a lot of work and effort went into it. I would recommend this to my fellow residents."

—*Medicine-Pediatrics Resident, Los Angeles County—USC Medical Center, Los Angeles, California*

"*The Philadelphia Guide: Inpatient Pediatrics* has a different, more clinically useful approach than other books. It gives clear directions for making a diagnosis, and good emphasis on differential diagnosis. One of the things that a resident has to learn to do is to rule in a diagnosis, and so this is a crucial addition to any book of this kind. There are sections here that are not found in other texts of this type (at least that I am aware of), so this will be seen as a valued resource."

—*Class of 2004, Tulane University, New Orleans, Louisiana*

"*The Philadelphia Guide: Inpatient Pediatrics* will be a wonderful addition to any med student or pediatric resident's collection. The information is easily accessible and the format style is terrific. I like the fact that each disease/section is broken down into epidemiology, etiology, differential diagnosis, pathophys, etc.

At the attending level, this book may serve as a quick reference guide during rounds on the inpatient ward. The topics and information in this book would have been useful during rounds as a pediatrics resident. In fact, when it comes out I will definitely purchase this book even though I will be in fellowship."

—*Pediatrics Resident, The University Children's Hospital, University of Medicine and Dentistry, New Jersey, Newark, New Jersey*